D0531952

Urology *for* Primary Care Physicians

Urology *for* Primary Care Physicians

Unyime O. Nseyo, M.D., F.A.C.S.
Professor
West Virginia University
Department of Urology
Morgantown, West Virginia

Chief, Urology Section
Veterans Affairs Medical Center
Clarksburg, West Virginia

Edward Weinman, M.D.
Professor
West Virginia University
Department of Medicine
Morgantown, West Virginia

Donald L. Lamm, M.D.
Professor and Chairman
West Virginia University
Department of Urology
Morgantown, West Virginia

W.B. SAUNDERS COMPANY
A Division of Harcourt Brace & Company
Philadelphia London Toronto Montreal Sydney Tokyo

W.B. SAUNDERS COMPANY
A Division of Harcourt Brace & Company

The Curtis Center
Independence Square West
Philadelphia, Pennsylvania 19106

Library of Congress Cataloging-in-Publication Data

Urology for primary care physicians / editors, Unyime O. Nseyo, Edward Weinman,
Donald L. Lamm.—1st ed.

p.   cm.

ISBN 0–7216–7148–9

1. Genitourinary organs—Diseases.   2. Urology.   3. Primary care
   (Medicine)   I. Nseyo, Unyime O.   II. Weinman, Edward.   III. Lamm,
   Donald L.
   [DNLM: 1. Urogenital Diseases.   WJ 140 U785 1999]

RC871.U766 1999

616.6—dc21

DNLM/DLC   98–40584

UROLOGY FOR PRIMARY CARE PHYSICIANS   ISBN 0–7216–7148–9

Printed in the United States of America.

Last digit is the print number: 9   8   7   6   5   4   3   2   1

Contributors

Emmanuel O. Abara, M.B., F.R.C.S.(C), F.A.C.S.
Consultant Urologist; Chief, Division of Urology, Department of Surgery, York Central Hospital, Richmond Hill, Ontario, Canada
Pediatric Enuresis and Voiding Dysfunction

Kevin R. Anderson, M.D.
Assistant Professor of Surgery and Urology and Director of Endourology and ESWL, Yale University School of Medicine, New Haven, Connecticut
Benign Prostatic Hypertrophy

John Battin, M.D.
Chief Resident, West Virginia University and Ruby Memorial Hospital, Morgantown, West Virginia
Uncommon Infections of the Genitourinary Tract

Filitsa H. Bender, M.D.
Assistant Professor, West Virginia University School of Medicine; Attending Neurologist, West Virginia University Hospital, Morgantown, West Virginia
Acute Renal Failure

Mitchell C. Benson, M.D.
George F. Cahill Professor of Urology, Columbia University College of Physicians and Surgeons; Director, Urologic Oncology, Columbia-Presbyterian Medical Center, New York, New York
Prostate-Specific Antigen

Robin E. Blum, B.A.
Project Coordinator; Harvard School of Public Health, Boston, Massachusetts
The Role of Primary Health Care Providers in Cancer Prevention

Gregory A. Broderick, M.D.
Associate Professor of Urology, Mayo Clinic; Attending Surgical Staff, St. Luke's Hospital at Jacksonville, Jacksonville, Florida
Genitourinary Tract Trauma

Virgilio Centenara, M.D.
Chief Resident, West Virginia University Department of Urology, Morgantown, West Virginia
Systematic Approach to Urologic Evaluation

Graham A. Colditz, M.D., Dr.P.H.
Professor of Medicine, Harvard Medical School, and Professor of Epidemiology, Harvard School of Public Health; Epidemiologist, Brigham and Women's Hospital, Boston, Massachusetts
The Role of Primary Health Care Providers in Cancer Prevention

Janet Colli, M.D.
Resident, West Virginia University Department of Urology and Ruby Memorial Hospital, Morgantown, West Virginia
Urologic Emergencies

Sakti Das, F.A.C.S.
Professor of Urology, University of California, Davis School of Medicine, Sacramento, California
Principles of Imaging Studies of the Genitourinary System

Joseph J. Del Pizzo
Chief Resident, University of Maryland
Department of Urology, Baltimore, Maryland
Management of Male Infertility

Melanie Fisher, M.D., M.Sc.
Associate Professor, West Virginia University
Department of Medicine and Robert C. Byrd
Health Sciences Center, Morgantown, West
Virginia
*Upper Urinary Tract Infections; Urinary Tract
Infections in Children*

Grant Franklin, Jr., M.D.
Resident, West Virginia University Hospitals
Department of Urology, Robert C. Byrd
Health Science Center, Morgantown, West
Virginia
Anatomic Basis of Common Urologic Diseases

Norman P. Gebrosky, M.D.
Staff Physician, Westmoreland Regional
Hospital, Greensburg, Pennsylvania
Sexually Transmitted Diseases

Leonard G. Gomella, M.D.
Bernard W. Godwin, Jr. Associate Professor
of Prostate Cancer, Kimmel Cancer Center,
Thomas Jefferson University Department of
Urology, Philadelphia, Pennsylvania
Hematuria: Evaluation and Management

David M. Hall, M.D.
Resident in Urology, West Virginia
University, Robert C. Byrd Health Sciences
Center, Morgantown, West Virginia
Urologic Problems in Pregnancy

Robert Hoeldtke, M.D., Ph.D.
Professor and Chief, Department of
Medicine, Section of Endocrinology and
Metabolism, West Virginia University
Medical School, Morgantown, West Virginia
Endocrine and Metabolic Disorders

Ossama Hozayen, M.D.
Nephrology Fellow, West Virginia University
Medical School, Morgantown, West Virginia
Renal Function in Pregnancy

Mohamed Ismail, M.D.
Assistant Lecturer of Urology, Cairo
University, Cairo, Egypt; Resident in General

Surgery, Thomas Jefferson University
Hospital, Philadelphia, Pennsylvania
Hematuria: Evaluation and Management

Jonathan P. Jarow, M.D.
Associate Professor, Bowman Gray School of
Medicine Department of Urology, Winston-
Salem, North Carolina
Management of Male Infertility

Ashish M. Kamat, M.D.
Resident, West Virginia University
Department of Urology, Robert C. Byrd
Health Sciences Center, Morgantown, West
Virginia
Laboratory Investigations in Urology

John J. Keizur, M.D.
Resident, Kaiser Permanente Hospital
Department of Urology, Oakland, California
*Principles of Imaging Studies of the
Genitourinary System*

Donald L. Lamm, M.D.
Professor and Chairman, West Virginia
University Department of Urology,
Morgantown, West Virginia
Carcinoma of the Genitourinary System

Dennis R. La Rock, M.D.
Clinical Assistant Professor of Urology, Tufts
University School of Medicine, Boston; Staff
Urologist, Charlton Memorial Hospital and
St. Anne's Hospital, Fall River,
Massachusetts
Lower Urinary Tract Infections in Men

Karen MacKay, M.D.
Associate Professor of Medicine, West
Virginia University Section of Nephrology,
Morgantown, West Virginia
Renal Function in Pregnancy

Daniel C. Merrill, M.D.
Urologist, Veterans Affairs Northern
California Health Care System, Martinez,
California
Sexual Dysfunction in the Male

Unni M. M. Mooppan, M.D., F.A.C.S.
Clinical Associate Professor of Urology,
Health Science Center of Brooklyn, State
University of New York (SUNY); Associate
Director, Department of Urology, Brookdale
University Hospital and Medical Center,
Brooklyn, New York
*Superficial Lesions of the Male External
Genitalia*

Michael E. Moran, M.D.
Clinical Associate Professor of Urology,
Albany Medical College; Medical Director,
St. Peter's Kidney Stone Center, St. Peter's
Hospital, Albany, New York
Urinary Calculus Disease

**Margaret Moyo, M.B., Ch.B., M.R.C.P.(Ire),
D.C.H.(UK), F.R.C.P.(C)**
Consultant Pediatrician, Timmins District
Hospital, Timmins, Ontario, Canada
Pediatric Enuresis and Voiding Dysfunction

Perinchery Narayan, M.D., F.A.C.S.
Professor and Chief of Urology, University
of Florida College of Medicine
Health Science Center, Gainesville, Florida
*Voiding Dysfunction in Men with Lower
Urinary Tract Symptoms and Benign Prostatic
Hyperplasia*

Farhad B. Nowzari, M.D.
Resident in Urology, West Virginia
University Hospital, Robert C. Byrd Health
Sciences Center, Morgantown, West Virginia
Genitourinary Malignancies in Children

Unyime O. Nseyo, M.D., F.A.C.S.
Professor, West Virginia University
Department of Urology, Morgantown; Chief,
Urology Section, Veterans Affairs Medical
Center, Clarksburg, West Virginia
*Anatomic Basis of Common Urologic Diseases;
Systematic Approach to Urologic Evaluation;
Laboratory Investigations in Urology; Urologic
Emergencies; Sexually Transmitted Diseases;
Uncommon Infections of the Genitourinary
Tract; Urologic Problems in Pregnancy;
Endocrine and Metabolic Disorders*

Raul C. Ordorica, M.D.
Assistant Professor, Division of Urology,
University of South Florida College of
Medicine; Chief, Urology Section, James A.
Haley Veterans Hospital, Tampa, Florida
*Lower Urinary Tract Infections in Women;
Voiding Dysfunction and Urinary Incontinence
in Women*

John L. Phillips, M.D.
Fellow, Urologic Oncology, National Cancer
Institute, National Institutes of Health,
Bethesda, Maryland
Benign Prostatic Hypertrophy

Pramod P. Reddy, M.D.
Fellow in Pediatric Urology, University of
Toronto Children's Hospital, Toronto,
Canada
Urinary Calculus Disease

Eric S. Rovner, M.D.
Assistant Professor of Urology, University of
Pennsylvania School of Medicine and
Hospital of the University of Pennsylvania,
Philadelphia, Pennsylvania
Genitourinary Tract Trauma

Grannum R. Sant, M.D.
Professor and Chairman, Department of
Urology, Tufts University School of
Medicine; Urologist-in-Chief, New England
Medical Center Hospitals, Boston,
Massachusetts
Lower Urinary Tract Infections in Men

Emmanuel M. Schenkman, M.D.
Attending Urologist, Arden Hill Hospital,
Goshen, New York
Congenital Anomalies

Michael Stifelman, M.D.
Chief Resident in Urology, Columbia
University College of Physicians and
Surgeons and Columbia-Presbyterian
Medical Center, New York, New York
Prostate-Specific Antigen

William F. Tarry, M.D.
Associate Professor, Departments of Urology
and Pediatrics, West Virginia University

School of Medicine; Director of Pediatric Urology and Renal Transplantation, West Virginia University Hospitals, Morgantown, West Virginia
Urinary Tract Infections in Children; Perinatal Urologic Consultation; Congenital Anomalies; Genitourinary Malignancies in Children

Ashutosh Tewari, M.D.
Josephine Ford Urinary Scholar, Josephine Ford Cancer Center and Department of

Urology, Henry Ford Hospital, Detroit, Michigan
Voiding Dysfunction in Men with Lower Urinary Tract Symptoms and Benign Prostatic Hyperplasia

Edward Weinman, M.D.
Professor, West Virginia University Department of Medicine, Morgantown, West Virginia
Acute Renal Failure

Preface

The intent of this primer is to present from the urologist's vantage point the most cost effective and appropriate approaches for the primary care physician to evaluate, treat, and/or triage patients with urologic problems in the office and/or emergency department. The systematic problem-oriented approach and the capsular presentation of highlights or "take home messages" make the book a practical quick reference for the practicing primary care practitioner, the resident/trainee in primary health care, and the medical student. Each author has been selected because of his or her expertise in the specific urologic problems. However, each chapter has been painstakingly written to suit as well as to be useful to the intended user. Each author has attempted to define and explain urologic terms succinctly from the perspective of the urologist.

The editors wish to express great gratitude to the contributors for their hard work and concise presentations of their topics. Their diligent efforts should ensure that this book remains a useful and practical companion to the primary care physician. We thank our clerical staff of Suzanne Dixon and Stephanie McInturff.

UNYIME O. NSEYO
EDWARD WEINMAN
DONALD L. LAMM

Contents

1 Anatomic Basis of Common Urologic Diseases 1
Grant Franklin, Jr.
Unyime O. Nseyo

2 Systematic Approach to Urologic Evaluation 11
Virgilio Centenera
Unyime O. Nseyo

3 Laboratory Investigations in Urology 17
Ashish M. Kamat
Unyime O. Nseyo

4 Principles of Imaging Studies of the Genitourinary System 35
John J. Keizur
Sakti Das

5 Urologic Emergencies 47
Unyime O. Nseyo
Janet Colli

6 Hematuria: Evaluation and Management 59
Mohamed Ismail
Leonard G. Gomella

7 Genitourinary Tract Trauma 75
Eric S. Rovner
Gregory A. Broderick

8 Urinary Calculus Disease .. 93
Michael E. Moran
Pramod P. Reddy

9 Sexually Transmitted Diseases 109
Norman P. Gebrosky
Unyime O. Nseyo

10 Upper Urinary Tract Infections 131
Melanie Fisher

11 Urinary Tract Infections in Children 145
Melanie Fisher
William F. Tarry

12 Lower Urinary Tract Infections in Women 151
Raul C. Ordorica

13 Lower Urinary Tract Infections in Men 163
Dennis R. La Rock
Grannum R. Sant

14 Uncommon Infections of the Genitourinary Tract 171
John Battin
Unyime O. Nseyo

15 **Voiding Dysfunction and Urinary Incontinence in Women** 183
Raul C. Ordorica

16 **Voiding Dysfunction in Men with Lower Urinary Tract Symptoms and Benign Prostatic Hyperplasia** 197
Ashutosh Tewari
Perinchery Narayan

17 **Benign Prostatic Hypertrophy** 209
John L. Phillips
Kevin R. Anderson

18 **Urologic Problems in Pregnancy** 217
David M. Hall
Unyime O. Nseyo

19 **Renal Function in Pregnancy** 223
Karen MacKay
Ossama Hozayen

20 **Perinatal Urologic Consultation** 233
William F. Tarry

21 **Congenital Anomalies** 243
Emmanuel M. Schenkman
William F. Tarry

22 **Pediatric Enuresis and Voiding Dysfunction** 251
Emmanuel O. Abara
Margaret Moyo

23 **Genitourinary Malignancies in Children** .. 263
Farhad B. Nowzari
William F. Tarry

24 **Prostate-Specific Antigen** ... 273
Michael Stifelman
Mitchell C. Benson

25 **Carcinoma of the Genitourinary System** 285
Donald L. Lamm

26 **The Role of Primary Health Care Providers in Cancer Prevention** 303
Robin E. Blum
Graham A. Colditz

27 **Acute Renal Failure** 311
Filitsa H. Bender
Edward Weinman

28 **Endocrine and Metabolic Disorders** 325
Robert Hoeldtke
Unyime O. Nseyo

29 **Management of Male Infertility** 335
Joseph J. Del Pizzo
Jonathan P. Jarow

30 **Sexual Dysfunction in the Male** 349
Daniel C. Merrill

31 **Superficial Lesions of the Male External Genitalia** 359
Unni M. M. Mooppan

Index 379

1 Anatomic Basis of Common Urologic Diseases

Grant Franklin, Jr.
Unyime O. Nseyo

A textbook about diseases of the genitourinary system would be incomplete without an overview of the anatomy of the genitourinary system and how that, practically, relates to some of the common pathophysiologic conditions. Gross anatomy of the urogenital system is reviewed. The microanatomy and embryology are discussed only as they pertain to specific disorders. This chapter is neither an exhaustive look at the anatomy nor a complete list of urologic disorders. For that, the reader is referred to the major texts, the respective chapters in this book, or the suggested readings. However, this chapter represents an inventory of certain urologic disorders regarded in their anatomic perspectives.

Adrenal Glands

ANATOMY AND PHYSIOLOGY

The adrenal glands are paired organs that lie atop the kidneys. The right adrenal is triangular in shape, while the left is rounded. Each adrenal is contained with its respective specialized retroperitoneal connective tissue called *Gerota's fascia.* In cases of congenital absence or ectopic location of the kidney, the ipsilateral adrenal can be found in its anatomic location. However, the adrenal can be ectopically located near the kidney, celiac axis, testis, or spermatic cord. On the right, the adrenal lies in close proximity to the liver, inferior vena cava, kidney, duodenum, and renal vasculature. The left adrenal is closely related to the body of the pancreas, the splenic vessels, the omental bursa of the

cardia of the stomach, the crus of the diaphragm, and the kidney (Fig. 1–1). The adrenals contain a yellow cortex that is composed of three specific layers: the outer zona glomerulosa, the middle zona fasciculata, and the inner zona reticularis. These layers are mesodermally derived and constitute 80% to 90% of the gland by weight. The brown medulla is composed of polyhedral cells. These chromaffin cells are derived from the neural crest and relate intimately with the sympathetic nervous system.

ARTERIES, VEINS, LYMPHATICS, AND NERVES

The blood supply of each adrenal is derived from three arterial branches from the inferior phrenic, aorta, and renal arteries. The right adrenal is drained by a short vein directly into the inferior vena cava, whereas the elongated left adrenal vein empties into the left renal vein. The lymphatics follow the venous drainage to empty into the para-aortic lymph nodes. The splanchnic nerves and celiac ganglion (T10 to L1) send abundant sympathetic innervation along the veins to the adrenal medulla. The sympathetic fibers synapse with the chromaffin cells. The adrenal cortex has no innervation.

PATHOPHYSIOLOGIC CONDITIONS

Cushing's syndrome of truncal obesity, purple skin striae, hypertension, hypokalemia, and plethoric facies results from hypersecretion of cortisol by the zona fasciculata and

1

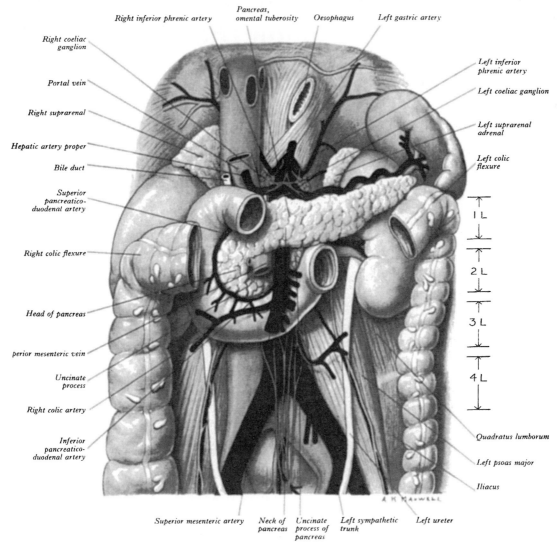

Figure 1-1

Organs of the anterior retroperitoneum, showing relations of the duodenum, pancreas, spleen, and colic flexures to the adrenals (suprarenals), kidneys, and upper ureter. The liver has been removed. Note also the slightly higher position of the right adrenal (suprarenal) gland in the retroperitoneum relative to the left adrenal gland. (From Williams PL, Warwick R [eds]: Gray's Anatomy, 36th ed. Philadelphia, WB Saunders, 1980.)

zona reticularis, which are regulated by adrenocorticotropic hormone (ACTH) from the pituitary. Cushing's disease is a result of ACTH hypersecretion by a pituitary adenoma. Carcinomas of the lung, breast, ovary, kidney, and other organs may cause ectopic ACTH production. The zona glomerulosa is the only source of aldosterone, which is the major mineralocorticoid regulating sodium reabsorption in the kidney, gut, salivary, and sweat glands. Adrenal adenoma results in autonomous hypersecretion of cortisol and low serum ACTH;

Conn's syndrome, which is characterized by hypertension, hypokalemic alkalosis, and low plasma renin activity, results from aldosterone hypersecretion secondary to either adrenal adenoma or hyperplasia.

Adrenal cysts are rare and usually incidental findings. Adrenal carcinomas are highly malignant and present most commonly with Cushing's syndrome or virilization. Functional adrenal tumor must be excluded in women with hirsutism, elevated serum testosterone, and dehydroepiandrosterone.

Pheochromocytomas are usually benign tumors arising from chromaffin cells of the adrenal medulla. Symptoms are due to hypersecretion of norepinephrine and epinephrine. The patient may present with anxiety, heart palpitation, and hypertension with accompanying severe headache. Pheochromocytomas are associated with multiple endocrine neoplasia Type 2, which may include medullary carcinoma of the thyroid, von Hippel-Lindau disease, and neurofibromatosis. The adrenals are favored sites for metastases from melanoma (50%), cancer of the breast, kidney (40%), and lung, as well as the contralateral adrenal, bladder, colon, esophagus, gallbladder, liver, pancreas, prostate, stomach, and uterus, in order of diminishing frequency.

Kidneys

ANATOMY

The kidneys weigh approximately 135 to 150 g each and lie obliquely along the medial border of the ipsilateral psoas muscle and in relation to the region of the back called the *costovertebral angle*. Each is contained in a unique retroperitoneal fat cushion with condensation of connective tissue called *Gerota's fascia*. This fascia also contains the ipsilateral adrenal gland. Gerota's fascia often keeps renal infections, extravasation, early malignancy, and bleeding from reaching adjacent peritoneal structures. The right kidney rests lower than the left owing to the position of the liver. The right kidney is in close proximity to the duodenum, the liver, and the hepatic flexure of the colon, while the left kidney is close to the stomach, the pancreas, the splenic flexure, and the jejunum (see Fig. 1–1). Inferiorly, Gerota's fascia forms a thin envelope that contains the ureters and the gonadal vessels. In the male, the tail of Gerota's fascia follows spermatic vessels and vas deferens into the scrotum as part of the condensation called the *gubernaculum*. Intrascrotal or inguinal infection or bleeding can ascend along this connective tissue pathway into the retroperitoneum. Such an ascending process does not occur in females because the distal Gerota's fascia and the gubernaculum condense into a fibrous tissue called the *round ligament*, which inserts into the labium.

In its macrosectional anatomy each kidney is composed of a fibrous capsule, outer cortex, central medulla, calyces, and pelvis. Each kidney contains about 1 million functional units called *nephrons.* Projections of cortex toward the pelvis between the papillae are called *columns of Bertini.* The collecting tubules of the papillae drain into the calyces, which drain into the renal pelvis. The apex of the calyx is called the *fornix* and is the most frequent site of extravasation secondary to acute rise in intrarenal pressure due to ureteral obstruction or iatrogenically induced high pressure during a retrograde pyelogram.

ARTERIES, VEINS, LYMPHATICS, AND NERVES

The renal artery is usually a single vessel arising from the aorta and entering the hilum between the posteriorly located renal pelvis and the anteriorly located renal vein. The artery divides into an anterior branch supplying the upper and lower poles and the anterior surface of the kidney. The posterior branch supplies the middle pole and the posterior aspect. The primary and secondary intrarenal subdivisions, that is, the intralobar and interlobular arteries, do not communicate. The intralobular forms the afferent arterioles of Bowman's capsule, or glomerular capsule. The glomerular arterial flow exits the glomerulus via the efferent arteriole, which either forms cortical capillary networks or descends into the medulla as vasa recta (straight arterioles). The renal medulla has less arterial blood than the cortex; hence the medulla tends to be more hypoxic under vascular stress and increased intrarenal pressure. Final urinary concentration takes place primarily in the renal medulla. This important function is one of the first to be deranged with pressure due to obstructive uropathy. The veins are paired with the corresponding arteries, but unlike the arterial system, intrarenal veins form profuse anastomoses and eventually unite to form one ipsilateral renal vein that empties into the inferior vena cava.

Renal nerves arise from the renal plexus, which overlies the aorta and the preganglionic fibers from the T8 to L2 spinal segments. These sympathetic fibers enter the kidney at the renal hilum. The parasympathetic innervation is from the vagus nerve and provides vasodilatory function. The sympathetic fibers produce vasoconstriction. Pain due to distention and stress of the renal capsule, renal pelvis, or upper ureter is transmitted via the sympathetic fibers.

The renal lymphatics are abundant and follow the renal blood vessels to exit in large trunks within the renal sinus. These large lymphatic trunks drain into the para-aortic lymph nodes on the left and on the right into the interaortocaval and right paracaval nodes. Some lymphatic drainage reaches retrocaval nodes. These may be the permissive routes for renal malignancies that commonly metastasize to the lungs.

PATHOPHYSIOLOGIC CONDITIONS

The array of neoplasms arising from the parenchyma of the kidneys is quite extensive. Benign tumors include renal cortical adenomas, angiomyolipomas, fibromas, leiomyomas, neurofibromas, and angiomas. Renal cortical adenomas arise from the renal cortex. Although they are classified as benign neoplasms, they are believed to represent an early stage of renal carcinoma and are thus treated as malignant. Renal hamartomas (angiomyolipomas) are noted on histology to contain blood vessels, fat cells, and smooth muscle cells. They are often associated with tuberous sclerosis. Malignant tumors include renal cell carcinoma, renal sarcomas, renal oncocytomas, and hemangiopericytomas, as well as metastatic renal neoplasms. Renal cell carcinoma is the most common renal malignancy. It arises from the cells of the proximal convoluted tubule. They often invade or displace the collecting system. Frequently, extension of tumor thrombus into the renal vein occurs. Paramount to differentiating renal tumors from benign cysts is the use of ultrasonography. However, computed tomographic scanning with contrast medium is the gold standard in the evaluation of renal masses. The kidney is also a common metastatic site for nonhematologic malignancies such as lung cancer, breast cancer, uterine cancer, and melanoma.

Hematuria is the most common (80%) presentation of urinary tract malignancy and renal parenchymal disease. Hematuria due to renal parenchymal disease is usually reddish brown and hazy secondary to formation of acid hematin in low pH urine. Severe proteinuria further supports a renal parenchymal source for hematuria, although some degree of proteinuria will be seen anyway as a result of red blood corpuscle degradation.

Pyelonephritis, characterized by fever, chills, and flank pain, is the result of infection of renal parenchyma with *Escherichia coli, Proteus, Klebsiella,* and, to a lesser extent, other organisms. Infrequently this occurs via hematogenous spread. Usually it results from the ascension of bacteria from the lower urinary tract. *Pyonephritis* refers to acute pyelonephritis with obstructive hydronephrosis. Emphysematous pyelonephritis is an infrequent complication of pyelonephritis in which parenchymal gas is produced by *E. coli* or other glucose-fermenting organisms. Perinephric abscesses lie between Gerota's (perirenal) fascia and the renal capsule and are usually the result of rupture of an intrarenal abscess into the perirenal space. Renal abscesses result usually from focal pyelonephritis or by hematogenous spread from cutaneous infection by *Staphylococcus aureus,* particularly in intravenous drug users and immunocompromised patients. Chronic pyelonephritis results in a small contracted kidney on imaging studies, the result of cortical scarring from long-standing infection.

Renovascular hypertension is the result of increased renin secretion secondary to any significant decrease in renal blood flow, commonly caused by renal arterial stenosis (5% to 15%) due primarily to atherosclerosis or fibromuscular disease (60% to 70%). This entity represents a small but important surgically correctable cause of hypertension. Typically, the patient is a white male with the following characteristics:

25 years of age or younger or older than 45 years

No family history of hypertension

Moderate to severe hypertension with an abrupt onset

A history of cigarette smoking

Mild to moderate azotemia as well as coexistent coronary or carotid artery disease

The finding of abdominal bruits in addition to these clinical features warrants a referral for evaluation.

Renal Calyces, Pelvis, and Ureter

The renal calyx, pelvis and ureter constitute the renal collecting system, which starts out microscopically at the level of the glomerulus. Here the filtrate, the precursor of urine, enters Bowman's capsule and flows through into various segments of the nephrons into the collecting system via the distal convoluted tubules (Fig. 1–2). The renal pelvis results from a confluence of 2 or 3 major calyces, the result of 8 to 12 minor calyces from the tips of the renal pyramids. The renal pelvis may be entirely intrarenal or a combination of intrarenal and extrarenal. It tapers to form a ureter. The ureter is approximately 30 cm long in the adult. Areas of anatomic narrowing occur at the levels of the ureteropelvic junction, at the crossing over the iliac vessels, and at the ureterovesical junction. These are three common anatomic sites for urinary stones to lodge during passage, resulting in urinary obstruction. In females the pelvic ureter travels close to the ovary and in between the uterine artery above and its vaginal branch below, before piercing the bladder at the level of the uterine cervix, making the ureter prone to injury during obstetric or gynecologic surgery. The ureter traverses the bladder wall obliquely through the specialized fibromuscular sheath of Waldeyer. The intramural ureter measures 1.5 to 2 cm in length. The ureteral orifice opens into the bladder base in the interureteric ridge of the trigone. Waldeyer's sheath and the posterior muscular layer of the intramural ureter provide a sphincteric

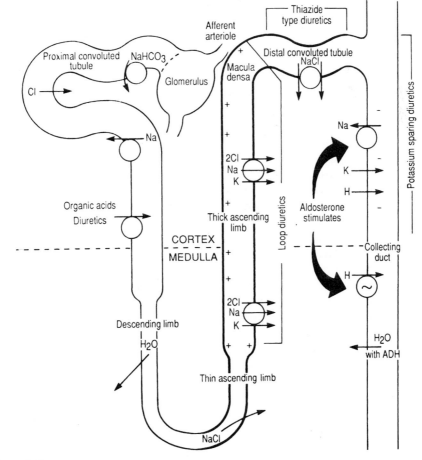

Figure 1–2

Model of major transport processes in the nephron, with sites of diuretic action. (From Pecker MS: Pathophysiologic effects and strategies for long-term diuretic treatment of hypertension. *In* Laragh JH, Brenner BM [eds]: Hypertension: Pathophysiology, Diagnosis, and Management. New York, Raven, 1990, pp 2143–2167.)

mechanism to prevent vesicoureteral reflux. The trigone is of müllerian embryonic origin and responds to estrogenic influence, as does the vagina, hence the characteristic squamous metaplasia common on cystoscopy in females. The ureteral orifice that is abnormally located laterally results in a shorter intramural ureter and a predisposition to vesicoureteral reflux. The ureteral orifice that is ectopic and distally located can lead to obstruction of the renal unit or urinary incontinence in females.

ARTERIES, VEINS, LYMPHATICS, AND NERVES

The blood supply to the renal pelvis and upper ureter is derived from the renal arteries; the blood supply to the mid ureter (abdominal/retroperitoneal ureter) is from the gonadal artery, aorta, and common iliac; and the lower pelvic ureter is supplied by the iliac and its branches (internal, superior vesical, uterine, middle rectal, vaginal, and inferior vesical). Innervation to the ureter is autonomic: sympathetic fibers are from the T10 to L2, and the parasympathetic fibers are from the S2 to S4 spinal segment. However, visceral pain fibers travel with sympathetic nerves, and visceral pain from distention (renal capsule, collecting system) or reflex muscle spasm (e.g., ureteral obstruction by calculi or blood clot) is referred to the somatic branches relating to the spinal segments. These branches typically include the subcostal (renal and upper ureter) and iliohypogastric (abdominal ureter) in the flank; and the ilioinguinal and genitofemoral nerves (pelvic ureter) in the groin, scrotal, and labial areas.

Physiologically, urine moves as a bolus by peristalsis from the renal pelvis through the ureter into the bladder and delivers a volume of about 30 mL/hr. The pacemaker for this autonomous process is located in the minor calyx or renal pelvis and is independent of innervation.

Bladder

ANATOMY

With a capacity of approximately 400 to 500 mL in the adult, the urinary bladder is a muscular reservoir for the storage and elimination of urine. The median umbilical ligament is a fibrous cord anchoring the bladder from the dome to the umbilicus; this cord represents the obliterated urachus. The urachus is embryonically derived from the urogenital sinus. Rarely, this remains patent in the adult as a sinus tract and may give rise to malignancy, typically adenocarcinoma. The nondistended bladder is usually a pelvic organ in the adult. When full, the bladder becomes an abdominal organ; it comes in contact with the lower abdominal wall and may be easily palpated and percussed (Fig. 1–3). This relationship makes it possible to perform percutaneous cystotomy on a full, distended bladder without risk of peritoneal injury. Traumatic perforation of the bladder in the dome causes intraperitoneal extravasation, while posterior bladder perforation leaks urine extraperitoneally and is contained in the deep pelvis below the peritoneum. In females the bladder shares a superior relation to the uterus, which presses and displaces the bladder severely during pregnancy, hence the high incidence of gestational voiding dysfunction. The base of the bladder and urethra are contiguous with the anterior vaginal wall. This relation predisposes to vesicovaginal fistula from trauma or cancer as well as damage during child delivery. The trigone of the bladder represents that area between the bladder neck and the interureteric ridge that separates the ureteral orifices. The internal sphincter is at the bladder neck but is not a true sphincter. It is formed by a convergence of detrusor fibers of the bladder neck (internal sphincter), which ultimately become the smooth muscle of the proximal urethra.

ARTERIES, VEINS, LYMPHATICS, AND NERVES

The arterial supply is extensive, receiving contributions from the anterior branch of the hypogastric artery, the obturator arteries, and the inferior gluteal arteries. Additionally, in females, branches come from the uterine and vaginal arteries. The aforementioned arteries contribute blood supply to the inferior, middle, and superior vesical arteries. Venous return is via a rich plexus that empties into the hypogastric veins. The perivesical lymphatics

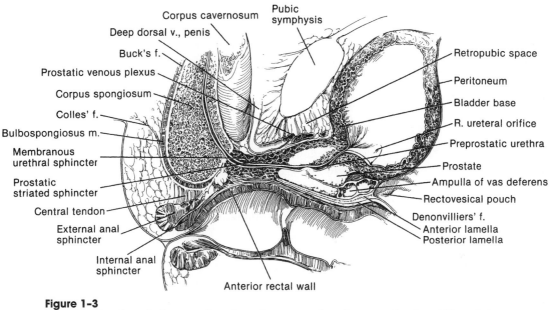

Figure 1-3
Sagittal section through the prostatic and membranous urethra, demonstrating the midline relations of the pelvic structures. (From Hinman F Jr: Atlas of Urosurgical Anatomy. Philadelphia, WB Saunders, 1993, p 356.)

drain into the external iliac lymph nodes. The sympathetic neural innervation to the bladder is from the T10 to T12 spinal segment via the splanchnic nerve, while the parasympathetic innervation to the bladder is from the S2 to S4 spinal cord segment via the pelvic nerve. The parasympathetic nerves predominate in the body of the bladder and are active during urine storage and compliance. The sympathetic fibers, alpha and beta, predominate in the base of the bladder and are active during micturition.

PATHOPHYSIOLOGIC DISORDERS

The specialized impervious transitional cell epithelium (mucosa), which covers the interior surface of the renal collecting system and ureter, lines the inside surface of the bladder. This specialized mucosa is subject to inflammation and cystitis (bacterial or nonbacterial), and malignancy typically is transitional cell carcinoma (90%). Other types of bladder cancer include squamous cell carcinoma (5%), adenocarcinoma (1%), and sarcoma and others (4%). The bladder is a favored metastatic site from the prostate, penis, kidney, breast, and lung. Dysfunction of the autonomic neurons to the bladder detrusor

(smooth) muscle results in dysfunction of the bladder in urine storage and micturition.

Prostate

The prostate gland lies inferior to, and its base wraps around, the urinary bladder outlet. The prostate is approximately 2 to 3 cm in length and contains the posterior urethra and the verumontanum, which marks its caudal end. It weighs approximately 20 g in the adult. Just proximal to the external striated sphincter, the ejaculatory ducts empty through the verumontanum into the prostatic urethra. The prostate contains five distinct anatomic zones: peripheral, central, transition, anterior, and preprostatic sphincter. The transition zone commonly contains benign hyperplasia, which predisposes to bladder outlet obstruction and lower urinary tract dysfunction. This zone also has a 25% incidence of adenocarcinoma of the prostate. The peripheral zone is palpable on digital rectal examination and contains the so-called lateral lobes with a central sulcus. Seventy-five percent of prostate cancer occurs in the peripheral zone, which is also the most common site of prostatitis. Prostatic stones also abound in the peripheral zone.

ARTERIES, VEINS, LYMPHATICS, AND NERVES

Arterial blood supply is derived from the inferior vesical artery. Venous drainage occurs via a periprostatic plexus that drains into the hypogastric veins. Nerve supply is via sympathetic as well as parasympathetic nerve plexuses. The lymphatics drain into the obturator and internal iliac nodes. In addition to cancer and infection, the prostate has potential for hemorrhage, abscess formation, and cystic dilation—conditions that predispose to bladder outlet obstruction.

Urethra

The bladder neck opens into the proximal urethra, which is also called the *prostatic urethra* in males. The proximal urethra ends at the level of the external sphincter, which contains the membranous urethra (2.0 to 2.5 cm in length). In females the urethra is short (4 cm) and exists primarily as the anterior urethra; it terminates at the meatus in the introitus. In males the anterior urethra contains the bulbar urethra at the level of the penoscrotal junction and the pendulous penile or anterior urethra, which terminates in the glans penis at the urethral meatus. The urethra is lined proximally by stratified and pseudostratified columnar epithelium and distally by stratified squamous epithelium.

ARTERIES, VEINS, LYMPHATICS, AND NERVES

Blood supply to the posterior urethra is from the prostatic artery, and the anterior urethra is supplied by a branch of the pudendal artery (bulbourethral artery). Venous drainage is via prostatic and penile venous systems into the internal iliac vein. The lymphatics drain into deep and superficial inguinal nodes from the anterior urethra and from the posterior urethra in men into the pelvic nodal chains.

Inflammation, bacterial infection, sexually transmitted disease, stricture (congenital/iatrogenic), and squamous cell cancer are common pathologic conditions of the urethra. These conditions, except cancer, inflammation, and urethral meatal stenosis, are rare in women. However, urethral caruncle is primarily a disease of the female urethra.

Penis

ANATOMY

The penis contains three spongelike tissue compartments: the nonerectile ventral corpus spongiosum, which contains the urethra and terminates as the glans penis, and the paired dorsal erectile bodies called *corpora cavernosa*. The penile artery, which arises from the internal pudendal artery (branches of the hypogastric), divides into the superficial and deep branches. Blood supply to the glans penis is from the external pudendal (branches of the femoral artery). Erection occurs with increased arterial inflow and engorgement of lacunae/sinusoids of the corpora, with compression of the venous outflow leading to increased penile girth and rigidity. Detumescence occurs with increased venous outflow and decreased arterial inflow resulting in a flaccid phallus. Both the superficial and deep penile veins drain into the dorsal venous complex of the anterior prostate. The primary lymphatics from the prepuce and skin of the penile shaft drain into the superficial inguinal lymph nodes. The lymphatic drainage of the glans penis and corpora is to the superficial and deep inguinal nodes, and then to the external iliac nodes. Parasympathetic activity causes relaxation of the cavernosal smooth muscle and arterial smooth muscle during erection. The sympathetic neural activity inhibits erection.

PATHOLOGIC DISORDERS

Balanitis, phimosis, paraphimosis, squamous cell cancer, fibrosis such as Peyronie's disease, fracture, and angulation/curvature are common pathologic afflictions of the penis. In examination of the uncircumcised male, the foreskin (prepuce) must be fully retracted to visualize the glans penis and the preputial mucosa to ensure the absence of occult cancer. Causes of organic erectile dysfunction (impotence) include impaired arterial inflow (e.g., arteriosclerosis, embolism, trauma), impaired engorgement of the cavernosal sinusoids (fibrosis) and dysfunctional venous outflow (venous leaks), and impairment of autonomic neural function (e.g., diabetes, pelvic surgery, or medications).

Vas Deferens and Seminal Vesicles

The vas deferens emerges from the head of the epididymis and runs posteriorly to the spermatic cord at the inguinal canal and along the lateral pelvic wall to the posterior aspect of the base of the prostate. The tortuous terminal portion is called the *ampulla of the vas* and stores spermatozoa. The seminal vesicles are the lateral outpocketings of the vas that lie at the base of the prostate just cephalad to and contiguous with the bladder base. The seminal vesicles do not store spermatozoa, but they add volume to the ejaculate that is released via the ejaculatory ducts into the posterior urethra. Ejaculation occurs with the rhythmic contractions of the bulbospongiosus muscle and the striated muscles of the membranous urethra.

ARTERIES, VEINS, LYMPHATICS, AND NERVES

The vas and seminal vesicles derive their blood supplies from the deferential artery (a branch of the superior vesical artery) as well as the inferior vesical artery. Venous drainage goes into the pelvic plexus. Nerve supply is sympathetic, which arises from the sympathetic pelvic plexus, and its excitation causes seminal emission. Lymphatics from the vas and seminal vesicles drain into the external and internal iliac nodes.

PATHOLOGIC CONDITIONS

The vas deferens and seminal vesicle may be pathologically obstructed (e.g., diabetes, tuberculosis, schistosomiasis), inflamed, and rarely involved with primary or secondary cancer. The seminal vesicle remains a prime site for extension of prostate cancer.

Spermatic Cord

Each spermatic cord contains the internal and external spermatic arteries, the pampiniform plexus of veins, the vas deferens, the artery of the vas, as well as lymphatics and nerves. The external spermatic artery supplies blood to the coverings of the cord while the internal spermatic artery courses its way to the testis. The pampiniform plexus converges to become the spermatic vein at the internal inguinal ring. Lymphatics from the cord empty into the external iliac nodes. The engorgement or enlargement of the pampiniform plexus results in varicocele, which afflicts the left side more often than the right. This phenomenon occurs because of high venous pressure in the left gonadal vein, which empties into the left renal vein at a right angle near the tributaries of the large left adrenal vein and the left lumbar vein.

Testes and Epididymis

The epididymis is connected to the testes by the efferent ducts. The epididymis is markedly coiled and ultimately forms the vas deferens. A small vestigial cystic structure at the upper pole of the epididymis is known as the *appendix* of the epididymis. An appendix testis occupies the upper pole of the testis and occasionally is associated with torsion.

ARTERIES, VEINS, LYMPHATICS, AND NERVES

Blood supply of the testes and epididymis is from the internal spermatic and deferential arteries. The internal/spermatic artery arises from the ipsilateral renal artery. Venous drainage is into the pampiniform plexus and the spermatic vein, which drains into the renal vein on the left and directly into the inferior vena cava on the right. In females the gonadal vessels arise and drain similarly as the spermatic vessels. The lymphatics drain into the hypogastric and external iliac nodes.

PATHOLOGIC CONDITIONS

The testis is subject to malignancy, inflammation, infection, abscess, and infarction second-

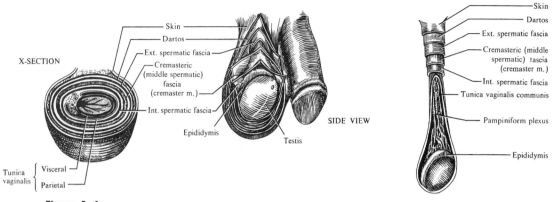

Figure 1–4

The scrotum and its layers. (From Pansky B: Review of Gross Anatomy, 6th ed. New York, McGraw-Hill, 1997, p 483. Reproduced with permission of The McGraw-Hill Companies.)

ary to torsion or trauma. The epididymis is subject to infection, inflammation, and abscess. The testis is cushioned in a bilayered covering called *tunica vaginalis,* with a potential space between its visceral and parietal layers. The potential space contains fluid that overaccumulates to cause hydrocele. The efferent ducts of the epididymis have potential for cystic dilation to form a spermatocele.

Scrotum

The scrotum ("leather-like sac") contains the testes and the epididymis. Its generously wrinkled wall contains six distinct layers: skin, dartos, external spermatic fascia, cremasteric fascia (middle spermatic fascia and cremaster muscle), and internal spermatic fascia (Fig. 1–4). The scrotum is highly vascularized, remains resistant to infection, and is quite responsive to healing after trauma or reconstruction.

SUGGESTED READINGS

1. Brooks JD: Anatomy of the lower urinary tract and male genitalia. *In* Walsh PC, Retik AB, Vaughan ED Jr, Wein AJ (eds): Campbell's Urology, 7th ed. Philadelphia, WB Saunders, 1998, pp 89–128.
2. Kabalin JN: Surgical anatomy of the retroperitoneum, kidneys, and ureters. *In* Walsh PC, Retik AB, Vaughan ED Jr, Wein AJ (eds): Campbell's Urology, 7th ed. Philadelphia, WB Saunders, 1998, pp 49–88.
3. Redman JF: Anatomy of the urogenital tract. *In* Hanno PM, Wein AJ (eds): Clinical Manual of Urology, 2nd ed. New York, McGraw-Hill, 1994, pp 1–51.
4. Redman J: Anatomy of the genitourinary system. *In* Gillenwater JY, Grayhack JT, Howards SS, et al (eds): Adult and Pediatric Urology, 3rd ed. St. Louis, Mosby-Year Book, 1996, pp 1–61.
5. Tanagho EA: Anatomy of the genitourinary tract. *In* Tanagho EA, McAninch JW (eds): Smith's General Urology, 14th ed. Norwalk, CT, Appleton & Lange, 1995, pp 1–16.
6. Tanagho EA: Embryology of the genitourinary tract. *In* Tanagho EA, McAninch JW (eds): Smith's General Urology, 14th ed. Norwalk, CT, Appleton & Lange, 1995, pp 17–30.

2 Systematic Approach to Urologic Evaluation

Virgilio Centenera
Unyime O. Nseyo

A urologic complaint or abnormality is the primary reason 15% to 20% of patients seek medical attention. The patient is most likely to present to the primary care physician initially with a "medical disorder" of the genitourinary tract. Often the patient is referred to the urologist with either a specific diagnosis such as an incidental finding of a mass in the kidney or symptoms such as pain and/or hematuria. However, the referring primary care physician should begin the patient's initial evaluation with a complete history of the present illness, past medical history, review of systems, and social and family history and confirm any abnormality, if any, on physical examination. This standard systematic approach to clinical data acquisition should facilitate the decision-making process. The urologic consultation may involve performing only a few specific diagnostic studies to confirm a presumptive diagnosis and to initiate treatment.

Urologic History

As in diagnosing any type of illness, a careful history and physical examination are crucial in determining the etiology of urologic diseases. The character, onset, duration, and progression of each symptom are carefully identified. Many urologic problems are of a highly personal nature and are indirectly hinted at, especially sexual dysfunction. Urologic symptoms can usually be related to four specific categories: pain, changes in urination, changes in the gross appearance of urine, and abnormal-appearing or -functioning external genitalia.

PAIN

Pain originating from the genitourinary tract can arise from two different processes: distention or inflammation of the respective organ. Pain can also be felt locally or referred to other organ systems or other areas of the body, thereby clouding the diagnosis.

Renal Pain

As mentioned previously, renal pain can occur as a result of distention of the renal collecting system, increased intrarenal pressure, or swelling and stretching of the renal capsule caused by inflammation, as in pyelonephritis. Renal pain is usually felt in the costovertebral angle, just below the 12th rib. The pain experienced can be either colicky in nature or a dull ache, depending on the etiology of the disease process. Pain in this area may also sometimes be referred to the ipsilateral groin or testicle. This occurs because of the common innervation of the testicles (or labia in females) and the kidneys. Renal diseases that are relatively slow growing may be painless. An example would be a staghorn calculus or a renal mass. Systemic symptoms (e.g., fever and chills) or gastrointestinal symptoms (e.g., nausea and vomiting) may constitute the initial presentation of these slow-growing processes.

Ureteral Pain

The most common cause of ureteral pain is sudden ureteral obstruction, with ureteral distention from a stone and peristalsis in the ureter as it tries to overcome the obstruction. A careful history usually will pinpoint the location of a ureteral obstruction. Pain from an upper ureteral stone is similar in distribution to that of renal pain, with pain radiating to the ipsilateral testicle in the male patient or labium in the female patient. Stones in the midureter send pain sensations to the lower abdomen. A stone in the lower ureter is felt in the suprapubic area, bladder, and urethra. Bladder symptoms of irritability or urinary frequency may also be present. The hallmark finding for renal colic, no matter the site of the obstruction, is the continuous wriggling that patients demonstrate as they attempt to find a comfortable position that relieves the pain.

Bladder Pain

Pain within the bladder is usually caused by acute urinary retention and overdistention, with an intense desire to, but inability to, urinate. Patients with a history of chronic urinary retention usually do not feel any pain, despite a massive postvoid residual, because the bladder has learned to accommodate that large amount of urine. Pain secondary to bladder inflammation or infection may be referred to the tip of the penis in males or to the tip of the urethra in females.

Prostate Pain

Prostate pain is usually an ache that is felt in the perineum, lower back, or rectum. It can also result in voiding problems such as dysuria, frequency, or urgency. These types of symptoms may mask the prostate as the true source of the pain.

Testicular Pain

Testicular pain is usually experienced as a dull ache, resulting from infection, torsion, or trauma, the severity of which is directly related to the etiology of the pain. A physical examination inconsistent with the severity of pain felt in that testicle should lead one to entertain the possibility of referred pain from the ureter or kidney.

VOIDING SYMPTOMS

Voiding symptoms can usually be broadly classified into two groups: irritative and obstructive.

Irritative symptoms include urinary frequency, urgency, dysuria, and nocturia. Urinary frequency can be a result of a decrease in the functional capacity of the bladder. If the bladder retains a large amount of urine after voiding, it will feel full shortly after voiding. Disease processes that cause bladder inflammation can also cause urinary frequency. If any portion of the bladder wall lining is inflamed, then even mild stretching will cause the bladder to contract. Similarly, bladder compliance also is diminished with inflammation. Fibrosis of the bladder, as seen with interstitial cystitis or radiation cystitis, can also result in a decrease of bladder compliance with subsequent urinary frequency. All of the just-mentioned processes also result in urinary urgency. This is manifested as a strong, sudden desire to urinate. The patient who complains of pain with urination usually has an inflammatory etiology of the urethra, bladder, prostate, or testicle. The pain is present only during voiding and disappears soon after. The patient usually is able to postpone micturition only temporarily. Nocturia can be attributed to the same disease processes. Renal dysfunction and the loss of urine-concentrating ability also can result in nocturia. The patient's recumbent position at night causes an increase in cardiac output as well as mobilization of fluid leading to nocturia. Lifestyle habits such as drinking coffee late at night can cause nocturia.

Obstructive symptoms may result from either a decrease in the force needed to initiate voiding, as in a neurogenic bladder, or the presence of obstruction in the lower urinary tract, as in benign prostatic hypertrophy or stricture. *Hesitancy* refers to the prolonged interval necessary to start the urinary stream. *Straining* refers to the need to use abdominal pressure to void. A decreased force and caliber of stream usually indicate the presence of obstruction within the urethra. *Terminal dribbling* refers to prolonged dribbling after voiding. A *sense of residual urine* refers to the feeling that the bladder is not completely empty following voiding. *Urinary retention* refers to the inability to empty the bladder. When it occurs acutely, it is extremely painful but can be totally asymptomatic when it occurs gradually and chronically owing to progressive obstruction from increasing prostatic hypertrophy and subsequent bladder distention. The sudden, painful interruption of the urinary stream may be caused by a bladder stone. A split urinary stream is usually due to urethral stricture.

INCONTINENCE

There are many reasons for incontinence, and it is not sufficient to know simply that a patient leaks urine. A careful history and quantification of the leakage usually lead to the proper diagnosis before any formal testing is scheduled.

Total incontinence is a constant dribbling of urine. The leakage occurs without any warning, and it may occur continuously or periodically. The more likely causes are damage to the urethral sphincter (prior surgery or irradiation), vesicovaginal or ureterovaginal fistulas, and ectopic ureters in females.

Overflow incontinence occurs in the patient with a chronically distended bladder. When the pressure within the bladder finally overcomes urethral closing pressure, urine will leak.

Urge incontinence results when the sensation to void becomes so severe that involuntary bladder emptying occurs. The patient usually complains of not making it to the bathroom in time. Any disease process that decreases bladder compliance can result in urge incontinence. This is commonly seen with urinary tract infections; however, an upper motor neuron lesion or even bladder cancer may also cause urge incontinence.

Stress urinary incontinence is the leakage that occurs with an increase in intra-abdominal pressure, as in sneezing and coughing. These patients usually have weakened muscles supporting the bladder neck and urethra. A consequence of this is that intra-abdominal pressure is not transmitted to the urethra and bladder equally. The resultant obtuse angle of the bladder neck leads to urinary leakage; this is common in multiparous women. Leakage is not seen without activity or physical straining.

APPEARANCE OF URINE

Pneumaturia is the presence of gas within the urine. Unless instrumentation has recently been performed, this is a good indicator of a fistula between the urinary and gastrointestinal tracts. Carcinoma of the sigmoid colon, diverticulitis, and trauma are common causes of these fistulas.

Cloudy urine can be the result of a urinary tract infection or of an alkaline urine with the precipitation of phosphates (phosphaturia). A urinalysis helps in distinguishing the cause of the cloudiness.

Bloody urine is an ominous sign. Asymptomatic hematuria warrants an evaluation of the entire urinary tract to rule out malignancy as the source of the bleeding. The other symptoms that may present concomitantly with the hematuria will reveal its source and/or cause. Renal colic with hematuria is usually associated with a renal stone. The other infrequent causes are blood clot and sloughed renal papilla. Hematuria with dysuria and urgency results often from an infection in the genitourinary tract. Bleeding that occurs during different phases of micturition provides important clues. The presence of blood throughout urination points to the bladder or the upper urinary tract as the source. Bleeding that occurs at the initiation of urination suggests an anterior urethral lesion. Terminal hematuria is likely to originate from the prostatic urethra, bladder neck, or trigone.

Urologic Physical Examination

The standard techniques of inspection, palpation, percussion, and auscultation are employed during the urologic examination. Patients with genitourinary problems are usually quite apprehensive. They want to feel confidence in the physician's assessments, sincerity in wanting to help them, and gentleness in the examination.

EXAMINATION OF THE KIDNEYS

Physical examination begins with the patient seated on the examination table for inspection of the back and flanks. Then gentle percussion using the heel of the hand over the area of the costovertebral angle is used to elicit tenderness due to underlying inflammation of the kidney. The patient should then lie supine on the examination table for bimanual palpation of the flanks. The examiner should then lift the flank by placing one hand beneath this area and use the other hand to palpate deeply beneath the costal margin. Because of the position of the liver, the right kidney is lower than the left. For this reason it is usually easier to palpate the lower pole of the right kidney, but the left kidney usually cannot be felt. Auscultation of the costovertebral areas and the upper abdomen should also be performed. Systolic bruits associated with aneurysms or stenosis of the renal artery may be discovered this way.

EXAMINATION OF THE BLADDER

The empty bladder is a pelvic organ; therefore, the bladder usually cannot be felt unless it is moderately distended. In a situation of urinary retention the bladder may be palpable at the level of the umbilicus. In this instance the bladder may be visualized as well as palpated.

EXAMINATION OF THE EXTERNAL GENITALIA

The Penis

A complete examination of the penis requires the foreskin to be retracted, if the patient is uncircumcised, so that the glans and urethral meatus may be inspected. Phimosis is the inability to completely retract the foreskin. Paraphimosis occurs when a tight constricting foreskin cannot be returned to its normal anatomic covering of the glans. The glans is inspected for suspicious lesions. The urethral meatus must be inspected for urethral discharge or areas of irritation. The meatus should be in the central area of the glans penis. If the urethral meatus opens on the ventral surface of the penis, this is called a *hypospadias.* If the opening occurs dorsally, then it is an epispadias. The prepuce should also be examined, because it may not encircle the glans completely. When it forms a dorsal hood over the glans, a hypospadias penis is likely. The penis is palpated from the shaft to the glans. Fibrous plaques along the shaft of the penis may represent Peyronie's disease. This can also be accompanied by curvature, or chordee, of the penis. Surgical intervention may or may not be warranted.

The Testes and Scrotum

The testes are palpated gently and in an orderly fashion, beginning with the testicle, then the epididymis and the cord structures, and then the area of the external ring, for the presence of an inguinal hernia (Fig. 2–1). The testes are palpated using the thumb and forefingers of both hands. Normal testes have a firm, rubbery consistency. The head, body, and tail of the epididymis should be palpated. Any scrotal swelling or mass should be transilluminated. The room should be darkened. and a light source should then be applied to the side of the scrotal swelling. Fluid-filled masses should transmit a red glow. These are usually hydroceles or spermatoceles. Any solid mass within the scrotum should be considered as a malignancy unless proven otherwise. Care must be taken to ensure that the testes of men in their 20s and 30s are carefully examined, because this is the appropriate age group for testicular tumors. A hydrocele should not prevent one from examining the testes in this age group, and other studies (e.g., ultrasonographic studies) may be warranted if a satisfactory testicular examination is not possible. About 10% of tumors are associated with a reactive hydrocele.

If a testicle is not palpated within the scrotum, then the groin should be searched. Palpation of the ipsilateral spermatic cord may be useful in localizing the testicle. One must distinguish between a true cryptorchidism and a retractile testis (one that can be brought down into the scrotum with gentle manipulation).

The epididymis is usually easily palpable separately from the testicle. Tenderness or induration should be noted because this may

Figure 2–1
Systematic approach to the examination of the external genitalia (the left hemiscrotum in this figure) begins with observation of the gross appearance of the skin with generous rugae. Palpation of the scrotal contents (preferably employing the thumb and the index and middle fingers) should be performed systematically in the sequence shown: testis, epididymis (head, body, and tail), spermatic cord, and external ring. (Adapted from Hanno PM, Wein AJ [eds]: Clinical Manual of Urology, 2nd ed. New York, McGraw-Hill, 1994. Reproduced with permission of The McGraw-Hill Companies.)

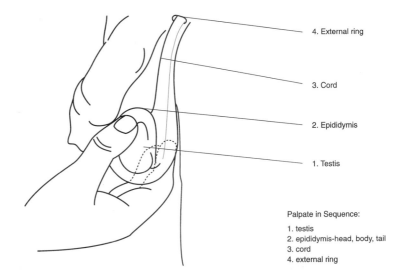

4. External ring

3. Cord

2. Epididymis

1. Testis

Palpate in Sequence:

1. testis
2. epididymis-head, body, tail
3. cord
4. external ring

indicate infection or tumor, although tumor of the epididymis is rare.

RECTAL EXAMINATION

A rectal examination can be performed in a number of positions. The patient may be in a fetal position facing the examiner; he may lean over with his elbows resting on the examining table; or he may be on all fours while on top of the examination table. The generously lubricated finger is placed at the anal verge. This maneuver gives a good approximation of sphincter tone. Laxity of the muscle strongly suggests some type of neurologic disease. The finger should not be jammed into the rectum but gently advanced to the level of the prostate. The prostate is then palpated but not massaged unless this is the intention of the examination and the patient had been previously informed about such a procedure. The examiner should refrain from excess prostatic manipulation if acute prostatitis is suspected. The prostate is usually about 4 cm in length from its apex (inferiorly above the anal verge) to its widest portion at the level of the bladder neck (base). The size of the palpated gland may only loosely correlate with the patient's voiding symptoms or level of obstruction. The consistency of the gland should then be determined. The examining finger is placed laterally and superiorly and rolled toward the midline. The entire gland is examined in this way. The normal gland usually feels rubbery and fleshy. A mushy or congested gland is felt if infection is present. A hard nodule, or indurated gland, can be found with carcinoma or prostatic calculi. The presence of any abnormality (e.g., nodularity, bogginess, or tenderness) warrants further work-up by the urologist.

EXAMINATION OF THE LYMPH NODES

Inflammatory and malignant lesions of the penis, scrotum, and vulva may involve the inguinal and subinguinal lymph nodes. These nodes should be carefully palpated. Tumors of the testis and prostate may involve the left supraclavicular nodes, the so-called Virchow's nodes.

NEUROLOGIC EXAMINATION

If neurologic disease is suspected, then an examination of the sensation of the perineal area, the anal sphincter tone, and the bulbocavernosus reflex should be performed. The bulbocavernosus reflex is performed by placing a finger within the rectum and squeezing the glans penis or clitoris; gently pulling on an indwelling urethral catheter is another method. The anal sphincter and bulbocavernous muscles normally contract when this maneuver is performed. If these tests are being performed in a child, one should examine the child's sacrum for a tuft of hair, dimpling, or other manifestations of sacral malformation.

SUGGESTED READINGS

1. Bushman W, Wyker JAW: Standard diagnostic considerations. *In* Gillenwater JY, Grayhack JT, Howards SS, et al (eds): Adult and Pediatric Urology, 3rd ed. St. Louis, Mosby-Year Book, 1996, pp 63–77.
2. McAninch JW: Symptoms of disorders of the genitourinary tract. *In* Tanagho EA, McAninch JW (eds): Smith's General Urology, 14th ed. Norwalk, CT, Appleton & Lange, 1995, pp 31–40.
3. MacFarlane MT: Urology for the House Officer. Baltimore, Williams & Wilkins, 1988, pp 7–10, 11–14, 25–26, 37–38.
4. Tanagho EA: Physical examination of the genitourinary tract. *In* Tanagho EA, McAninch JW (eds): Smith's General Urology, 14th ed. Norwalk, CT, Appleton & Lange, 1995, pp 41–49.
5. Van Arsdalen KN: Signs and symptoms: The initial examination. *In* Hanno PM, Wein AJ (eds): Clinical Manual of Urology, 2nd ed. New York, McGraw-Hill, 1994, pp 53–88.

3 Laboratory Investigations in Urology

Ashish M. Kamat
Unyime O. Nseyo

Approximately 1 in 5 patients visiting a primary physician's office has a urologic problem. The primary caregivers who have a broad knowledge of the laboratory methods available to test these patients are able to diagnose and treat these problems more effectively. In this chapter we attempt to provide an easy reference for primary care physicians so as to enable them to start the diagnostic process and speed up care of the patient. We provide the basic information needed for requesting the appropriate laboratory investigations. A brief mention of the ancillary diagnostic procedures is made, and a full discussion can be found in the relevant chapters.

Uroscopy

Uroscopy is the science and art of diagnosing disease by the observation and examination of urine. Hippocrates wrote, "One can obtain considerable information concerning the general trends by examining the urine." He believed that the urine was filtered off from blood by the kidneys and hence was a reflection of the general status of the patient's health. Urinalysis was, and remains, a most valuable and important means of diagnosis in clinical medicine.

COLLECTION

The method of collecting, transporting, and storing a sample of urine is of prime importance. The patient should wash his or her hands before voiding, wash the genitalia with a mild soap solution or commercial preparation kit, and rinse with water. Men should be instructed to retract the foreskin and direct the cleansing process from the meatus backward. After voiding for a few seconds and without interrupting the stream, the patient places the cup in the path of the stream and collects the specimen without contaminating the inside of the container.

Women should manually clean the labia and area around the meatus with a mild soap solution, again directing flow away from the meatus. Squatting over the toilet seat, the patient should then separate the labia with one hand and place the collection cup in the urine stream after a few seconds of voiding without interrupting the stream. If this proves unsatisfactory, physicians may need to place the patient in a lithotomy position and collect a midstream specimen themselves.

TIMING

There are three main types of urine samples: first morning, random, and timed. The first-morning sample is usually an 8-hour collection that offers valuable information about the ability of the kidney to concentrate fluids and gives a higher yield of sediments. The random sample is convenient since it is obtained at the time the patient visits the physician or laboratory and can be examined immediately. A fresh-voided specimen taken a few hours after the patient has eaten and examined within the hour after voiding is the most reliable. It should be obtained prior to any genital or rectal examination to prevent contamination from expressed secretions. The timed samples are used for special tests and require detailed instructions to the patient regarding method of collection, storage, and dietary restrictions, if any.

The midstream urine reflects the urine composition in the bladder accurately and is the preferred sample for routine analysis. The terminal urethra or vagina contains a large number of microorganisms, and these can contaminate the urine specimen. The first few seconds of voiding help wash out these organisms and the midstream specimen may be used for culture.

STORAGE AND TRANSPORT

Urine is an unstable fluid that, after voiding, undergoes several changes. The color darkens and the numbers of crystals and bacteria increase, resulting in increased turbidity. Cells lyse, nitrite increases, and glucose, bilirubin, and urobilinogen decrease. Immediate examination of urine is imperative to avoid these changes.

Studies have shown that urine may be left up to 2 hours at room temperature without significantly affecting the outcome of analysis. A delay of more than 2 hours should be avoided. Refrigeration of urine can be used, but it precipitates urate or phosphate crystals, and these may obscure the other cells and casts. Chemical preservation of urine with buffers or acidifying agents may be used in certain situations such as for mail-in specimens.

Urinalysis

Before we proceed to outline a symptom-oriented guide to urologic laboratory investigations, let us start with a synopsis of the various elements of urinalysis.

MACROSCOPIC EXAMINATION

Macroscopic examination involves visual inspection as well as the increasingly popular dipstick testing. Although many physicians are relying solely on the dipstick, this is only an initial means of assessing the urine.

Color and Appearance

Normal urine is clear and yellow. Various factors such as concentration, foods, and dyes can discolor urine and make it darker.

Red urine does not always mean hematuria. It can result from myoglobinuria, porphyria, beet ingestion, numerous food dyes such as rhodamine B and drugs such as phenolphthalein, and hemoglobinuria from hemolysis. Also, infection with *Serratia marcescens* can cause red diaper syndrome.

Cloudy urine may signify infection, or it may be a result of excess phosphates or urates in urine. These can be differentiated by the addition of acid or alkali, respectively, in which they dissolve.

Specific Gravity

Normal urine has a specific gravity that ranges from 1.003 to 1.030. This test remains the easiest and best method for rapid estimation of fluid status in surgical patients. Dilute urine can result from diabetes insipidus, overhydration, or renal concentrating failure. Concentrated urine can result from dehydration, spillover of glucose or proteins, or gross infections.

pH

If the pH is greater than 7.0, this suggests the presence of urea-splitting organisms such as *Proteus* and certain strains of *Klebsiella, Pseudomonas, Providencia,* and *Staphylococcus.* Urine obtained after a large meal or left standing longer than 2 hours tends to be alkaline.

The pH also gives a clue as to the type of stone present. An acid environment favors the formation of uric acid and cystine crystals. Patients with uric acid stones rarely have a urinary pH higher than 6.5. Calcium phosphate forms at a pH of 6.6 or higher. Patients with a urine pH greater than 7.0 are more likely to have struvite stones because magnesium ammonium phosphate precipitates at pH 7.2 or higher.

Renal tubular acidosis can be suggested by an inability to acidify urine below pH 5.5 in spite of an acid load or fasting.

Protein

Normally, less than 20 mg of protein is excreted daily, of which 50% is albumin. The dipstick is more reactive to albumin as compared with mucoproteins, Bence Jones proteins, or globulins. The dipstick reads positive if the protein content is more than 10 mg/dL and hence is negative in a normal specimen. The 3% sulfosalicylic acid test is the gold standard and has a higher specificity and sensitivity. It is used to confirm any proteinuria detected on screening dipstick testing.

Positive results can be seen in orthostatic proteinuria, after prolonged exercise, or with fever. Persistent high proteinuria (> 150 mg/day) may indicate disease, including cancer.

The protein:creatinine ratio in an early-morning voided specimen can be as useful as a quantitative assay and is less time consuming. A normal ratio is 0.2, whereas a ratio of 3.5 mg of protein per 1 mg of creatinine indicates significant proteinuria (> 1 g/day).

Glucose

Usually seen when the blood glucose is more than 180 mg/dL, urinary glucose is generally indicative of diabetes mellitus. False-positive results may be seen in large-dose aspirin, vitamin C, or cephalosporin intake. The urologic importance of diabetes lies in its many ramifications, including impotence, infections, papillary necrosis, balanitis, and neurogenic bladder.

Hemoglobin

The dipstick test is not specific for hemoglobin and hence should serve only as a screening test.

Positive results are due to hematuria with more than 5 to 10 red blood cells (RBCs) per high-power field (hpf), hematuria with lysis of RBCs due to hypotonic (specific gravity <1.008) or alkaline urine, hemoglobinuria from intravascular hemolysis, and myoglobinuria from muscle injury. False-positive results may be obtained in the presence of heavy infection (peroxidase) or bleach in the container. Also, negative results may be obtained with heavy vitamin C ingestion or intake of drugs that produce formaldehyde in urine.

The sensitivity of the dipstick test has been routinely quoted at 90%, whereas the specificity is more variable owing to a higher incidence of false-positive readings. The important factor to remember is that confirmation of the dipstick reading by microscopy is mandatory.

Nitrites

Normal urine does not contain nitrites. The nitrite test is based on the ability of several gram-negative organisms to reduce nitrates in urine. When positive, it suggests the presence of more than 10^5 organisms per milliliter. Since the nitrite test positive for only the coagulase-splitting bacteria, it is accurate only in 50% to 60% of cases when used alone (sensitivity can be increased to 90% when a first-morning specimen is used). A false-negative nitrite test result can occur in the following circumstances: (1) the bacteria do not contain nitrate reductase, (2) urine is not present in the bladder for more than 4 hours, (3) absence of dietary nitrite, (4) dilute urine, (5) acidic (pH < 6) urine, (6) presence of urobilinogen, or (7) ingestion of ascorbic acid. False-positive results can be seen owing to specimen contamination.

Leukocytes

The leukocyte esterase test identifies white blood cells (WBCs) even after they have been lysed, and a positive result indicates 10 to 12 WBCs per hpf. This is a good indicator of pyuria. A false-negative leukocyte esterase reaction can be produced by the following circumstances: (1) glucosuria and (2) the presence of urobilinogen, vitamin C, nitrofurantoin, phenazopyridine (Pyridium), or rifampin. False-positive results are caused by specimen contamination.

Overall the sensitivity ranges from 70% to 95% and the specificity from 65% to 86%. It has been suggested that these numbers may be improved by reading the test at 1 minute and again at 5 minutes.

MICROSCOPIC EXAMINATION

Microscopy to look for cellular constituents (Fig. 3–1) remains the gold standard and must

Cells

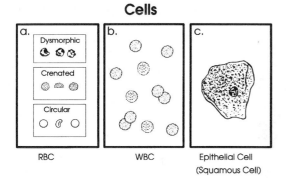

Figure 3-1
High-power magnification (×400) drawing of cells in the urinary sediment. *a*, Red blood cells (RBC): dysmorphic, crenated, and circular. *b*, White blood cells (WBC). *c*, Epithelial cell. (From Walsh PC, Retik AB, Vaughan ED Jr, Wein AJ [eds]: Campbell's Urology, 7th ed. Philadelphia, WB Saunders, 1998, p 154.)

be used to confirm the dipstick and macroscopic findings.

Red Blood Cells

Significant hematuria is defined as more than 3 RBCs per hpf in a voided specimen from an adult male. Dilute urine can lyse RBCs and give a false-negative or subthreshold microscopic impression.

To determine the origin of the RBCs, phase-contrast microscopy may be performed. In the absence of a phase-contrast microscope the condenser of a regular microscope can be lowered to produce sufficient contrast. If 90% or more cells are eumorphic, that is, regular with smooth rounded or crenated membranes and an even distribution of hemoglobin, this suggests an epithelial origin or nonglomerular source of bleeding. If more than 20% cells are dysmorphic with irregular shapes and minimal or uneven hemoglobin distribution and an uneven cytoplasmic distribution, then a glomerular source of bleeding is likely. It is

presumed that the passage of erythrocytes through the nephron causes the dysmorphism.

Leukocytes

A finding of 5 to 8 WBCs per hpf in a clean-voided specimen from men and clean catheterization in women is considered significant pyuria. This is considered to be presumptive evidence of infection, but other sources such as sterile urolithiasis must be excluded. Sixty-one percent of women with pyuria may not show bacterial growth as identified by culture of the urine. In addition, only 50% of patients with bacterial infections have pyuria, thus making it a poor test.

A careful study of the urine can often reveal "old" leukocytes (small, wrinkled cells), which are present in the vagina of women and thus may indicate contamination. "Fresh" leukocytes indicate acute urinary tract injury.

Bacteria

The identification of bacteria (Fig. 3–2) or yeast in an uncontaminated specimen is pathognomonic for urinary tract infection (UTI). It has been shown that approximately 5 bacteria per hpf is equivalent to a colony count of 100,000 organisms per milliliter. The microbiologist can differentiate between different types of bacteria and yeast on the basis of Gram or acid-fast stain, thus giving an early clue as to the type of infection and the appropriate choice of antibiotic. Formal culture and sensitivities further direct the choice of antibiotics.

Epithelial Cells

Squamous epithelial cells found in a urine specimen may indicate contamination of the

Bacteria

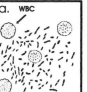
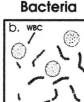

Figure 3-2
High-power magnification (×400) drawing of bacteria in the urinary sediment. *a*, Bacilli. *b*, Streptococci. *c*, Staphylococci. (From Walsh PC, Retik AB, Vaughan ED Jr, Wein AJ [eds]: Campbell's Urology, 7th ed. Philadelphia, WB Saunders, 1998, p 155.)

specimen and are often found in specimens obtained from women.

If large numbers of transitional cells are seen, especially in clumps with abnormal histology such as increased nucleus:cytoplasm ratio or multiple nucleoli, a malignant lesion should be suspected. The Papanicolaou stain can help in identifying these uroepithelial tumors.

Crystals and Casts

The significance of crystals and casts (Figs. 3–3 and 3–4) is often overrated. In brief, RBC casts are diagnostic of glomerular bleeding, whereas casts of other elements are nonspecific indicators of renal tubular and nephron damage. Granular or waxy casts are nothing but a result of further breakdown of the cellular casts and have no special meaning.

CULTURES

The presence of bacteria in a urine specimen that has been obtained correctly warrants a provisional diagnosis of bacterial infection and should be confirmed by culture. The culture is used to estimate the number of bacteria in the urine, identify the specific organisms, and predict the sensitivity to antimicrobials. Different methods and culture agents are detailed in Chapters 10, 11, and 12.

Crystals

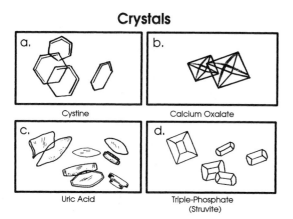

Figure 3-3
Urinary crystals. *a*, Cystine. *b*, Calcium oxalate. *c*, Uric acid. *d*, Triple-phosphate (struvite). (From Walsh PC, Retik AB, Vaughan ED Jr, Wein AJ [eds]: Campbell's Urology, 7th ed. Philadelphia, WB Saunders, 1998, p 155.)

Casts

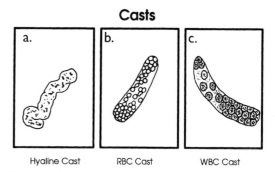

Figure 3-4
High-power magnification (×400) drawing of urinary casts. *a*, Hyaline cast. *b*, Red blood cell (RBC) cast. *c*, White blood cell (WBC) cast. (From Walsh PC, Retik AB, Vaughan ED Jr, Wein AJ [eds]: Campbell's Urology, 7th ed. Philadelphia, WB Saunders, 1998, p 155.)

OTHER STUDIES

Prostatic Massage Specimen

Prostatic massage specimen forms an essential part of the investigation in males with lower urinary tract symptoms. Macrophages and clumps of WBCs indicate inflammation and can differentiate between prostatitis and prostatodynia. The prostatic secretion should be cultured whenever there is any question of infection.

Stone Analysis

A formal stone analysis is recommended to establish the type of stone disease whenever an intact stone can be recovered. Otherwise, the presence of large amounts of calcium, uric acid, oxalate, magnesium, or citrate in urine can offer valuable clues.

Vaginal Exudate

Vaginal exudate forms an essential part of the investigation in females with lower urinary tract symptoms. Macrophages and clumps of WBCs indicate inflammation. An inspection of the secretion under the microscope can show yeast or trichomonads, giving an instant clue to treatment. The secretion should be cultured whenever there is any question of recurrent infection.

Cultures of the Genital Tract

Genital tract infection has been linked to infertility through epidemiologic studies, although no specific organism has been identified.

It is important to culture patients with clinical evidence of inflammatory or infectious processes and to test them for *Mycoplasma* and *Chlamydia*. In addition, semen may be cultured for bacterial organisms. Patients with no evidence of disease do not require a routine culture.

RENAL FUNCTION TESTS

A brief summary of the various indicators of renal function useful for the primary care physician is given in the following sections. Details may be found in Chapter 27.

Serum Creatinine

The normal range of serum creatinine is 0.8 to 1.2 mg/dL for adults and 0.4 to 0.8 mg/dL for children. Serum creatinine is a good indicator of renal function because it is seldom affected by dietary intake or fluid status. The values remain relatively normal, however, until about 50% of renal function has been lost.

Creatinine Clearance

The creatinine clearance test is currently the most accurate and reliable noninvasive method to determine renal function. Since creatinine production is a stable process and creatinine is largely excreted by filtration, its clearance reflects the glomerular filtration rate.

It is determined by obtaining a timed 24-hour collection of urine and serum values and calculated by the following formula:

$$\text{Clearance} = UV/P$$

where U = urine creatinine in milligrams per deciliter, V = volume of urine in milliliters per minute, and P = creatinine in plasma in milligrams per deciliter. The normal value is 90 to 110 mL/min. The creatinine clearance is commonly used to assess renal function and to adjust dosages of medications.

Blood Urea Nitrogen

The blood urea nitrogen (BUN) level is related to the glomerular filtration rate. However, it is affected by protein intake, fluid status, and bleeding in absorptive areas. It is less specific than creatinine, and requires that about 60% of renal function be affected before a significant rise is seen. However, the BUN-to-creatinine ratio is still commonly used to give diagnostic information. The normal ratio is 10:1. A rise in ratio to 20 to 40:1 indicates dehydration or bilateral urinary obstruction or extravasation. A low ratio may be seen in overhydrated patients and also in cases of impaired protein catabolism or hepatic failure.

Hematuria (Table 3–1)

Hematuria is a common problem facing the primary care physician and a common presenting symptom of many urologic diseases. The question often arises as to what should be considered significant hematuria and how extensive the work-up should be prior to prudent referral. Hematuria should be considered a red flag and should never be ignored. Most urologists have a low threshold for working up significant hematuria owing to the danger of missing a tumor and the benefit of an early diagnosis to the patient.

CAUSES

The causes of hematuria can be stratified according to age. In children the common causes include glomerulonephritis (50%) and UTIs. No cause may be seen in 9% to 22% of pediatric cases. In people younger than 40 years of age, UTI, stones, and glomerulonephritis are common causes. The prevalence of microscopic hematuria increases with age, and this fact must be tempered by the increased incidence of malignancy among the elderly. As age increases, the incidence of tumors makes this the common most cause in men, along with benign prostatic hypertrophy (BPH). No cause may be found in 5% to 50% of cases.

HISTORY AND PHYSICAL EXAMINATION

It is important to elicit any associated symptoms such as pain, timing of hematuria, and

Table 3-1
Key Laboratory Tests for Hematuria

Finding	Clinical Implication
Dipstick	
Blood	Use only for screening—must confirm by presence of RBCs on microscopy
Leukocytes	Signifies infection or inflammation
Nitrites	Infection with urease-producing organisms
Heavy proteinuria	Suggests glomerulopathy
Microscopy	
RBCs	Hematuria is defined as presence of >3 RBC/hpf
Eumorphic RBCs	Implies epithelial origin of bleeding
Dysmorphic RBCs	Implies glomerular origin of bleeding
WBCs	Signifies infection or inflammation
Casts	Favor medical cause of bleeding
Crystals	Seen early in stone formation
Cytology	Aids in diagnosis of urothelial cancer
Culture	Needed to confirm suspected infection
Blood	
CBC	May see anemia, thrombocytopenia, or leukocytosis
Serum creatinine	Marker of renal function; required for IVP
Others (based on history)	Sickle cell panel
	Coagulation parameters
	Tumor markers

CBC, complete blood count; RBC, red blood cell; WBC, white blood cell; IVP, intravenous pyelogram.

symptoms of bladder irritability. The diagnostic work-up can then be tailored to meet specific needs. Silent hematuria must be regarded as a symptom of tumor unless otherwise proven. This type of hematuria is usually intermittent, and complacency because the bleeding has stopped can have disastrous consequences.

ASSESSMENT

Urinalysis

DIPSTICK

The dipstick test is simple, can even be performed at home by the patient, and can offer considerable information. This test is not specific for hemoglobin, however, and should serve only as a screening tool.

Positive results are associated with hematuria greater than 5 to 10 RBCs per hpf, hematuria with lysis of RBCs due to hypotonic or alkaline urine, hemoglobinuria from intravascular hemolysis, and myoglobinuria from muscle injury. False-positive results may be obtained by the presence of heavy infection (peroxidase) or bleach in the container. Also, negative results may be obtained with heavy vitamin C ingestion or intake of drugs that produce formaldehyde in urine.

The presence of leukocytes and nitrites would point toward cystitis as the cause for hematuria. Heavy proteinuria, in conjunction with hematuria, often points to a medical source of the hematuria.

GROSS EXAMINATION

The timing of the hematuria in relation to the urinary stream is important in defining the anatomic location of the bleeding. Initial hematuria suggests bleeding in the anterior urethra, whereas terminal hematuria suggests bleeding in the posterior urethra near the bladder neck or prostate. If the hematuria persists throughout the urinary stream, it indicates bleeding at or above the level of the bladder.

Bright red, or macroscopic, hematuria with or without clots is usually of lower tract origin, whereas smoky, hazy, or reddish-brown urine is usually from the renal parenchyma due to formation of acid hematin.

MICROSCOPY

Blood. Red urine does not always mean hematuria; it can result from myoglobinuria, porphyria, beet ingestion, numerous food dyes such as rhodamine B and drugs such as phenolphthalein, and hemoglobinuria from hemolysis. Hence the first step is to establish the presence of RBCs by microscopic examination of the urine. The presence of RBCs in the urine is the true definition of hematuria.

Significant hematuria is defined as more than 3 RBCs per hpf in a voided specimen from an adult male. Dilute urine can lyse RBCs and give a false-negative or subthreshold microscopic impression. To determine the origin of the RBCs, phase-contrast microscopy may be performed. If 90% or more cells are eumorphic, this suggests an epithelial origin or nonglomerular source of bleeding. If more than 20% cells are dysmorphic, then a glomerular source of bleeding is likely.

WBCs. If WBCs are present, an inflammatory process should be high in the differential diagnosis. This is a good presumptive evidence of infection, but other sources must be excluded, including urolithiasis, hemorrhagic cystitis, foreign body reaction, and nephritis.

Casts. Non-RBC casts favor a medical cause for the hematuria. RBC casts indicate bleeding from the renal parenchyma.

Crystals. Crystals can be present in early stone formation and reflect nephrolithiasis.

Other. Urine cytology can help diagnose transitional cell carcinoma but is not useful in evaluating renal cell or prostate cancer. If large numbers of transitional cells are seen, especially in clumps with abnormal histology such as an increased nucleus:cytoplasm ratio or multiple nucleoli, a malignant lesion should be suspected. The Papanicolaou stain can help in identifying these uroepithelial tumors

CHEMICAL

Proteinuria out of proportion to the degree of hematuria suggests a renal parenchymal origin for the hematuria.

CULTURE

A culture should be performed if infection is suspected, as is indicated by pyuria or bacteriuria.

Blood
COMPLETE BLOOD COUNT

A complete blood count is useful to evaluate the extent of anemia that may be associated with cancer or prolonged bleeding. The presence of leukocytosis may indicate an infectious cause.

CHEMISTRIES

Routine chemistries are not needed, but if there is a clinical suspicion of renal impairment, serum potassium and serum creatinine may be measured. Serum creatinine determination is also required by most radiologists prior to performing any further studies such as the intravenous pyelogram (IVP) and offers a good preprocedural baseline. If the patient has significant proteinuria, serum albumin levels may be checked.

OTHER

Depending on the history and physical examination, other ancillary tests may be ordered as clinically indicated. In African Americans, it is important not to forget the possibility of sickle cell disease, and a sickle cell panel should be obtained.

Coagulation studies may be obtained to rule out anticoagulation as a cause of bleeding.

Tumor markers and prognostic indicators such as ferritin and haptoglobin in renal cell carcinoma may be needed if a specific diagnosis is entertained and further work-up is indicated.

Imaging Studies
PLAIN FILM

The plain film (kidney, ureter, and bladder [KUB]) should be the first radiologic study to be obtained. The presence or absence of calcification is of importance and can indicate a stone. The renal parenchymal shadow can be evaluated.

INTRAVENOUS PYELOGRAM

An IVP is the principal diagnostic test for hematuria in surgical patients. It should be performed before cystoscopy in case the upper tracts need further delineation by retrograde ureteropyelography. The IVP can demonstrate small lesions in the urinary tract, such as uroepithelial tumors and papillary necrosis.

COMPUTED TOMOGRAPHIC SCAN

The value of computed tomographic (CT) scan in hematuria is mainly to help in the staging of tumors or, in acute cases, to evaluate the renal parenchyma in situations such as trauma. An ultrasound or CT scan is done to evaluate any mass found or even missed on IVP. Cysts may be aspirated under CT guidance, and if the fluid is bloody or contains calcium crystals or malignant cells, further work-up is mandated.

ARTERIOGRAPHY

Arteriography may be done to assess renal vein involvement; to diagnose tumors, atherosclerotic lesions, and arteriovenous malformations; and to provide a road map of the vasculature and aid surgery in some cases.

Cystoscopy

Cystoscopy and bladder washings are an essential part of the evaluation of surgical hematuria. Cystoscopic evidence of infection, tumors, or stones may be seen, and biopsies can be performed. Retrograde urograms may be required if the IVP is unsatisfactory or inconclusive or the patient has an allergic reaction to the IVP dye.

Biopsy

Renal biopsy is indicated in patients suspected of having medical hematuria. The renal biopsy may be done if the physician has ruled out malignancy and needs a diagnosis of glomerulonephritis to be confirmed; however, in adults, this adds little to the management of the patient.

Other

After a surgical cause of hematuria is ruled out, then further work-up with renal biopsy

and measurement of C3, C4, antinuclear antibody, and antistreptolysin O titers may be performed. If no diagnosis is established at this time, it may be that the patient has a small calculus that has passed, a missed malignancy, coagulopathy, or a vascular abnormality.

Stones (Table 3–2)

Often in stone disease the overwhelming feature is the excruciating pain. As clinicians, we often rush to make a diagnosis and then concentrate on treatment of the pain and the stone. However, a thorough metabolic evaluation directing appropriate medical therapy and lifestyle changes is of prime importance since, without such follow-up and medical intervention, stone recurrence rates can be as high as 55% within 5 years.

HISTORY AND PHYSICAL EXAMINATION

Pain is the leading symptom in 75% of cases. Pain associated with renal calculi is localized to the affected flank and is commonly associated with costovertebral tenderness. Ureteral calculi cause a typical agonizing, colicky pain that radiates toward the ipsilateral groin and may be felt in the testis or labium. Nausea and vomiting often accompany ureteral colic. If the stone is in the bladder, severe irritative symptoms such as stranguria may be present.

The presence of fever or chills raises a red flag and suggests that infection is present, a serious and potentially life-threatening complication.

ASSESSMENT

Urinalysis

DIPSTICK

pH. The pH of the urine can offer clues as to the type of stone present. An acid environment favors the formation of uric acid and cystine crystals. Patients with uric acid stones rarely have a urinary pH higher than 6.5. Calcium phosphate forms at a pH of 6.6 or higher. Patients with calcium stones, nephrocalcinosis, or both may have renal tubular

Table 3-2
Key Laboratory Tests for Renal Stones

Finding	Clinical Implication or Type
Dipstick	
pH	Gives a clue as to the type of stone present:
	Acidic—uric acid or cystine crystals
	Alkaline—phosphates, struvite
Blood	Must confirm by microscopy
Leukocytes	Signifies infection or inflammation
Nitrites	Infection with urease-producing organisms
Microscopy	
RBCs	May not have hematuria with complete obstruction
WBCs	Signifies infection or inflammation
Crystals	Oxalate—bipyramids or dumbbells
	Phosphate—splinter-like
	Struvite—"coffin lids"
	Uric acid—amorphous powder
	Cystine—hexagonal
Culture	Definitive diagnosis of associated infection
24-hour urine—calcium, magnesium, oxalate, phosphate, creatinine	Determine etiology in recurrent stone formers
Blood	
CBC	Leukocytosis—infection
Serum creatinine	Marker of renal function; required for IVP
Other (order selectively)	Calcium
	Uric acid
	PTH
	Magnesium

RBC, red blood cell; WBC, white blood cell; CBC, complete blood count; IVP, intravenous pyelogram; PTH, parathyroid hormone.

acidosis, which is characterized by an inability to acidify urine below 5.5 in spite of an acid load or fasting.

If the pH is higher than 7.0, this suggests the presence of urea-splitting organisms such as *Proteus.* These patients are more likely to have struvite stones because alkaline urine makes the inorganic salts less soluble; ammoniomagnesium phosphate precipitates at a pH of 7.2 or higher.

Other. The presence of RBCs can be detected as detailed in the earlier section on hematuria. Nitrites and leukocytes may be found if there is superimposed bacterial infection.

GROSS MICROSCOPY

Blood. Patients with calculi nearly always have hematuria—gross or microscopic. As always, this should be confirmed by microscopy. Rarely, there may not be any RBCs in the urine if the calculus is causing complete obstruction. Persistent hematuria after stone passage, especially in elderly patients, should prompt a search for an alternate source.

WBCs. The inflammatory response caused by the presence of a calculus within the urinary tract often leads to WBCs in the voided specimen. If WBCs are present out of proportion, this may suggest associated infection. Although struvite stones are most indicative of infection, any stone may be associated with infection secondary to obstruction and stasis.

Crystals. Crystals may have a characteristic appearance but in reality are not seen as often as in commonly believed. If present, they can often give clues as to the type of stone and possible causative factors.

CHEMICAL

Chemical studies are helpful in determining and treating the underlying factors involved in the formation of a calculus. A thorough metabolic evaluation is of paramount importance in directing appropriate medical therapy to help reduce recurrent stone disease. A stone analysis must be performed to help direct the work-up, and the laboratory tests may be directed by the composition of the stone.

Hypercalciuria is the most common abnormality and may be differentiated into Types I, II, and III. Type II (dietary dependent) can be excluded by placing the patient on a sodium- and calcium-restricted diet and measuring the urinary calcium, which should fall to less than 250 mg/day. Type I (absorptive) hypercalciuria is characterized by a 50% drop in urinary calcium and normal parathyroid hormone (PTH) levels after the patient is placed on a calcium binder, and urinary calcium and serum PTH levels are checked before and after.

A metabolic evaluation for calcium, magnesium, oxalate, cystine, and uric acid excretion in urine should be performed. This should preferably be done in an outpatient 24-hour urine collection.

Based on these findings, the appropriate intervention can be suggested as outlined in Chapter 8.

CULTURE

A urine culture should be performed if infection is suspected or as indicated by pyuria or bacteruria. Repeated urine cultures must be obtained in patients with infectious calculi. This forms an important part of the diagnostic work-up.

STONE ANALYSIS

A formal stone analysis is recommended to establish the type of stone disease whenever an intact stone can be recovered. Otherwise, the presence of large amounts of calcium, uric acid, oxalate, magnesium, or citrate in urine can offer valuable clues.

Blood

COMPLETE BLOOD COUNTS

An elevated WBC count can be indicative of acute-phase response or infection as dictated by the clinical situation. Infection accompanying obstruction is a potentially life-threatening event.

CHEMISTRIES

Routine chemistries should include electrolytes, calcium, phosphorus, uric acid, and estimation of serum albumin. Serum creatinine is helpful in gauging renal function and is also required by radiologists prior to performing studies such as the IVP or CT scan.

A systematic metabolic evaluation must be undertaken after the patient has recovered from the acute episode to prevent recurrence of the stone.

OTHER

Serum PTH studies are useful in determining the presence of a parathyroid adenoma in patients with urolithiasis and an elevated serum calcium level. Serum uric acid levels are often elevated in patients with uric acid stones

IMAGING STUDIES

PLAIN FILM

A plain film or KUB is the first radiologic test ordered and can offer a lot of information. Ninety percent of the stones are radiopaque. Pure calcium oxalate monohydrate and calcium phosphate stones are very dense, smooth, and rounded as compared with calcium oxalate dihydrate stones, which are less dense, irregular, and spiculated. Struvite stones are less radiopaque, often have laminations, and commonly occur as staghorn calculi. Cystine calculi are faintly radiopaque and may present as staghorn calculi. Uric acid stones are nonopaque but may show eggshell calcification from calcium deposition.

INTRAVENOUS PYELOGRAM

The IVP is useful in a number of ways. It may reveal nonopaque calculi as filling defects. It serves to detail the renal pelvis and ureteral anatomy and to differentiate acute versus chronic obstruction. It can serve as an indicator of function as well as reveal contralateral pathologic conditions.

Retrograde pyelography may be used to supplement the initial examination in cases where the distal tract is not seen.

COMPUTED TOMOGRAPHIC SCAN

CT scan is rarely used in the evaluation of urolithiasis but may be useful in rare instances where differentiation between a nonopaque calculus and a tumor, clot, or cholesteatoma is an issue or determination of the anatomic relationship of the kidneys is necessary.

ULTRASONOGRAPHY

The renal architecture can be assessed using ultrasonography. It is useful in patients unable to undergo IVP; it helps in the evaluation of hydronephrosis, associated renal masses or nonradiopaque filling defects; and it gives a picture of the renal parenchyma.

Urinary Tract Infection

(Table 3–3)

UTI is the most common bacterial infection seen in humans.

HISTORY AND PHYSICAL EXAMINATION

It has been shown that the history and physical examination alone cannot reliably differentiate between renal infection and lower UTI or between bladder infection and urethral syndrome.

ASSESSMENT

Urinalysis

It is of vital importance that the urine collected for diagnosis of UTI be sterile and obtained in an exact manner. (See the section on methods of collection of a urine sample.)

DIPSTICK

The test strips that detect nitrites (bacteria) and leukocyte esterase (WBCs) are accurate predictors of bacteriuria. When the nitrite is positive, it suggests the presence of more than 10^5 organisms per milliliter. Many of the bacteria responsible for UTIs such as the enterobacteria are detected by this test, but, being positive for only the coagulase-splitting bacteria, it is accurate only in 50% to 60% cases when used alone. The leukocyte esterase test identifies WBCs even after they have been lysed, and a positive result indicates 10 to 12 WBCs per hpf. This is a good indicator of pyuria. Used together, the two tests are as

Table 3–3
Key Laboratory Tests for Urinary Tract Infection

Finding	Clinical Implication
Dipstick	
pH	>7.0 implies urea-splitting organisms
Nitrites	Infection with urease-producing organisms
	Accuracy 50–60% when used alone
Leukocytes	Sensitivity: 70–95%
	Specificity: 65–86%
Glucose	Diabetes
Microscopy	
RBCs	May be seen in severe infections or with a stone or tumor acting as nidus of infection
WBCs	5–8 WBC/hpf is considered significant
Casts	Leukocyte casts may imply pyelonephritis
Bacteria/organisms	Presumptive therapy may be started
	5 bacteria/hpf implies 100,000 colonies
Culture	Definitive diagnosis and antibiotic sensitivity
Blood	
CBC	Leukocytosis implies tissue infection
Blood culture	Required in cases of urosepsis
Serum creatinine	Marker of renal function; required for IVP
Other	
Expressed prostatic secretions	Useful for differential diagnosis in men with lower tract symptoms

RBC, red blood cell; WBC, white blood cell; CBC, complete blood count; hpf, high-power field; IVP, intravenous pyelogram.

predictive of UTI as is microscopic analysis. A false-negative nitrite test can result if the bacteria do not contain nitrate reductase, if urine is not present in the bladder longer than 4 hours, or if there is an absence of dietary nitrite or ingestion of ascorbic acid. Glucosuria, vitamin C, nitrofurantoin, phenazopyridine, or rifampin can produce a false-negative leukocyte esterase reaction.

If the pH is higher than 7.0, this suggests the presence of urea-splitting organisms such as *Proteus* and certain strains of *Klebsiella, Pseudomonas, Providencia,* and *Staphylococcus.* It must be remembered, however, that urine obtained after a large meal or left standing longer than 2 hours tends to be alkaline.

The presence of glucose in urine could indicate diabetes mellitus, which predisposes patients to UTIs.

GROSS EXAMINATION

Although cloudy urine has traditionally been thought to represent pyuria, it more often results from large amounts of amorphous phosphates or urates. This can be verified by the addition of acid or alkali, which dissolves the phosphates or uric acid, respectively.

MICROSCOPY

Blood. RBCs may be present in large amounts in cases of severe infection such as hemorrhagic cystitis or in cases of urolithiasis or tumors acting as a nidus for infection.

WBCs. In the sediment from a clean-catch specimen from men or a catheterized specimen from women, 5 to 8 WBCs per hpf is considered as abnormal and indicates pyuria. Female patients can have pyuria and symptoms of UTI without bacteria in the urine. Sterile pyuria, the presence of pyuria without bacteria, may indicate renal tuberculosis and, if persistent, should prompt acid-fast staining to detect the organism.

A careful study of the urine can often reveal "old" leukocytes (small, wrinkled cells), which are present in the vagina of women and thus indicate contamination. "Fresh" leukocytes indicate acute urinary tract injury.

Casts. Leukocyte casts have been considered suggestive of pyelonephritis and can be easily differentiated from epithelial casts by the addition of acetic acid.

Bacteria. The identification of bacteria or yeast in an uncontaminated specimen is pathognomonic for UTI. It has been shown that approximately 5 bacteria per hpf are equivalent to a colony count of 100,000 organisms per milliliter. The microbiologist can differentiate between different types of bacteria and yeast on the basis of Gram or acid-fast stain, thus giving an early clue as to the type of infection and the appropriate choice of antibiotic. Formal culture and sensitivities further direct the choice of antibiotics.

Other. Squamous epithelial cells in the urine suggest contamination of the specimen. The presence of trichomonads or yeast in the urine can establish the diagnosis and define the treatment.

Chemical

CULTURE

The presence of bacteria in a urine specimen that has been obtained correctly warrants a provisional diagnosis of bacterial infection and should be confirmed by culture. The culture is used to estimate the number of bacteria in the urine, to identify the specific organisms, and to predict the sensitivity to antimicrobials.

It has been considered a standard that 10^5 organisms per milliliter of midstream urine are needed to diagnose a UTI. This has been challenged by several authors, and it has been shown in one study that only 51% of women with symptomatic UTIs were correctly identified using this criterion. The concentration of urine can alter the colony count, and in a dilute specimen, fewer bacteria may be significant.

For routine UTIs, identification of the offending microorganism and its sensitivity may not be necessary, but this is important in cases of recurrent or persistent infections.

If renal tuberculosis is suspected, special methods for growth of *Mycobacteria* should be used. These organisms grow slowly, taking 6 to 8 weeks or longer.

In males, a special method of specimen collection can be employed in the diagnosis of UTI. Four sterile containers are used. The genitalia are prepared in the usual manner. The patient then begins to void. The first 15 mL is collected in container A. The next 15 mL is collected in container B. A prostatic massage is performed and the secretions are collected in container C. The final voiding specimen is then collected in container D. Urine from each container is then tested for nitrite-leukocyte and microscopy. Positive results only in A indicate anterior urethritis. If all specimens are positive, this indicates cystitis or an upper UTI. If only C and D are positive with a colony count ten times that in A, this is indicative of prostatitis.

COMPLETE BLOOD COUNT

Upper UTIs result in significant neutrophilic leukocytosis. The WBC count is used to monitor the response to treatment.

CHEMISTRIES

Routine chemistries should include electrolytes, calcium, phosphorus, and uric acid and an estimation of serum albumin. Serum creatinine is helpful in gauging renal function and is also required by radiologists prior to performing studies such as the IVP and CT scan.

BLOOD CULTURES

Blood cultures are frequently positive in renal parenchymal infections or infections secondary to seeding from remote sites.

Imaging Studies

PLAIN FILM

The KUB is important to identify radiopaque stones or unusual gas patterns, as in emphysematous pyelonephritis. Findings suggestive of a perirenal abscess include absent psoas shadow or altered renal contour.

INTRAVENOUS PYELOGRAM

The IVP may show renal enlargement, impaired contrast secretion, cortical striation, or ureteral striations—all indicative of acute pyelonephritis. It is required in cases of complicated UTI and may demonstrate possible complicating factors such as stones or obstruction or urinary tract anomalies.

COMPUTED TOMOGRAPHIC SCAN

A CT scan is helpful when a renal abscess or postoperative infectious complications are suspected. It is the best method to delineate anatomic detail because it shows the various planes and is sensitive for the detection of attenuated parenchyma, compression of the collecting system, or renal enlargement. It may also be used to place a drain or for other interventional modalities.

ULTRASONOGRAPHY

Renal ultrasound demonstrates stones, abscesses, cysts, or hydronephrosis. It is easy and noninvasive and is rapidly performed. It can be used to follow renal growth in children who have had severe infections in early childhood.

VOIDING CYSTOURETHROGRAM

The voiding cystourethrogram is an imaging study that is useful in children to document and diagnose reflux disease such as vesicourethral reflux. It can also be used to evaluate neurogenic bladder or urethral or cystic diverticula, which often lead to repeat infections.

OTHER

Radionuclide scans with gallium or indium are helpful in patients in whom an intra-abdominal abscess is suspected but localizing signs are absent and the ultrasonogram or CT scan is noninformative.

Prostate Cancer

SERUM PROSTATE-SPECIFIC ANTIGEN

Since its introduction in 1986, prostate-specific antigen (PSA) testing has revolutionized the treatment and screening of prostate cancer. PSA is a protease with a half-life of 3 days that is secreted by prostatic cells and serves to liquefy semen.

Total PSA

The "normal" values of PSA range between 0 and 4 ng/mL. In BPH, the estimated rise in PSA level is about 0.3 ng/mL for every 1 g of BPH. In prostate cancer, the rise in PSA varies with the degree of differentiation of the cancer cells. About 30% of patients with PSA levels higher than 4 ng/mL have prostate cancer, regardless of rectal examination findings. An age-adjusted measurement scale can increase the sensitivity and specificity of PSA. Various studies quote the upper limit of normal as 2.5 ng/mL for men between 40 and 49 years of age, 3.5 ng/mL for men 50 to 59 years of age, 4.5 ng/mL for men 60 to 69 years of age, and 6.5 ng/mL for men 70 years of age and older. Fewer than 5% of patients with prostate cancer have a normal PSA, and even in this group, age-specific PSA levels are able to identify the subgroup that will benefit from a biopsy.

PSA Velocity

The Baltimore Longitudinal Study of Aging gives a guideline for following the serial measurement of PSA levels in men with elevated PSA levels but negative biopsies. If the PSA level rises by 0.75 ng/mL per year or faster, repeat biopsies are indicated. Most authors recommend following a trend of PSA levels over 6 months to detect this change early.

PSA Density

PSA density (serum PSA/prostate volume) is another method to determine which patients need biopsy. A PSA density of between 0.1 and 0.15 is associated with a 15% incidence of cancer, whereas a density higher than 0.15 is associated with a 60% incidence of cancer.

Free PSA

PSA exists in several forms, including free PSA, which is unbound to proteins. The ratio of free to total PSA has been proposed as a new indicator to improve the specificity of this marker. A ratio of less than 0.15 is associated with prostate cancer. This is most useful in the range of total PSA between 2 and 10 ng/mL.

The greatest value of PSA lies in its ability to detect recurrences. The PSA level should drop below 0.1 ng/mL after radical prostatectomy. Failure to do so reflects residual disease. A rising PSA level after surgery also indicates recurrence of disease. This recurrence is a microscopic recurrence in the prostate bed in 42% of patients and is systemic disease in the remaining 58% of patients.

PSA also seems to be an effective marker to monitor patients with advanced prostate cancer and to monitor response to therapy in these patients. A relation between disease-free survival and serially measured PSA levels as well as a relation between the rate of fall of PSA after chemotherapy and survival has been reported.

DIGITAL RECTAL EXAMINATION

The only sign of prostate cancer may be an abnormal rectal examination. Any irregular, firm, or hard nodule palpable on digital rectal examination (DRE) should be biopsied. Needless to say, the DRE should be a standard part of any routine physical examination performed by the primary care physician who, more and more, is becoming the only physician a patient is likely to see.

TRANSRECTAL ULTRASOUND

Transrectal ultrasound (TRUS) can identify up to 55% of cancers that may be nonpalpable. The highly cellular, compact nature of the cancerous region makes it hypoechogenic in 60% of cases. TRUS also allows the urologist to perform directed sextant biopsies of the prostate, ensuring that adequate sampling is obtained. TRUS can also be used to gauge the extracapsular extent of the disease and for real-time biopsy of seminal vesicles. However, TRUS has a high false-positive rate due to lesions such as BPH and prostatitis and a high false-negative rate due to the 40% of cancers that are hyperechoic or isoechoic.

NEEDLE BIOPSY

Needle biopsy of the prostate gives tissue for examination and definitive diagnosis of the presence of cancer as well as the grade of cancer.

INTRAVENOUS PYELOGRAPHY

IVP is no longer required in the evaluation of prostate cancer, because the positive findings are nonspecific and occur late in the disease process. Prostate cancer, like BPH, can obstruct the bladder outlet and produce bladder hypertrophy, trabeculation, and residual urine that can be seen on IVP. Infrequently, prostate cancer may invade the bladder and cause ureteral obstruction.

COMPUTED TOMOGRAPHIC SCAN

The role of CT scanning in prostate cancer is limited to when extensive nodal involvement is suspected. It is useful in patients with a rising PSA after surgery to evaluate adenopathy but has a sensitivity ranging from 50% to 75%, and the disease has to be extensive for it to be detected by CT scanning.

MAGNETIC RESONANCE IMAGING

Magnetic resonance (MR) imaging has limited usefulness in the staging or evaluation of patients with prostate cancer. Although this study is more accurate than TRUS (75% compared to 65%), most patients already have undergone TRUS and do not need MR imaging. MR imaging is useful in younger patients, where it serves to delineate the neurovascular bundle along its entire course, thus aiding nerve-sparing operations. In cases where radiographic lymph node staging is to be performed, MR imaging is the choice over CT scan.

BONE SCANNING

The most accurate method to identify and delineate bony metastasis in patients with prostate cancer is technetium 99m–labeled methylene diphosphonate bone scanning. The false-positive rate of bone scintigraphy is quoted at less than 2%. False-positive results may result from previous bony trauma, Paget's disease, or arthritis. Plain films may aid to differentiate these lesions, followed by CT scanning or MR imaging if needed. A bone biopsy may be required in some cases.

OTHER TUMOR MARKERS

Acid phosphatase was formerly used as the classic marker for prostate cancer. It is elevated in 70% of patients with extracapsular and metastatic prostatic disease. The sensitivity and specificity values of PSA are better than those of acid phosphatase, and most physicians have abandoned acid phosphatase determination for uncomplicated prostate cancer.

Semen Analysis

SAMPLE COLLECTION

At least two samples of semen at 1-week intervals are required to make any valid deductions. Two to 3 days of sexual abstinence prior to specimen collection is required. The specimen can be collected by masturbation, coitus interruptus, or intercourse using a special condom without spermatotoxic agents and placed in a clean, wide-mouthed container. No more than 2 hours should elapse before the specimen is examined.

COMPOSITION OF SEMINAL FLUID

Normal values for semen* are the following:
  Ejaculate volume 1.5–5.0 mL
  Sperm concentration >20 million/mL
  Motility >60%
  Forward progression >2.0
  Morphology >60% normal
  In addition, there should be no significant pyospermia, hyperviscosity, or significant agglutination.

Volume

The normal volume of semen per ejaculate is 1.5 to 5 mL. Less than 1.5 mL signifies either absence or dysfunction of the seminal vesi-

---

*Macleod J: The semen examination. Clin Obstet Gynecol 8:115–121, 1965.

cles, obstruction of ejaculatory ducts, androgen deficiency, or retrograde ejaculation. A volume that is greater than 5 mL can cause dilution of the sperm with low concentration.

Concentration

Various studies have shown that unless the sperm count falls below 20,000,000/mL, there is no effect on male fertility. If the semen volume is less than 1.5 mL or more than 5.0 mL, then fertility may be affected, per se, regardless of count.

Motility

Sperm motility is the most important factor in considering individual factors of semen composition. *Motility* refers to the number (in percentage) of sperm having flagellar motion.

Normalcy is the presence of at least 60% motile cells with a scale greater than 2.

Morphology

The normal spermatozoon is 3 to 5 μm long and 2 to 3 μm wide. The normal specimen contains 60% or more normal forms with fewer than 3% immature forms.

Additional Parameters

pH

The normal pH of seminal fluid is 7.05 to 7.80. The pH of seminal vesicles is higher than 7. The pH of prostatic secretions is less than 7. Hence, pH is lower in patients with absent or dysfunctional seminal vesicles.

FRUCTOSE

The normal range of fructose in semen is 120 to 450 mg/dL. Values less than 120 mg/dL are seen in inflammation of the seminal vesicles, androgen deficiency, partial obstruction of the ejaculatory ducts, or incomplete ejaculation. Fructose is absent in patients with absent seminal vesicles and vas deferens or in case of obstructed seminal vesicles.

WBC STAINING OF SEMEN

WBC staining of semen is a test that is recommended in patients with more than 10 to 15 round cells per hpf or more than 1 to 3 million round cells per milliliter. If most of the cells are WBCs and the concentration is greater than 1 to 3 million WBCs per milliliter, the patient should be evaluated for a genital tract infection.

SUGGESTED READINGS

1. Brendler CB: Evaluation of the urologic patient. *In* Walsh PC, Retik AB, Vaughan ED Jr, Wein AJ (eds): Campbell's Urology, 7th ed. Philadelphia, WB Saunders, 1998, pp 131–157.
2. Bushman Ward Wyker JAW: Standard diagnostic considerations. *In* Gillenwater JY, Grayhack JT, Howards SS, et al (eds): Adult and Pediatric Urology, 3rd ed. St. Louis, Mosby-Year Book, 1996, pp 63–77.
3. Shock NW, Greulich RL, Andres R, et al: Normal Human Aging: The Baltimore Longitudinal Study of Aging. NIH Publication No. 84-2450. Washington, DC, U.S. Government Printing Office, 1984.
4. Williams RD: Urologic laboratory examination. *In* Tanagho EA, McAninch JW (eds): Smith's General Urology, 14th ed. Norwalk, CT, Appleton & Lange, 1995, pp 48–60.

4 Principles of Imaging Studies of the Genitourinary System

John J. Keizur
Sakti Das

Radiologic imaging studies play an integral role in the diagnostic evaluation, therapeutic procedures, and overall management of urologic disorders. These tests help define the structural anatomy of the urinary tract as well as its functional status and thereby aid in characterizing the disease process. Quite often, however, the physician is overwhelmed by a myriad of available tests to evaluate a particular condition. A basic understanding of the individual tests can help develop a rational selection of the tests, which would limit injudicious use of imaging studies, minimize morbidities of exposure to radiation and contrast agents, and reduce health care costs.

To better define the urinary tract, iodinated radiopaque contrast agents are used that attenuate and block x-rays to create opacification. Following intravenous (IV) administration, these relatively inert contrast agents are neither secreted nor reabsorbed by the proximal tubule. They are exclusively excreted by the kidneys, reaching a final concentration 50 to 100 times greater than the fluid first filtered at the glomeruli. Hypertonicity of these otherwise inert agents can cause a variety of toxic reactions mediated by hyperostosis and direct hemotoxicity. It is important for the primary physician to know about the contraindication of contrast studies and how to prevent and treat potential reactions to contrast agents.

Common Urologic Imaging Studies

INTRAVENOUS PYELOGRAPHY

There has been a steady decline in the use of intravenous (excretory) pyelography (IVP) during the last two decades owing to the proven utility of ultrasonography as the initial study for determining the presence or absence of a kidney, localizing renal masses and assessing their cystic or solid nature, and identifying hydronephrosis. In patients with significant renal trauma, computed tomography (CT) is frequently used as the initial study instead of IVP.

Despite the trend in its limited use, IVP is a historical cornerstone study in urologic imaging and remains as the primary modality for assessment of calculi, the pyelocalyceal collecting system, and the ureter.

Technique

There are differences in opinion about the need for catharsis and fluid restriction prior to IVP. Decision for such preparations should be individualized depending on the urgency for the study and associated medical conditions. Ordinarily we prefer to give a dose of magnesium citrate as a light bowel preparation to minimize intestinal gas and feces that may obscure fine details of the study.

Before injection of contrast agent, a scout film of the abdomen including the kidney, ureter, and bladder (KUB) must be obtained. The KUB offers valuable information about factors such as the soft tissues, skeletal structures, calculus diseases, and abnormal calcifications. Interpretation of a pyelogram could be deceptive without a KUB film.

Iodinated contrast agent is hand-injected through the IV line or a butterfly cannula. The dose used depends on the contrast agent, the patient's size, and the physician's preference. The average adult dose is 200 mg of iodine per kilogram of body weight. In most instances we rapidly inject the contrast agent as a bolus using two 50-mL syringes.

Our usual postinjection filming sequences include exposures at 1, 5, 10, and 20 minutes. A postvoid film is obtained at the end. An ideal study is actively monitored by the physician. Additional films, depending on the clinical situation, may include delayed films, oblique or prone views, films obtained with abdominal compression, and nephrotomograms.

Intravenous Pyelography Findings

A properly performed IVP provides detailed information of the upper urinary tract. On the KUB, any suspicious calcifications, soft tissue masses, or skeletal abnormalities should be noted (Fig. 4–1A). The 1-minute postinjection film shows bilateral equal

nephrograms without calyceal filling. This nephrogram phase provides an excellent opportunity to note renal contour, size, position, axis, and function and any abnormal mass effects. The kidneys should be symmetric, approximately three or four vertebral bodies in length, with the upper pole just beneath the 11th or 12th rib. The right kidney typically is lower than the left because of the liver. By the follow-up 5-, 10-, and 20-minute films, contrast filling of the calyces and ureter should be apparent. Any calyceal deformity, distention, or filling defects should be noted. Similarly, the ureteral course and lie are traced with attention to any medial or lateral deviation or filling defects. Contrast agent is typically visible in the distal ureter by 10 minutes. Delay in contrast medium excretion denotes ureteral stasis and obstruction. The IVP provides only marginal information about the bladder; however, any calculi, filling defect, diverticula, or extreme compression require attention. The postvoid film de-

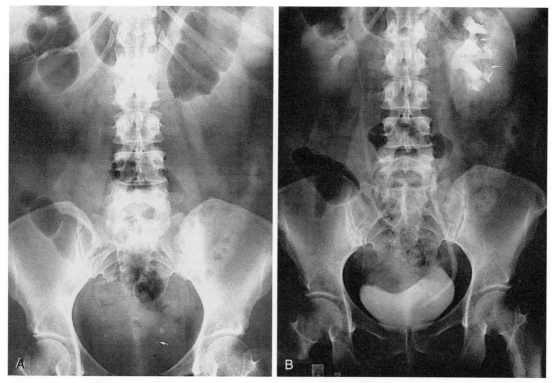

Figure 4-1
A, Plain radiograph (kidneys, ureter, and bladder) taken before contrast medium administration for an intravenous pyelogram shows a small radiopaque calculus shadow *(arrow)* at the left ureterovesical junction (UVJ). *B,* Subsequent delayed film at 40 minutes shows extravasation of the dye at the calyceal fornices *(arrows)* and columnization of the dye up to the left UVJ calculus.

termines bladder-emptying capability and also exposes the distal ureter.

PEARLS

- Acute ureteral obstruction requires delayed films until the contrast agent columns down to the level of obstruction. High-grade obstruction may be suspected when it takes longer than 2 hours for the contrast agent to reach the site of obstruction. Contrast extravasation near the renal sinus and calyces indicates high-grade acute distal obstruction (Fig. 4–1B).
- Oblique films often help establish whether a radiopaque shadow lies within the kidney-ureter. A right oblique film enhances the right kidney and left distal ureter and the left oblique film enhances the opposite.
- Abdominal compression can aid in filling and visualizing the upper collecting system. A film immediately after release of compression maximizes filling of the distal ureter. Compression should not be used if obstruction is suspected.

VOIDING CYSTOURETHROGRAPHY

Ideally performed under fluoroscopic monitoring, voiding cystourethrography (VCUG)

provides information regarding the anatomy of the bladder, antegrade voiding function, and integrity of the ureterovesical valve mechanism.

Technique

After a precontrast KUB is obtained, the bladder is filled with contrast agents under gravity pressure through a urethral catheter until the patient complains of fullness and desires to void. The catheter is then removed and the patient is instructed to void. Under fluoroscopic monitoring the entire study may be recorded, with intermittent spot films obtained during voiding (Fig. 4–2A and B).

Normal Findings

The bladder should appear smooth and ovoid, with adequate capacity. The bladder on voiding should be completely emptied with no vesicoureteric reflux. The urethra should be smooth without abnormal narrowing or dilation.

PEARLS

- Bladder capacity in children can be estimated by the following formula:

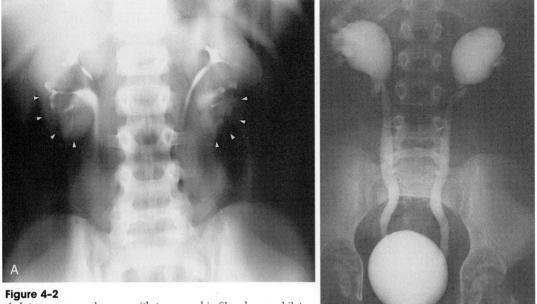

Figure 4–2
A, Intravenous pyelogram with tomographic film shows a bilateral duplicated system with scarring and atrophy of the lower renal segments. B, Voiding cystourethrogram showing vesicoureteric reflux into both lower renal segments.

Age in years + 2 = capacity in ounces

- Oblique and postvoid views can unmask low-grade reflux hidden behind a full bladder.
- In situations where the patient cannot void on the imaging table, a straining film should be obtained. After the patient has voided in privacy, an immediate postvoid film should be taken.
- Vesicoureteral reflux can manifest with only a small amount of contrast agent in the kidneys.
- Gas in the rectum can mimic a filling defect in the bladder. True filling defects in the bladder can be differentiated by lack of gas on the scout film and its persistence in different positions.

RETROGRADE URETHROGRAM

A retrograde urethrogram is necessary in the evaluation of strictures or anterior urethral disease in males.

Technique

The patient is positioned 45 degrees obliquely with the dependent thigh flexed. A small Foley catheter is inserted in the distal urethra, and its balloon is inflated in the fossa navicularis with 1 to 2 mL of saline. The penis is gently stretched out to eliminate redundancy of penile urethra. About 30 mL of radiopaque contrast material is hand injected and a film is obtained of the distended urethra. Often the bladder is distended with injected dye and a voiding film can be obtained to delineate the proximal urethra.

Findings

The pendulous and bulbar urethra should be of smooth outline and uniform caliber. Urethral strictures appear as irregular, narrow areas with proximal dilation (Fig. 4–3). Natural narrowing is noted at the level of the membranous and prostatic urethra.

PEARLS

- Compression of the proximal bulbar urethra by prominent bulbocavernosus muscles in

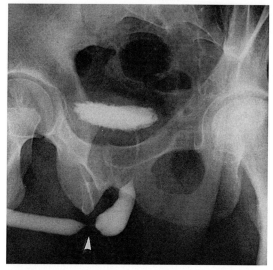

Figure 4–3
Retrograde urethrogram showing a 2-cm-long narrow stricture *(arrow)* at the distal bulbar urethra.

young males may be mistaken for urethral stricture.
- Excessive injecting pressure can cause contrast medium extravasation into corpus spongiosum.
- Retrograde filling of Cowper's duct and gland often indicates the presence of a bulbar urethral stricture.

ULTRASONOGRAPHY

Ultrasonography is probably the most commonly performed imaging technique used in the evaluation of the genitourinary tract. In this study, high-frequency sound waves (ultrasounds) are transmitted to the area of anatomic interest. Sound waves meeting tissues and structures of different densities are reflected back to the transducer, which processes the information by digital computing techniques and displays the image on a monitor. Many advantages of ultrasonography include safety, noninvasiveness, and lack of ionizing radiation. In addition, there is no need for contrast agents and the examination is not affected by renal function and the speed of obtaining real-time dynamic images in different planes. Ultrasound machines are less expensive, widely available, and easily portable to the bedside of seriously ill patients. Ultrasonographic monitoring is extremely useful in guiding percutaneous punctures for drainage, access to renal collecting system, and organ biopsies. More recent color-coded duplex Doppler ultrasonography has made a major impact on the definition of vascular anatomy and blood flow studies of renal, testicular, prostatic, and penile disorders.

The disadvantages are that shadowing by gas, bone, or calculi often obscures the views behind the acoustic shadowing. The field of view is narrow and limited. Ultrasonographic studies are operator dependent.

Despite the limitations, however, because of the clear advantages mentioned earlier, ultrasonography is a common screening technique for patients suspected of a particular ailment. It often provides a diagnosis in an inexpensive manner or, in equivocal situations, leads to supplemental tests such as CT scanning.

Renal Ultrasound

Pathologic distention of the renal pelvis, calyces, and ureter due to ureteropelvic junction or ureteral obstruction is often evident as an echo-free dilated collecting system. Prenatal ultrasonography has become a valuable tool in the diagnosis of antenatal hydronephrosis of the fetus.

Renal calculi appear as echogenic areas casting acoustic shadows. Renal ultrasonography is of special value in demonstrating radiolucent calculi.

Ultrasonography depicts simple renal and peripelvic cysts as echo-free, smooth-walled areas. Renal abscesses have cystic characteristics with low-level internal echoes. Diagnostic confirmation as well as therapeutic drainage is often accomplished by percutaneous puncture under ultrasonic guidance.

Renal cell carcinoma typically appears as an echogenic or relatively echo-poor solid mass (Fig. 4–4A). Angiomyolipomas of the kidney have a characteristic bright appearance on ultrasound due to high reflectivity of the contained fatty elements.

Various medical renal diseases appear with increased echogenicity of the cortex and medulla in a focal or diffuse manner, depending on the pathologic condition. Renal ultrasound is commonly used to screen for renal scarring in children with vesicoureteric reflux.

PEARLS

- If a kidney is not detected in the renal fossa during ultrasonography, one must examine the abdomen and pelvis, looking for an ectopic kidney.
- In addition to obstructive causes, neonatal hydronephrosis on ultrasound may be physiologic or secondary to vesicoureteric reflux or a distended bladder. Further studies with methods such as nuclear scan and VCUG are often necessary with serial follow-up to determine the exact cause of progress of hydronephrosis.
- During pregnancy, hydroureteronephrosis

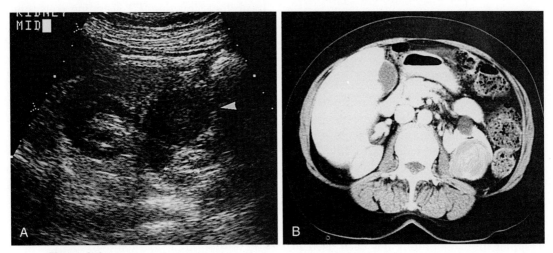

Figure 4–4
A, Renal ultrasound shows a solid echo-poor mass in the lower half of the left kidney. B, Computed tomography delineates the solid left renal neoplasm and a small cortical cyst.

may be observed on ultrasonography, especially on the right side, owing to the pressure of the gravid uterus. This appearance may mimic an acute ureteral obstruction from a calculus.

Bladder Ultrasound

Ultrasonographic evaluation of the bladder as part of the pelvic ultrasound studies sometimes reveals intravesical lesions such as carcinoma, calculi, and ureteroceles with their own characteristic appearances. It is the least invasive method for determination of post-void residual urine.

Prostate Ultrasound

With increasing interest in the early detection of cancer of the prostate, transrectal ultrasound evaluation of the prostate has become a common urologic imaging study in the office to examine the prostate and to guide needle biopsy of the gland. The prostate is scanned in both the transverse and longitudinal axes. The zonal anatomy of the different lobes of the prostate is easily discernible. Benign prostatic hyperplasia often appears as a symmetric echogenic enlargement affecting mostly the transition zone. Carcinomas appear usually as hypoechoic areas in the peripheral zone.

In patients with obstructive azoospermia, prostatic ultrasound may reveal cystic dilation of the ejaculatory duct as evidence of distal obstruction.

Scrotal Ultrasound

- High-frequency, high-resolution ultrasound scanning is helpful in the diagnostic assessment of various chronic and acute scrotal ailments. Testes and epididymis are visible as homogenous echogenic structures. Intratesticular swelling with irregular echoes may denote neoplasm, abscess, or infarction (Fig. 4–5). Clinical correlation helps in establishing the diagnostic suspicion. Colored Doppler ultrasonography has been used in differentiating testicular torsion from acute orchitis.

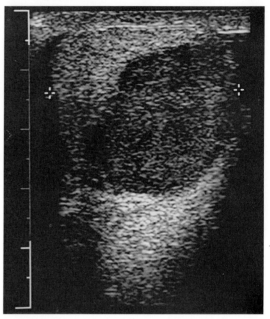

Figure 4-5
Testicular ultrasound showing an intratesticular solid neoplasm.

PEARL

- Because ultrasonography is operator dependent, it is important for the physician and/or patient to point out small testicular swellings for critical evaluation by the sonographer.

COMPUTED TOMOGRAPHY IN UROLOGIC IMAGING

In urologic imaging, CT scanning constitutes the most definitive diagnostic modality. It can illustrate the anatomic features of the urinary tract and retroperitoneal structures in exquisite detail. With dynamic scanning using IV contrast agents, the vascular anatomy of renal lesions is well depicted. Therefore, CT has mostly replaced the more invasive arteriographic studies for diagnosis.

The kidneys and their surrounding structures in the upper abdomen are studied with contiguous 1-cm slices. Oral contrast agents consisting of commercially available water-soluble barium solutions are used to differentiate contrast-filled intestinal tract from renal and retroperitoneal structures.

The initial study is done before IV contrast agent administration. This nonenhanced scan

can reveal features such as calcifications and hemorrhage and provides the baseline CT density (Hounsfield units) for comparison. The study is then repeated following administration of IV contrast medium in a bolus.

Space-occupying lesions in the kidney and retroperitoneum appear in great detail on CT (see Fig. 4–4B). Solid renal tumors are homogenous or have irregular density whose CT numbers are enhanced in the postcontrast study. In comparison, renal cysts do not enhance and have postcontrast density readings near that of water. This feature of nonenhancement becomes significant in differentiating high-density complex cysts or hemorrhagic cysts from renal neoplasms.

For the purpose of staging malignant genitourinary neoplasms, CT is used to scan the liver and examine the retroperitoneum and pelvis for metastatic adenopathy. Suspicious lesions can be aspirated or biopsied with CT-guided needles. In this regard CT has more precision than does ultrasonography guidance.

CT lacks sensitivity in the diagnosis and staging of urologic cancers in the pelvis such as that of the bladder and prostate. We often use CT guidance for needle-aspiration biopsy of large pelvic lymphadenopathy.

Agents for Urologic Imaging

Use of iodinated contrast media is prevalent and is incorporated into many of the previously described studies. Clinicians who request and monitor these tests should have a working knowledge of the properties and toxicities of these agents.

PROPERTIES

Contrast agents are classified into two categories: high-osmolar contrast media (HOCM) and low-osmolar contrast media (LOCM). Conventional agents (HOCM)—diatrizoate and iothalamate—are ionic monomeric salts of tri-iodinated substituted benzoic acids. The hypertonicity and high-osmolar load delivered is responsible for many of the adverse reactions observed. In an attempt to reduce the relative risks of these agents, low-osmolar agents have been developed: Iohexol and io-

pamidol are nonionic benzoic rings with methylated side chains, and ioxaglate is an ionic dimer of two benzoic rings. Although these newer agents are still hypertonic, the reduced osmolar load lessens the risk of adverse reactions while providing quality images. Currently, the universal use of LOCM is limited by the greater expense of these agents.

Contrast media have a number of physiologic effects attributed to the hypertonicity of the agents as well as to direct chemical interactions. Infusion of hypertonic contrast media expands the vascular space, increases cardiac output, and reduces peripheral resistance. Peripheral vasodilation in turn stimulates a reflex tachycardia. Hypertonic influences can result in leakage across the blood-brain barrier, stimulating vagal and emetic centers. In the kidney, contrast media cause initial vasodilation followed by a unique vasoconstriction. Ultimately, the glomerular filtration rate is decreased.

Direct chemotoxic effects of contrast media and its additives depress myocardial contractility and lower the threshold of ventricular fibrillation. Furthermore, contrast media inhibit the coagulation cascade, interfere with platelet aggregation, and cause deformation of red blood cell morphology. In the kidney, evidence supports probable direct chemotoxicity to the renal tubules.

Most of the physiologic properties attributed to the hypertonicity as well as chemotoxic reactions can be attenuated with the use of LOCM. The physiologic effects are transient and rarely of clinical consequence. The risk of contrast-induced nephrotoxicity and anaphylactoid reactions, however, is of clinical significance.

NEPHROTOXICITY

Radiopaque contrast media–induced nephrotoxicity usually manifests with serum creatinine levels starting to rise 24 to 48 hours after exposure and peaking by 3 to 5 days. In most cases, these effects are subclinical and transient, with levels returning to baseline by 10 to 14 days. The occurrence of contrast media–induced nephrotoxicity is usually underestimated unless actively measured. It is estimated to be the third most common cause of hospital-acquired renal insufficiency. In hos-

Table 4-1
Anaphylactoid Reactions

Mild	Moderate	Severe
Local injection pain	Vomiting	Hypotension
Oral metallic taste	Extensive urticaria	Severe bronchospasm
Generalized warmth sensation	Headaches	Laryngeal edema
Sneezing	Facial edema	Pulmonary edema
Coughing	Mild dyspnea, bronchospasm	Myocardial arrhythmia
Limited urticaria	Faintness	Loss of consciousness
	Abdominal or chest pains	

pitalized patient groups, the general incidence of nephrotoxicity is approximately 4.6%. In high-risk groups, this rate may climb to 93%. Since symptoms are delayed and subclinical, identification of these high-risk patients is essential to limit the occurrence of contrast media nephropathy.

The most important predictive risk factor for contrast media–induced nephrotoxicity is pre-existing renal insufficiency. Rates as high as 55% to 61% have been reported in studies of nondiabetic patients with azotemia. The presence of diabetes and azotemia accentuates this risk even further. In diabetic patients with serum creatinine levels higher than 5 mg/dL, contrast media–induced nephrotoxicity occurs in 93%; 56% of these patients will have irreversible changes. Of note, diabetes by itself is not a risk factor. Diabetic patients with normal renal function have rates of contrast media–induced nephrotoxicity equal to those of the general population. Any underlying conditions that may herald the presence of renal insufficiency, such as advanced age, hypertension, proteinuria, and vascular disease, should signal a cautious approach to the use of contrast media. In these cases, a pretest serum creatinine determination is obtained.

Typical radiology departmental protocol involves a preliminary bowel preparation and induction of relative dehydration state to optimize visualization. Healthy kidneys tolerate these effects well; however, diseased kidneys with less reserve are more susceptible to these changes. High-risk patients scheduled to receive contrast media should have alternative studies considered. If that is unavoidable, excessive and repetitive dosing should be restricted, hydration maintained, and LOCM used. Use of LOCM in high-risk groups significantly lowers the incidence of nephrotoxicity.

ANAPHYLACTOID REACTIONS

Intravascular exposure to iodinated contrast media can stimulate an allergy-like reaction.

Table 4-2
Risk Factors for Contrast Media Anaphylactoid Reactions

Strong	Relative
Prior incidence of anaphylactoid reactions	History of asthma
	History of cardiovascular disease
History of strong allergic diathesis	Advanced age
	High anxiety state
Shellfish allergy	Large intravenous bolus of contrast medium

Table 4-3
Commonly Used Medications in Anaphylactoid Resuscitation

Agent	Dosage
Epinephrine	1:1000 0.1–0.3 mL SQ or IM
	1:10,000 1–3 mL IV
Diphenhydramine	50 mg IM or IV
Cimetidine	300 mg IV
Ranitidine	50 mg IV
Famotidine	20 mg IV
Beta-agonist inhalers (albuterol, metaproterenol)	2 puffs
Terbutaline	0.25–0.5 mg IM or SQ
Aminophylline	250 mg IV load, then 0.4–1 mg/kg/hr
Hydrocortisone	200–1000 mg IV load, then 100 mg every 6 hr IV
Ephedrine	10–25 mg IV
Atropine	0.5–1 mg IV
Dopamine	2–20 mg/kg/min IV
Isoproterenol	2–20 mg/min IV

IM, intramuscular; IV, intravenous; SQ, subcutaneous.

These reactions do not seem to be mediated by the classic Type 1 IgE-mediated hypersensitivity cascade and thus are termed *anaphylactoid*. Reactions observed can vary in a wide spectrum of symptoms from mild to severe or life threatening (Table 4–1). Anaphylactoid reactions can occur in any person exposed to iodinated contrast media. Pretesting with a small dose of contrast media is unreliable and has been abandoned. The presence of certain risk factors, however, can help identify a subgroup of patients predisposed to contrast agent reactions (Table 4–2).

Constant diligence is essential whenever iodinated contrast media is used. Since symptoms usually occur within 5 to 10 minutes of injection, rapid recognition of anaphylactoid reactions is imperative to optimize a successful outcome. Trained personnel and a prop-

erly stocked crash cart should be readily available (Table 4–3). Minor reactions usually require no treatment other than reassurance and the occasional antiemetic. Vomiting and sneezing, however, may be a precursor and a warning of an impending severe reaction. In situations of symptomatic urticaria or limited facial edema, antihistamines such as diphenhydramine (Benadryl) can be used alone. More significant and severe reactions, however, require the use of epinephrine. When a patient is showing signs of a severe reaction, epinephrine should be administered immediately after an emergent assessment of patient airway, breathing, and circulation. Epinephrine reverses bronchospasm and maintains cardiovascular support. Administration can be by intramuscular (IM), subcutaneous (SQ), or IV route. Dilutional strength is critical to

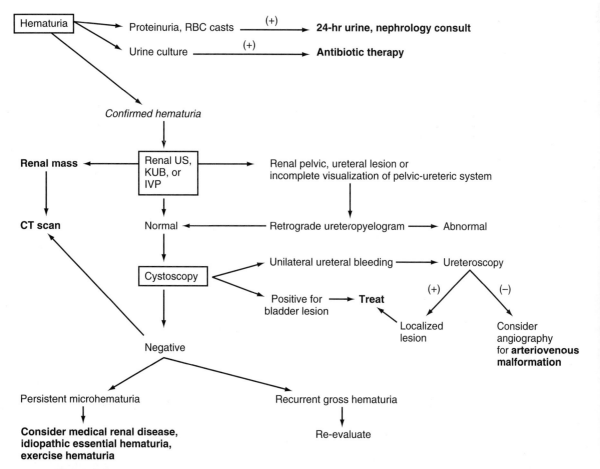

Figure 4–6
Approaches for radiologic evaluation of hematuria are outlined. RBC, red blood cell; US, ultrasound; KUB, kidney, ureter, and bladder; IVP, intravenous pyelogram.

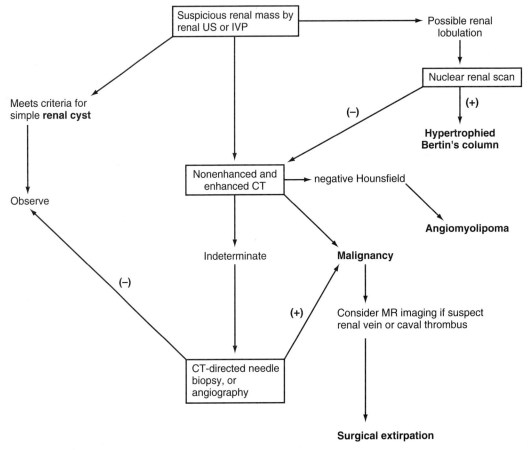

Figure 4-7
This is a suggested scheme for evaluating a renal mass. US, ultrasound; IVP, intravenous pyelogram.

the route administered: Doses recommended for IM or SQ are 0.2 to 0.5 mL of 1:1000 diluted epinephrine (0.2 to 0.5 mg). Doses are repeated as necessary to a maximum of 2 to 3 mL. Alternatively, 1 to 3 mL of 1:10,000 diluted epinephrine IV (0.1 to 0.3 mg) can be used. In frank cardiac arrest, 5 to 10 mL of 1:10,000 epinephrine IV is used. Epinephrine can induce ventricular arrhythmia, myocardial ischemia, and hypertensive crisis. Patients on long-term beta-agonist therapy may become desensitized to the effects of epinephrine and require higher doses. Moreover, patients with hypertension chronically on alpha antagonists may have paradoxical hypotension secondary to unopposed beta-activity effects of the epinephrine. Use of bronchodilators such as albuterol, metaproterenol, and terbutaline can help alleviate bronchospasm. H_1 and H_2 antagonists can soothe cutaneous

reactions. Coincident with pharmacologic therapy, aggressive volume expansion should also be considered.

Vagal reactions characterized by severe bradycardia and hypotension are distinct from anaphylactoid reactions. Treatment consists of IV hydration with incremental doses of atropine, 0.5 to 1 mg IV, to a total of 2 mg. Alternatively, 10 to 25 mg of ephedrine IV may be used.

Prevention of anaphylactoid reactions can be enhanced with pretreatment corticosteroid use and LOCM. Corticosteroids administered 12 to 48 hours prior to a scheduled test in divided doses of 30 to 150 mg of prednisone can significantly reduce the incidence of anaphylactoid reactions in high-risk patients. Of note, corticosteroids given immediately prior to the test (within 2 hours) provide no protective benefit. Use of LOCM also clearly reduces the incidence of anaphylactoid reactions: The incidence of severe reactions is reduced 10-fold with the use of LOCM. LOCM used alone is superior to corticosteroid pretreatment; however, additional protection is gained when the two strategies are used in combination.

Algorithms

Suggested approaches for the radiologic evaluation of hematuria are outlined in Figure 4–6. The approach for evaluation of a renal mass is outlined in Figure 4–7.

SUGGESTED READINGS

1. Bush WH: Treatment of systemic reactions to contrast media. Urology 25:145, 1990.
2. Katholi RE, Taylor GJ, Woods WT, et al: Nephrotoxicity of nonionic low-osmolality versus ionic high-osmolality contrast media: A prospective, double-blind, randomized comparison in human beings. Radiology 186:183, 1993.
3. Keizur JJ, Das S: Current perspectives on intravascular contrast agents for radiologic imaging. J Urol 151:1470, 1994.
4. Novelline RA: Abdomen: Nontraumatic emergencies. *In* Harris JH, Harris WH, Novelline RA (eds): The Radiology of Emergency Medicine. Baltimore, Williams & Wilkins, 1993, p 819.
5. Taveras JM, Ferrucci JT (eds): Radiology: Diagnosis, Imaging, Intervention. Volume 4: Gastrointestinal, Abdominal, and Pelvic Genitourinary. Philadelphia, Lippincott-Raven, 1997.

5

Urologic Emergencies

Unyime O. Nseyo
Janet Colli

Overall, the incidence of urologic emergencies is low; however, the primary care physician needs to be aware of and able to seek appropriate urologic consultations and to do so in a timely manner.

This chapter concerns the following common urologic emergencies that may present either in the office or the emergency department (ED): acute urinary retention, gross hematuria, acute renal colic and flank pain, and acute scrotum, which includes a discussion on torsion and epididymitis. The less common but important urologic emergencies—priapism, Fournier's gangrene, and renal infarction—are also discussed. Early recognition and prompt treatment of each condition can prevent morbidity and mortality. Some of these conditions are discussed in more detail in related chapters. We intentionally exclude from this chapter a discussion of acute urologic injuries, which are presented in detail in the chapter on genitourinary trauma.

Acute Urinary Retention

Urinary retention, whether chronic or acute, has underlying causes, including intravesical or urethral obstruction, impaired detrusor function from neurologic conditions, or psychogenic factors (Table 5–1). Occult neurogenic disease must be ruled out in young males and females who present with acute urinary retention. In men 55 years of age or younger, prostate cancer must be excluded as a cause of their acute urinary retention.

EVALUATION AND MANAGEMENT OF ACUTE URINARY RETENTION IN THE EMERGENCY DEPARTMENT

Diagnosis

Evaluation of a patient experiencing acute urinary retention begins with a thorough history, including a history of trauma, prior lower genitourinary tract disease, instrumentation, or malignancy. A complete physical examination with particular attention to the abdomen, genitalia, and perineum should be performed.

Physical Examination

Physical examination of the abdomen begins with looking for asymmetry, abdominal distention, or a palpable bladder. Examination of the genitalia should reveal the presence or absence of swelling, laceration, or blood at the urethral meatus. Perineal examination should exclude swelling, ecchymosis, or tenderness that would indicate urethral trauma.

Management

A history of urethral stricture, prior transurethral resection of the prostate, lower urinary tract instrumentation, or lower urinary tract trauma should alter the approach. Catheterization should be performed with a smaller ($\leq$ 14 French) catheter. If the catheter fails to advance freely into the bladder, a urologic consultation should be considered. A patient with blood at the urethral meatus should not be catheterized; the patient must be evaluated by a urologist. A patient in acute urinary

Table 5-1
Acute Urinary Retention:
Etiologic Classifications

Classification	Etiologic Factors
Anatomic	Urethral stricture
	Benign prostatic enlargement
	Acute prostatic hematoma
	Prostate cancer
	Bladder neck contracture
	Urethral stone
	Foreign body (iatrogenic)
Functional	Neurogenic
	Neurogenic bladder
	Neurologic diseases
	Multiple sclerosis, Parkinson's disease
	DESD, tabes dorsalis, Alzheimer's disease
	Spinal cord injury, stroke, brain tumor
	Spinal bifida occulta
	Abdominal pelvic resection
	Posterior pelvic exenteration
	Spinal anesthesia
	Postoperative pain
	Viral infection
	Echovirus (primarily in female children)
	Encephalitis
	Lower urinary tract instrumentation
	Pregnancy
	Drug toxicity
	Alcohol toxicity
	Traumatic pain
Psychogenic	Hinman's syndrome
	Emotional derangement

DESD, detrusor external sphincter dyssynergia.

retention secondary to acute prostatitis may be managed best with suprapubic cystotomy drainage.

The following steps are suggested in managing patients in acute urinary retention:

1. Have available a wide range of catheter sizes (10 to 24 French).

2. Instill 10 mL of lubricating jelly, preferably mixed with 2% viscous lidocaine, into the urethra.

3. Attempt urethral catheterization with an average-sized catheter of 18 French.

4. Consider a coudé-tip Foley catheter, 20 to 24 French, which has the push-strength to push aside the lateral lobes of benign prostatic enlargement.

5. At the most, three fruitless attempts at bladder catheterization should warrant a urologic consultation.

6. Use of metal sound dilators such as van Buren sounds or filiform with followers by nonurologists to dilate urethral stricture should be discouraged and is not recommended.

7. Should a catheter meet an obstruction in the anterior urethra or if there is a history of urethral stricture disease, a member of the urology service should pass a filiform through the stricture into the bladder. If the filiform is successfully placed into the bladder, a follower could be successfully threaded onto the filiform and advanced into the bladder to dilate the urethral stricture. It is important to soak the filiform and followers in warm sterile saline or water to keep them soft and pliable during use. Filiform and followers that have not been soaked and softened in warm saline or water should not be used to dilate a urethral stricture.

8. When an attempted blind transurethral drainage of the bladder fails, the urologist most likely will elect to perform percutaneous suprapubic cystotomy under local anesthesia. An alternative approach in the ED or office is the use of flexible cystoscopy to insert a guidewire through a narrow urethral lumen under direct vision into the bladder. If in doubt, a fluoroscopy with the C arm is used to confirm the proper placement of the guidewire into the bladder. A Hayman dilator is passed over the guidewire to dilate the urethral stricture. After adequate dilation to at least 18 French, a coudé-tip Councill catheter is passed over the guidewire into the bladder for drainage.

9. A patient who has a complicated urethral catheterization should receive an immediate broad-spectrum parenteral antibiotic followed by an oral antibiotic for a few days.

10. There is no contraindication to draining the bladder rapidly.

11. Urologic consultation must accompany every patient treated for urinary retention in the ED or office. The role of the urologist remains to identify the underlying condition and/or precipitating events that contributed to the urinary retention.

Potential Complications of Acute Relief of Bladder Outlet Obstruction

Urinary bleeding (hematuria) is usually caused by rapid decompression of the distended bladder with resultant mucosal venous oozing.

POSTOBSTRUCTIVE DIURESIS

Etiology. Clinical postobstructive diuresis (continuous urine output > 200 mL/hr) occurs if bladder outlet obstruction results in bilateral ureteral obstruction. Patients have retention of sodium and water. The diuresis, which is often transient and self-limited, is an attempt to achieve fluid and electrolyte balance. The rare pathologic significant diuresis may occur when the following conditions are present: (1) impaired urine-concentrating ability; (2) impaired sodium reabsorption; and (3) solute diuresis caused by retained sodium or administered glucose.

Management. Thirst mechanisms correct any water loss in the conscious patient. However, daily weights should be monitored and frequent blood pressure measurement must be made. Pathologic sodium loss should be replaced with 0.5 normal saline at 50% of total urine output to avoid sodium overload. Pathologic diuresis from nephrogenic diabetes insipidus has a urine specific gravity ranging from 1.000 to 1.004. The patient who has impaired sodium reabsorption has isotonic urine.

HYPOTENSION

Hypotension is a complication that may occur as a consequence of vasovagal response to the rapid relief of distention or relief of chronic pelvic venous stasis caused by the bladder distention. This is often transient and self-limiting and should be treated symptomatically.

Gross Hematuria

Hematuria in general has been discussed extensively in Chapter 6; however, this chapter contains outlines of the management of gross hematuria in the ED.

COMMON CAUSES OF GROSS HEMATURIA

Table 5–2 lists the common causes of hematuria.

Table 5–2
Hematuria: Common Causes

Infection: cystitis, pyelonephritis, prostatitis, urethritis
Stone: renal, ureteral, bladder
Malignancies: renal, ureteral, bladder, prostatic, urethral
Benign prostatic enlargement
Trauma
Postoperative conditions
   Prostatectomy
   Resection of bladder tumor

DIAGNOSTIC EVALUATION

An evaluation should include a complete history; physical examination; laboratory tests, including urinalysis, coagulation profile, platelets, and creatinine; and imaging studies. All diagnostic tests should be individualized according to the patient's age, gender, and clinical presentation.

MANAGEMENT OF GROSS HEMATURIA IN THE EMERGENCY DEPARTMENT

The most important principle of ED management of gross hematuria associated with multiple trauma is that the hematuria must be evaluated and treated in the context of other associated injuries.

All patients with gross hematuria evaluated in the ED must have a urologic follow-up. Bladder tumors tend to bleed intermittently; therefore, a delay in diagnosis is quite common. Patients must be counseled properly. The patient with associated injuries, hypotension, and clot retention needs immediate intervention. The trauma team must be available to evaluate and manage any associated injuries. Hypotension must be treated by replacement of intravascular volume with crystalloids and colloids; consider blood transfusion if indicated.

The patient with bladder clot retention must be evaluated by the urology service immediately. The initial action may be the insertion of a large-bore (22 to 24 French) Foley catheter, and irrigation, till clear of clots, with sterile water, which lyses the clots better because of its hypotonicity. The urology service will subsequently proceed with cystoscopy, clot evacuation, and examination for the source of the bleeding. Hematuria from acute cystitis in a healthy young male or female does not call for hospitalization.

Acute Renal Colic and Flank Pain

Pain in the urinary tract can be either locally felt in or near the affected organs or referred from a distant involved organ because of common innervation of both the involved site and the location of the perceived pain. However, the ED physician must consider other possible gastrointestinal or gynecologic causes of similar presentation of pain.

Involvement of the upper ureter (i.e., ureteropelvic junction) might elicit the referred pain to the loin and lower flank or testis (in males) or vulva (in females); obstruction at the level of the mid-retroperitoneal ureter refers the pain to the lower quadrants or suprapubic region; and the distal pelvic ureter refers the pain to the scrotum (in males) or vulva (in females) or groin.

DIFFERENTIAL DIAGNOSIS

Urolithiasis is the most likely cause of renal colic and flank pain. However, the other common urologic sources of pain such as pyelonephritis must be ruled out. One must consider also the less common conditions outlined in Table 5–3.

Table 5–3
Urolithiasis: Primary Differential Diagnosis

Renal colic secondary to noncalculus etiology
  Passage of blood clot
  Passage of necrotic material (sloughed papilla)
  Stricture or compression of ureter (extrinsic) or
    excessive angulation of ureter
Other causes of abdominal/flank pain
  Gastrointestinal: appendicitis (retrocecal), terminal
    ileitis, diverticulitis, cholecystitis, cholelithiasis,
    duodenal or ventricular ulceration, pancreatitis
  Vascular: infarction of kidney, spleen, or bowel, renal
    vein thrombosis, abdominal aortic aneurysm
  Gynecologic: ovarian cysts, adnexitis, ectopic
    pregnancy, endometriosis
Rare causes: psoas abscess, retroperitoneal masses,
  cardiac infarction, porphyria, heavy metal
  intoxication, diabetes mellitus, pheochromocytoma,
  Addison's disease, metastatic breast cancer

PHYSICAL EXAMINATION AND HISTORY

In a patient presenting with an upper urinary tract stone, a thorough history would elicit a classic acute onset of the renal colic. Pain is intermittent with ureteral contractions and resultant increased intrarenal pelvic pressure. Change in the position does not ameliorate the pain. It is commonly associated with nausea and vomiting. Depending on the site of ureteral obstruction, the pain can be referred to the groin, scrotum, or testis in men and to the groin or vulva in women. History must also include any comorbid medical conditions. The physical examination should include palpation of the neck for parathyroid tumor or adenoma.

Flank pain due to pyelonephritis often has a gradual onset and an unrelenting course; it worsens by movement and is associated with high fever. There is often an associated history of cystitis. However, a patient with an infected stone can present with acute obstructive pyelonephritis associated with high fever, costovertebral angle tenderness, and bacteriuria.

LABORATORY AND DIAGNOSTIC STUDIES

Urinalysis. The important confirmatory laboratory test typically shows red blood cells, fewer white blood cells, and no bacteria except in the case of an infected stone. Infected urine has red blood cells, lots of white blood cells, and bacteria; the presence of white blood cell casts is diagnostic of pyelonephritis. Crystals in the urine may suggest the composition of stones.

Serum Chemistries. An elevated serum creatinine level, particularly in a patient with a solitary kidney or obstructing urolithiasis, warrants an emergent urologic consultation and renal drainage to relieve the obstruction. An elevation in serum creatinine contradicts obtaining an intravenous pyelogram. Serum calcium, phosphorus, or uric acid determination is not indicated in the ED; however, any abnormal result must be considered in triaging the patient.

Serum Complete Blood Count. This test is necessary in the differential diagnosis and in triaging the patient whose diagnosis of urinary tract stone is not straightforward.

Urine Culture. A urine specimen for culture should be obtained in every patient with renal colic.

Plain Abdominal Radiograph (Kidney, Ureter, and Bladder [KUB]). A large percentage (85% to 90%) of kidney stones are radiopaque and can be visualized on a plain radiograph. Watch out for "hidden stones" overlying the sacrum or lateral spinal processes and "false stones" in the pelvis mimicked by phleboliths with characteristic uniform roundness and central lucency.

Intravenous Pyelogram. This remains the most important diagnostic study in the detection and treatment of urinary tract calculi. The test is contraindicated in the patient with an elevated serum creatinine level (> 2 ng/dL) or history of contrast allergy. A renal ultrasound should be the preferred study in this patient, and any evidence of obstructive uropathy should warrant an emergency urologic consultation.

MANAGEMENT

Indications for admission of the patient with renal colic include the following:

1. Obstructing stone associated with fever and urinary tract infection, (i.e., obstructive pyelonephritis)
2. Obstructing stone in a patient with a solitary kidney
3. Pain controllable only by continuous parenteral analgesics and/or narcotics
4. Intolerance to oral hydration
5. A large (>1 cm) stone too large to pass spontaneously
6. Comorbid medical conditions such as diabetes mellitus; debilitating illness such as spinal cord injury; advanced age; and steroid-dependent chronic obstructive pulmonary disease

Most patients presenting with acute renal colic and flank pain due to calculi are young and healthy and can be treated for their acute symptoms in the ED. Hydration to initiate diuresis and parenteral or oral narcotics are the immediate therapeutic options. Subsequent management should include pain control with nonsteroidal anti-inflammatory drugs and/or oral analgesics, and oral hydration. All patients evaluated and/or treated in the ED for renal colic or flank pain must have follow-up urologic consultation.

Acute Scrotum

The most common causes of acute scrotum are torsion and epididymitis. However, Table 5–4 contains the clinical features to be considered in the differential diagnosis of acute scrotum.

Table 5–4
Acute Scrotum: Differential Diagnosis

	Torsion*	Epididymitis	Tumor
AGE	Birth to 20 yr	Puberty to old age	15–35 yr
PAIN			
Onset	Sudden	Rapid	Gradual
Degree	Severe	Increasing severity	Mild or absent†
NAUSEA/VOMITING	Yes	No	No
EXAMINATION			
Testis	Swollen together and both tender	Normal early	Mass
Epididymis		Swollen, tender	Normal
SPERMATIC CORD	Shortened	Thickened, often tender as high as inguinal canal	Normal
URINALYSIS	Normal	Often infection	Normal

*Testis and appendices of testis and epididymis.
†Present in 30% of patients with testis tumor.

TORSION

Background and Incidence

Torsion of the spermatic cord occurs in 1:4000 men 25 years of age or younger. Two thirds of the cases of torsion occur in boys between 12 and 18 years of age.

Etiology

Etiology of torsion is not fully understood; however, putative factors include abnormal anchoring of the testis to a narrow mesorchium or loose attachment of the epididymis to the testis. The so-called bell-clapper deformity is depicted in Figure 5–1. This deformity is usually bilateral. A majority of torsions are intravaginal. Neonates often have extravaginal torsion.

Diagnosis

Torsion of the spermatic cord remains one of the most serious pediatric emergencies and demands urgent and accurate diagnosis. In the history, torsion is characterized by a sudden onset of an acute, severe pain that may be associated with nausea, without voiding symptoms, urethral discharge, or fever. One third of patients have had a history of previous scrotal pain due to incomplete torsion and detorsion. On physical examination the involved testis rides high in the scrotum with a horizontal line (Fig. 5–2); the cremasteric reflex may be absent; and there is no relief of pain on elevation of the testis. A bell-clapper deformity may be palpable on the contralateral side.

Laboratory and Special Studies

Urinalysis is often normal; and a complete blood count may show mild leukocytosis. An imaging study, such as color Doppler ultrasound or testicular scan, may show a decrease or lack of blood flow with a cold spot. Torsion of 720 degrees (two complete twists) is necessary for a complete stoppage of blood flow.

Treatment

Testicular survival or germ cell viability is directly related to the duration of torsion. Therefore, aggressive surgical intervention is mandatory. Delay in surgical intervention is often caused by inappropriately ordered tests. Manual detorsion may be performed in the ED and used only as a temporary measure.

Bilateral orchidopexy should be performed to prevent retorsion. Orchiectomy is indicated only when the affected testis appears clinically ischemic and nonviable, that is, after a prolonged duration of more than 12 hours or in the absence of a rapid return of blood flow following intraoperative detorsion. Surgical excision of the nonviable (affected) testis minimizes adverse effect, probably immunologic, on the contralateral testis.

Clinical Outcome

Permanent germ cell injury occurs after 4 to 6 hours of torsion. There are 70% to 90% salvage rates if detorsion occurs within 12 hours or less after the onset of torsion.

EPIDIDYMITIS

Etiology

In the age group in which torsion is common, epididymitis is the other important condition that must be considered. In boys, epididymitis is more common in those with a history of urinary tract infections, genitourinary

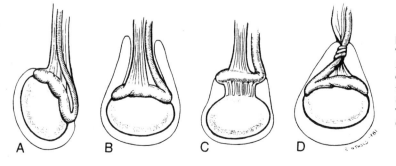

Figure 5–1
Testicular suspensions: *A,* Normal; *B,* bell-clapper deformity; *C,* loose epididymal attachment to testis; *D,* torsed testis with transverse lie. (From Ransler CW III, Allen TD: Torsion of the spermatic cord. Urol Clin North Am 9[2]:245–250, 1982.)

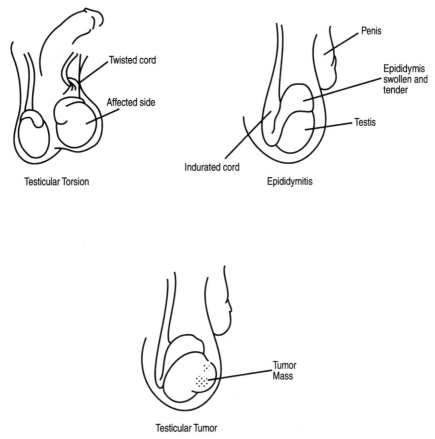

Figure 5–2
Physical findings in acute scrotum: *Upper left,* Testicular torsion; *Upper right,* epididymitis; *Lower,* testicular tumor. Scrotal examination, which begins with palpation of the scrotal contents, should be performed in the following order: (1) testes; (2) epididymides; (3) spermatic cord structures; and (4) inguinal ring.

anomalies, indwelling catheters, and a history of genitourinary surgery. Epididymitis causes 8% to 40% of cases of acute scrotum and is more common in adolescents. Uncircumcised boys have three times higher risk than circumcised boys.

Diagnosis

Onset of scrotal swelling associated with epididymitis is often gradual, with or without fever or chills. A physical examination reveals swelling and tenderness of the involved hemiscrotum. Prehn's sign (relief of scrotal pain with elevation of the testis) may be positive in epididymitis but not with torsion. This finding is unreliable in young children.

Associated signs include fever, leukocytosis, pyuria in 46%, and bacteriuria in 60%. Increased edema and erythema of the in-

volved scrotum are noticeable findings on examination. Epididymitis in young children or infants warrants a complete genitourinary work-up with renal ultrasound and voiding cystourethrogram. An intravenous pyelogram or renal ultrasound should be obtained in adults. Laboratory tests should include urinalysis, complete blood count, urine culture with sensitivity, and determination of postvoid residual bladder urine volume either by bladder scan or urethral catheterization with a 14 French or smaller catheter.

Treatment

The patient with acute epididymitis should be treated with broad-spectrum antibiotics until a urine culture report is available. Scrotal elevation and limited activity are recommended until significant clinical improvement occurs.

Indications for hospitalization include the following:

1. Elevated temperature ($>101°$ F)
2. Clinical evidence of urosepsis
3. Associated acute urinary retention
4. Clinical evidence of evolving epididymo-orchitis
5. Comorbid conditions such as diabetes mellitus, immunosuppression, and advanced age

Priapism

BACKGROUND AND EPIDEMIOLOGY

Priapism (a derivative of Priapus, the Greek god of fertility and lasciviousness endowed with an overzealous phallus) is a painful, prolonged erection, not necessary associated with sexual stimulation (Table 5–5). The erection does not subside after sexual intercourse or masturbation. The two erectile spongy tissues are affected in the following way: the corpora cavernosa become rigid and painful, while the corpus spongiosum remains unaffected. This condition often results in erectile dysfunction (impotence); hence, it is considered a urologic emergency. Priapism can occur in any age group, including neonates. However, there are two characteristic incidence peaks: (1) children 5 to 10 years of age—in this group most cases (64%) are associated with sickle cell disease; and (2) men aged 20 to 50 years, with the apex of the peak occurring at age 20

to 25 years. Most cases in this age group as well as in the neonates are idiopathic.

DIAGNOSIS

The diagnosis of priapism is often made on the basis of history and physical examination. Precipitating factors of priapism include mild acidosis associated with hypoventilation during sleep, erection during the rapid-eye movement phase of sleep, sexual intercourse, masturbation, concomitant infection, and local trauma. The ED physician must elicit any history of an underlying systemic condition such as sickle cell disease or trait, malignancy (e.g., leukemia), polycythemia, or medications. The medications include intracavernosal erectogenic agents, psychotropics, antidepressants, hypnotics, alcohol, cannabis, antihypertensives, anticoagulants, or psychedelic street drugs. In children priapism usually starts during sleep. In a subset of young persons there is a history of frequent recurrent, prolonged erections.

The patient may complain of difficulty with urination; however, associated acute urinary retention is rare. On physical examination, the penis is erect and tender to palpation and manipulation. The dorsal corpora cavernosa are turgid and tense, in contrast with the soft ventral corpus spongiosum and glans penis.

TREATMENT

Priapism is a true urologic emergency. The immediate goal of treatment is to facilitate venous drainage of corpora cavernosa, allowing detumescence of the penis and preventing resultant ischemia, fibrosis, and im-

Table 5–5
Comparison of Normal Erection and Priapism

Factor	Normal Erection	Priapism
Portion of penis involved	Corpora cavernosa and corpus spongiosum and glans	Corpora cavernosa
Cause	Vasodilation of penile arteries	Obstruction of venous outflow
		Disturbance of neuroarterial mechanism (imbalance between it and adrenergic activity)
		Increased viscosity
Sexual desire	Present	Absent
Pain	Absent	Present
Duration	Minutes to hours	Hours to days

potence. The sooner the therapy is offered, the greater the chance of resolving the priapism and minimizing any impotence. Therefore, the ED physician should consult the urologist immediately when the diagnosis of priapism is suspected. The conservative treatment protocol outlined in Table 5–6 should be initiated, and efforts should be made to correct the underlying cause while the urologic team is being contacted.

Percutaneous aspiration and irrigation with saline and injection of epinephrine (10 to 20 μg) or phenylephrine (250 to 500 μg) and manual massage often result in detumescence. If tumescence persists, then surgical intervention is indicated. Venous shunting by whichever means results in a high success rate if it is instituted within 12 hours of onset of priapism. The shunts include percutaneous corpora-to-glans shunt; surgical corpora-to-glans shunt; corpora-to-spongiosum shunt; corpora-to–saphenous vein shunt; and corpora-to–dorsal vein shunt. The other surgical maneuvers include proximal ligation of the internal pudendal artery, embolization of the internal pudendal artery, and division of the pudendal nerve and ischiocavernous muscle.

Priapism secondary to sickle cell disease accounts for 2% to 5% of the cases, and important aspects of management ought to be addressed. If erection persists in the patient with sickle cell disease after implementation of the conservative measures (see Table 5–6), transfusion or supertranfusion with packed red blood cells should be performed. This treatment increases the hematocrit and reduces abnormal forms of hemoglobin. Red blood cell exchange pheresis (erythropheresis) is also recommended. This procedure with normal red blood cells (containing HbAA) results in dilution of sickle cells and increase in oxygen pressure in the general as well as peripheral circulation, including the penile vasculature. If, despite these measures, penile blood gases after 12 hours of observation show marked hypoxia, priapism must be treated aggressively with shunts. The prognosis in boys (7 to 18 years old) is better than in men.

CLINICAL OUTCOME

In general, fibrosis of the corpora cavernosa results in impotence in 50% of affected men. Persistence of the therapeutic shunts could contribute to this posttherapy erectile dysfunction. However, the first and often incomplete erection should occur not later than 3 months after therapy for priapism. Permanent erectile failure can be managed with a penile prosthesis.

Fournier's Gangrene

Fournier's gangrene was initially described in the 1800s as a fulminant, necrotizing infection or fascitis involving the male genitalia. However, this condition now presents often with a more indolent clinical course, with an identifiable source in most of the patients. Associated conditions include local trauma (including operations such as circumcision or inguinal herniorrhaphy), steroid medications, immunosuppression (e.g., acquired immunodeficiency syndrome, renal transplant, hemodialysis, malignancy, or systemic chemotherapy), diabetes mellitus, alcoholism, periurethral extravasation, paraphimosis, and perianal or perirectal infection.

CLINICAL PRESENTATION

Patients often present with generalized symptoms of malaise, genital or perianal discomfort, fever, and chills or sweats for days. The classic triad of sepsis with high fever (>101° F), confusion, and hypotension may herald

---

Table 5–6
Priapism: Conservative Management Protocol

Pain relief: analgesics / narcotics
Sedation: lorazepam may be helpful
Hydration: intravenous fluid and nothing orally until surgical intervention is considered unnecessary
Bladder drainage: with Foley catheter or suprapubic catheter (if patients develop urinary retention)
Reduction of blood pressure may be considered with nitroprusside
Thrombolytic/anticoagulant therapy: given only to those patients with thrombosis of pelvic veins or when priapism occurs during a course of thromboembolic disorder
Discontinue alpha-blocking drugs
Perform specific tests to find cause

impending catastrophe. The genital, perianal, or rectal discomfort is out of proportion to the physical examination. Dysuria, hematuria, pyuria or a history of obstructive micturition, or urethral stricture may suggest a urinary source.

In addition, pain, bleeding with defecation, and a history of anal fissures or fistula may suggest a gastrointestinal source of the problem. Sites of origin include the urinary tract (25%), genitalia (25%), anorectal area (10%), retroperitoneum (10%), and others (30%).

DIAGNOSIS

Clinical presentation, history, and findings of impending necrosis and crepitus in the involved organ often lead to the unmistakable diagnosis of Fournier's gangrene. Laboratory abnormalities include anemia secondary to the overwhelming or evolving sepsis, elevated serum creatinine level, hyponatremia, and hypocalcemia. A plain radiograph of the abdomen, particularly in the presence of crepitus, may be helpful in identifying and delineating the extent of air.

TREATMENT

Immediate diagnosis is crucial in aborting the 50% mortality rate associated with this condition, which progresses rapidly in most cases. Cellulitis, a less aggressive condition, may present with local pain, edema, and erythema and delay the diagnosis of Fournier's gangrene. However, only Fournier's gangrene can present with exaggerated systemic signs and symptoms of sepsis. Patients need to be stabilized clinically and hemodynamically with parenteral hydration. Because wound and tissue cultures grow multiple aerobic and anaerobic organisms, triple broad-spectrum antibiotics must be initiated. The ED physician must consult the urologic team to initiate surgical interventions that include drainage and débridement, with or without urinary diversion. A general surgical consultation should be sought if there is evidence of perianal or perirectal involvement.

CLINICAL OUTCOME

The clinical outcome of Fournier's gangrene depends on early aggressive treatment, co-morbid medical conditions such as diabetes, alcoholism, immunosuppression, and colorectal involvement. Mortality ranges from 7% to 75%; however, the rate averages 20% when management is aggressive.

Renal Infarction

Acute renal arterial occlusion is a rare embolic problem but an important cause of renal failure and hypertension. The common sources of arterial embolism are the heart and an aneurysm. Cardiac arrhythmias are a causative factor in 55% of the cases; 30% of patients have underlying coronary artery or valvular heart disease. More than 90% of emboli originate either in the left atrium due to atrial fibrillation, atrial myxoma, or left ventricular mural thrombus following myocardial infarction. Any aneurysm—thoracic or abdominal aorta—has embolic potential. The kidneys are affected by embolization in 2% to 3% of all arterial embolic. Renal artery thrombosis has been associated with trauma, complications of angioplasty or angiography, oral con-

Table 5-7
Renal Infarction:
Clinical and Laboratory Features

Feature	Prevalence (%)
Clinical	
Cardiac disease (all causes)	90
Fever >37.5°C	83
Pain	82
Hematuria	80
Atrial fibrillation	59
Nausea and vomiting	50
Nonradiating flank pain	50
CVA tenderness	35
Decreased urine output	24
Gross	17
Hypertension	13
Laboratory	
Elevated LDH	100
Albuminuria 1+ to 4+	93
Elevated SGPT	83
WBC > 15,000	71
Hematuria > 7 hpf	80
Elevated SGOT	66
Elevated alkaline phosphatase	33

CVA, costovertebral angle; LDH, lactose dehydrogenase; SGPT, serum glutamate pyruvate transaminase; WBC, white blood cell; hpf, high-power field; SGOT, serum glutamate oxalic transaminase.

traceptives, syphilis, cocaine use, and pheochromocytoma.

CLINICAL PRESENTATION

There are no consistent or pathognomonic signs of renal infarction; however, acute sharp, nonradiating flank pain is the most common complaint. Other commonly reported clinical features are summarized in Table 5–7. Hematuria, leukocytes, and elevated lactate dehydrogenase isoenzymes 1 and 2 levels are the most prevalent laboratory abnormalities (see Table 5–7).

DIAGNOSIS

The differential diagnosis of renal arterial occlusion includes nephrolithiasis, pyelonephritis, myocardial infarction, and acute cholecystitis. The diagnosis of renal infarction is often suggested on the finding of partial or complete renal ischemia on computed tomographic scan or a defect or nonvisualization in the nephrogram phase of the intravenous pyelogram. Arteriography remains the most accurate test of diagnosis and localization of

the infarct. The angiogram should allow assessment of the status of contralateral kidney and evidence of thrombus or embolic source(s).

TREATMENT

Warm ischemic time of the human kidney is approximately 3 hours; however, aggressive therapy is advocated beyond 24 hours of infarction. Renal revascularization may be accomplished by percutaneous transcatheter thrombolysis with fibrinolytic agents (e.g., streptokinase, urokinase, and recombinant tissue plasminogen activator), or surgical thrombectomy. Treatment endpoints are renal salvage with minimal morbidity and mortality.

SUGGESTED READINGS

1. Fry RE, Fry WJ: Renovascular emergencies. Urol Clin North Am 9:209–214, 1982.
2. Payne CK: Emergency room urology. *In* Hanno PM, Wein AJ (eds): Clinical Manual of Urology. New York, McGraw-Hill, 1994, pp 247–264.
3. Ransler CW III, Allen TD: Torsion of the spermatic cord. Urol Clin North Am 9:245–250, 1982.
4. Sagalowsky AI: Priapism. Urol Clin North Am 9:255–258, 1982.

6

Hematuria: Evaluation and Management

Mohamed Ismail
Leonard G. Gomella

Hematuria is a commonly encountered problem in clinical practice. *Hematuria* is defined as the presence of blood in urine, which can either be gross (visible) or microscopic. Although gross hematuria has been described since antiquity, microscopic hematuria was first described in 1837. The clinical difference between these two types of hematuria is purely quantitative, not qualitative, and it is a matter only of the degree of pathology rather than the type of pathology that differentiates them. In other words, *any lesion that can cause gross hematuria can cause microscopic hematuria.*

Most of the investigations of hematuria have been written by either urologists or nephrologists. Because the two specialists' approaches to hematuria are sometimes different, this chapter attempts to combine the general approaches to hematuria and note where areas of controversy may exist.

Definitions

Gross hematuria occurs when a sufficient amount of blood is contained within the urine to change its color to pink, red, or brown. Only a small quantity of blood (1 mL of blood in 1000 mL of urine) is necessary to make urine appear red. The patient usually detects and reports the gross hematuria. It may be associated with painful voiding or irritative symptoms, or the patient may develop blood clots and be unable to void (so-called clot retention). Asymptomatic microscopic hematuria (AMH), the presence of blood on urinal-

ysis in the absence of any complaints, is a common clinical situation.

The distinction of gross hematuria must be made from other causes of red urine (Table 6–1). First, a determination (microscopic examination) must be made that there are truly red blood cells (RBCs) in urine. If there are none, then the differential diagnosis must be made between other causes of red urine such

Table 6-1
Causes of Red Urine

With a Positive Dipstick
1. Hematuria
2. Hemoglobinuria: negative urinalysis
3. Myoglobinuria: negative urinalysis

With a Negative Dipstick
DRUGS
  Aminosalicylic acid
  Deferoxamine mesylate
  Ibuprofen
  Phenacetin
  Phenolphthalein
  Phensuximide
  Rifampin
  Anthraquinone laxatives
  Doxorubicin
  Methyldopa
  Phenazopyridine
  Phenothiazine
  Phenytoin

DYES
  Azo dyes
  Eosin

FOODS
  Beets, berries, maize
  Rhodamine B

METABOLIC
  Porphyrins
  Serratia marcescens (red diaper syndrome)
  Urate crystalluria

as drugs, vegetables, dyes, or pigments that may lead to pseudohematuria.

Microscopic hematuria is a much more problematic entity, and currently there is no consensus on its exact definition. This is partly due to the fact that normal urine contains a small number of RBCs. The upper limit of what number of RBCs in the urine is "normal" lacks clear definition. In clinical practice, a concise definition of significant microscopic hematuria is needed because various studies have shown that serious urologic disease is present in 5% to 20% of adult patients referred to a urologic clinic for the diagnostic work-up of microscopic hematuria. These studies, however, used broad parameters to define hematuria (ranging from 1 to more than 30 RBCs per high-power field [hpf]), making interpretation of data difficult. In addition, different investigators use different methods for urine collection, handling, and analysis. *For practical purposes, a working definition of microscopic hematuria can be considered to be more than 3 RBCs per hpf in a man and more than 5 RBCs per hpf in a woman.*

Detection of Hematuria

Fresh urine is usually the best sample; if the sample cannot be tested immediately, it should be refrigerated. Urine left standing at room temperature longer than 2 hours is generally not acceptable for urinalysis. Referrals for investigation of microscopic hematuria are often based on a positive urine dipstick test. The test is based on the peroxidase activity of heme. The test can be positive with RBCs, free hemoglobin, or myoglobin in the urine. Thus, a positive dipstick test *must* be confirmed by a microscopic examination. The urine dipstick pattern and the intensity of the color change have been correlated with the number of RBCs or hemolyzed RBCs present and thus provide a semiquantitative analysis.

Myoglobinuria is usually associated with extensive crush injuries or severe burns. Hemoglobinuria in the absence of RBCs on microscopy can be seen in transfusion reaction and paroxysmal nocturnal hemoglobinuria or with extensive systemic hemolysis seen in parasitic infections, drugs, or chemical exposure. Free hemoglobin can be seen in a sample with RBCs that have undergone lysis from improper handling of the specimen.

Several studies have compared dipstick to microscopic urinalysis for RBCs. The sensitivity has been reported to range from 86% to 100%, whereas the specificity has been in a wider range, from 65% to 99%. Today, many clinical laboratories perform a dipstick urinalysis, reserving the microscopic evaluation for those samples that demonstrate an abnormal dipstick.

Using a dipstick, false-positive results can occur when the urine is contaminated by oxidizing agents such as hypochlorite, povidone, or bacterial peroxidases. In women, menstrual flow can contaminate the specimen and make interpretation of the dipstick difficult. False-negative results occur in the presence of reducing agents such as vitamin C at high levels and in urine pH of less than 5.1.

Etiology

There are many causes of hematuria and variations in the frequency with which hematuria is attributed to different conditions. However, in the adult population, neoplasms, urinary tract infections, stones, and benign prostatic hypertrophy (BPH) are the most common causes of hematuria. In children, glomerulonephritis accounts for about half the cases of hematuria, with urinary tract infection as the second most common cause.

With gross hematuria the source in adults is as follows: kidney, 15%; ureter, 6%; bladder, 40%; prostate, 25%; and urethra, 4%. From a practical standpoint, the causes of hematuria are best categorized into the following areas: congenital, traumatic, inflammatory, neoplastic, metabolic, and miscellaneous. These are summarized in Table 6–2 and are discussed further in the following sections.

CONGENITAL

Cystic Renal Disease. Included in the category of cystic renal disease are polycystic kidney disease, medullary sponge kidney, medullary cystic disease, and occasionally simple renal cysts. Ultrasound examination often establishes the diagnosis. Medullary sponge

Table 6-2
Etiology of Hematuria

Congenital
Cystic renal disease
Vascular malformations
Inherited renal tubular disorders
Hematologic abnormalities
Ureterovesical reflux
Pelvic-ureteric obstruction
Benign familial hematuria
Alport syndrome
Posterior urethral valves
Ureterocele

Traumatic
Urinary tract injury
Exercise-induced hematuria
Foreign bodies of bladder or urethra

Inflammatory
Urinary tract infections
Specific infections
Glomerulonephritis
Radiation nephritis or cystitis

Metabolic
Urinary calculi
Hypercalciuria

Neoplasm

Miscellaneous
Urethral disease
Drugs
Anticoagulation-associated hematuria
Nutcracker syndrome
Loin pain–hematuria syndrome
Iatrogenic
Benign prostatic hyperplasia
Renal vessel disease
Obstructive uropathy
Idiopathic urethrorrhagia
Endometriosis

kidney may be associated with the development of urolithiasis.

Primary Ureteropelvic Junction Obstruction. Hematuria can often result after minor trauma. These patients may have flank pain after ingesting large volumes of fluids.

Other Conditions. Posterior urethral valves, vesicoureteric reflux, ureteroceles, and ureteral duplications commonly present in the infant or child as a urinary tract infection.

Vascular Malformations. Hemangiomas and other vascular anomalies are rarely the cause of hematuria. Lower urinary tract vascular lesions are rare. The diagnosis is usually made with urethroscopic evaluation of the upper tract when blood is seen coming from

one ureteric orifice and there is no other more common identifiable cause (i.e., stone or tumor).

Benign Familial Hematuria or Thin Basement Membrane Nephropathy (TMN). TMN is a relatively common condition, with an estimated incidence between 2.5% and 9.2% in the general population. The condition is three to five times more common in females than in males and is a benign condition. The diagnosis is only made on renal biopsy, where the glomerular basement membrane is often seen to be uniformly thinned.

Alport's Syndrome. This syndrome is characterized by recurrent or persistent microscopic hematuria, occasional gross hematuria, proteinuria, progressive renal insufficiency, and high-frequency hearing loss. The mode of inheritance is X-linked dominant with incomplete penetrance.

Inherited Renal Tubular Disorders. This category includes renal tubular acidosis Type I (characterized by hypokalemic, hyperchloremic, non-anion gap metabolic acidosis, and a urinary pH consistently < 6.0), cystinuria, and oxalosis. These conditions may result in stone formation with secondary hematuria.

Hematologic Abnormalities. Bleeding dyscrasias and sickling disorders, especially sickle cell trait, account for 4% and 12%, respectively, of cases of hematuria. Hematuria due to sickle hemoglobinopathies is usually considered only in African Americans, but may occur in whites, especially of Mediterranean origin. (Anticoagulation-related hematuria is discussed in a later section.)

TRAUMATIC

Urinary Tract Injuries. Blunt or penetrating injuries can involve the urinary tract. The degree of hematuria is a poor indicator of the severity of injury to the kidney; severe hematuria may be seen only with minor contusions as well as with massive lacerations. Depending on the type of trauma, one can suspect where the injury to the urinary tract occurs. If the trauma involves the abdomen and the patient has hematuria, renal or ureteral injury is likely. If the patient has a pelvic fracture, injury to the bladder or the urethra is probable.

Exercise-Induced Hematuria. This condition is defined as hematuria, either gross or microscopic, that occurs following strenuous exercise and resolves with rest in people with no underlying urinary tract abnormality. Because the early reports of this condition almost exclusively involved men, some investigators believed that the condition occurred only in male athletes. However, recent evidence in a population of men and women runners suggests a 15% to 30% incidence without a sex bias. Fortunately, the incidence of serious disease in patients with exercise-induced hematuria is extremely low in both men and women, especially in athletes younger than 40 years of age. The cause of exercise-induced hematuria is not completely understood, but it appears to be multifactorial. The various causes have been subdivided according to the anatomic sites of injury and the nature of the sport activity in which the injury occurs. A traumatic renal source of exercise-induced hematuria, whether from a direct blow or from shaking and jolting, is believed to originate from the renal vasculature. Nontraumatic renal injury during exercise is believed to result from hypoxic damage to the nephron as a consequence of decreased renal blood flow as a result of the preferential shift of blood to the heart, skeletal muscles, and lungs. The bladder was implicated as the source of exercise-induced hematuria in one study. Other causes to consider for exercise-induced hematuria are the prostate and the urethra because hematuria has been reported in cyclists and in children riding bicycles with banana-style seats.

Foreign Bodies. Foreign bodies of the bladder or urethra, including a Foley catheter, can cause hematuria.

INFLAMMATORY

Urinary Tract Infections. Infection anywhere in the urinary tract (pyelonephritis, cystitis, prostatitis, urethritis) can give rise to hematuria. The microscopic analysis performed initially should alert the physician to this possibility, since pyuria and/or bacteruria are often present. In most cases, however, there are associated symptoms of the primary process.

Specific Infections. Schistosomiasis, tuberculosis, toxoplasmosis, and malaria are common causes of hematuria in some parts of the world but not in the United States, except in the immigrant population from the endemic areas and in patients with acquired immunodeficiency syndrome.

Glomerulonephritis. Glomerulonephritis is a common cause of hematuria in children and young adults. Several histologic types may be observed, and a brief discussion of this group is included here. With secondary forms of glomerulonephritis, the cause may be obvious on clinical grounds. Such is the case in children, in whom a common cause of hematuria is acute glomerulonephritis secondary to streptococcal pharyngitis or impetigo. In this instance the appearance of gross hematuria 2 or 3 weeks after the infection, low complement levels, and other typical features are usually sufficient to make the diagnosis. Similarly, glomerular involvement by systemic diseases such as Henoch-Schönlein purpura, systemic lupus erythematosus (SLE), hemolytic-uremic syndrome, or bacterial endocarditis can often be recognized from the clinical picture. In contrast with primary forms of glomerulonephritis, a renal biopsy is necessary to make a definitive diagnosis. Different types of glomerulonephritis can cause hematuria; however, IgA nephropathy is by far the most common form in the world and may affect as many as 4% of the population. It is often an indolent form of inflammatory glomerulonephritis that has microscopic hematuria as a constant feature. Taking a careful history will reveal episodes of gross hematuria in 35% to 50% of patients. This may be associated with infections of the upper respiratory tract and other mucosal surfaces where IgA is the protective immunoglobulin. It has a potential to cause progressive renal failure in 25% to 40% of patients. The condition shows a 3:1 male-to-female predilection and is most common between the ages of 15 and 25 years.

Radiation. Radiation nephritis is likely to occur in an adult when the dose to the kidney exceeds 23 Gy. Manifestations of radiation nephritis may appear, after a latency period lasting from months to years, as proteinuria, hypertension, renal insufficiency, and microscopic hematuria. Radiation nephritis is currently uncommon because of proper shielding and advances in radiation therapy techniques. On the other hand, radiation cystitis is relatively more common in patients receiving pelvic irradiation for the treatment of pelvic malignancies.

METABOLIC

Urinary Calculi. Hematuria has been considered helpful in diagnosing urinary calculi. However, hematuria is not universal in patients with urinary calculi at various sites, whether symptomatic or not. Approximately 15% of patients may not have blood in the urine, especially with upper tract stones. It has been speculated that with increasing obstruction, it is less likely that urine can pass to the bladder to demonstrate hematuria from the calculus. In the series evaluating microscopic hematuria, renal calculi have been one of the most common diagnoses, occurring in 5.5% of patients. Although calculi have been found in all series and can be considered to be a cause of microscopic hematuria, a full evaluation should be completed, even after finding a calculus, to rule out neoplasm.

Hypercalciuria. An association between hematuria and hypercalciuria was first noted in 1981. In these studies, patients had increased urinary excretion of calcium despite normal serum calcium levels, with some patients developing urolithiasis. One study involving the evaluation of 83 children with asymptomatic hematuria found 23 with hypercalciuria and suggested that hypercalciuria is the most common definable cause of hematuria in children who do not have urinary infection or proteinuria. Hypercalciuria can occur as a result of many conditions, including hyperparathyroidism, immobilization, vitamin D intoxication, and idiopathic hypercalciuria. Idiopathic hypercalciuria may result from a tubular leak of calcium (renal hypercalciuria) or from increased gastrointestinal absorption of calcium (absorptive hypercalciuria). The mechanism whereby hypercalciuria causes hematuria remains unclear, but it is assumed that hematuria is the result of irritation of the uroepithelia by microcalculi or that microscopic areas of nephrocalcinosis cause bleeding. There is often a family history of renal stone, and some authors recommend evaluation of parents and siblings for hypercalciuria. In contrast with benign essential hematuria, gross bleeding and occasional blood clots may be seen in patients with hypercalciuria. Symptoms may include dysuria, suprapubic pain, or renal colic.

NEOPLASTIC

Neoplastic Lesion. Any neoplastic lesion within the urinary tract can present with hematuria. Although there are a few benign neoplasms of the urinary tract, most lesions are malignant. Cancers commonly seen in the urinary tract can involve the urethra, bladder, ureter, or kidney. Microscopic hematuria, sometimes intermittent, may be the only presenting sign of an underlying cancer of the urinary tract. In several studies urologic cancer was found in 20% to 40% of patients with gross hematuria, with most of the neoplasms in the bladder. In microscopic hematuria, urologic cancer is found in an average of 5.1%, again with most being located in the bladder. Several factors influence the diagnostic yield of cancer in a given patient with hematuria (see later).

MISCELLANEOUS

Urethral Diseases. Urethral strictures are most often seen in men. While sexually transmitted diseases (gonococcal infection) or trauma can result in stricture formation, iatrogenic causes (instrumentation, prolonged or traumatic urethral catheterization) are the most common. Urethral caruncles and diverticulum are seen almost exclusively in women.

Drugs. The pathophysiology of renal damage and hematuria caused by most nephrotoxic agents (aminoglycoside, cyclosporine, cytotoxic cancer drugs, and heavy metals) is similar. These agents cause tubular necrosis and altered membrane permeability. The acute renal failure or tubular necrosis secondary to nephrotoxins is generally reversible. Other drugs can also be incomplete toxins. In abnormal doses or after prolonged use, they may become complete toxins. Hypersensitivity to these drugs may develop and cause interstitial nephritis, particularly in case of penicillin, sulfa drugs, nonsteroidal anti-inflammatory agents, analgesics, cephalosporins, and furosemide. Analgesic abuse can result in analgesic nephropathy, particularly if the lifetime ingestion of the analgesic exceeds 8 to 9 kg. Hematuria occurs in 30% of patients who abuse analgesics. Papillary necrosis is the hallmark lesion, and most patients treated for as brief a period as 12 to 17 years with nonsteroidal anti-inflammatory agents have developed papillary necrosis. Occasional aspirin usage or daily use of low-dose aspirin is unlikely to result in hematuria. Another mechanism by which drugs can cause hematuria is hemorrhagic cystitis, which has been described following administration of cyclophosphamide, mitotane, and methicillin. Finally, certain drugs can indirectly result in hematuria through either urolithiasis (triamterene and carbonic anhydrase inhibitors) or induction of urothelial malignancy (cyclophosphamide and phenacetin).

Hematuria in Anticoagulated Patients. Bleeding in association with anticoagulation has been reported to occur in as many as 40% of patients and is related to the intensity of anticoagulation. In the last few years there has been a decrease in anticoagulation intensity. As a consequence, the bleeding episodes in anticoagulated patients have become rarer. In most cases of macroscopic hematuria an underlying disease is present. A recent prospective study investigated the risk of microscopic hematuria in patients anticoagulated with warfarin (Coumadin). The incidence of microscopic hematuria in the anticoagulated and the control groups was 0.05 and 0.08 per 100 patient-months, respectively. Most anticoagulated patients with microscopic hematuria were found to have an underlying genitourinary tract disease. The data demonstrate that maintaining anticoagulation within accepted parameters (i.e., INR of 2 to 3), anticoagulation does not predispose to hematuria. Thus,

persistent microscopic hematuria or an episode of macroscopic hematuria in an anticoagulated patient warrants screening of underlying genitourinary disease.

Nutcracker Syndrome. This syndrome is caused by compression of the left renal vein between the aorta and the superior mesenteric artery, with consequent venous stasis and parenchymal congestion that may be responsible for the hematuria. The hematuria is usually gross but occasionally may present with microscopic hematuria.

Loin Pain Hematuria Syndrome. This syndrome is mainly described in young women taking oral contraceptives but can also affect young and middle-aged men. The syndrome is characterized by renal colic, which may be unilateral or bilateral and usually does not radiate. Low-grade fever may be present. In most cases the loin pain is associated with isolated dysmorphic hematuria, sometimes with gross hematuria. Blood pressure and renal functions are normal; mild proteinuria may be present. The diagnosis is one of exclusion but may be facilitated by renal arteriography and/or renal biopsy. Arteriography may reveal narrowing and tortuosity of terminal branches and segmental ischemia. Renal biopsy may show mild mesangial proliferation, arteriolar thickening, and hyalinosis with complement deposits in the arterioles. Areas of cortical ischemia and cortical infarcts resulting from microemboli can be seen in nephrectomy specimens. It has been hypothesized that the syndrome is caused by renal vasospasm, which may lead to local hypercoagulability.

BPH. BPH, although one of the most common causes of hematuria in men older than 60 years of age, should never be considered as a cause of hematuria except after more serious urologic pathology has been excluded. The presence of gross or microscopic hematuria in a patient with clinical evidence of BPH is an indication for a full urologic evaluation.

Renal Vessel Disease. Complement 3 arteriolar deposition, arterial emboli or thrombosis, or renal vein thrombosis can present with gross or microscopic hematuria.

Obstructive Uropathy. Hydronephrosis from any cause (e.g., extrinsic compression of ureter from tumors) can present with hematuria, particularly after minimal trauma.

Idiopathic Urethrorrhagia. This is a disease seen in prepubertal boys who see a physician for blood spotting on their underwear between voiding. The cause is unknown, and the course may be protracted. Urethrorrhagia is almost always accompanied by dysuria. Microscopic hematuria can be seen in 57% of patients. Bacterial cultures are always negative. The condition is usually self-limited. A viral cause is suspected but not proven. Meatitis is usually seen in the circumcised boy who is still in diapers. Presumably, the meatitis is caused by an ammonia dermatitis in the area of the meatus, with subsequent ulceration and bleeding. Urethral prolapse in girls may cause blood spotting of the undergarments. It is seen more commonly in African American girls than in whites and is suggested by the appearance of a friable mass at the urethral meatus.

Endometriosis of the Urinary Tract. Endometriosis of this type is a rare cause of hematuria that should be suspected in a woman with cyclic hematuria.

Acute Tubular Necrosis. In addition to the drug causes noted earlier, prolonged periods of hypotension and poor renal perfusion can result in acute tubular necrosis and hematuria in addition to other cellular elements in the urinalysis.

Iatrogenic Causes. Surgical procedures on the urinary tract can result in transient hematuria. Cystoscopy and prostate biopsy may be associated with blood in the urine that tends to clear quickly. Transurethral resection of the prostate or laser prostatectomy may have persistent hematuria, often as long as 3 months. Hematuria after a gynecologic procedure should raise the suspicion of a complication involving the urinary tract.

Work-Up of Hematuria

The diagnosis in patients with hematuria may be readily apparent at the first visit or may require extensive investigation. The sequence and techniques used to evaluate hematuria remain somewhat unsettled. One issue is the value of different imaging modalities and invasive procedures as cystoscopy or renal biopsy in patients presenting with hematuria. More important, the threshold of AMH warranting investigation is still undefined. The follow-up patients with no identifiable cause for AMH after an initial evaluation remains unclear. In the following section, information is presented to identify areas of controversy and highlight the relative value and importance of different imaging modalities in the diagnosis of the cause of hematuria. A reasonable algorithm is then presented.

HISTORY

Personal History. Two points that help to narrow the diagnostic possibilities are the age and sex of the patient. The most frequent causes of hematuria in men and women of different age groups are given in Table 6–3. A history of tobacco smoking should be obtained owing to its strong association with urothelial tumors. Occupational carcinogen exposure to compounds such as naphthyla-

Table 6–3
Most Frequent Causes of Hematuria by Age and Sex

0–20 yr
Acute glomerulonephritis
Acute urinary tract infections
Congenital urinary tract anomalies with obstruction
20–40 yr
Acute urinary tract infection
Bladder cancer
Urolithiasis
40–60 yr (women)
Acute urinary tract infection
Bladder cancer
Urolithiasis
40–60 yr (men)
Acute urinary tract infection
Bladder cancer
Urolithiasis
60 yr and older (women)
Acute urinary tract infection
Bladder cancer
60 yr and older (men)
Acute urinary tract infection
Benign prostatic hyperplasia
Bladder cancer

From Gillenwater JY, Grayhack JT, Howards SS, et al (ed): Adult and Pediatric Urology, 3rd ed. Chicago, Mosby-Year Book, 1996.

mine, benzidine, and 4-aminodiphenyl, often found in rubber or dye industries, predisposes to transitional cell carcinoma and should be verified. Cytoxan chemotherapy may cause acute hemorrhagic cystitis or increase the risk of transitional cell carcinoma 10 years or longer after treatment. In women a menstrual history is helpful because vaginal bleeding is often mistaken for hematuria.

Presenting Complaint. The timing of blood during urinary stream is useful: Initial hematuria suggests prostatic or urethral pathology; terminal hematuria may indicate a bladder calculus irritating the trigone as the bladder empties; hematuria throughout the stream is more often of vesical or upper urinary tract origin. Painless gross hematuria is the hallmark of bladder cancer. Any pain and associated urologic symptoms must be carefully ascertained. The site of pain associated with bleeding may be related to the site of the pathology. Classically, flank pain with hematuria and a palpable abdominal mass are pathognomonic of renal cell carcinoma. Ureteral colic is most often caused by calculi but can also be due to a tumor or blood clot. Symptoms of urinary tract infection and prostatitis should be sought. Symptoms of outflow tract obstruction are relevant because a vascular prostate gland may bleed, whereas incomplete bladder emptying predisposes to infection. Details of factors provoking hematuria, such as exercise and trauma, should be sought. Upper respiratory tract infections are associated with proliferative glomerulonephritis or IgA nephropathy.

Past Medical History. A history of previous nephrourologic disease or surgery must be sought. Details of sexually transmitted diseases or urethral instrumentation (including catheterization) are significant because these predispose to urethral stricture. Past history of tuberculosis, pelvic irradiation, and bleeding diatheses is also relevant.

Family History. There are a number of familial conditions that may cause hematuria, including benign familial hematuria, Alport's syndrome, sickle cell disease or trait, polycystic kidney disease, and coagulation abnormalities. In addition, family history of hypertension, nephrolithiasis, cancer, or chronic renal failure may be relevant.

Drug History. A detailed drug history is mandatory in patients with hematuria. In addition to the variety of drugs that can cause hematuria that were detailed earlier, phenytoin, rifampicin, and ibuprofen and a number of other drugs can lead to pseudohematuria (see Table 6–1).

PHYSICAL EXAMINATION

The physical examination is often normal; however, positive findings in the presence of hematuria, if present, are often significant.

Hypertension may signify renal parenchymal disease, renal failure, renal cystic disease, and renal vascular disease. Hearing loss may suggest Alport's syndrome. Heart murmurs may be associated with subacute bacterial endocarditis. Pallor indicating anemia is associated with several abnormalities, including hemolytic anemia, SLE, and renal failure. Rashes are associated with Henoch-Schönlein purpura and SLE. Generalized edema is associated with severe forms of glomerulopathies (nephrotic syndrome) or renal failure.

Palpable abdominal or flank masses are consistent with hydronephrosis, renal cystic disease, renal tumors, and renal vein thrombosis. Flank tenderness is suggestive of pyelonephritis or urolithiasis. The flank should be examined for evidence of lacerations, contusions, or rib fractures in cases of trauma. Examination of the genitalia may reveal urethral prolapse, meatitis, or meatal stenosis.

Pelvic examination is essential in women, as is assessment of the prostate in men. The pelvic examination in women may identify a urethral caruncle or vaginal prolapse and may exclude misinterpreted vaginal bleeding.

INDICATIONS FOR EVALUATION

In symptomatic hematuria the indications for full evaluation are sometimes dictated by the associated symptoms. On the other hand, a full evaluation in patients with painless gross total hematuria is mandatory because significant urologic lesions are present in approximately 90% of patients. Urologic cancer has been found in approximately 20% to 40%

of these patients, with the majority having bladder pathology. Nephrolithiasis is found in another 11% of these patients.

Microscopic hematuria is somewhat more problematic to evaluate. The difficulty has been to determine what level of microscopic hematuria should be evaluated and which studies should be included. Some authorities recommend the investigation of anyone with microscopic hematuria, irrespective of age, sex, or association with any symptoms. Population-based studies to determine the prevalence of AMH suggest a prevalence of 2.5% to 20%. As many as 38.7% of young men between 18 and 33 years of age had microscopic hematuria at some point over a 15-year follow-up period. If everyone with AMH were to be investigated, then there would be considerable cost involved.

An important discriminating factor in the decision to proceed with a full evaluation is the presenting age. In children, urinalysis should be repeated several times, since at least 20% of cases of microscopic hematuria are transient. Apart from the first set of investigations, in cases of nonglomerular bleeding, it is useful to evaluate the daily urine quantitative excretion of calcium and/or the ratio of urine calcium to creatinine. Ultrasonography may be used to evaluate the upper tract, and, if an abnormality is detected, a radionuclide study may be used to exclude reflux or other congenital anomaly such as ureteropelvic junction obstruction. In children with glomerular hematuria, it is useful to investigate the urine of the parents and relatives to detect a possible familial nephropathy such as benign essential hematuria or Alport's disease. Laboratory tests (discussed later) may be abnormal, pointing to a particular cause for glomerular bleeding. Although only the renal biopsy may provide the final diagnosis, the procedure is optional in patients with isolated microscopic hematuria for whom no therapeutic measures are adopted. Many clinicians prefer to follow the patients regularly to postpone biopsy until proteinuria develops.

In adults the problem is more complex since microscopic hematuria may be the only sign of an underlying malignancy. Previous studies have shown that patients with AMH have incidences of malignancies ranging from 2% to 22%. The chances of those younger than 50 years of age having an underlying urologic malignancy are low. Additionally, in women with microscopic hematuria, the risk of underlying malignancy is considerably lower. In a prospective study, no case of neoplasia was found in 177 women older than 50 years of age followed for more than 6 years. Thus, the risk of cancer in men older than 50 years of age with microscopic hematuria is significant, while it seems negligible in younger men and in women. Of importance, in most patients there is no relationship between the severity of the microscopic hematuria and that of the underlying pathology. An additional factor that may be considered is a history of tobacco use, because this may increase the incidence of urothelial cancers in younger patients of either sex.

Another approach in patients with AMH who are at low risk of cancer may be changing the algorithm of investigations by using less invasive procedures because the incidence of urologic neoplasms is low. Erythrocyte morphology (see later), urine cytology, and an abdominal ultrasound may help the general practitioner in deciding which patients require further evaluation. Further large population-based studies of the prevalence of AMH and its relationship with age and sex are needed before any definitive recommendations, which could have considerable implications for human resources, are formalized into guidelines.

BASIC LABORATORY TESTS

The urinalysis is the cornerstone of diagnosis. All aspects of the urinalysis are important, especially careful microscopic examination of the sediment. The color of urine gives diagnostic clues: Bright red bleeding often suggests a surgically treatable lesion, whereas brown or tea-colored urine generally indicates glomerulonephritis. Specific gravity is a measure of the kidneys' ability to concentrate the ultrafiltrate. Poorly concentrated urine with low specific gravity may suggest hydronephrosis with renal impairment or impaired renal function secondary to nephrologic disease. Urine protein elevations are often present in the presence of gross hematuria. Hemoglobin and plasma protein alone can account for protein of as much as 2+; however, heavy

(3+ to 4+) proteinuria greatly in excess of the degree of hematuria is a frequent feature of the various forms of glomerulonephritis. RBC casts, when present, are pathognomonic of a glomerular source of bleeding. The presence of crystalluria may point to underlying urolithiasis. The urine should be cultured for bacteria when white blood cells, often suggested by a positive leukocyte esterase on the urinary dipstick, are present and if there is microscopic hematuria without RBC casts.

Blood tests such as serum urea, creatinine, and electrolyte estimations identify patients with gross renal impairment. A complete blood count is needed to exclude anemia, especially with macroscopic hematuria. Microscopic hematuria itself is usually not the cause of anemia.

URINE CYTOLOGY

Cytology is particularly helpful to detect high-grade urothelial tumors. Low-grade tumors are much less commonly detected by cytology since they tend to shed microscopically recognizable fragments less often. Atypical cells may also appear as a reaction to calculi or inflammation. Urinary cytology does not normally permit the diagnosis of solid renal masses such as renal cell carcinoma.

Positive urine cytology may precede grossly detectable lesions. In a study of nine patients who had positive urine cytology but normal excretory urograms and cystoscopic findings, eight were found to have urologic neoplasms within 22 months of follow-up. Therefore, any patient with positive urinary cytology on an otherwise negative evaluation for microscopic hematuria should be reevaluated after a several-month interval.

Recently, other tests such as BTA (Bard, Redmond, WA) have been used to detect bladder tumor–associated antigen in voided urine through a type of dipstick analysis. Although several studies have shown that the BTA test may be more sensitive than urine cytology in detecting the presence and/or recurrence of bladder tumors, these tests are not yet considered part of routine clinical practice.

SUPPLEMENTAL LABORATORY TESTING

If a high index of suspicion is present for a glomerular etiology of bleeding, further laboratory measurements should include the following:

- Streptozyme (antistreptolysin O titer)—to evaluate for poststreptococcal syndromes
- Serum complement and antinuclear antibody—to evaluate collagen and vascular disorders
- Total serum proteins and albumin:globulin ratios—to evaluate nephrotic syndrome
- Urine calcium:creatinine ratio should be obtained in cases of microscopic hematuria without other cellular elements—if measured in the first-morning voided specimen, the result correlates with quantitative 24-hour excretion of calcium. A ratio of more than 0.18 is significant and usually means that the 24-hour calcium excretion is 4 mg/kg per day or higher.

Other laboratory tests may include a complete blood count and examination of the peripheral smear for sickling if sickle cell disease or trait is suspected. A skin test and urinary mycobacterial cultures may be performed to exclude tuberculosis.

ADVANCED URINE STUDIES IN DETERMINING THE SOURCE OF URINARY RED BLOOD CELLS

The distinction between glomerular and nonglomerular hematuria may be significant for the diagnosis and the treatment options. Although this can be suggested by the presence of RBC casts and proteinuria or by the clinical setting itself, all these are nonspecific.

Erythrocytes may undergo several morphologic changes in the urine. In patients with glomerulonephritis, urine erythrocytes are distorted, whereas they have normal morphology in patients with urologic pathology. The sensitivity of erythrocyte morphometrics was 95% and specificity 100%. These findings were confirmed in a larger series of patients by the same authors as well as by a number of other investigators. However, in some clinical conditions the analysis of RBC morphology may be unreliable. For example, isomorphic hematuria can be found in glomerulonephritis patients with gross hematuria, with renal insufficiency, or with forced diuresis. Moreover, a mixed morphologic pattern of urinary erythrocytes has been reported in IgA nephritis, which is the most frequent cause of glomerular hematuria.

Recently, the identification of acanthocytes as a marker of glomerular bleeding has been proposed. These cells are ring formed, with one or more protrusions of different size and shape. Their identification is earlier than that of "traditional" dysmorphic erythrocytes and is less subjective. When acanthocytes represent at least 5% of total erythrocytes, an underlying glomerular disease can be diagnosed with a sensitivity of 52% to 99% and a specificity of 98% to 100%. Using a 4% cut-off, in 216 urine sediments from 172 patients, acanthocytes were found in 71% of the samples of patients with glomerulonephritis, which is a 98% specificity and a 96% reproducibility.

Coulter counters, currently employed to count and differentiate peripheral blood cells, can also help differentiate glomerular from nonglomerular hematuria. With a Coulter counter, two clear-cut volume curves can be obtained according to the origin of erythrocytes. In fact, in glomerular bleeding the mean volume of urine erythrocytes is about 50 μm^3 or less and in urologic disorders it is about 90 to 100 μm^3. The method is faster than microscopy, does not require trained personnel, and does not raise any problem of interpretation. A number of investigators confirmed the usefulness of this approach. However, it was found to have lower sensitivity in mild hematuria. Moreover, the presence of cellular and noncellular debris may give unreliable curves. Comparisons with phase-contrast microscopy showed equivocal results, and it was suggested that, whenever possible, both methods should be used.

IMAGING STUDIES

The first-line radiologic investigation of hematuria remains the excretory urography (intravenous pyelogram is considered an "older" term). The scout film of the abdomen may identify potential calculi (Fig. 6–1). Contrast agent is excreted via the urinary system, giving rise to the nephrogram, pyelogram,

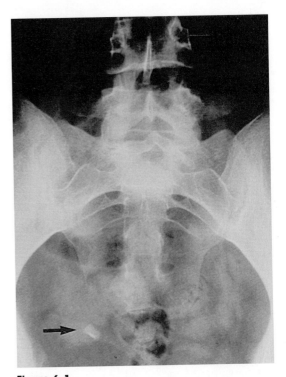

Figure 6-1
Kidney, ureter, and bladder (KUB) radiograph in a patient presenting with hematuria shows a radiopaque shadow (*arrow*) along the course of the distal right ureter that proved to be a calculus.

and cystogram phase of the examination. The nephrogram is usually seen on the immediate film, showing the size, shape, and position of the kidneys. A compression band is usually put around the lower abdomen to delay the flow of contrast agent from the renal pelvis, leading to improved outlining of any filling defect, such as a stone or tumor (Fig. 6–2). Following release of the band, contrast agent flows freely down the ureters. Normally, the ureter is only seen in segments as it peristalses. A standing column of contrast agent within the ureter, delayed excretion, or ureteric dilation may suggest ureteric obstruction. The cystogram image outlines the size and shape of the bladder, with the postmicturition film giving a broad indication of the completeness of bladder emptying. The cystogram phase of the excretory urogram does not provide enough detail of the bladder to exclude intravesical pathology. For this purpose, cystoscopy is needed (see later).

There is continuing debate over the relative merits of excretory urography versus ultrasound scan of the abdomen with a plain ra-

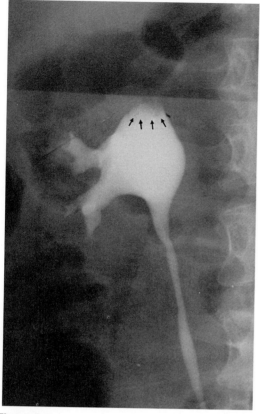

Figure 6-2
Excretory urography in a patient presenting with hematuria that shows a filling defect *(arrows)* in the upper pole calyx. A ureteroscopic biopsy confirmed the presence of a transitional cell carcinoma.

example, renal sonography may be particularly advantageous in a patient who is allergic to intravenous contrast media or who is pregnant.

Computed tomography scanning and magnetic resonance imaging are not a routine part of the initial evaluation of hematuria and are generally reserved for when the initial evaluation reveals the presence of a renal mass.

CYSTOSCOPY AND RELATED TECHNIQUES

Cystoscopy has been the mainstay for evaluating the lower urinary tract. The entire urethra and bladder can be visualized to detect even tiny or subtle lesions. The development of flexible fiberoptic cystoscopes has afforded the patient considerably less discomfort, and in adults this is typically an outpatient procedure using topical local anesthesia. Cystoscopy has been an integral part of the evaluation of hematuria, both gross and microscopic. It is extremely valuable in the presence of gross hematuria to evaluate the lower urinary tract visually, since the source of bleeding may be detected directly. Benign lesions that may be overlooked when bleeding has stopped may be defined as the source. For instance, vessels on the surface of the

diograph. Proponents of ultrasound state that it is less costly and safer than excretory urography. However, with ultrasound there is difficulty in visualizing renal pelvic, and particularly ureteropelvic junction, calculi. In addition, ultrasound cannot detect lesions within the mid-ureter unless the lesion causes obstruction and ureteral dilation. Conversely, ultrasound is more sensitive for imaging parenchymal renal masses, which represent 80% to 90% of adult primary upper tract malignancies (Fig. 6–3). This is particularly important in patients with AMH who may have proportionately smaller renal tumors, most of which are renal cell carcinomas. Several studies conclude that routine excretory urography should not be routinely performed in patients with AMH, particularly in those younger than 40 years of age. Finally, specific risks or benefits of any modality may promote or restrict its use in an individual patient. For

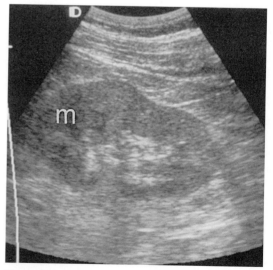

Figure 6-3
Ultrasound image of the right kidney showing a mass (m) in the upper pole that proved later to be a renal cell carcinoma. This mass was treated by radical nephrectomy. (Courtesy of Dan Merton.)

prostate or telangiectatic lesions in the bladder may be seen to bleed. Hematuria emanating from the upper tract may be lateralized as bloody urine streaming from one ureteric orifice. There is additional potential benefit of visualizing a neoplasm within the bladder or the urethra (Fig. 6–4).

Microscopic hematuria also warrants cystoscopic evaluation. Much of the yield in terms of significant lesions found in series of patients with microscopic hematuria has been from cystoscopy. For example, lucent bladder calculi not large enough to produce visible filling defects on the cystogram can be easily seen cystoscopically. Small bladder tumors can be seen in the same way.

Retrograde pyelograms can be performed in conjunction with a cystoscopic examination. Here, contrast agent is injected under direct vision into the ureteral orifice to opacify the ureter and renal pelvis. This is useful in patients who have contrast allergy that precludes intravenous administration of contrast agent but who need an examination of the collecting system.

In patients with a filling defect in the collecting system or in whom the evaluation has localized the bleeding to one kidney without any obvious abnormality detected, ureteroscopy is useful. Here, a tiny fiberoptic scope is passed through the urethra into the ureter and into the renal pelvis and kidney. It allows

biopsy and identification of unusual lesions for hematuria such as hemangioma or arteriovenous malformation of the renal pelvis.

Cystoscopy is not usually recommended in the pediatric population owing to the rarity of tumors and the need for general anesthesia. In addition, at least two studies have suggested only limited value of cystoscopy in specific groups of patients with microscopic hematuria. In a study of 100 men younger than 40 years of age with microscopic hematuria who were evaluated with excretory urography and cystoscopy, the cystoscopy did not detect any lesion not seen with excretory urography. A study of 177 women undergoing similar evaluation for microscopic hematuria also found a low yield from cystoscopy.

RENAL BIOPSY

Needle biopsy of the kidney should be considered in some cases of hematuria. Renal biopsy is a local procedure in adults usually performed using ultrasound guidance. Formal surgical renal biopsy, typically performed laparoscopically, is reserved for patients who are not suited for the ultrasound approach (small kidney, unacceptable body habitus). A recent study from England in patients with AMH demonstrated that the results from renal biopsy were much higher than cystoscopy in all age groups. In this study in which renal biopsy was used routinely to assess patients with AMH, approximately 50% of patients were found to have glomerular disease. This was particularly the case in those younger than 45 years of age (69.2% in those < 20 years), but also in the elderly (40% of the biopsies were abnormal in the seventh decade).

Although renal biopsy is a routine and extremely safe procedure in experienced hands, it is not mandatory in every case. Indeed there may be specific contraindications, such as single or atrophic kidneys. In each case, the merits of obtaining renal histology must be considered. Specific histology may provide a diagnosis but need not necessarily influence management. Many systemic diseases can be diagnosed by blood tests (e.g., lupus nephritis) or are clinically apparent (e.g., Henoch-Schönlein purpura). Classic postinfectious glomerulonephritis can often be confidently

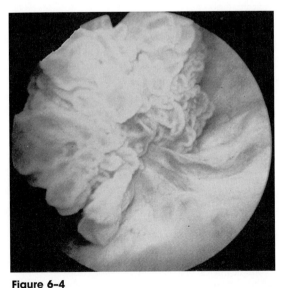

Figure 6–4
Cystoscopic view of a typical transitional cell carcinoma of the bladder.

diagnosed by typical clinical presentation, early fall in the C3 component of complement, raised antistreptolysin O titer, and hemolytic streptococci cultured from a throat swab. More often the clinical picture is less clear, and the absence of renal histology may lead to overinvestigation. The clinical presentation of macroscopic hematuria as part of a nephritic syndrome with deteriorating renal functions demands urgent renal biopsy and frozen section. The finding of a crescentic nephritis then necessitates immunosuppressive

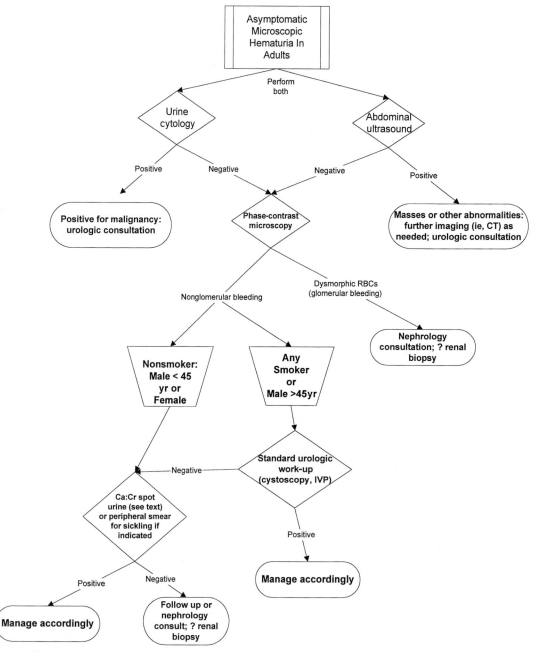

Figure 6–5
Suggested algorithm for the evaluation of adult asymptomatic microscopic hematuria. These patients must have no symptoms referable to the hematuria and a negative urinalysis except for red blood cells (RBC). Adults with gross hematuria require a full urologic evaluation. Ca:Cr, calcium:creatinine ratio; IVP, intravenous pyelogram.

therapy. In a less acute situation, renal biopsy may be sought to reassure the clinician or the patient or to indicate the prognosis in various chronic glomerular conditions.

FOLLOW-UP SURVEILLANCE

Studies indicate that even after a complete evaluation the cause of hematuria remains undiagnosed in as many as 35% of patients. Opinion is divided on the need to follow these patients. Based on a large study evaluating microscopic hematuria that has shown that 19% of the patients with life-threatening lesions had at least one urinalysis with less than 3 RBCs per hpf within 6 months of diagnosis, some recommend periodic urinalysis and cytology. However, how often these patients need to have a standard urologic evaluation is unclear. A long-term follow-up suggests that only patients who become symptomatic should be reinvestigated. Conversely, in another study urologic neoplasms developed within 2 years in 9% of patients who had an initial negative evaluation but had persistent microscopic hematuria.

Recommendations for Evaluation

As can be seen from the earlier discussion, the standard work-up for hematuria cannot be easily generalized. Clinical history, physical findings, physician preferences, and resources available all can alter the evaluation for hematuria. As mentioned earlier, gross hematuria dictates a complete urologic evalua-

tion. On the other hand, the indications and work-up of AMH are less clear. In Figure 6–5 we provide a general guideline for the work-up of AMH in adults, supported by the available contemporary literature. This approach should minimize the risks and cost of the evaluation and optimize the diagnostic process.

Conclusions

Hematuria is a common clinical finding prompting further evaluation. In adults, neoplasm, stones, and infections are the most common causes. In children, glomerulonephritis, infection, and congenital anatomic abnormalities are the most common causes. A careful history, supplemented by the physical examination, may provide insight into the etiology. However, most patients do require formal evaluation for microscopic hematuria, with the extent and techniques used in the evaluation dictated by the clinical setting.

SUGGESTED READINGS

1. Bagley DH: Hematuria in the adult. *In* Coe FL, Favus MJ, Pak CYC, et al (eds): Kidney Stones: Medical and Surgical Management. Philadelphia, Lippincott-Raven, 1996, pp 521–528.
2. Cilento BG Jr, Stock JA, Kaplan GW: Hematuria in children: A practical approach. Urol Clin North Am 22:43, 1995.
3. Clarkson AR: Microscopic hematuria—whom to investigate. Aust NZ J Med 26:7, 1996.
4. Fogazzi GB, Ponticelli C: Microscopic hematuria: Diagnosis and management. Nephron 72:125, 1996.
5. Sultana SR, Goodman CM, Byrne DJ, Baxby K: Microscopic hematuria using a standard protocol. Br J Urol 78:691, 1996.

7

Genitourinary Tract Trauma

Eric S. Rovner
Gregory A. Broderick

Trauma is the leading cause of death for males between the ages of 1 and 40 years. Approximately 10% to 15% of all patients with abdominal trauma have an associated injury to the genitourinary tract. The majority of these injuries are due to blunt trauma (<90%), with the remainder resulting from penetrating injuries. The vast majority of injuries to the genitourinary tract are not immediately life threatening; however, if not recognized they may result in significant morbidity. Failure to identify and appropriately treat urologic injuries at the time of initial evaluation may result in urinoma, abscess, fistula, and/or sepsis. Because of the retroperitoneal position of the kidneys and ureters, injury may not be readily apparent on the initial examination. Thus, a high index of suspicion must be maintained for occult urologic injuries in the patient with trauma. Clues to the presence of urologic injury include gross or microscopic hematuria, pelvic fracture, rib fracture, spinal cord injury, scrotal enlargement or hematoma, and difficulty placing a Foley catheter.

Evaluation of the Patient with Suspected Urologic Injury

A thorough and systematic initial trauma evaluation begins with assessment of the ABCs of trauma (airway, breathing, and circulation). Following resuscitation and stabilization, the injured patient should be evaluated with regard to the urinary tract. A history and physical examination are critical in estab-

lishing the mechanism of trauma, which will often guide subsequent evaluation and management. The conscious patient will be able to provide valuable information regarding the circumstances of the trauma as well as details of personal medical and surgical history, medications, and allergies. The unconscious patient will be unable to provide any information; however, witnesses at the scene of the accident can provide valuable information. For example, the police may be able to provide a characterization of the weapon in cases of penetrating trauma. This characterization may be invaluable in determining the potential extent of injury in gunshot wounds (e.g., in comparison with low-velocity bullets, high-velocity bullets result in a greater transfer of energy and greater immediate trauma as well as a greater potential for delayed necrosis from a blast effect to surrounding tissues) and stab wounds (e.g., longer knives may potentially injure deeper body cavities). In addition, details of an accident scene from the police may be helpful in determining the potential injuries from blunt trauma (e.g., extent of vehicular damage and use of seat belts). Important information obtained from the paramedics at the scene includes the presence of significant hypotension (shock), loss of consciousness, or severity of blood loss.

Physical examination should be expeditious yet complete. Urologic injury may result in flank hematoma, abdominal pain or distention, lower abdominal bruising, midline infraumbilical mass, scrotal enlargement, discoloration of the external genitalia, or blood at the external urethral meatus. After unstable spine injury has been ruled out, the patient with penetrating trauma should be rolled and examined for entry and exit wounds. Rectal examination may disclose a "high-riding" prostate suggestive of posterior urethral disruption or heme-positive stool indicating hemorrhage into the gastrointestinal tract. A urine specimen, voided or catheterized, is essential.

Several points should be stressed at the initial evaluation. Although urinary drainage is essential in the patient with multiple injuries, a Foley catheter should never be placed immediately in the setting of pelvic fracture, blood at the urethral meatus, or scrotal hematoma or in cases of suspected urethral trauma. These patients should undergo retrograde urethrography to determine continuity of the urethra prior to Foley catheter placement. Urethral injury may be indicated by extravasation of contrast medium on retrograde urethrography and will necessitate placement of a suprapubic cystostomy tube for temporary urinary drainage.

Dipstick urinalysis is considered both sensitive and specific in detecting the presence of blood in urine, especially helpful in the hectic setting of a trauma bay. Microscopic urinalysis showing more than five red blood cells per high-power field is a reasonable sign for urologic injury. Conversely, the degree of microhematuria and even gross hematuria does not always correlate with the severity of injury: a subcapsular renal hematoma may produce worrisome gross hematuria without requiring renal exploration, and renal injury may occur without gross hematuria. In a series of more than 1000 trauma patients, McAninich noted gross hematuria in only 30% of patients with renal pedicle injuries, no hematuria in 40% of renal injuries, and no hematuria in 24% of traumatic renal vascular occlusions.

When urinary tract injury is suspected, radiographic evaluation of the urinary tract must follow. The lower urinary tract is best evaluated with contrast studies such as retrograde urethrography to image the anterior and posterior urethra followed by cystography to examine for bladder injury. The bladder may be filled retrograde through the urethra, but most commonly, once the urethra is cleared, the catheter is advanced into the bladder for formal cystography. The upper urinary tracts are evaluated with intravenous urography or computed tomographic (CT) scan. In rare cases, ultrasound or angiography may be indicated. Thorough radiographic evaluation permits identification and staging of suspected urologic injury. Staging of urologic injury allows the surgeon to formulate a rational and effective treatment plan and to avoid unnecessary operative exploration, minimizing morbidity.

Urologic trauma is classified by the damaged organ (e.g., bladder, kidney) as well as the mechanism of injury (e.g., penetrating vs. blunt trauma). Those patients with penetrating trauma, especially abdominal wounds, likely require surgical exploration. In the San Francisco General Hospital series fewer than 10% of blunt renal injuries required surgical exploration, whereas 42% of stab and 76% of gunshot wounds involving the kidney required surgery. In this same series the authors reported an overall renal salvage rate of 88%, which they attributed in part to appropriate staging by imaging.

HIGHLIGHTS

- Accurate details surrounding the circumstances of the injury are critical and should be obtained from the patient when possible or from witnesses (such as the police and paramedics) at the scene of the trauma.
- Physical examination of the patient with urologic trauma includes inspection of the flanks, abdomen, external genitalia, and rectum.
- The degree of hematuria is *not* an accurate indicator of the degree of urologic injury.
- A Foley catheter should *not* be placed in the setting of gross or microscopic hematuria, pelvic fracture, or blood at the urethral meatus unless a retrograde urethrogram has been performed and shows no evidence of urethral injury.
- Most cases of urologic injury are completely staged radiographically prior to surgical intervention. This may include retrograde urethrography, cystography, intravenous pyelogram, CT scan, and in some cases, angiography.

Renal Injuries

The kidney is the most commonly injured organ in the urogenital system. Despite the relatively protected positions of the kidneys in the retroperitoneum, blunt or penetrating abdominal and thoracic trauma should always raise the suspicion of renal injury. Hematuria is the most specific indicator of renal trauma but may also indicate injury elsewhere in the urinary tract.

Historically, renal injuries are classified according to the primary mechanism of injury: blunt trauma accounts for 80% to 90% of reported renal injuries, and penetrating trauma accounts for 10% to 20%—these percentages are a reflection of the predominance of motor vehicle accidents. Unfortunately, in many major urban centers the proportion of penetrating injuries is changing, probably related to the proliferation of automatic weapons.

BLUNT RENAL TRAUMA

Evaluation

Blunt renal trauma results following a direct forceful blow (to the abdomen, flank, or thorax) or rapid deceleration. Commonly this occurs as a result of a motor vehicle accident, sports injury, occupational injury, or assault. Injury from blunt trauma can be explained by three mechanisms: A direct blow to the flank may result in the kidney's being directly compressed against adjacent musculature or bone, producing parenchymal disruption. A fractured rib or lateral vertebral process may lacerate the adjacent parenchyma. Sudden deceleration injury results in stretching and/or shearing of the renovascular pedicle with consequent intimal tearing and arterial thrombosis, or avulsion of a vessel. The clinical stigmata of significant blunt renal trauma include contusions, seat belt marks, lower rib fractures, fractures of vertebral bodies, and/or vertebral processes.

Once a blunt renal injury is suspected, radiographic imaging is indicated. Large retrospective series have shown that an absolute indication for renal imaging in the adult is microscopic hematuria associated with shock (systolic blood pressure <90 mm Hg). In pediatric patients, however, any degree of he-maturia is an indication for radiographic staging. Unfortunately, children (<16 years old) do not consistently show signs of shock (systolic blood pressure <90 mm Hg) with significant renal bleeding. Several characteristics may put children at greater risk for significant renal injury from blunt abdominal or flank trauma: their kidneys are relatively larger in size and less protected by fat and back muscle, and their pedicles are more mobile. The presence of congenital renal abnormalities identified during trauma work-up in children has been reported at 23%. Thus, radiographic imaging in pediatric patients with blunt renal trauma and any degree of hematuria is essential.

All patients with gross hematuria following blunt trauma, regardless of the presence of shock, should undergo immediate imaging of the urinary tract. Multiple studies have shown that in the absence of other clinical stigmata suggestive of renal trauma (rib fracture, flank hematoma, or other significant intra-abdominal trauma such as liver laceration) and with consistently stable blood pressure, the likelihood of major renal injury in adults with blunt trauma and microhematuria is less than 1%. Despite the lack of immediacy for imaging of these patients, they should all undergo repeat urinalysis in follow-up. If the hematuria is persistent, it may signify a urologic source unrelated to the traumatic event (e.g., urologic malignancy).

Once the need for radiologic evaluation of the kidneys has been established, selecting the appropriate studies requires coordination with the trauma team and an assessment of the patient's clinical stability. When associated abdominal injuries are suspected, CT scanning is the initial study of choice. If only renal injuries are suspected and the patient is stable without indication for other abdominal imaging, an intravenous pyelogram with nephrotomography may be adequate. The pyelogram is up to 96% accurate in establishing the presence or absence of renal injury. An abnormal pyelogram or incomplete visualization of the kidneys mandates further studies. Suspicious findings on intravenous pyelography may include contrast extravasation, renal contour deformity, or nonvisualization of one or both renal units. These findings should prompt further imaging, which may include

CT scanning and/or arteriography to define the extent of renal injury.

When the injured patient requires emergent operative exploration, a two-shot "on-table" pyelogram provides valuable information. Radiographic contrast material is given as a bolus of 2 mL per kg (maximum 150 mL) and plain abdominal films are taken at 1 and 5 minutes after injection. This two-shot pyelogram provides an essential piece of information: Is the contralateral renal unit present and functional? The decision to undertake renal exploration and repair of the injured unit should be made with an understanding of contralateral renal integrity. Nonvisualization of one or both renal outlines may signify bilateral renal trauma, congenital absence of one kidney, vascular avulsion, arterial thrombosis, pelvic kidney, or nonperfusion secondary to systemic hypotension (systolic blood pressure <80 to 90 mm Hg).

HIGHLIGHTS

- Blunt renal trauma is exceedingly more common than penetrating renal trauma.
- All pediatric patients with blunt abdominal trauma and any degree of hematuria should undergo urographic imaging.
- All adult patients with blunt abdominal trauma and hemodynamic compromise (e.g., shock) should undergo urographic imaging. All adults with gross hematuria after blunt abdominal trauma should be imaged. Adults with blunt trauma and microhematuria and no evidence of hemodynamic compromise do not require immediate imaging, but routine follow-up should be scheduled.
- Intravenous pyelography and/or CT scan are the most useful imaging modalities for examination of the upper urinary tract after blunt abdominal trauma. The importance of accurate radiographic staging is twofold: determining the extent of renal injury as well as establishing the presence of a functioning contralateral renal unit.
- Important findings suggestive of renal injury on intravenous pyelography include contrast extravasation, renal contour deformity, and nonvisualization of one or both renal units.

Management

Blunt renal trauma has been classified by the extent of parenchymal damage and the presence or absence of collecting system involvement (Table 7–1). Minor renal injuries (Grades I through III) account for the vast majority (85%) of cases (Fig. 7–1). The majority of these patients are managed nonoperatively with bedrest, hydration, serial hemoglobin counts, frequent monitoring of vital signs, and repeat imaging. Patients with more severe renal injuries (Grades IV and V), including shattered kidney, significant urinary extravasation and/or renal pedicle injury, require surgical exploration (Fig. 7–2). The low rate of surgical exploration for isolated renal trauma at major trauma centers (<2%) underscores the success of CT staging and conservative management of blunt renal trauma. These guidelines are certainly dependent on the availability of sophisticated imaging; however, they are not compulsory. For example, in selected cases of Grade IV injury, nonoperative therapy may be adequate even in the face of a small devitalized fragment or urinary extravasation. If there is no other intra-abdominal injury requiring laparotomy, the injury does not involve the renovascular pedicle and has been completely defined radiographically, then observation may be sufficient. Similarly, a Grade III renal injury should be explored in the pres-

Table 7–1
Classification of Renal Injuries

Grade	Injury
I	Renal contusion or subcapsular hematoma
II	Renal cortical laceration or perirenal hematomas
III	Renal parenchymal laceration through the corticomedullary junction or thrombosis of a segmental renal artery
IV	Renal lacerations resulting in a devascularized fragment or collecting system injury with urinary extravasation *or* renal pedicle injury with contained hemorrhage
V	Avulsion of the renal hilum, arterial thrombosis of the main renal artery, or multiple lacerations resulting in a "shattered" kidney

Adapted from Moore EE, Shackford SR, Pachter HL, et al: Organ injury scaling: Spleen, liver, kidney. J Trauma 29:1664, 1989.

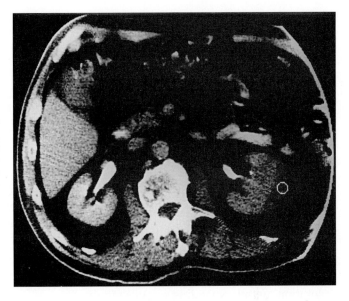

Figure 7-1
Left-sided renal subcapsular hematoma. CT scan with contrast medium shows a smooth, flat indentation of the lateral aspect of the left kidney suggestive of hematoma (indicated by the cursor) with diminished parenchymal enhancement when compared with the contralateral side.

ence of other intra-abdominal injuries requiring laparotomy. Immediate renal exploration and repair in patients with blunt renal trauma and simultaneous intraperitoneal injuries considerably reduce morbidity when compared with simple observation alone.

Indications for emergent renal exploration include an expanding hematoma or a pulsatile hematoma seen at laparotomy, life-threatening hemodynamic instability due to renal hemorrhage, and known Grade V renal injury. Transfusion requirement is not uncommon after renal injury and should not, in isolation, prompt renal exploration. When the need for exploration has been determined, the preferred approach is a midline transabdominal incision. The midline approach allows simultaneous intra-abdominal exploration and retroperitoneal access. Choice of surgical therapy is dependent on a number of factors, including the extent of injury, the salvageability of the kidney, the presence of a functional contralateral renal unit, the hemodynamic stability of the patient, and associated abdominal injuries. Early vascular control through a midline incision reduces renal blood loss and allows for a controlled renal exploration. Renal lacerations can be oversewn using Gelfoam bolsters, Dexon mesh, or retroperitoneal fat if necessary to reapproximate the renal

Figure 7-2
Left-sided renal parenchymal laceration with extension into the collecting system resulting in urinary extravasation. CT scan with contrast medium shows extravasation of the medium into the left perinephric space lateral and anterior to the kidney.

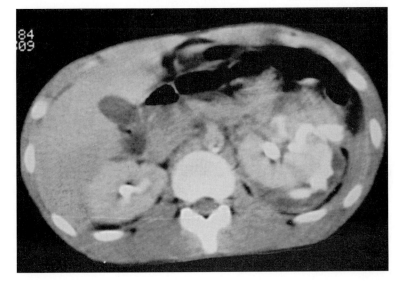

capsule. Devitalized tissue is débrided, collecting system injuries are closed in a watertight fashion, and well-vascularized tissue such as omentum can be laid into the perirenal field to absorb urinary extravasation, preventing the formation of urinomas and urinary fistulas. Nephrectomy or partial nephrectomy is reserved for shattered kidneys or for those patients too unstable to undergo definitive repair.

HIGHLIGHTS

- The vast majority of blunt renal injuries (≤85%) are minor injuries that do not require surgical exploration.
- Absolute indications for emergent renal exploration are an expanding or pulsatile hematoma, life-threatening hemodynamic instability due to a known renal hemorrhage, and a known, radiographically staged Grade V renal injury.
- Principles of surgical exploration for renal trauma are midline incision, early vascular control, débridement of devitalized tissue, and adequate drainage.

PENETRATING RENAL TRAUMA

Evaluation

Penetrating abdominal injuries from stab or gunshot wounds are associated with significant renal injury in 8% of cases. The mechanism of injury in penetrating trauma may be due to the knife or missile itself, fragmentation of the missile, or blast effect of the missile. Blast effect results from the dissipation of energy from high-velocity missiles as they traverse the tissues in the form of heat. This may result in devascularization, devitalization, and necrosis of tissue adjacent to the path of the bullet after the acute injury. Thus, when gunshot wounds are evaluated, careful attention must be paid to the viability of the surrounding and adjacent tissues, with aggressive débridement reserved for tissues whose viability is questionable (Table 7–2).

All patients with penetrating abdominal, flank, or thoracic trauma—regardless of the presence or absence of hematuria—should be considered to have a urinary tract injury until proven otherwise. Lack of hematuria does not

Table 7–2
Indications for Radiographic
Evaluation of Suspected Renal Injuries

Adult penetrating trauma
All pediatric blunt and penetrating trauma
Blunt trauma with microhematuria and hypotension
Blunt trauma with gross hematuria
Suspected associated abdominal injuries

exclude urinary tract injury; up to 14% of patients with major renal trauma (major lacerations or vascular injury) present without hematuria. Since there are no reliable clinical signs of major renal injury secondary to penetrating trauma, all patients who have suffered penetrating injury to the abdomen, thorax, or flank require radiographic surveillance. In the past all penetrating renal injuries came to exploration. Modern imaging techniques, especially CT scanning, can obviate exploration in some instances. For patients undergoing open operative staging for associated intra-abdominal injury or hemodynamic instability, the two-shot on-table intravenous pyelogram may be performed to establish the presence and function of the contralateral renal unit.

Management

As in blunt trauma, a range of options exists for surgical repair of renal trauma depending on several factors, including the extent of injury, the salvageability of the kidney, the presence of a contralateral functioning renal unit, the hemodynamic stability of the patient, and associated intra-abdominal injuries. In the properly staged, hemodynamically stable trauma patient without other intra-abdominal injuries, serial CT scanning has resulted in significant renal salvage with conservative, nonoperative management.

HIGHLIGHTS

- All patients with penetrating abdominal, flank, or thoracic injuries should be radiographically evaluated for urologic injury, regardless of the presence or absence of hematuria.
- "Blast effect" from high-velocity weapons results in devitalization and necrosis of tissues adjacent to the path of the missile.

- As in blunt renal trauma, accurate radiographic staging is essential in the management of penetrating renal injuries.
- Modern radiographic imaging techniques have permitted selective nonoperative management of certain penetrating renal injuries that previously were universally explored.

RENOVASCULAR PEDICLE INJURY

Evaluation

Renovascular injuries are predominantly due to rapid deceleration trauma such as a motor vehicle accident or a significant fall, and much less commonly are due to penetrating trauma. Deceleration injuries may include renal artery or vein thrombosis secondary to stretching and tearing of the vessel intima and thrombus formation over the exposed media. Blunt trauma with vascular injury involves the renal artery in 70% of cases, the vein in 20% of cases, and both vessels in 10% of cases. Rarely, penetrating trauma results in a renal pedicle injury (Grade V) that may cause acute life-threatening hemorrhage.

A high index of suspicion should be maintained for renovascular injury. In many cases hematuria is not seen. Presentation may include unilateral or bilateral nonfunction of the kidneys on contrast media–enhanced radiographic imaging, life-threatening hypotension, or pulsatile retroperitoneal hematoma. Unfortunately, 70% of trauma victims with abdominal or thoracic arterial injuries present in shock, and 30% of the patients with abdominal arterial injuries die. In the case of renovascular injury CT scan may show an absent nephrogram with cortical rim enhancement due to retrograde filling of renal capsular vessels with abrupt cut-off of the main renal artery; a wedge-shaped defect of renal parenchyma is seen if a segmental branch is lost. In the case of renal venous injury there may only be a large retroperitoneal hematoma. Angiography may be used to confirm renal artery thrombosis or to embolize significant hemorrhage.

Management

Early diagnosis and vascular reconstruction are the only hope for preserving renal function. Revascularization can be performed with some salvage of renal function in kidneys with less than 10 hours of warm ischemia time. In large series, 25% to 55% of renovascular injuries result in immediate nephrectomy, and morbidity and mortality rates are high because of associated injuries. Expeditious nephrectomy may be life-saving in many cases of penetrating trauma because severe hemorrhage and associated injuries may mitigate against complex vascular reconstructive efforts of the injured pedicle.

HIGHLIGHTS

- Renovascular injuries are primarily due to deceleration injuries and involve the artery more than twice as often as the vein.
- Nonvisualization of one or both kidneys on radiographic imaging suggests a vascular injury.
- Emergent angiography may confirm vascular injury, and subsequent angiographic embolization may be life-saving in cases of significant hemorrhage.
- Surgical exploration may be attempted in select cases of arterial injury when associated with minimal concomitant intra-abdominal injury and a short warm-ischemia time.

Ureteral Injuries

Evaluation

Ureteral injuries usually occur as a result of iatrogenic or penetrating abdominal trauma. Iatrogenic injuries may occur in gynecologic surgery during hysterectomy, vascular surgery during aortic aneurysm repair, and urologic surgery, especially during endoscopic ureteral manipulation for stone disease or tumor. With the exception of hyperextension/flexion injuries in children that may result in disruption of the ureteropelvic junction, blunt trauma is only rarely responsible for ureteral injury. Ureteral injuries due to external trauma commonly are difficult to diagnose owing to the lack of significant hemorrhage and few early signs and symptoms. One third of patients with penetrating ureteral injuries do not present with hematuria. A high degree of suspicion is required to diagnose ureteral injuries in the acute setting. Diagnosis is often made days or weeks after the acute event by follow-up intravenous urography or CT scanning performed for the evaluation of abdominal pain or fever. Radiographic findings indicative of a missed ureteral injury may include abdominal ascites due to urinoma, hydronephrosis, urinary extravasation, or perirenal abscess (Fig. 7–3). In the acute setting, intraoperative administration of intravenous indigo carmine or methylene blue may confirm ureteral injury by demonstrating urinary extravasation in the operative field.

Management

Treatment of ureteral injuries depends on the anatomic level of trauma (upper, middle, or lower third segment of the ureter), degree of ureteral damage sustained (contusion, partial or complete laceration), time of recognition (intraoperative or delayed recognition), and associated injuries. Isolated, discrete partial ureteral lacerations or perforations at any level can be managed with internal ureteral stenting. Short- and long-term follow-up imaging ensures the resolution of extravasation and the absence of stricture. The options for managing significant distal ureteral injuries include primary reanastomosis over a stent (ureteroureterostomy); mobilization of the upper ureteral segment and anastomosis to the contralateral ureter (transureteroureterostomy); and ureteral reimplantation into the bladder with or without a bladder flap, depending on the amount of ureteral gap that

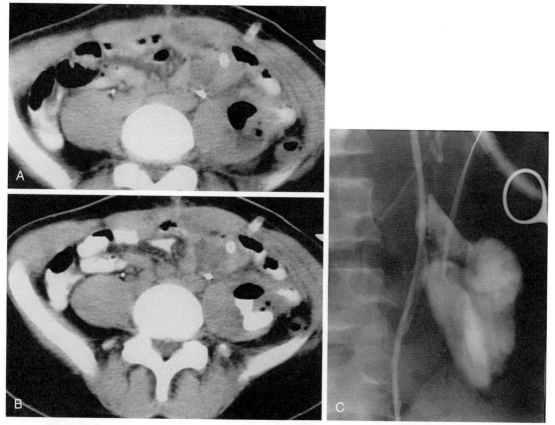

Figure 7–3
These films were obtained for evaluation of gross hematuria after a stab wound to the left flank. *A,* CT scan demonstrates air and blood within the soft tissues of the left flank and psoas muscles, with normal-appearing contrast medium–filled ureters anterior and somewhat medial to the psoas. *B,* Repeat CT scan several hours later for continued abdominal pain and fever demonstrates extravasation of contrast material into the previously air-filled soft tissues, presumably from a ureteral laceration. *C,* Antegrade pyelogram shows extravasation of contrast medium from the ureter into the soft tissues. A contrast medium–filled ureteral stent can be seen traversing the injured segment of ureter.

needs to be bridged. Options for more proximal ureteral injuries include ureteroureterostomy, transureteroureterostomy, ureterocalycostomy (ureteral anastomosis directly to the lower pole renal calyx after performing a lower pole partial nephrectomy), and ureteropyelostomy (ureteral anastomosis directly to the renal pelvis). Interposition of small bowel segments acting as functional "neoureters" and renal autotransplantation are reconstructive options limited to those patients with a long segment of devitalized ureter. Ureteral injuries not immediately recognized later present as urinoma, abscess, sepsis, and/or obstruction. In these delayed presentations initial treatment is proximal urinary diversion (usually percutaneous nephrostomy) and drainage of collections. Reconstructive efforts can then be attempted when the patient is stable and the inflammatory response is resolved. Finally, in the multiply injured trauma patient or in cases of ureteral transection during aortic graft surgery, nephrectomy may be indicated for expediency in the former and prevention of prosthetic graft infection due to urinary extravasation in the latter.

HIGHLIGHTS

- Most ureteral injuries result from penetrating trauma. Blunt ureteral injury is rare except in the pediatric age group.
- A high degree of suspicion is required to diagnose ureteral injuries because many do not present with hematuria.
- Treatment options in the setting of ureteral injury range from internal stenting and drainage to complex urinary tract reconstruction, depending the location (level) and extent of injury.

Bladder Injuries

Evaluation

Bladder injury is uncommon, accounting for only 2% of abdominal injuries requiring repair. Blunt trauma accounts for the majority of bladder injuries; 80% to 90% of bladder ruptures are associated with pelvic fracture. From the orthopedic perspective, only 5% to 10% of pelvic fractures have a concomitant bladder or urethral injury. Bladder ruptures occur in the setting of motor vehicle accidents, falls, and industrial crush injuries. Mortality rates in these cases are high (22%) because of associated injuries, hemorrhage from pelvic bleeding, and other late complications such as sepsis. Bladder rupture from blunt trauma without associated pelvic fracture is typically due to a direct blow to the abdomen (a kick) or sports injury in the presence of a full bladder.

Bladder ruptures are classified as either intraperitoneal or extraperitoneal, with extraperitoneal rupture approximately two or three times more common than intraperitoneal rupture. In 5% to 10% of cases of bladder rupture both intraperitoneal and extraperitoneal injuries are noted. Intraperitoneal ruptures are the result of a tear in the dome—the most cephalad portion of the bladder, which is also considered to be the weakest portion of the urinary bladder. This results in extravasation of urine into the peritoneal cavity. Extraperitoneal bladder rupture results in contained extravasation of urine into the perivesical fat.

Some degree of hematuria is found in all cases of bladder rupture, with gross hematuria being noted in most cases (>90%). Patients may present with severe lower abdominal pain and the inability to urinate in some instances. Radiographic analysis of suspected bladder rupture includes the abdominal plain film, retrograde urethrogram, and cystogram with postdrainage films. Intravenous urography or CT scan with only intravenous contrast agent is nondiagnostic in many cases of bladder rupture because of inadequate filling or lack of distention due to the presence of a Foley catheter. As stated earlier, any patient with gross hematuria, blood at the urethral meatus, pelvic fracture, and/or perineal trauma should be evaluated first with a retrograde urethrogram to rule out a concomitant urethral injury. Cystography with postdrainage films is then the procedure of choice to evaluate suspected bladder injury. Postdrainage films are necessary; 10% of patients will have the diagnosis of urinary extravasation based on this one image. Well-performed cystography is highly accurate (85% to 100%) as compared with the pyelogram (15%) in defining bladder injury (Fig. 7–4). Bladder distention is critical during the cystogram to adequately demonstrate extravasation (Fig. 7–5). A minimum of 250 mL of radiographic contrast material should be instilled to ensure adequate bladder distention.

Radiographic characterization of the bladder rupture as intraperitoneal or extraperitoneal is important. Intraperitoneal bladder ruptures are characterized by filling of the paracolic gutters with contrast medium outlining bowel loops. Extraperitoneal ruptures typically reveal a starburst pattern over the pelvis and diffuse retention of contrast medium in the pelvis below the acetabular line on postdrainage films (Fig. 7–6).

Management

Bladder rupture with pelvic fracture may be associated with large pelvic hematomas and/or urethral injury precluding placement of a Foley catheter for drainage. In these unfortunate cases, an open or percutaneous suprapubic cystostomy may be required for urinary drainage. In many cases extraperitoneal bladder ruptures can be managed nonoperatively with large-bore catheter drainage, antibiotics, and follow-up cystography in 7 to 10 days. Exceptions to this include tears of the bladder neck or large extraperitoneal ruptures that should be repaired in the acute setting, especially if the patient is to have surgical explora-

tion for other associated injuries. The repair should be transvesical to avoid possible pelvic hematomas, and closure should be effected with multiple layers of absorbable suture material. For intraperitoneal bladder rupture, a transperitoneal approach with closure of the bladder in multiple layers and suprapubic tube drainage is preferred. Penetrating bladder injuries should be surgically explored, débrided, and repaired in conjunction with a thorough assessment of other associated intra-abdominal trauma.

HIGHLIGHTS

- Most bladder injuries are due to blunt trauma, associated with hematuria, and occur in the setting of a pelvic fracture.
- Adequate radiographic evaluation of bladder trauma must include images of a well-distended bladder as well as postdrainage films.
- Extraperitoneal bladder rupture may be managed nonoperatively in many cases with Foley catheter drainage.

Male Urethral Injuries

The urethra in males can be divided anatomically into posterior and anterior segments. The posterior, or more proximal, portion consists of the prostatic and membranous ure-

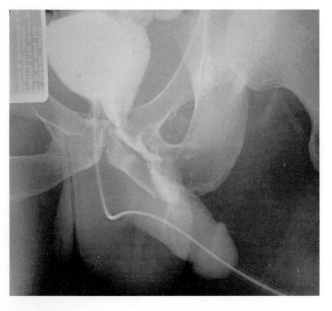

Figure 7–4
Extraperitoneal rupture of bladder. The cystogram demonstrates a contrast medium–filled catheter entering the bladder with gross extravasation of contrast medium overlying the inferior pubic ramus. This injury had an associated pelvic fracture not seen on this film.

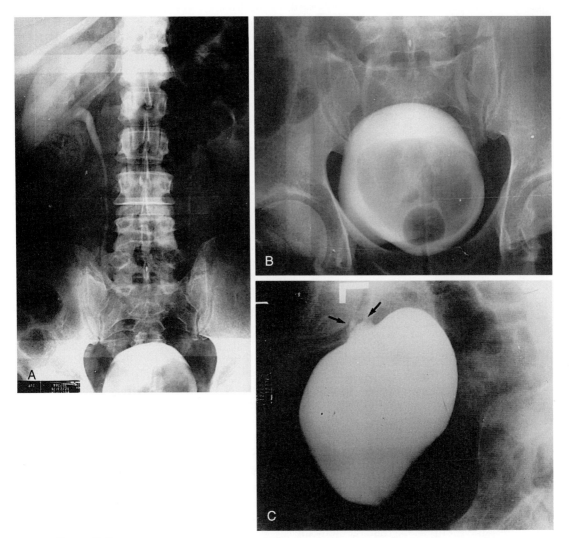

Figure 7-5

These films, obtained for evaluation of gross hematuria in a woman found unconscious after a severe physical beating, show air in the large bowel somewhat obscuring the normal left nephrogram. *A,* The 15-minute film from the intravenous urogram shows normal upper tracts. *B,* Prevoiding film of the urogram shows a filling defect in the bladder suggestive of a blood clot but no clear evidence of extravasation of contrast medium to suggest lower tract injury. *C,* Cystogram obtained several days later demonstrates resolution of the clot, but extravasation of contrast medium is seen *(arrows).* This underscores the importance of adequately filling the bladder during cystography to definitively rule out extravasation.

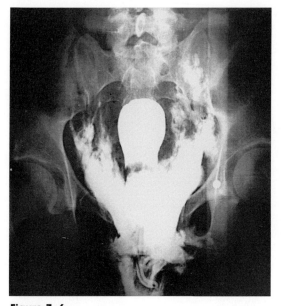

Figure 7-6
Cystogram demonstrating classic extraperitoneal bladder rupture and "tear-drop"–shaped bladder suggesting pelvic hematoma.

thra. The anterior or more distal urethra consists of the bulbar and pendulous (or penile) urethra.

POSTERIOR URETHRAL INJURIES

Evaluation

Injuries to the posterior urethra most often result from blunt trauma and associated pelvic fractures. As many as 95% of posterior urethral disruptions are associated with pelvic fractures that typically involve the pubic rami or diastasis of the symphysis pubis. Posterior urethral injuries can be classified as either complete or incomplete disruptions, which may have important management implications.

The posterior urethra is fixed in place by the urogenital diaphragm and the puboprostatic ligaments. In cases of complete posterior urethral disruption the urethra is typically sheared off proximal to or at the level of the urogenital diaphragm. In incomplete posterior urethral injuries the urethra is stretched or partially torn, but continuity remains between the bladder and the urethra.

The presence of a severe pelvic fracture with hematuria, blood at the urethral meatus, or the inability to void suggests posterior ure-

thral injury and must be evaluated. All patients should undergo digital rectal examination because the displaced or high-riding prostate may suggest posterior urethral trauma. Retrograde urethrography is the study of choice in all cases of suspected urethral injury. In cases of complete urethral disruption, retrograde urethrography demonstrates extravasation of contrast medium in the region of the urogenital diaphragm and disruption of the urethra with no contrast medium entering the bladder (Fig. 7–7). In cases of incomplete urethral disruption, contrast medium is seen extravasating in the region of the urogenital diaphragm, with some of the medium entering the bladder.

Management

Urologic treatment is directed toward preservation of continence and potency with minimization of long-term complications such as urethral stricture, impotence, and urinary incontinence (Fig. 7–8).

Incomplete posterior urethral injuries are managed by placement of a suprapubic cystostomy tube in the acute setting and observation. Many times incomplete injuries heal without stricture formation, obviating the need for additional surgery. A Foley catheter is never blindly placed per urethra in incomplete posterior urethral injuries because it can convert a partial injury into a complete disruption. A voiding cystourethrogram (VCUG) is obtained 2 to 4 weeks later, and if a dense urethral stricture or urinary extravasation is not noted, the tube is removed. Short, diaphanous strictures seen on VCUG can be treated with endoscopic incision and catheter drainage. Longer, dense, and recurrent strictures after failed endoscopic incision may require open surgical repair via posterior urethroplasty.

Traditionally, complete posterior urethral disruptions have been managed by acute suprapubic cystostomy tube placement and delayed urethral repair in 4 to 6 months. In many studies this method has been shown to be associated with the lowest rates of long-term complications such as impotence and incontinence. However, in the setting of complete urethral disruption, this approach is associated with a nearly universal rate of oblit-

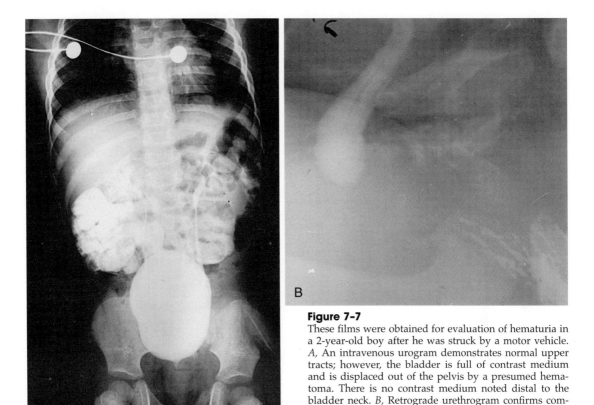

Figure 7-7
These films were obtained for evaluation of hematuria in a 2-year-old boy after he was struck by a motor vehicle. *A*, An intravenous urogram demonstrates normal upper tracts; however, the bladder is full of contrast medium and is displaced out of the pelvis by a presumed hematoma. There is no contrast medium noted distal to the bladder neck. *B*, Retrograde urethrogram confirms complete posterior urethral disruption with perineal and periurethral extravasation of contrast medium into the cavernosal tissues.

erative urethral stricture requiring open operative urethroplasty. In addition, concomitant bladder injuries may exist in up to 20% of cases of posterior urethral disruptions. Gross hematuria on placement of the suprapubic cystostomy catheter suggests a concomitant bladder injury and should be investigated with a cystogram through the suprapubic tube. When a severe bladder injury is noted on cystogram or a bladder neck tear is seen, immediate operative exploration may be indicated.

As opposed to suprapubic tube placement and delayed urethroplasty, some authors have advocated immediate repair or primary realignment over a Foley catheter. When successful, this aggressive approach obviates the need for a long-term indwelling suprapubic tube and has a decreased risk of urethral stricture requiring delayed operative urethroplasty. Primary urethral repair in the acute setting has been associated with higher rates of impotence and incontinence and risks additional hemorrhage and infection of the

pelvic hematoma. Many times these patients are hemodynamically unstable owing to associated injuries and pelvic hemorrhage and pelvic exploration is contraindicated owing to the risk of uncontrolled bleeding. An alternative method of management in the acute setting involves primary urethral alignment. When pelvic exploration is indicated for repair of bladder rupture, internal bone fixation, or exploration of associated abdominal injuries, primary urethral alignment may be attempted. After a transperitoneal opening of the bladder, Foley catheters are passed antegrade down the bladder neck and retrograde through the urethra. If urethral continuity can be achieved, the urethral Foley is left indwelling for a period of 4 to 6 weeks. Care must be taken to avoid extravesical periprostatic dissection or disruption of the pelvic hematoma. An intermediate approach has also been taken at some trauma centers, delaying repair for a period of several weeks with suprapubic drainage and then performing definitive urethral repair transperineally with

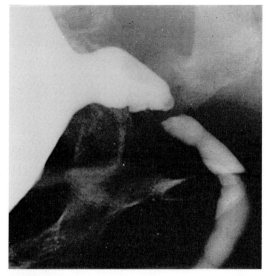

Figure 7-8
Simultaneous retrograde urethrogram and suprapubic
cystogram demonstrate complete urethral obliteration
several months after posterior urethral disruption. This is
a virtually universal occurrence after complete posterior
urethral disruptions managed by suprapubic cystostomy
tube drainage alone. This condition requires open urethroplasty for definitive repair.

evacuation of the organizing pelvic hematoma.

Recent data suggest that 35% to 60% of
patients with pelvic fracture and complete
posterior urethral disruption are rendered impotent by the injury alone. Of those patients
who regain potency in the intervening
months prior to definitive repair, none are
made impotent by delayed repair via the perineal approach. The traditional approach of
immediate suprapubic cystotomy and delayed urethral repair at 4 to 6 months has
historically been associated with the least
morbidity due to infection of pelvic bleeding,
incontinence, and impotence; it remains the
urologic standard. When impotence results
following pelvic fracture, it requires sophisticated investigation to determine if the insult
is neurogenic, vasculogenic, or both.

HIGHLIGHTS

- Most posterior urethral injuries occur in the
  setting of a pelvic fracture.
- Diagnosis of posterior urethral injury is confirmed by retrograde urethrography.
- A Foley catheter placement should not be

attempted in the setting of a posterior urethral injury.
- Temporary urinary diversion using a suprapubic cystostomy tube is the gold standard for the initial treatment of posterior
  urethral injury.
- Complications of posterior urethral injuries
  such as impotence and urinary incontinence
  usually occur as a result of the injury itself.

ANTERIOR URETHRAL INJURIES

Evaluation

Anterior urethral injuries are less frequent
and typically less morbid than posterior urethral injuries. The most common cause of anterior urethral trauma is a straddle injury,
crushing the bulbar urethra upward against
the inferior arch of the symphysis pubis. Penetrating trauma from gunshot or stab wounds
may also injure the anterior urethra with or
without simultaneous injury to the corpora
cavernosa. Many times additional injuries to
the scrotum, testes, and/or rectum are noted
when evaluating anterior urethral injuries
due to a similar mechanism of injury.

Patients with anterior urethral injury may
present with a butterfly-shaped perineal hematoma, a penile shaft hematoma in a sleeve-
like distribution, blood at the urethral meatus,
gross hematuria, or an inability to void. All
patients with suspected anterior urethral injuries should undergo retrograde urethrography. This is the study of choice to define the
site and extent of injury (Fig. 7–9). Anterior
urethral injuries may result in complete or
partial urethral disruption. Complete disruptions are characterized by urinary extravasation and a lack of contrast medium entering
the posterior urethra or urinary bladder. Retrograde urethrography of a partial injury reveals extravasation with some contrast medium entering the posterior urethra or
bladder.

Management

Unlike posterior urethral disruptions, long-
term complications such as impotence and
incontinence are uncommon in anterior urethral injuries. Instead, prevention of urethral
stricture is the primary concern because it is

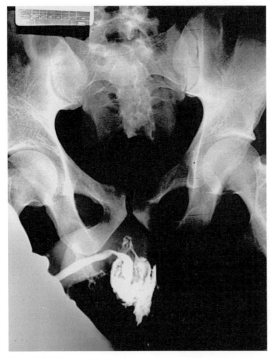

Figure 7-9

Retrograde urethrogram demonstrates complete rupture of the bulbar (anterior) urethra with extravasation of contrast medium following a straddle injury against the handlebars of a motorcycle. No contrast medium is seen entering the bladder, confirming the diagnosis of complete disruption.

responsible for most of the morbidity associated with anterior urethral injury. A Foley catheter should never be passed blindly in suspected urethral injury because it may convert an incomplete disruption into a complete disruption.

Complete disruption of the anterior urethra from blunt trauma—a crush or straddle injury—is best managed with suprapubic cystostomy tube placement followed by radiographic evaluation in 4 to 6 weeks and delayed urethral repair for stricture, if necessary. This approach allows temporary urinary diversion and resolution of the hematoma and inflammation before repair. Incomplete anterior urethral disruption due to blunt trauma is also best managed by temporary urinary diversion with a suprapubic cystostomy tube. In these cases follow-up imaging at 4 to 6 weeks is less likely to reveal a urethral stricture, and thus patients will usually require no further surgery.

In contrast, immediate surgical repair is ad-

vocated for gunshot and stab wounds to the urethra. In these cases secondary injury to the scrotum or testes is commonly found that requires immediate exploration, and the urethral injury can be explored and surgically repaired as necessary at the same time. Minimal débridement of the spongiosum and corpus cavernosum is advocated because these spongy tissues are highly vascularized and have a reduced risk of postoperative infection and stricture. Contraindications to immediate exploration in penetrating trauma include hemodynamic instability, contaminated or dirty wounds, and a large urethral defect requiring extensive reconstruction. These patients are best served by suprapubic cystostomy and radiographic re-evaluation in several weeks.

HIGHLIGHTS

- Anterior urethral injuries most commonly occur in the setting of blunt trauma as a result of a straddle injury.
- Anterior urethral injury is indicated by urinary extravasation seen on retrograde urethrography.
- Urethral stricture is the most common long-term sequela.
- Temporary urinary diversion with a suprapubic cystostomy may be adequate therapy in cases of blunt trauma; however, surgical exploration, débridement, and primary repair should be performed in the setting of penetrating anterior urethral trauma.

Female Urethral Injuries

Most female urethral injuries are due to iatrogenic causes such as gynecologic (anterior colporrhaphy), obstetric (childbirth), and/or urologic (e.g., urethropexy, urethral dilation) manipulation and not external trauma. These types are not further considered here. Other causes of female urethral trauma are exceedingly rare and are usually seen in the setting of pelvic fracture, straddle injury, or penetrating trauma. Commonly, urethral injuries in the female are associated with bladder neck and/or vaginal injury because the female urethra is quite short (3 to 4 cm) and for most of its course lies anatomically beneath the anterior vaginal wall. Diagnosis is usually made by inspection, although VCUG detects proximal urethral and bladder neck injuries that are not otherwise suspected.

Treatment guidelines for female urethral injury are less clear because of its uncommon occurrence. However, several generalizations can be made. In most cases attempts at urethral stenting with a Foley catheter are less likely to result in inadvertent injury in the female patient with pelvic trauma as opposed to the male patient because of the short urethra and its relatively straight course into the bladder. Furthermore, if urethral catheterization is unsuccessful, suprapubic cystostomy and urinary diversion in the acute setting of blunt trauma are always an option. Elective radiographic re-evaluation can then be performed weeks later when the patient is stable. Finally, open pelvic fractures with associated injury of the vagina or rectum merit an operative approach and primary repair, during which a suprapubic catheter is easily inserted if necessary.

Male External Genitalia Injuries

The penis, the testes, and the scrotum can be injured by a variety of mechanisms involving blunt and penetrating forces. The goal of initial interventions is to control hemorrhage and preserve vital tissues of sexual and reproductive function. Complex surgical reconstruction is required in many of these cases.

PENIS

Lacerating or avulsing injuries to the penis are usually the result of motor vehicle accidents, industrial accidents, or self-inflicted trauma. These may result in degloving injuries of the penis in which the skin is traumatically torn from the penile shaft. These injuries require thorough wound cleansing followed by primary closure if the native penile skin is available or split-thickness skin grafting from a hairless donor site if the penile shaft skin is lost. Split-thickness and full-thickness skin grafts from non–hair-bearing areas allow for normal skin expansion during erection, which is essential in the potent patient. With a cir-

cumferential loss of penile skin, the distal penile shaft skin must be débrided to the level of the coronal sulcus of the penis to prevent later sloughing due to ischemia.

Most penetrating penile injuries are gunshot wounds. A high degree of suspicion for concomitant urethral injury should prompt retrograde urethrography if blood is seen at the meatus or the patient is unable to void. Prompt surgical exploration remains the best way to stage and manage these injuries.

Penile amputation is a rare injury, and successful reanastomosis depends on receiving a distal fragment that has been well preserved in the trauma field. Reconstruction has as the primary goal re-establishing urethral continuity and reanastomosing the corporal bodies. Microvascular anastomosis of one dorsal artery and at least one deep dorsal vein is needed to preserve the glans. Microvascular anastomosis of the corporeal arteries is more difficult. Circumferential closure of the tunica surrounding the corporeal spaces should permit sexual rehabilitation with a penile prosthesis at a later date.

Trauma to the erect penis may result in a tear in the tunica albuginea covering of the corpus cavernosum and a "fracture" of the penile shaft. Typically the injury occurs laterally to one corporeal body of the erect penis during coitus. The injury usually results during pelvic thrusting, with the penis inadvertently striking the perineum, resulting in an abrupt forceful deflection followed by a popping or cracking sound and rapid detumescence. A large hematoma develops on the injured side as a result of a tear or fracture in the tunica albuginea. The patient presents with the hematoma deflecting the penis to the opposite side of the injury. Concurrent urethral injury is rare, but blood at the meatus, gross hematuria, or the inability to void should be assessed by retrograde urethrography. The goal of therapy is the preservation of sexual function, which is best accomplished by immediate surgical exploration, evacuation of the hematoma, and primary repair of the tunica.

SCROTUM AND TESTES

The scrotum and its contents may be injured in penetrating or blunt trauma. Approximately one half of testicular injuries are due to blunt trauma and may result in testicular rupture. Large hematomas may form in the scrotum, precluding physical examination of the scrotal contents, but high-resolution color Doppler ultrasonography has come to play a major role in evaluating traumatic scrotal and testicular pathology when scrotal contents are not palpable (Fig. 7–10). Scrotal ultrasonography with color Doppler not only delineates the anatomy of testicular and/or epididymal injury but also demonstrates symmetry or asymmetry of blood flow within the testes. Associated urethral trauma should be ruled out by use of the retrograde urethrogram when indicated.

Once injury to the testes and spermatic cord has been ruled out, hematomas of the skin and dartos layer may be managed conservatively. Open lacerations or gunshot wounds should be explored, débrided, irri-gated, and drained. Superficial scrotal lacerations can be closed primarily with absorbable suture after sufficient irrigation. Large areas of scrotal skin must be lost to preclude primary reapproximation because of the intrinsic nature and redundancy of the scrotal sac. Split-thickness skin grafts can be fashioned to cover the testes when necessary. When the entire scrotum is lost but the testes are still viable, such as in cases of severe burns, the testes can be temporarily placed in subcutaneous thigh pockets, with scrotal reconstruction scheduled at a later date.

Testicular ruptures should be explored immediately with débridement of extruded tubules and primary closure of the tunica with absorbable sutures. In cases of bilateral testicular trauma, every effort should be made to ensure the viability of at least one testicle not only for fertility reasons but for the continued production of testosterone.

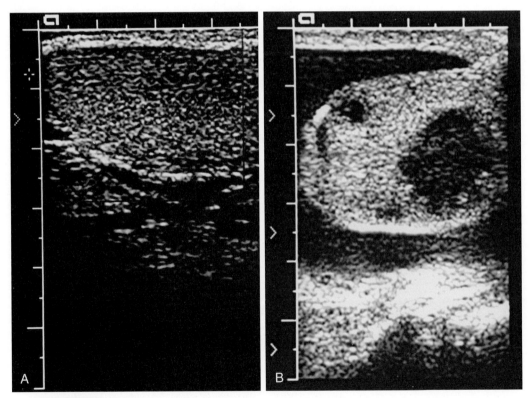

Figure 7–10
Ultrasonogram obtained in a young male 2 weeks after he was struck by a golf ball in the scrotum. His right hemiscrotum was enlarged and tender, and a testicle could not be definitively palpated. *A,* Normal left testicle with homogenous echotexture of testicular parenchyma. *B,* Right testicle with surrounding hematocele and intratesticular hypoechoic regions suggestive of hematoma. Scrotal exploration confirmed testicular rupture, which was not well seen on the ultrasonogram.

HIGHLIGHTS

- Injury to the penis or scrotum, whether blunt or penetrating, may be associated with concomitant urethral injury. If urethral injury is suspected, retrograde urethrography should be performed.
- Ultrasonographic examination of the scrotum is usually adequate in delineating the nature and extent of testicular trauma.
- Rupture of the tunica albuginea of the penis or testicles requires surgical evaluation and exploration.

SUGGESTED READINGS

1. Carlin BI, Resnick MI: Indications and techniques for urologic evaluation of the trauma patient with suspected urologic injury. Semin Urol 13:9–24, 1995.
2. McAninch JW, Carroll PR, Jordan GH (eds): Traumatic and Reconstructive Urology. Philadelphia, WB Saunders, 1996.
3. Sagalowsky AI, Peters PC: Genitourinary trauma. *In* Walsh PC, Retik AB, Vaughan ED Jr, Wein AJ (eds): Campbell's Urology, 7th ed. Philadelphia, WB Saunders, 1998, pp 3085–3118.
4. Weigel JW: Management of trauma of the external genitalia and urethra. *In* Seidmon EJ, Hanno PM (eds): Current Urologic Therapy 3. Philadelphia, WB Saunders, 1994, pp 426–430.
5. Wessells H, McAninch JW: Update on upper urinary tract trauma. AUA Update Series 15:110–116, 1996.

8

Urinary Calculus Disease

Michael E. Moran
Pramod P. Reddy

Epidemiology

Urinary calculi are a complex group of biomaterials that can and do occur anywhere within the urinary tract. Stones have afflicted humans since the first recorded histories of medicine. Over the centuries bladder stones have become less common than upper urinary tract stones owing to dietary changes. This trend still persists and can be shown to be true if one were to compare the incidence of urinary calculi in the industrialized nations with that in the developing nations. This change to upper tract development of urinary calculi necessitated a change in the management strategies of urolithiasis.

One of the sentinel medical developments of the twentieth century has been the introduction of extracorporeal shock-wave lithotripsy (ESWL). The impact on our ability to manage urolithiasis represents the combined benefits of the surgical and medical advances in understanding the pathophysiology, diagnosis, and treatment of urolithiasis. Metabolic or environmental causes of nephrolithiasis can be found in approximately 97% of patients evaluated for their stone disease.

Within the United States the eastern half of the country tends to have a higher stone incidence than the western half. The same increased risk is noted for the South versus the North. The southeastern region of the United States has long been known to be the "stone belt" of this country. Using the Southeast as the comparison region, a decreased risk of having a kidney stone was found from 13% lower in the Mid-Atlantic region and 31% lower in the Northwest. This geographic variability has been evaluated to assess whether race, age, education, body mass, or diet affects the frequency data, but ambient temperature and sunlight levels remain the greatest risks.

African Americans have about one third to one fourth the incidence of stones as compared with their white counterparts; however, they demonstrate a higher infectious stone rate. Given the fact that approximately 12% of all people experience calculus disease in their lifetime, urolithiasis represents a considerable factor in terms of the health care dollars spent on its management and also the cost to society as a result of working days and wages lost.

In this chapter we attempt to address the current rationale of diagnosis and treatment modalities in patients with urolithiasis.

EMERGING INCIDENCE

Stone disease has long plagued humankind; however, prior to the Industrial Revolution the bladder was the primary repository of these concretions. In the United States and most developed counties upper tract stones predominate (97% in the calyx, pelvis, and ureter vs. 3% in the bladder or urethra). The incidence of stone disease has been estimated at 0.1% to 0.3%, or 240,000 to 720,000 cases in the United States yearly. Urolithiasis accounts for 7 to 10 of every 1000 hospital admissions in the United States and has an annual incidence of 7 to 21 cases per 10,000 persons. The prevalence of stone disease is 5% to 12%; that

93

is, essentially 12 to 24 million Americans will develop a stone in their lifetime, which is a conservative estimate. It has been classically known that 80% of patients with stones are men, and the onset of disease is during the most productive years (age 30 to 40 years). Mounting data suggest that this gender difference in stone disease incidence is decreasing further, supporting a rapid expansion of new cases within the United States.

STONE TYPES

The majority of stones (70% to 80%) are composed of calcium oxalate (Table 8–1). The remainder contain calcium phosphate salts, uric acid, ammoniomagnesium phosphate hexahydrate (struvite), and (rarely) the amino acid cystine. Calcium oxalate stones dominate modern stone series in incidence in two primary forms, often admixed: whewellite (WH) is calcium oxalate monohydrate and is more common; weddellite (WE) is calcium oxalate dihydrate and is the crystal moiety that is commonly seen in urinalysis specimens. The calcium oxalate type is crucially important to urologists treating calculus because WH stones are more likely to fail ESWL than are WE stones. There is no preoperative modality to identify which type of stone is present in a given patient. In pooled stone series, calcium oxalate stone may be present in 65% to 80% of all stones.

Calcium phosphate stones are much more heterogeneous. They are rarely pure components within stones, most commonly complexed with calcium oxalate. The exception is brushite (BR), calcium hydrogen phosphate. Stones composed predominantly of calcium

Table 8–1
Comparative Incidence of Forms of Urinary Lithiasis in the United States

Form of Lithiasis	Incidence (%)
Pure calcium oxalate	33
Mixed calcium oxalate and phosphate	34
Pure calcium phosphate	6
Magnesium ammonium phosphate (struvite)	15
Uric acid	8
Cystine	3
Artifacts and other	1

phosphate approximate 10% of the total. These patients should have a full metabolic evaluation by the treating physician because calcium phosphate stones represent a harbinger of active stone disease and significant underlying medical disorders. BR in particular should be a trigger to further investigations to identify distal renal tubular acidosis, primary hyperparathyroidism, or sarcoidosis. In addition, pure BR calculi represent the second most difficult stone to fragment with ESWL, predisposing to secondary interventions.

Magnesium ammonium phosphate hexahydrate (struvite) are the bacteria-induced or infectious stones. These stones are often heterogeneous, with varying amounts of other mineral (carbonate apatite) or proteinaceous matrix present. These stones represent 2% to 20% of the total stone population and are twice as common in women as in men. These stones are classically associated with urease-producing infections, most commonly due to *Proteus mirabilis*. Struvite calculi account for most of the staghorn stones encountered in clinical practice.

Purines and their salts (uric acid, uric acid dihydrate, monosodium urate, and rarely xanthine or 2,8-dihydroxyadenine) account for 5% to 10% of stones. The calculi occur because humans lack the enzyme to convert uric acid into the freely soluble allantoin. Since human urine is predominantly acidic, depending on the saturation, normally between 500 and 600 mg/L, precipitation is always possible. In addition, another capability of uric acid crystallization is its ability to propagate crystal deposition with calcium oxalate, termed *heterogeneous nucleation*. About 10% of calcium oxalate stone formers have only hyperuricosuria as the principal metabolic abnormality. Uric acid stones and their salts are truly radiolucent, which underlies the difficulties with diagnosis and therapy. Standard radiographs are not helpful, so ultrasonography, intravenous pyelography, or, in difficult cases, nonenhanced renal computed tomography (CT) must be used to follow these patients. Secondary uric acid lithiasis should always be evaluated to rule out primary pathologic processes such as gout and myeloproliferative disorders.

Cystine stone disease is the least common, occurring in 1% of patients, and results from an autosomal recessive disorder affecting membrane transport of dibasic amino acids. Cystine stones are radiopaque secondary to their disulfide bonds. There is a propensity for these stones to occur in younger people, in their second or third decade; two thirds of the stones are pure, whereas one third contain a mixture with a mineral content.

Triamterene-containing stones constitute a class of iatrogenically induced urolithiasis and are rare. Triamterene, a potassium-sparing diuretic, is often used in combination with thiazides to treat hypertension. Should a patient pass a stone while taking this drug, the stone should be analyzed and the drug discontinued. Silicate is another rare compound found in human stones. It is used in many pill-forming processes but is found in largest concentration in some antacids (magnesium trisilicate). Sulfonamides were a concern three decades ago when poorly soluble, high-dose regimens were popular and stone formation was a problem. The protease inhibitors such as indinavir used to treat acquired immunodeficiency syndrome–related complications have been increasingly associated with stone formation. Indinavir is known to be poorly soluble in urine, and rapid precipitation with symptomatic stone formation has been reported in at least 3% of patients on this drug.

Rare stone types may result from inborn errors of metabolism of nucleic acids on the pathway to uric acid production. Two such stones are xanthine and 2,8-dihydroxyadenine, which are both radiolucent and exceedingly rare, and occur more commonly in children. Stones suspected of being uric acid that do not respond to chemodissolution by alkali should be considered as one of these two types.

PATHOGENESIS OF UROLITHIASIS

The initiation and growth of urinary calculi involve a chemical precipitation of dissolved ions or molecules from urine that is supersaturated with those components as the glomerular filtrate traverses the nephron. This rather simplistic explanation leads us to the prevailing theories of lithogenesis. The process of earliest crystal precipitation is referred to as *nucleation*. In the urinary tract this process is believed to occur predominantly on existing surfaces, either epithelium or other crystals (heterogeneous nucleation). Once formed, the crystal growth process is by aggregation. This process generally occurs in waves because the urine is rarely saturated by the stone-forming salts continuously. There exist both promoters and inhibitors of stone formation. Promoters are those substances that may predispose to stone precipitation. Inhibitors are those substances that interact with the crystallization process of a given stone type. Many of the current specific medical therapies today take advantage of these inhibitory interactions to reduce the risk of stone recurrence (such as potassium citrate, magnesium oxide, and others). Some drugs act as complexing agents promoting the solubility of stone-forming ions (potassium citrate). There exists no widely used method that is capable of preventing stone recurrence by inhibiting matrix production.

The mechanisms of stone formation are essential to understanding current evaluation and management of patients with urolithiasis. The most common abnormality identifiable on evaluating a stone former is hypercalciuria. Daily excretion of more than 300 mg calcium in men or 250 mg in women is termed *hypercalciuria*. Classification of hypercalciuria by measurable differences in response to calcium challenge is as follows:

Absorptive hypercalciuria Type I—non–dietary-responsive intestinal absorption of calcium (parathyroid hormone suppressed)
Absorptive hypercalciuria Type II—dietary-responsive intestinal absorption of calcium (parathyroid hormone suppressed)
Absorptive hypercalciuria (phosphate leak, Type III)—absorptive hypercalciuria associated with renal wasting of phosphorus
Renal hypercalciuria—renal leak of calcium (parathyroid hormone stimulated)
Resorptive hypercalciuria—secondary to increased bone demineralization (primary hyperparathyroidism)

The primary defect in absorptive hypercalciuria is an increased passive mucosal absorption of calcium and oxalate in the jejunum. There are strong indications that this is an autosomal dominant defect, making a family history of calcium stone disease a risk factor. This may be a vitamin D_3–mediated process, because as many as 50% of patients with absorptive hypercalciuria have elevated 1,25-dihydroxyvitamin D levels. Clinical stratification of hypercalciuria shows that 20% have Type I, 28% have Type II, 2.5% have the renal type, and 3.5% have the resorptive type; however, not all hypercalciurias are derived from intestinal calcium reabsorption disorders.

Hypocitruria is another physicochemical abnormality associated with stone formation in 15% to 63% of patients. Urinary citrate levels should typically be greater than 320 mg daily. Conditions associated with hypocitruria include distal renal tubular acidosis, chronic diarrhea, and laxative abuse. Hyperoxaluria is noted in 5% to 15% of patients. Eighty percent of urinary oxalate is from endogenous rather than dietary sources. Primary hyperoxaluria Type I is caused by a deficient liver enzyme. Type II, or L-glycericaciduria, is a much rarer variant. Enteric hyperoxaluria occurs in patients with derangements of small bowel absorption such as jejunoileal bypass and small bowel resection (short gut syndromes) with or without steatorrhea. Idiopathic hyperoxaluria makes up the remainder of patients with elevated urinary oxalate (levels higher than 40 mg daily) and probably represents most patients with slight elevations in urinary oxalate excretion. Hyperuricaciduria has been noted alone or in combination with one of the aforementioned metabolic abnormalities in 10% to 50% of stone formers. The increased urinary excretion of acid (>600 mg per 24 hours) on restricted diets is diagnostic.

Clinical Presentation

As discussed earlier, 97% of all urinary stones in the United States occur in the upper urinary tract (parenchyma, papilla, calyces, pelvis, or ureter). Consequently, most patients present with symptoms of renal colic or flank pain. Only 3% occur in the lower urinary tract (bladder or urethra). The physician, once notified, has to decide whether to see the patient in the office, send the patient to the emergency department, and/or contact a urologist. Primary consideration should be given to the nature of the patient's symptoms

regarding the severity of colic, associated fever, and any comorbid medical conditions.

COLIC

The most common presentation of stone disease is renal colic. The pain associated with urinary stone passage is generally ascribed to the following mechanisms:

1. Dilation of the musculopropulsive urinary tract with stretching of the pain receptors
2. Local irritation in the wall of the ureter or pelvis with edema and release of pain mediators

Colic has seasonal variability. Hot, humid months have classically been the most frequent times for presentation to emergency departments.

OBSTRUCTIVE PYELONEPHRITIS

There is a significant correlation between urinary tract obstruction and urinary tract infections. Acute pyelonephritis with high fever, costovertebral angle tenderness, and bacteremia with all the consequences associated with the septic syndrome can occur quickly with obstructing stone and infection. Prompt intervention with proximal urinary drainage can convert such patients to a much more stable condition such that surgical stone ablation can be performed electively when such patients are at less risk.

HISTORY

The nature of the colic varies with the location of the stone. Renal colic usually begins suddenly and intensifies in a crescendo fashion over a period of 15 to 30 minutes until it becomes a steady, unbearable pain that localizes to the ipsilateral flank. The pain radiates down along the course of the ureter as the stone makes its way toward the bladder—this distribution of the pain is due to the innervation of the ureter by the branches of the genitofemoral nerve. As the stone descends in the ureter the pain may radiate to the umbilicus and subsequently to the ipsilateral groin and genitalia. The exact pathophysiologic explanation for the pain is unclear; however, it is probably secondary to a combination of increased intraluminal pressure, local distention of the ureteral wall, and release of proinflammatory mediators secondary to local ureteral ischemia or irritation. The patient who presents with a stone in the right ureter can pose a diagnostic challenge because the pain of an acutely inflamed appendix lying in contact with the right ureter can easily be confused with ureteral colic. Careful consideration and appropriate evaluation for other causes of flank pain (Table 8–2) should yield the correct diagnosis.

As the stone progresses downward into the distal ureter it can cause urinary frequency, urgency, dysuria, and stranguria. The pain is often associated with nausea, vomiting, and costovertebral angle tenderness on the ipsilateral side. The shared segmental innervation between the intestine and ureter is the basis for the disordered intestinal motility that results in nausea and vomiting by means of a viscero-visceral reflex.

Patients with calculi in the urinary tract can present with hematuria, which might be either gross or microscopic. In some instances hematuria may be absent (approximately 15%), as in those cases with total obstruction or stones attached to the renal pelvic epithelium, that is, calyceal stones or stones in calyceal diverticula.

If the patient presents with a fever and/or chills, this would be highly indicative of an infection. Low-grade fevers may be present in the absence of an infection and are believed to be due to the release of endogenous pyrogen from the obstructed kidney.

Patients with bladder stones present with a different set of symptoms and their complaints are rarely acute. Most patients report symptoms of severe dysuria with or without obstructive voiding symptoms, a sense of incomplete voiding, stranguria, and pain radiating to the tip of the urethra. Additionally, some patients present with a sense of ballottement in their bladder; this sensation is usually more pronounced when the patient is descending stairs. Another symptom unique to bladder stone patients is sudden, usually painful obstruction of the urinary stream caused by the sudden propulsion of the stone into the bladder neck during micturition.

It is not unusual to discover clinically silent stones during a work-up for microscopic hematuria or during a radiographic evaluation for disease processes separate from the urinary tract.

PAST MEDICAL HISTORY

The numerous medical conditions that predispose to the development of urolithiasis are summarized in Table 8–3.

PHYSICAL EXAMINATION

The patient should be examined initially in a supine position with the right-handed physician on the patient's right side.

Inspection

Examine the patient for any signs of trauma such as bruises because injury to the underlying ribs can often masquerade as renal pain. Evaluate the inguinal regions and scrotum for any swellings or masses to rule out hernias or a primary scrotal lesion as the cause of pain.

Auscultation

Auscultation may demonstrate hypoactive bowel sounds secondary to a viscero-visceral

Table 8-2
Differential Diagnosis for Ureteral Calculus Colic

Renal colic secondary to noncalculus etiology
  Passage of blood or clot
  Passage of necrotic material (sloughed papilla)
  Stricture or compression of ureter (extrinsic) or
    excessive angulation of ureter
Other causes of abdominal/flank pain
  Gastrointestinal: appendicitis (retrocecal),
    terminal ileitis, diverticulitis, cholecystitis,
    cholelithiasis, duodenal or ventricular
    ulceration, pancreatitis
  Vascular: infarction of kidney, spleen, or bowel,
    renal vein thrombosis, abdominal aortic
    aneurysm
  Gynecologic: ovarian cysts, adnexitis, ectopic
    pregnancy, endometriosis
  Rare causes: psoas abscess, retroperitoneal
    masses, cardiac infarction, porphyria, heavy
    metal intoxication, diabetes mellitus,
    pheochromocytoma, Addison's disease,
    metastatic breast cancer

Table 8–3
Past Medical History Significant for Urolithiasis

Diseases associated with disturbances of calcium metabolism: primary hyperparathyroidism, Wilson's disease, medullary sponge kidney, osteoporosis, immobilization, sarcoidosis, osteolytic metastases, plasmacytoma, neuroendocrine tumors, Paget's disease

    Dietary history: purine gluttony, calcium excess, milk alkali, oxalate excess, sodium excess, low citrus fruit intake

    Medications: uricosurics, diuretics, analgesics, vitamins C and D, antacids (especially phosphorus-binding agents), acetazolamide, calcium channel blockers, triamterene, theophylline, protease inhibitors (indinavir), sulfonamides

Diseases associated with disturbances of oxalate metabolism: primary hyperoxaluria Types I and II, Crohn's disease, ulcerative colitis, intestinal bypass surgery (especially jejunoileal bypass), ileal resection

Diseases associated with disturbances of purine metabolism

    Intrinsic metabolic disorders—anemia, neoplastic disorders (especially leukemias), intoxication, myocardial infarction, irradiation, cytotoxic chemotherapy

    Enzyme deficiency—primary gout, Lesch-Nyhan syndrome

    Altered excretion—renal insufficiency, metabolic acidosis

Infectious history: organisms (particularly *Proteus* and *Klebsiella*), febrile upper tract involvement and dates if hospitalized.

reflex causing an ileus. Additionally there may be some atelectasis in the lower lung fields on the ipsilateral side secondary to limited diaphragmatic excursions due to the pain.

Palpation

Palpation of the abdomen may reveal tenderness and some guarding, but no true rigidity. In ureteric colic the discomfort caused by deep palpation is relieved when the examining hand is removed as opposed to the examination of acute appendicitis where the pain is accentuated on releasing the hand (rebound tenderness). Signs of peritoneal irritation are usually not present. Proper attention should be paid to the inguinal regions to rule out an incarcerated hernia as the cause of the symptoms.

Once the patient has been examined in the supine position, he or she should sit up and the examiner should perform the costovertebral angle test (Murphy's kidney punch), which when positive is indicative of deep-seated pain.

A digital rectal examination should be performed to evaluate the prostate gland for enlargement or masses, because this is a predisposing factor for the development of bladder calculi.

The physical examination would be incomplete if the neck were not palpated for the rare yet possible presence of a palpable parathyroid tumor/adenoma.

EMERGENCY DEPARTMENT VERSUS OFFICE EVALUATION

There are four comorbid conditions that should immediately cause concern to the practitioner and probably would be best evaluated within an emergency department and expeditiously involve a urologist. First is any evidence of obstructive pyelonephritis. Patients with obstructing stones and concurrent infections can become unstable from sepsis rapidly. Simple proximal drainage is the least aggressive modality to rapidly ensure hemodynamic stability in critically ill patients with obstructive pyelonephritis. Second is any diabetic patient passing a calculus. Because diabetics have associated disturbances of renal function and immune compromise, they may tolerate stone passage poorly and are at increased risk for complications. Papillary necrosis and xanthogranulomatous pyelonephritis are more common in diabetic patients with stones. Third are patients with solitary kidneys. For obvious reasons, if the stone should obstruct the only ureter, acute renal failure could ensue. Finally, debilitated patients such as those with spinal cord injury, the very aged, and steroid-dependent chronic obstructive pulmonary disease and asthma all represent more complex scenarios that should probably be managed in the hospital with urologic consultation.

Most acute stone patients are younger and healthier than those just discussed. If on initial contact patients are not experiencing progressive, crescendo colic, they can be seen and evaluation commenced in the office. Many emergency departments have begun to observe patient with refractory colic in the departments for 23 hours. Most patients with smaller calculi (<4 mm in diameter) spontaneously improve overnight and can be discharged without formal hospitalization.

Clinical Evaluation and Diagnosis

IMAGING STUDIES

The patients passing a calculus usually require some documentation of the location and size of the calculus. In addition, a number of other key bits of information that aid in patient management would include the presence of normal versus abnormal renal anatomy, presence of nephrocalcinosis, contralateral (bilateral) disease, degree of renal obstruction, severity of associated ileus, and any other abdominal processes to be ruled out in the differential diagnosis. As previously mentioned, most stones (about 70%) pass spontaneously. There are compelling data that spontaneous passage of upper tract stones is size dependent. Stones between 5 and 6 mm in diameter have a greater than 50% spontaneous passage. Not only stone size but its location at presentation are also predictive of passage. Calculi in the distal third of the ureter have a spontaneous passage rate of 45% versus 20% in the middle third and only 12% for those in the proximal third. Patients should know that these statistics do not apply to all individuals; the asymptomatic stones that show continued progression down the ureter without colic or infection can be followed without intervention.

Ultrasonography is a simple examination and can be repeated without irradiation. Stones in children and pregnant women should be studied with ultrasound initially.

Ultrasonography loses its specificity in following ureteral stones and correctly predicting the degree of obstruction. Ultrasonography cannot discriminate between radiopaque and radiolucent stones. The quality of the examination has been shown to be user dependent with a sensitivity of 93%, positive predictive value of 93%, specificity of 83%, and a negative predictive value of 83%. The intravenous pyelogram remains the gold standard and provides accurate size, shape, location, and functional data regarding the calculus and the kidney.

Non–contrast medium helical computed tomographic (CT) scanning represents another method for the emergency evaluation of colic. The signs of obstruction on such scans include the following: stranding of perinephric fat, dilated collecting system, dilated ureter, and stone localization.

Renal scanning can be used when patients are allergic to one or more intravenous contrast agents. It provides information on renal function, morphology, and blood flow. Diuretic isotope renal scanning may add further to the sensitivity and specificity of the diagnosis of acute renal obstruction caused by stones; however, it lacks diagnostic accuracy. Obstruction can be demonstrated as well as reduced function, but the cause cannot be determined.

LABORATORY TESTS

Urinalysis, serum chemistries, and complete blood count are routinely done in patients with urolithiasis. For the first-time stone-forming patient with no identifiable risk factors, an abbreviated approach to identify metabolic risk factors is warranted (Fig. 8–1). Important aspects of the automated serum chemistry panel are the calcium, creatinine, uric acid, phosphorus, sodium, potassium, bicarbonate, chloride, and magnesium levels. More controversial but of added value would be the inclusion of the ionized calcium and serum parathyroid hormone levels. A microscopic urinalysis and stone composition are necessary, but a urine culture and sensitivity need be performed only if clinically indicated by white blood cells or bacteria seen on urinalysis. The significance of abnormal screening studies is indicated in Table 8–4.

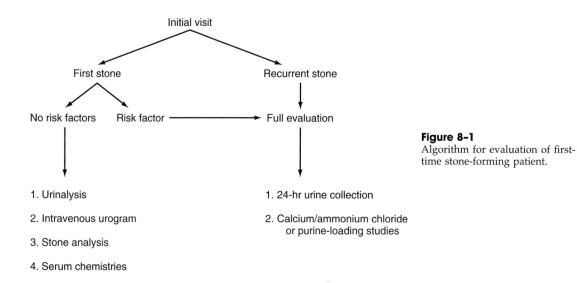

Figure 8-1
Algorithm for evaluation of first-time stone-forming patient.

In patients with recurrent or synchronous bilateral stone disease, patients presenting at a young age (<20 years), or those with identifiable risk factors, more extensive metabolic evaluation should be performed (Table 8–5). The normal values are listed in Table 8–6. Calcium stone–forming patients represent the vast majority of patients, and screening studies are normal in most. To identify the metabolic abnormality takes more detailed chemical analysis of these patients' urine. Hypercalciuria is the most common metabolic abnormality of patients with calcium oxalate stone disease. Stratification of these metabolically active patients requires 24-hour urine collection and quantification of calcium excretion after fasted and loaded evaluation.

Patient Management

The trend in patient management currently favors a balanced analgesic regimen combining the best of both the nonsteroidal and narcotic drugs.

Hydration has always been an uncertain variable in the management of acute ureteral colic. With dehydration, urine output is reduced and may result in less distention of the collecting system producing less pain. This has not been formally evaluated and is not considered standard practice. Other adjuncts to aid in stone passage and the alleviation of colic have been proposed, including acupuncture and intranasal vasopressin. Spasmolytic drugs and smooth muscle relaxants represent another modality to decrease the pain and improve stone passage. Remember that 60% to 80% of stones pass spontaneously. The

Table 8-4
Serum Chemistry Evaluation and Clinically Important Aberrations*

Item for Analysis	Relevance
SMA-20	
Increased Ca, decreased P	Primary hyperparathyroidism
Decreased K and CO_2	Renal tubular acidosis
Elevated uric acid	Gouty diathesis
Decreased P	Hypophosphatemic absorptive hypercalciuria
Urinalysis	
Crystal identification	Estimate of size and number
pH (by electrode if possible)	<5.5 gouty diathesis >7.5 infectious etiology (urea splitting)
Qualitative cystine	
Culture	

*Any abnormalities may warrant more extensive evaluation.

Table 8-5
Risk Factors for Full Metabolic Evaluation

Medical conditions identified in Table 8–3
Family history of stone disease
Nephrocalcinosis on radiographic studies
Bilateral stone disease
Chronic recurrent infections (recurrent infectious stones)

Table 8-6
Chemistry Evaluation of Stone-Forming Patients: Normal Values

Item for Analysis	Normal Values	
	Men	**Women**
Serum		
Creatinine (mg/100 mL)	1.01 ± 0.31	0.82 ± 0.19
Sodium (mEq/L)	139.6 ± 3.2	139.3 ± 3.3
Potassium (mEq/L)	3.89 ± 0.54	3.95 ± 0.60
Chloride (mEq/L)	104.3 ± 4.8	105.0 ± 4.5
Calcium (mg/100 mL)	9.59 ± 0.62	9.4 ± 0.70
Magnesium (mg/100 mL)	2.03 ± 0.28	1.97 ± 0.26
Phosphorus (mg/100 mL)	3.49 ± 1.19	3.55 ± 1.08
Uric acid (mg/100 mL)	5.66 ± 1.2	4.15 ± 0.83
Urine		
Volume (L/24 hr)	1.27 ± 1.04	1.27 ± 1.37
Creatinine clearance (L/24 hr)	187 ± 76	151 ± 66
Sodium (mEq/24 hr)	175 ± 133	126 ± 94
Potassium (mEq/24 hr)	64 ± 44	59 ± 34
Calcium (mg/24 hr)	169 ± 146	117 ± 123
Calcium/g of creatinine (mg/g)	92 ± 80	99 ± 106
Calcium/kg of body weight (mg/kg/24 hr)	2.4 ± 2.2	2.1 ± 2.1
Oxalate (mg/24 hr)	35 ± 17	26 ± 15
Citrate (mg/24 hr)	458 ± 440	593 ± 704
Magnesium (mg/24 hr)	97.7 ± 69.5	80.6 ± 51.4
Phosphorus (g/24 hr)	0.953 ± 0.554	0.687 ± 0.404
Uric acid (g/24 hr)	0.674 ± 0.330	0.527 ± 0.240

physician can aid the process by reassurance and pharmacotherapy.

OBSERVATION

Patients with known urolithiasis can be either symptomatic with colic or obstructive pyelonephritis or incidentally found during workup of microscopic hematuria. In the latter scenario patients are otherwise asymptomatic and observation can be considered. Several caveats apply to the selection of observation versus treatment. Concurrent infection and obstruction should be ruled out. Obstruction and infection can compromise renal function, and intervention should be considered. If no infection or obstruction exists, then stone-forming activity should next be considered. Active stone formation is suggested by documented stone growth, bilateral stones, nephrocalcinosis, or multiple, recurrent stones. Infectious stones (struvite) represent the greatest risk to the patient under observation. These stones can rapidly progress and fill the entire collecting system without causing symptoms. Untreated struvite staghorn calculi represent a constant threat to the function of the involved kidney as well as to the

life of the patient. If observation is chosen, it behooves the practitioner to be vigilant for both infection and obstruction. Stone growth should be evaluated routinely. Nonspecific metaphylactic measures should be instituted, and compliance should be checked at each scheduled follow-up visit. About 63% of asymptomatic patients with nonobstructing stones remain asymptomatic for 3 to 5 years.

RECURRENCE RATES

The extent to which stone formers should undergo more extensive evaluation depends on the severity of their disease. All stone-forming patients should be made aware of the risk for recurrence. Recurrence rates vary widely. A second stone occurs in about 50% of patients within 8 years. Another way of presenting this to a patient is that there is a 7% risk of recurrence per year after the first stone passage. This suggests that stone-forming activity does not wane with time. The average rate of new stone formation in patients who have previously formed stones is about one stone every 2 or 3 years if conditions are left untreated.

NONSPECIFIC PREVENTIVE STONE MEASURES (Table 8–7)

It has long been known that increased fluid consumption with its associated diuresis is beneficial in preventing stone recurrence. If the average patient's daily urine output is 800 to 1000 mL daily, then it is recommended that this should be doubled to 2 L daily. This is most critical during the summer months because of the increased risk imparted by dehydration. In addition, certain stone-forming conditions that are difficult to treat medically (such as cystinuria) benefit from drinking even larger fluid volumes. Fluid therapy should preferentially be based on water. In studies evaluating the water hardness and the risk of urolithiasis, there is little evidence that a given community's water would affect the incidence of stone formation. Even though distilled or low-mineral-content water is probably better, the axiom is that regardless of the source, more water is better than less.

Cranberries are relatively high in oxalate, and excessive consumption of cranberry juice is not believed to be a practical fluid therapy in patients with calcium oxalate stone disease. Lemonade, on the other hand, is known to be a good source of the major urinary inhibitor citrate, and should be liberally recommended to recurrent stone formers of all types. Eight glasses daily can produce rises in urinary citrate levels comparable to treatment with citrate medications.

Diet probably plays a significant role in the rate of stone formation. Nonspecific dietary and fluid therapies can result in a decreased incidence of new stone formation, from 0.54 to 0.25 stones per patient per year (61%). As many as 24 dietary elements have been implicated in the formation of a urinary calculus.

Dietary restriction of calcium is somewhat controversial. Calcium and oxalate compete for intestinal absorption, and severe restrictions in calcium may promote the absorption and renal excretion of oxalate. Absorptive hypercalciuria is the most identifiable metabolic abnormality identified in stone-forming patients. Dietary restriction of calcium from 600 to 300 mg daily can reduce significantly 24-hour calcium excretion in 40% of patients as well as reduce the number of recurrent episodes of stone passage. Patients with Type II hypercalciuria can be controlled with dietary restriction of calcium (400 to 600 mg daily). High calcium–containing foods include dairy products, yogurt, rhubarb, beets, broccoli, collards, dandelion, mustard greens and turnips, salmon, and sardines.

Dietary oxalate is also another method of reducing stone-forming substrate. The average diet has a wide variability in oxalate consumption, from 100 to 900 mg daily. The major common dietary sources of oxalate are dark-green leafy vegetables (spinach and rhubarb), cola, chocolate, nuts (peanut butter), seeds (especially sesame), tea, and pepper. Much of the consumed dietary oxalate is excreted unchanged, with estimates that bacteria within the intestines metabolize 50%. In addition, vitamin C may be restricted because it is a substrate for the endogenous formation of oxalate.

Dietary purine restriction is another nonspecific therapy used for calcium and uric acid stone–forming patients. Since uric acid is the breakdown product of purine metabolism, it has long been known that exogenous restriction of foods with high-purine content is capable of reducing uric acid levels. Excessive purine intake can come in the form of meat, fish, and poultry at the expense of breads, grains, and starches. The dietary sources of excessive purine are meats, especially the organs (such as liver and pancreas), seafood, and legumes. Recommendations currently are to reduce dietary consumption of protein in stone formers to 120 mg daily.

Table 8–7
Metaphylactic Measures to Institute in All Stone-Forming Patients

High fluid intake (recommend enough to maintain 2 L of urine production daily)

Avoidance of stone-provoking medications (as per Table 8–3)

Restrict dietary oxalate (avoid seeds, nuts, peanut butter, chocolate, tea, cola, spinach, excessive vitamin C)

Restrict ingestion of high sodium foods (canned, processed foods and table salt)

Decrease ingestion of animal proteins (purines)

Avoid excessive consumption of calcium (no more than 600–800 mg daily)

Increase consumption of fresh fruit (four servings daily)

Daily consumption of lemonade (glass with each meal; other citrus may be substituted, but not cranberry juice)

Other nonspecific measures considered effective are reducing the consumption of acid ash and sodium chloride and increasing the daily consumption of fiber and citrate. Acid ash is abundant in animal proteins and is known to acidify the urine and decrease the excretion of urinary citrate. The benefit of sodium restriction in reducing stone formation is controversial. However, without sodium restriction the benefit of thiazide administration in reducing calcium excretion is lost. Citrate is the most effective urinary inhibitor of calcium oxalate precipitation and is a chelator of calcium in the urine. Citrate is abundant in fresh fruits, especially citrus fruits and melons. It is also plentiful in fresh orange juice and lemonade.

SPECIFIC MEDICAL MANAGEMENT OF STONES

There are those patients with active stone disease or significant risk factors who benefit from specific medical therapy. The dominant problem with medical metaphylaxis is patient compliance. It is imperative for physicians dealing with recurrent stone-forming patients to be aware that lapses in compliance are common and improved surveillance and investigation into alternative practical methods of metaphylaxis need to be sought for some patients.

Hypercalciuria is the most identifiable metabolic abnormality in patients with calcium oxalate stone, occurring in 30% to 60%. Type I hypercalciuria persists despite dietary restriction. Classically, thiazides were considered the first-line therapy secondary to their hypocalciuric action that is augmented by dietary restriction. Although this approach is effective in reducing stone formation, there are concerns in this subgroup of patients that the efficacy is temporary and up-regulation of intestinal absorption can occur. The recommended doses of various thiazides for adults are trichlormethiazide 2 to 4 mg daily, hydrochlorothiazide 25 mg twice daily, or bendroflumethiazide 2.5 mg twice daily. The thiazide drugs have significant side effects, especially the development of hypokalemia and hypocitruria.

Other medical therapies for the treatment of absorptive hypercalciuria exist. Magnesium preparations have also been effective in decreasing the stone incidence in hypercalciuria. It probably is most effective in patients with hypomagnesuria. Doses and type of magnesium vary, with most studies reporting the efficacy with magnesium oxide from 650 to 1500 mg daily in divided doses. Diarrhea is the most common side effect that limits the upper dose range. Sodium cellulose phosphate is a nonabsorbable ion exchange resin capable of binding intestinal calcium. The usual dose is 10 to 15 g daily divided to each meal. Although urinary calcium excretion drops and stone recurrence rates are diminished, as many as 34% of the patients stop the drug because of side effects. In addition, hypomagnesuria, hyperoxaluria, and B vitamin depletion may need to be treated during therapy. Another medication widely used for absorptive hypercalciuria are the orthophosphates, which enhance pyrophosphate inhibitory levels in the urine with reduction in stone passage rates. The usual recommended starting dose is 1.5 g in divided doses with each meal. Diarrhea is the most common side effect, and soft tissue calcification has rarely been reported in patients with hypercalcemic states. These preparations are effective adjuncts in treating absorptive hypercalciuria Types I and II and renal phosphate leak variations. A newer preparation is a slow-release, neutral potassium phosphate salt (UroPhos-K), which may be as effective as the other orthophosphates with fewer side effects.

In patients with renal hypercalciuria the specific medical therapy is the thiazide class of drugs. Most patients with this condition have rapid, persistent return of metabolic derangements after starting on this regimen. Stone formation can be reduced dramatically, but development of hypocitruria and hypokalemia must be monitored. It is not advisable to add triamterene to reduce potassium excretion, since triamterene can cause stones, but potassium citrate can replace potassium and inhibit stone formation as well.

The treatment of patients with hyperuricosuria and calcium oxalate stone disease primarily is the reduction of the exogenous source (dietary purines). If this fails, the xanthine oxidase inhibitor allopurinol should be considered. Allopurinol at 300 mg daily induces an 81% reduction in stone formation.

Side effects are infrequent, with skin rash and elevated hepatic transaminase levels reported. Potassium citrate has also been shown to be efficacious in treating this metabolic derangement, with remission rate of 84% and reduced new stone formation rate of 75%. The dose is typically 1 mEq/kg per 24 hours in divided doses, but there is some support for a single bedtime treatment in metaphylaxis.

Hypocitruria is variably present in 19% to 63% of stone formers alone and in combination with other metabolic defects. Potassium citrate is the drug of choice starting at 40 to 60 mEq per day in divided doses. Alternative preparations available include liquid potassium and sodium citrate, crystalline potassium citrate, as a pill, and as a slow-release wax matrix tablet (Urocit-K). Potassium citrate is contraindicated in patients with hyperkalemia or moderate to severe renal insufficiency. Citrus fruits and fruit juices (both orange juice and lemonade) have been shown to be good dietary sources of citrate. Patients with gouty diatheses tend to have fixed acidic urinary pH and benefit from the oral citrate therapy. Although potassium citrate has become the mainstay therapeutic regimen, other alternative drugs are available, such as $KHCO_3$, sodium citrate, and $NaHCO_3$ in various preparations. In addition, acetazolamide is capable of alkalinizing the urine at the expense of reducing urinary citrate levels.

Hyperoxaluria may be present in 5% to 15% of patients. Pyridoxine (vitamin B_6) may reduce the production of oxalate by up-regulating the hepatic conversion of glyoxylate to glycine. A dose of 150 to 400 mg daily may be necessary. Magnesium oxide has also been noted to complex with oxalate in the urine, reducing the availability to precipitate with calcium. Beelith is a tablet of magnesium oxide (600 mg) and pyridoxine (25 mg) that provides both medications in a single tablet. Orthophosphates have also been shown to have beneficial actions by increasing urine pyrophosphate concentration, which inhibits calcium oxalate crystallization. In patients with enteric hyperoxaluria, calcium citrate supplementation may both bind intestinal oxalate as well as increase the amount of excreted urinary citrate. Calcium citrate (Caltrate) is usually commenced at 500 mg with meals, titrating carefully to upward of 4 g. It is important to follow the therapeutic effect by repeating 24-hour urine levels regularly. The goal is to adjust the dose to achieve decreased urinary oxalate excretion without significant rises in calciuria. Cholestyramine (4 g four times daily) has been shown to decrease diarrhea and lower oxalate excretion, especially in patients with steatorrhea. However, caution is advised since there are reported cases of this medication exacerbating both steatorrhea and calcium oxalate stone formation. Probably more important is to restrict dietary fat consumption to 40 to 60 g daily. In addition, medium-chain triglycerides can be substituted for some fat that limits the saponification of calcium in the intestine.

Cystinuria represents the most difficult recurrent stone disease to treat primarily because of the lack of safe medical therapeutics. D-Penicillamine (Cuprimine) was the drug of choice until this decade. Titration of this drug is necessary, starting at 250 mg and increasing to greater than 1000 mg daily in divided doses, if necessary, by following urinary levels. D-Penicillamine has numerous dose-limiting side effects consisting mainly of diarrhea, nausea, abdominal pain, impaired taste and smell, rashes, hypersensitivity reactions, hematopoietic impairment, and liver and renal complications (nephrotic syndrome). Approximately 50% of patients cease therapy with this drug secondary to side effects. Alpha-mercaptopropionylglycine (α-MPG, Thiola) has replaced D-penicillamine as the drug of choice in cystinuria. Its major advantage is the decreased incidence and severity of side effects. Dosage starts at 100 mg daily and is titrated upward in divided doses to achieve a reduction in urinary cystine levels to below 250 mg/L. Discontinuing this drug secondary to side effects has still been reported in as many as 30.6% of patients. In other words, from the multicenter trial, multiple adverse reactions to Thiola occurred in 43% of patients versus 67% to Cuprimine. Because of these toxicities, some have begun to evaluate captopril, which is a thiol angiotensin-converting enzyme inhibitor used in managing hypertension as an adjunctive agent. Doses of 75 to 100 mg daily have been shown to have some benefit.

Metaphylactic measures for struvite stone–forming patients are exceedingly complicated. Because these stones are induced by urease-producing infections, antibiotics are the first-line drugs of choice. The primary problem appears to be the microflora within the retained stone fragments that are rarely eliminated despite long-term suppressive antibiotic regimens such as sulfonamides, nitrofurantoins, and methenamine salts. Long-term, culture-specific antibiotics appear to be the most effective, such as penicillin, ampicillin, and tetracycline. Surveillance cultures are necessary when instituting long-term antimicrobial therapy. Urease inhibitors are another class of drugs that block the enzymatic cascade converting urea to ammonia and water. Hydroxamic acids are known to be inhibitors of the enzyme urease. Acetohydroxamic acid (AHA, Lithostat) can be given at a dose of 250 mg every 8 hours. Approximately 20% to 30% of patients are unable to tolerate AHA because of significant side effects (gastrointestinal upset, headache, tremulousness, loss of taste, hallucinations, and others). Lithostat is contraindicated in patients with azotemia (serum creatinine > 2.0 ng/dL). The combination of AHA and antibiotics is synergistic and may reduce the dose and hence the side effects of AHA, but prospective data are lacking. Urinary acidification has been attempted as another specific therapy to lower the saturation of urine with struvite and carbonate apatite. Vitamin C (ascorbic acid) has not been proven to effectively acidify urine. Ammonium chloride can successfully acidify the urine, but long-term effects remain unclear. Finally, two other medications have been shown to have some benefit for patients with struvite stones. Aluminum hydroxide gels (antacids), when combined with dietary phosphorus restriction, have been shown to reduce the urinary phosphorus level, which is the substrate for precipitation in patients with these stones. Although they are effective in reducing urinary phosphate excretion, side effects and compliance make current utilization limited.

Surgical Options

SHOCK WAVE LITHOTRIPSY

New improvements in the technology of treating patients surgically are best exempli-

fied by ESWL. The major risk of therapy is that the stone fragments must pass following their fragmentation. Approximately 10% to 15% of patients develop acute colic following ESWL during passage of these fragments. Depending on the initial stone size, location, and composition, large volumes of stone debris can pass, causing a unique type of obstruction referred to as *steinstrasse*. Success rates (65% to 85%) for ESWL of renal stones depend on stone size, composition, location, and degree of associated obstruction.

INTRACORPOREAL LITHOTRIPSY

Patients may require other endoscopic procedures to treat stones where ESWL is ineffective, when distal obstruction is present, or when the stone burden is too great to pass spontaneously. There are four basic methods for intracorporeal lithotripsy: electrohydraulic, ultrasonic, ballistic, and laser. The approaches are percutaneous nephroscopy (usually rigid endoscopes), percutaneous antegrade ureteroscopy, transurethral ureteroscopy, and laparoscopic ureterolithotomy. The availability of smaller ureteroscopes allows more options for the patients via the transurethral approach.

Other methods of stone removal include endoscopic-guided basketing, retrograde-catheter loop extraction, laparoscopic ureterolithotomy, and open ureterolithotomy. The first two methods are appropriate when the stones are small and the intact removal of the calculus is not likely to damage the ureter. The latter two methods, laparoscopic and open ureterolithotomies, are rarely necessary.

Conclusions

Stone disease continues to increase in prevalence in North America and represents a major health care issue. In 1993, urolithiasis represented 0.9% of discharge diagnoses with a mean hospital stay of 3 days. The cost to the health care system in 1993 was estimated to be $1.83 billion. If left alone, most patients who form stones experience a recurrence, and at least 20% of these recur several times. Given the complexity of this disease and the continued recent advances in the medical and surgical therapies, it is not surprising that some medical generalists and specialists defer to a urologist for both evaluation and therapy of stone disease. The more complex the stone-forming patient, or the more recalcitrant a patient is to metaphylactic measures, the more he or she requires such a center carefully focusing on outcomes. Children with stone disease are an exception to the management discussed previously. Dietary changes cannot be as harsh as they are for an adult because of requirements for growth. Pregnant women are another exception because standard radiographic evaluation and surgical interventions must be considered carefully because the fetus carries some risk. Finally, there is a group known as *fictitious stone formers* who use this disease for personal benefit, often for intravenous narcotics, and who from time to time present to the emergency department.

PEDIATRIC UROLITHIASIS

Children with urolithiasis present with all of the same stone types and metabolic derangements as afflict the adults, but anatomic variability must be a primary consideration. Both infectious stones and genitourinary tract anomalies are more common in pediatric stone-forming patients than in the adult population. The incidence of stone disease in children is 1 in 1000 to 7600 hospital admissions, with females and males being affected equally. One rather unique occurrence in children is hematuria associated with hypercalciuria, hyperoxaluria, and hyperuricosuria without an actual calculus. Cystinuria is more likely to present in children than in adults and should be screened for if a stone is present. The surgical modalities for treating symptomatic children are the same as with adults. The least invasive modality (ESWL) should be considered first. The absolute contraindication to this therapy would be an obstructed kidney. Open surgery may be required more often in children than in adults to synchronously correct anatomic aberrations if they coexist with stones.

PREGNANCY AND UROLITHIASIS

Pregnancy represents another unique condition in which urolithiasis can complicate the normal gestational process. Occurrence during pregnancy is estimated at 0.05% to 0.35% and is least common in the first trimester but rises throughout the second and third trimesters. Urolithiasis represents a major differential diagnostic dilemma during pregnancy. A high index of suspicion is necessary, and invariably a screening renal ultrasonographic examination is performed. Problems with this study are the mechanical and hormonal responses of the patient to her pregnancy with dilation of her upper urinary tracts (especially the right side). Limited intravenous pyelograms can be obtained, with limitation in the number of exposures, especially beyond the first trimester. Women of childbearing age with known asymptomatic renal calculi should consider treatment prior to becoming pregnant. Pregnancy remains a contraindication for SWL. All other modalities remain, with palliative diversion by percutaneous nephrostomy or ureteral stenting being the foremost alternatives because there is least risk to both mother and fetus. Approximately 50% of pregnant patients with urolithiasis pass the stone spontaneously during their pregnancy, and observation is a definite option. Nonspecific therapy can and should be recommended during the pregnancy by pushing oral fluid and adding citrus fruits four times daily, but restricting dietary calcium and multivitamins seems unwise. Full evaluation and therapy can proceed following delivery.

FICTITIOUS UROLITHIASIS

The most difficult subgroup of patients with potential urolithiasis are those with fictitious symptoms. These patients tend to be increasingly difficult to distinguish from patients with true stones, but several clues predispose to making an accurate diagnosis prior to the patient depleting the emergency department of narcotics. Often the patient will state that he or she forms "uric acid" stones, knowing that these are radiolucent and will not show up on screening kidney, ureter, and bladder films. The patient is usually "allergic" to intravenous contrast agents of all types. The severity of the patient's pain is out of proportion or overdramatized while lacking the visceral signs associated with severe ureteral colic, such as diaphoresis, nausea, and vomiting. The patients usually can manipulate their urinalysis to obtain microscopic hematuria. Several questions are essential when this scenario exists. First, where has the patient been treated for previous stones? (The typical response is out of state or that the patient just moved to this area.) Were the stones obtained and analyzed? Some fictitious stone formers go so far as to present with fake stones in their possession. There are many ways to evaluate and manage these patients. Initially, the pharmacologic therapy for colic worldwide is nonsteroidal anti-inflammatory medications such as ketorolac tromethamine (Toradol) parenterally. If the patients are allergic to this drug, indomethacin suppositories should next be tried. By this time the patients are suspicious that you are not feeding them narcotics and often will sign out of the emergency department against medical advice. Even in patients who are allergic to contrast media, nonenhanced spiral CT has good sensitivity and specificity in the setting of acute ureteral colic. If unavailable, then a regular CT with overlapping cuts approximates the sensitivity of the spiral machines. Ultimately a diuretic radioisotope renal scan can rule out significant obstruction in those patients for whom lingering concerns exist.

SUGGESTED READINGS

1. Atkinson RL Jr, Earll JM: Munchausen syndrome with renal stones. JAMA 230:89, 1974.
2. Clark JY, Thompson SA, Optenberg SA: Economic impact of urolithiasis in the United States. J Urol 154:2020–2024, 1995.
3. Coe FL, Moran E, Kavalach AG: The contribution of dietary purine overconsumption to hyperuricosuria in calcium oxalate stone formers. J Chron Dis 29:793–800, 1976.
4. Cordell, WH, Wright SW, Wolfson AB, et al: Comparison of intravenous ketorolac, meperidine, and both (balanced analgesia) for renal colic. Ann Emerg Med 28:151–157, 1996.
5. Drach GW: Acute stone episode. In Common Problems in Infections and Stones. Philadelphia, Mosby-Year Book, 1992, pp 139–142.
6. Ettinger B, Pak CYC, Citron JT, et al: Potassium-magnesium citrate is an effective prophylaxis against recurrent calcium oxalate nephrolithiasis. J Urol 158:2069–2073, 1997.
7. Jones WA, Corea RJ Jr, Ansell JS: Urolithiasis associated with pregnancy. J Urol 122:333–335, 1979.
8. Kizer KW, Moran ME, Vassar M: Apparent change in the male:female ratio of incidence of urolithiasis in California. Med J Aust 160:448, 1993.
9. Menon M, Parulkar BG, Drach GW: Urinary lithiasis: Etiology, diagnosis, and medical management. In Walsh PC, Retik AB, Vaughan ED Jr, Wein AJ (eds): Campbell's Urology, 7th ed. Philadelphia, WB Saunders, 1998, pp 2661–2734.
10. Moran ME, Calvano CJ, White MD, et al: Silent near-lethal ureteral calculi in the intensive care setting. J Endourol 11:S194, 1997.
11. Pak CYC, Ohata M, Lawrence EC, et al: The hypercalciurias: Causes, parathyroid functions, and diagnostic criteria. J Clin Invest 54:387, 1974.
12. Pak CYC, Peterson R, Sakhaee K, et al: Correction of hypocitraturia and prevention of stone formation by combined thiazide and potassium citrate therapy in thiazide-unresponsive hypercalciuric nephrolithiasis. Am J Med 79:284–288, 1985.
13. Preminger GM: Nephrolithiasis—solutions for emerging problems [Editorial]. J Urol 156:910–911, 1996.
14. Preminger GM, Harvey JA, Pak CYC: Comparative efficacy of "specific" potassium citrate therapy versus conservative management in nephrolithiasis of mild-moderate severity. J Urol 134:658–661, 1985.
15. Schneider HJ: Urolithiasis: Etiology, Diagnosis. New York, Springer-Verlag, 1985, pp 4–5.
16. Sharon E, Diamond HS: Fictitious uric acid urolithiasis as feature of Munchausen syndrome. Mt Sinai J 41:698–699, 1974.
17. Shepherd P, Thomas R, Harmon EP: Urolithiasis in children: Innovations in management. J Urol 140:790, 1988.

9 Sexually Transmitted Diseases

Norman P. Gebrosky
Unyime O. Nseyo

INCIDENCE AND BACKGROUND

Sexually transmitted diseases (STDs) have plagued humans since antiquity. With the advent of modern antibiotics, it was once believed that STDs would be completely eradicated. This view has certainly changed during the past several decades. Since the sexual revolution in the 1970s, the incidence and varieties of STDs have increased significantly. Diseases such as gonorrhea, previously quite susceptible to treatment with penicillin, have become increasingly resistant to antibiotic therapy. More recently, newer STDs such as hepatitis B, genital herpes, and acquired immunodeficiency syndrome (AIDS) have been identified as being sexually transmitted and have been found to be increasing in incidence at near pandemic rates.

The primary care physician is in a unique position when it comes to diagnosing and treating patients with STDs. They often are the initial health care provider seen for management of these illnesses. Unfortunately, owing to feelings of guilt or shame, the patient may be reluctant to present for treatment or may hide his or her true reasons for seeking medical attention. It is imperative that all personnel involved in the care of these patients put forward an open, caring, and nonjudgmental attitude. In this way patients are more likely to discuss frankly their symptoms and sexual practices, allow identification and treatment of sexual contacts, and feel motivated to follow through with their own treatment. Without adequate treatment of both the patients and their sexual contacts, control of STDs will remain unobtainable.

TRENDS AND POPULATION AT RISK

STDs occur among sexually active people. Traditionally, they have been most common among older adolescent and young adult males. STDs occur less frequently in older persons, women, and young teenagers. Men continue to have higher rates of infection than do women. These rates may be higher because men are more likely to seek medical attention owing to noticeable signs and symptoms. Additionally, men generally have more sexual partners than do women. Rates among women are increasing. This increase is believed to be related to women's sexual behavior becoming more like that of men. Women are becoming sexually active at a younger age and may have an increased number of sexual partners. The increased incidence of STDs among women carries significant consequences. Complications such as ectopic pregnancy, pelvic inflammatory disease (PID), and cervical carcinoma are also occurring more frequently. Finally, rates of infection among young teenagers and children are also on the rise. Again, this is believed to be related to an earlier age of first sexual activity and to a lack of understanding about methods of transmission and prevention of these diseases.

Race, socioeconomic level, and sexual preference also affect rates and type of sexually transmitted infection. In the United States, African Americans have the highest reported incidence of STDs, followed by whites and then Asian Americans. People of lower socioeconomic status still have the highest morbidity rates. Whites have been shown to be more commonly infected with genital herpes than are African Americans. In addition, homosexual men are more prone to certain STDs such as syphilis, hepatitis, gonorrhea, and human immunodeficiency virus (HIV) than are heterosexual men.

SPECIAL SEXUALLY TRANSMITTED DISEASE POPULATIONS

Pregnant Women

Pregnant women, adolescents, children, and HIV-infected patients are believed to represent unique populations of STD patients. Prenatal or perinatal transmission of an STD can have disastrous or fatal consequences to a fetus. During the initial prenatal visit, pregnant women and their sex partners should be questioned about a history of STDs and their risk factors for infection. The Centers for Disease Control and Prevention (CDC) recommend a number of screening tests for pregnant women (Table 9–1). In the early stages of pregnancy, all women should be screened for syphilis. If a patient is at high risk for syphilis, she should be retested during the third trimester and again at delivery. Testing at delivery is mandated in some states. Women having a spontaneous abortion after 20 weeks' gestation should also be tested for syphilis. Other recommended screening tests include a serologic test for hepatitis B surface antigen (HBsAg), cervical culture for *Neisseria gonorrhoeae,* and testing for *Chlamydia trachomatis.* Women younger than 25 years of age or with new or multiple sexual partners are believed to be at increased risk for *Chlamydia*

infection. They should therefore be screened and, if needed, treated during the first trimester. Retesting during the third trimester is also recommended to prevent infection of the infant and to prevent maternal postnatal complications. Testing for HIV infection is recommended for women with risk factors for HIV infection or with a high-risk sex partner. Some experts advocate HIV testing of all pregnant women. As with nonpregnant patients, pretesting and posttesting HIV counseling should be provided.

Women with their first case of genital herpes are at highest risk for transmitting the virus to their child. Transmission occurs at the time of delivery as the baby passes through an infected birth canal. If viral lesions are not noted during the third trimester, routine serial cultures for herpes simplex virus (HSV) are not indicated because the results of viral cultures during pregnancy have not been shown to predict viral shedding at the time of delivery. At the onset of labor, all women should be questioned about symptoms of genital herpes and carefully examined for viral lesions. If herpetic vesicles are noted, cesarean section should be performed. If no symptoms or vesicles are noted, the woman may deliver vaginally. Obtaining viral cultures at the time of delivery from a women with a history of genital herpes may be helpful in guiding neonatal management. The presence of genital warts is not considered to be an indication for prophylactic cesarean section. All pregnant women, particularly those at high risk for STDs, should be screened as detailed in Table 9–1.

Children

STDs among children and adolescents are becoming increasingly common. Investigation and management of children with STDs require a multiteam approach. The physician and child welfare authorities must work closely together. When acquired after the neonatal period, diseases such as gonorrhea, syphilis, and *Chlamydia* infection are almost universally acquired by sexual contact. If any of these illnesses are diagnosed or suspected, investigation for sexual abuse must be initiated.

Table 9–1
STD Screening of Pregnant Women

Recommended

Serologic tests for syphilis
Serologic test for hepatitis B surface antigen
Test for *Neisseria gonorrhoeae*
Test for *Chlamydia trachomatis*

Suggested

Serologic test for human immunodeficiency virus (if risk factors identified)
Viral cultures for herpes simplex virus at time of delivery (in patients with history of recurrent genital herpes)

STD, sexually transmitted disease.

Adolescents

Adolescents have been found to have the highest rates of infection with gonorrhea, *Chlamydia,* and possibly human papillomavirus (HPV). In the United States, parental consent is not required for an adolescent to receive treatment of an STD. All adolescents may consent to confidential diagnosis and treatment. In many states, adolescents may also consent to HIV counseling and testing. As with any health issues of a teenager, discussions and explanations must be directed to the patient's developmental and educational level. It is also particularly important to remain open, caring, and nonjudgmental throughout the evaluation, treatment, and counseling of these patients.

A diagnosis of HIV infection imparts a great deal of emotional and psychological distress on patients. They need help with learning to cope with the stigma attached to this illness and with the realization that they will probably have a shortened life span. These patients need to develop strategies for maintaining their physical and emotional health. Finally, aggressive counseling is required to help them initiate lifestyle changes needed to prevent HIV transmission.

PREVENTION

One of the cornerstones of treating STD is preventing the spread of disease to others. Prevention is based on four major concepts: education to reduce risk of transmission; diagnosis and treatment of infected persons not seeking medical attention; diagnosis and treatment of those persons infected and seeking medical attention; and identification, treatment, and education of partners of persons known to be infected. Physicians are in a unique position to work on each of the four concepts. They can interrupt transmission by identifying and treating symptomatically and asymptomatically infected patients, educating patients about their particular risks for infection, and identifying and treating sexual contacts of infected patients. As stated earlier, it is imperative that the physician put forth a caring, open, and nonjudgmental attitude to allow effective delivery of prevention messages.

Once the risk factors are identified, educational counseling can take place. Emphasize that the most effective way to prevent transmission of an STD is to avoid sexual intercourse with an infected partner. If the infection status of a partner is in question or the patient chooses to have intercourse with an infected partner, men should use a new latex condom with each act of intercourse. When used correctly, condoms provide an effective means of preventing a variety of STDs, including HIV infection. Although not nearly as effective as male condoms, female condoms act as a mechanical barrier to sperm, bacteria, and viruses.

Patients must be aware that nonbarrier forms of contraception such as oral contraceptive pills, hormonal implants, intrauterine devices, and surgical sterilization offer no protection against STDs. Spermicidals, vaginal contraceptive sponges, and diaphragms have been shown to decrease the risk for contracting some STDs, but none have been shown to prevent HIV infection or to prevent other STDs as well as a male condom.

Another important step in preventing further transmission of disease is treating not only symptomatic patients but also their sexual contacts. If, based on history alone, a partner is believed to have a treatable STD, that person should be treated. Appropriate antibiotics should be given even if no signs of infection are present and before confirmatory test results are complete.

Sexually Transmitted Diseases Associated with Genital Ulcers

Table 9–2 contains highlights of the clinical features, diagnosis, and recommended treatments of sexually transmitted genital ulcers.

Genital herpes, syphilis, chancroid, lymphogranuloma venereum, and granuloma inguinale are STDs associated with genital ulcers. In the United States, genital herpes occurs most commonly, followed by syphilis, chancroid, lymphogranuloma venereum, and granuloma inguinale. Up to 10% of patients with genital ulcers are infected by more than one organism. Each of these diseases has been

Table 9-2
Differential Diagnosis of Genital Ulcers: Highlights

Disease	Etiology	Incubation Time	Early Lesion	Local Pain	Diagnostic Test
Granuloma inguinale	*Calymmatobacterium granulomatis*	2–3 mo	Superficial ulcer of skin	Little	Stained organisms in scraping from ulcer or biopsy
Herpes progenitalis	Herpes virus Type 2	Unknown (often recurrent); systemic flulike symptoms in >50%	Multiple superficial vesicles on the foreskin or glans	Slight local burning or itching; more severe in women	Isolation of virus
Syphilitic chancre	*T. pallidum*	2–4 wk	Enlarging papule that finally ulcerates	Very painful	Serum tests, darkfield examination, direct immunofluorescence for *T. pallidum*
Chancroid	*H. ducreyi* (Ducrey's bacillus)	3–10 d	Macule or papule, then formation of ulcer	Very painful	Selective medium culture for *H. ducreyi*
Lymphogranuloma	*Chlamydia* bacterium	3–21 d	Transient, usually not seen; papule or macule heals rapidly	None	Culture for *C. trachomatis*

T. pallidum, Treponema pallidum; H. ducreyi, Haemophilus ducreyi; C. trachomatis, Chlamydia trachomatis.

associated with an increased risk of HIV infection.

Genital ulcers present a diagnostic dilemma. The differential diagnostic features are highlighted in Table 9–2. A diagnosis based solely on the physical appearance of the ulcer is often in error. Neoplastic disorders such as squamous cell carcinoma and erythroplasia of Queyrat (discussed elsewhere in this text) may also present as a penile ulcer. If malignancy is suspected, biopsy of the lesion is required. Figure 9–1 presents a strategy for evaluating patients with genital ulcers. Specific tests are often required to accurately diagnose the cause of genital ulcers (see Table 9–2). All patients with a genital ulcer should have a serologic test for syphilis. Other tests are employed based on clinical or epidemiologic suspicion. Viral culture or antigen testing is most useful in diagnosing genital herpes. Darkfield examination or direct immunofluorescence is used to confirm the presence of syphilis. Chancroid is diagnosed by selective medium culture of *Haemophilus ducreyi,* and culture of *C. trachomatis* is diagnostic of lymphogranuloma venereum (LGV). Histologic evaluation of a crush preparation from the ulcer base is used to identify granuloma inguinale. Finally, HIV testing should be offered to all patients with genital ulcers, especially those with syphilis or chancroid.

GENITAL HERPES

Background and Incidence

Genital HSV infection has been increasing in incidence for many years. It has been esti-

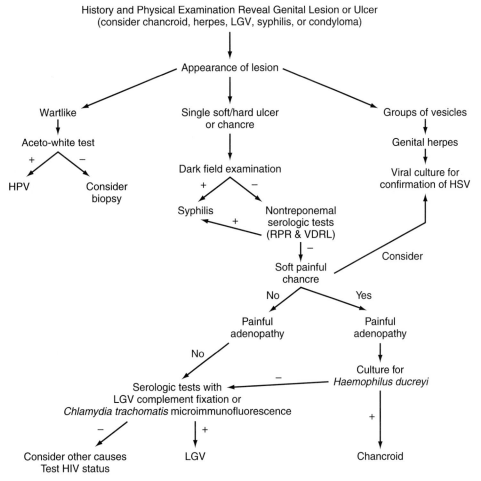

Figure 9–1

Evaluation of patients with genital lesions or ulcers. LGV, lymphogranuloma venereum; HSV, herpes simplex virus; HPV, human papillomavirus; RPR, rapid plasma reagin; VDRL, Venereal Disease Research Laboratory; HIV, human immunodeficiency virus.

mated that 30 million people in the United States are infected with genital herpes. HSV infection is the most common STD noted among college students. Infected patients may note genital ulcers, but most are asymptomatic. HSV may be recurrent and has been linked to significant neonatal morbidity and mortality and to cervical cancer. At present, no curative therapies are available.

An infected patient may never notice signs of HSV infection. When present, symptoms will occur 2 to 7 days after exposure. Generally the signs and symptoms of initial infection are much more severe than in recurrent disease. Isolated or groups of painful, erythematous vesicles may be noted. Dysuria, lymphadenopathy, and flulike symptoms may also occur.

Recurrent infections tend to be much less severe. A mild tingling, pain, or burning may be noted as a prodrome to clinical infection. The number and size of lesions are smaller, and they tend to be unilateral. Pain and lymphadenopathy are milder and less common. Systemic symptoms are uncommon, as is dysuria. Viral shedding also occurs less frequently and for a shorter period.

Diagnosis

Diagnosis of genital HSV infection is based on a history of exposure, visual appearance of the genital lesions, and confirmatory laboratory tests. Vesicles grouped on an erythematous base not following any neural distribution are pathognomonic for HSV infection.

Treatment

There is no curative therapy for genital herpes. Systemic acyclovir has been shown to decrease duration of viral shedding, time to crusting and healing of lesions, and duration of pain and itching noted with the primary infection. Dysuria, systemic symptoms, and the development of new lesions are also improved by systemic acyclovir. Topical acyclovir has been found to be much less effective, and its use is not recommended. The recommended treatment for initial infection is listed in Table 9–3.

Treatment of recurrent episodes has been found to be less effective. Oral acyclovir has been found to decrease the duration of viral shedding and time to crusting of recurrent lesions but has not been shown to decrease the duration of local pain or itching. Maximal effect is noted only if the drug is given during the prodrome. The recommended regimen for treating clinical recurrence is listed in Table 9–3.

Daily suppressive therapy has been found to be useful in patients with frequent recurrences (six or more episodes per year). Suppressive therapy does not eliminate viral shedding or the potential for viral transmission. Suppression should be discontinued after 1 year to allow assessment of the patient's rate of recurrent episodes. If needed, it may be reinstituted. Table 9–3 lists the recommended suppressive regimen.

Intravenous acyclovir should be given to those patients with severe disease or disseminated infection (i.e., encephalitis, pneumonitis, or hepatitis). The treatment regimen for severe infections is also listed in Table 9–3.

Prevention of Transmission

As with all STDs, the use of condoms should be encouraged with all sexual activity. Patients need to be advised to abstain from sexual relations while the disease is clinically active or lesions are present. They must be made aware of the potential for recurrent episodes and of their risk for sexual transmission, including asymptomatic viral shedding. Sex partners of patients with genital herpes should be evaluated. If indicated, treatment should be initiated as outlined earlier. Sex partners should also be instructed to perform self-examinations for lesions in the future.

Perinatal Herpes Infection. HSV also has the capacity to cause perinatal infections. The risk of transmission to the neonate is highest among women with their first episode of genital herpes occurring near the time of delivery. The risk of transmission is low ($\leq 3\%$) among women with recurrent herpes. Screening viral cultures during pregnancy are not recommended since they do not predict viral shedding at the time of delivery.

At the time of delivery, women without signs or symptoms of genital herpes or prodrome may deliver vaginally. If the mother or

Table 9-3
Treatment Recommendations for the Common STDs

Disease	Adults	Children	Neonates
Genital herpes First episode	Acyclovir 200 mg five times daily for 7–10 days		
Recurrence	Acyclovir 200 mg five times daily for 5 days or 400 mg three times daily for 5 days or 400 mg twice daily for 5 days		
Severe disease	Acyclovir 5–10 mg/kg IV every 8 hours for 5–7 days		Acyclovir 30 mg/kg/day for 10–14 days
Syphilis Primary, secondary, or early latent stages	*Recommended treatment* Benzathine penicillin 2.4 million units IM single dose	Benzathine penicillin 50,000 units/kg IM up to 2.4 million units	
	Alternative treatment Doxycycline 100 mg PO twice daily for 14 days *or* Tetracycline 500 mg PO four times daily for 14 days *or* Erythromycin 500 mg PO four times daily for 14 days		
Late latent or tertiary (nonneurosyphilis)	Ceftriaxone 250 mg IM daily for 10 days *Recommended treatment* Benzathine penicillin G 2.4 million U IM weekly for 3 weeks (7.2 million U total)	Benzathine penicillin G 50,000 U/kg IM weekly for 3 weeks (150,000/kg total up to adult dose)	
	Alternative treatment Doxycycline 100 mg PO twice daily for 28 days		
Neurosyphilis	*Recommended treatment* Aqueous crystalline penicillin 12–24 million U IV every 4 hours for 10–14 days		
	Alternative treatment Procaine penicillin 2.4 million U IM daily plus probenecid 500 mg PO daily, both for 10–14 days		
Chancroid	*Recommended treatment* Azithromycin 1 g PO as a single dose *or* Ceftriaxone 250 mg in as a single dose *or* Erythromycin base 500 mg PO four times daily for 7 days		

Table continued on following page

Table 9-3 Continued
Treatment Recommendations for the Common STDs

Disease	Adults	Children	Neonates
Lymphogranuloma venereum	*Alternative treatment* Amoxicillin 500 mg plus clavulanic acid 125 mg PO three times daily for 7 days *or* Ciprofloxacin 500 mg PO twice daily for 3 days *Recommended treatment* Doxycycline 100 mg PO twice daily for 21 days *Alternative treatment* Erythromycin 500 mg PO four times daily for 21 days *or* Sulfisoxazole 500 mg PO four times daily for 21 days		
Gonorrhea Uncomplicated	*Recommended treatment* Ceftriaxone 125 mg IM as a single dose *or* Cefixime 400 mg PO as a single dose *or* Ofloxacin 400 mg PO as a single dose *plus* doxycycline 100 mg PO twice daily for 7 days *Alternative treatment* Spectinomycin 2 g IM as a single dose	*Prophylaxis in newborns* Ceftriaxone 25–50 mg/kg IV or IM (not to exceed 125 mg)—single dose	Prophylaxis for ophthalmia neonatorum silver nitrate (1%) aqueous solution *or* Erythromycin (0.5%) *or* Tetracycline (91%)
Disseminated gonococcal infection	*Recommended treatment* Ceftriaxone 1 g IM every 24 hours *Alternative treatment* Cefotaxime 1 g IV every 8 hours *or* Ceftizoxime 1 g every 24 hours *or* Spectinomycin 2 g IM every 12 hours for 24 hours *Follow-up regimens* Cefixime 400 mg PO twice daily for 7 days *or* Ciprofloxacin 500 mg PO twice daily for 7 days	Ceftriaxone 25–50 mg/kg IV or IM every 24 hours for 7 days (10–14 days for meningitis) *or* Cefotaxime 25 mg/kg IV or IM every 12 hours for 7 days (10–14 days for meningitis)	Ophthalmia neonatorum: Ceftriaxone 25–50 mg/kg IV or IM (not to exceed 125 mg)—single dose
Gonococcal meningitis and endocarditis	Ceftriaxone 1–2 g IV every 12 hours		

Nongonococcal urethritis	*Recommended treatment* Erythromycin base 500 mg PO four times daily for 7 days; *or* Erythromycin ethylsuccinate 800 mg PO four times daily for 7 days; if high-dose erythromycin cannot be tolerated: erythromycin base 250 mg PO four times daily for 14 days; *or* Erythromycin ethylsuccinate 400 mg PO four times daily for 14 days	
Chlamydia infection	*Recommended treatment* Erythromycin base 500 mg PO four times daily for 7 days *Alternative treatment* Erythromycin base 250 mg PO four times daily for 14 days *or* Erythromycin ethylsuccinate 800 mg PO three times daily for 7 days *or* Amoxicillin 500 mg PO three times daily for 7–10 days	*Recommended treatment* Doxycycline 100 mg PO twice daily for 7 days Azithromycin 1 g PO; single dose *Alternative treatment* Ofloxacin 300 mg PO twice daily for 7 days *or* Erythromycin base 500 mg PO four times daily for 7 days *or* Sulfisoxazole 600 mg PO four times daily for 10 days
Sexually transmitted epididymitis		*Recommended treatment* Ceftriaxone 250 mg IM in a single dose plus doxycycline 100 mg PO twice daily for 7 days
Nonsexually transmitted epididymitis		*Alternative treatment* Ofloxacin 300 mg PO twice daily for 10 days Trimethoprim/sulfamethoxazole, one double-strength tablet PO twice daily for 10 days *or* Ofloxacin 300 mg PO twice daily for 10 days

Recommended treatment
Erythromycin 50 mg/kg/day PO in four divided doses for 10–14 days

IV, intravenous; IM, intramuscular; PO, oral.

sex partner has a history of genital herpes, cultures of the birth canal at delivery may aid in decisions relating to neonatal management. If active infection or vesicles are noted, cesarean section should be performed.

Infants delivered through an infected birth canal should be followed carefully. Viral cultures should be obtained 24 to 48 hours postpartum. Treatment with acyclovir is reserved for infants with positive viral cultures or evidence of clinical disease. Treatment of neonatal infection is listed in Table 9–3.

SYPHILIS

Background and Incidence

The incidence of syphilis is also on the rise, with close to 40,000 cases being reported per year. Syphilis is a systemic disease caused by the spirochete *Treponema pallidum.* Genital contact allows the organism to gain access through the skin or mucous membranes. Various stages of disease occur, and patients may present for treatment during any stage (see Tables 9–2 and 9–3).

The later stages of syphilis tend to be a reflection of systemic disease. Secondary syphilis occurs 2 to 10 weeks after the primary lesions. Fever, sore throat, generalized lymphadenopathy, headache, and a rash of the palms and soles of the feet are commonly present. Nephrotic syndrome, arthritis, and arthralgias may also be noted. After the last episode of secondary disease, the patient enters a stage of latent disease. Patients with latent syphilis who are known to have been infected within the past year are considered to have early latent syphilis. Those infected more than a year before have late latent syphilis. Patients with late latent disease, like those with tertiary syphilis, require longer courses of treatment.

Persons not treated during the primary, secondary, or latent stages of disease may develop tertiary syphilis. Three to 10 years after the last evidence of secondary disease, an immunologic reaction by the host may result in formation of nonprogressive, localized lesions of dermal elements or supporting structures of the body. These are called *gummas.* They are most commonly found in the liver, bones, skin, and testes. The central nervous system (CNS) may become involved 5 or more years after development of primary disease. This neurosyphilis may present as dementia, tabes dorsalis (locomotor ataxia due to disease of the posterior [sensory] columns of the spinal cord and sensory nerve roots), seizures, optic atrophy, and amyotrophic lateral sclerosis. Finally, 10 to 40 years after primary infection the cardiovascular system may become involved, resulting in cardiovascular syphilis. This most commonly involves the great vessels of the heart. The resulting arteritis of the aortic and pulmonary vessels may result in aneurysm formation, stenosis, angina, myocardial insufficiency, and death.

Syphilis can also be transmitted from an infected mother to her unborn child. Serologic screening for syphilis should be performed on all women during early evaluation of pregnancy. In patients believed to be at high risk for infection, testing should be repeated during the third trimester and again at delivery. Any women delivering a stillborn fetus after 20 weeks' gestation should also be tested for syphilis. Risk of transmission is greatest among untreated women with primary and secondary syphilis but may occur during any stage of disease. Early congenital syphilis is similar to the secondary stage of sexually acquired disease. Most infants are asymptomatic at birth. If left untreated, however, symptoms develop within several weeks or months. Congenital syphilis may involve multiple organ systems. Some of the common manifestations of this illness include hepatosplenomegaly, jaundice, lymphadenopathy, and osteochondritis of wrists, elbows, ankles, and knees. Late manifestations include saddle nose, Hutchinson teeth, and juvenile tabes. Infants should be serologically tested if they were born to seropositive mothers who were believed to be inadequately treated or who show physical evidence of congenital disease.

Diagnosis

Early syphilis may be diagnosed by darkfield examination and direct fluorescent antibody tests of scrapings obtained from the base of the chancre. Presumptive diagnosis may also be made using serologic tests. Two types of serologic tests exist: nontreponemal (Venereal Disease Research Laboratory [VDRL] and rapid plasma reagin [RPR]) and treponemal (fluorescent treponemal antibody absorption test [FTS-ABS] and microhemagglutination assay for antibody to *T. pallidum* [MHATP]). The use of one test alone is insufficient for diagnosis. Nontreponemal antibody titers are reported quantitatively and usually correlate with disease activity. Treponemal antibody titers correlate poorly with disease activity and, once positive, generally remain positive for life.

Treatment

Treatment for primary and secondary syphilis is summarized in Table 9–3.

Patients should be re-examined at 3 and 6 months after treatment. If a fourfold decline in antibody titers is not seen within 6 months of treatment, evaluation for neurosyphilis should be pursued. Retreatment should occur as indicated.

The later stages of syphilis require alternative therapies (see Table 9–3). Early latent syphilis is treated like primary syphilis. Late latent syphilis should be treated with three weekly doses of benzathine penicillin. Neurosyphilis requires more aggressive therapy with 10 to 14 days of intravenous aqueous crystalline penicillin G. If compliance with therapy can be ensured, daily intramuscular procaine penicillin plus oral probenecid, both for 10 to 14 days, may be used as an alternative regimen. Non–penicillin-based regimens have not proven to be effective. If penicillin allergy exists, desensitization should be performed.

Children with early disease should be treated with benzathine penicillin G 50,000 U/kg intramuscular, up to the adult dose of 2.4 million U in a single dose. Those patients with late latent syphilis or tertiary disease are treated with three doses of benzathine penicillin G.

As with other infections, patients with HIV infection may be more resistant to therapy, requiring more prolonged or aggressive treatment.

Prevention of Transmission

Sexual transmission of syphilis can occur only when a chancre or mucocutaneous lesions are present (i.e., during primary or secondary infection). Sexual activity should be avoided until after treatment is completed. As with other STDs, patients should be counseled to always use a latex condom, and if found to be infected, to consider being tested for HIV.

A partner of a patient with syphilis of any stage should be clinically and serologically evaluated or treated based on the following criteria. A person exposed to a patient with primary, secondary, or early latent syphilis within the preceding 90 days may be infected even if seronegative; such persons should be presumptively treated. Treatment should also be given to partners of a patient who has syphilis of unknown duration and who have high nontreponemal serologic test titers (>1:32). Finally, long-term sex partners of patients with late syphilis should be serologically and clinically tested.

CHANCROID

Background and Incidence

Although chancroid was infrequently diagnosed in the past, it is now endemic in many areas of the United States and appears to be increasing in incidence. Chancroid often occurs in conjunction with other STDs, particularly HIV and syphilis. It is caused by *H. ducreyi*. Clinical features, diagnosis, and treatments are summarized in Tables 9–2 and 9–3.

Diagnosis

Syphilis should be ruled out by darkfield examination of ulcer exudate or performance of serologic tests for syphilis 7 or more days after the development of ulcers. Similarly, HSV should be excluded by the clinical appearance of the ulcers, viral culture, or HSV antibody testing. Gram stain smear of the base of the chancre can be helpful if groups of intracellular and extracellular bacilli are noted.

Treatment

Recommended treatment regimens are summarized in Table 9–3. Successful treatment results in symptomatic improvement within 3 days and objective improvement within 7 days. Treatment also prevents transmission to others. If extensive lesions were present, scarring may result.

All treated patients should be re-examined 3 to 7 days after initiation of therapy. If clinical improvement has not occurred, re-evaluation is needed. The diagnosis of chancroid may be incorrect.

LYMPHOGRANULOMA VENEREUM

LGV occurs rarely in the United States. It is caused by C. trachomatis serotypes L1, L2, and L3. Like chancroid it is commonly associated with coinfection with other STDs. LGV is more common among African Americans than whites and among homosexuals. Differential diagnosis, clinical features, and treatment are summarized in Tables 9–2 and 9–3.

GRANULOMA INGUINALE

Granuloma inguinale is caused by the Donovan body, or *Calymmatobacterium granulomatis*. It occurs rarely in the United States. Males are predominantly affected. Sexual transmission results in chronic infection of the skin and subcutaneous tissue of the inguinal area, perineum, and genitalia. Several days to months after infection, a small papule or ulcer develops. Differential diagnosis, clinical features, and treatment are summarized in Tables 9–2 and 9–3.

Sexually Transmitted Disease Associated with Urethritis, Cervicitis, or Vaginal Discharge

Several STDs result in local infection of the urethra or cervix. Urethritis, or inflammation of the urethra, is generally characterized by a purulent discharge and dysuria. Cervicitis, inflammation of the cervix or endocervix, is characterized by a yellow exudate visible in the endocervical canal or on an endocervical swab specimen. Cervicitis is often asymptomatic but may result in abnormal vaginal discharge or bleeding. Both urethritis and cervicitis are most commonly caused by N. gonorrhoeae or C. trachomatis. Other agents

such as *Ureaplasma urealyticum, T. vaginalis, Gardnerella vaginalis,* and *Candida* species may also cause urethritis, cervicitis, and/or vaginitis. (Candidiasis is not considered to be sexually transmitted but is included because it is a common infection among women being evaluated for STDs.) Figure 9–2 presents a strategy for evaluating patients with dysuria or urethral/vaginal discharges.

GONORRHEA
Background and Incidence

Gonorrhea is one of the more well-known STDs. In the United States, it is estimated that 1 million new infections with N. gonorrhoeae occur each year. The bacterium is a gram-negative diplococcus. Symptoms of infection generally occur 3 to 10 days after exposure to an infected partner. Most cases are acquired during intercourse. A man has a 15% to 20% risk of acquiring gonorrhea during a single episode of unprotected intercourse with an infected partner. The risk of infection increases as the number of contacts with an infected partner increases. Transmission may also occur during oral or anal intercourse.

Most infections among men are symptomatic. Classically, infection in men results in urethritis that produces a profuse, purulent urethral discharge and severe dysuria. Up to 60% of infected men and many infected women are asymptomatic. Unfortunately, infections among women often do not produce recognizable symptoms until complications such as PID have occurred. PID may cause endometritis, salpingitis, tubo-ovarian abscess, or pelvic peritonitis. Asymptomatic infection may also induce tubal scarring, resulting in infertility or ectopic pregnancy. Because gonorrhea among women is often asymptomatic, screening of high-risk women is recommended.

Systemic infection and symptoms among men and women occur rarely. Disseminated gonococcal infection arises from gonococcal bacteremia. Petechial or pustular skin lesions, asymmetrical arthralgias, tenosynovitis, septic arthritis, hepatitis, endocarditis, or meningitis can result. Strains of N. gonorrhoeae causing disseminated infection have become uncommon. Gonococcal conjunctivitis may also be seen.

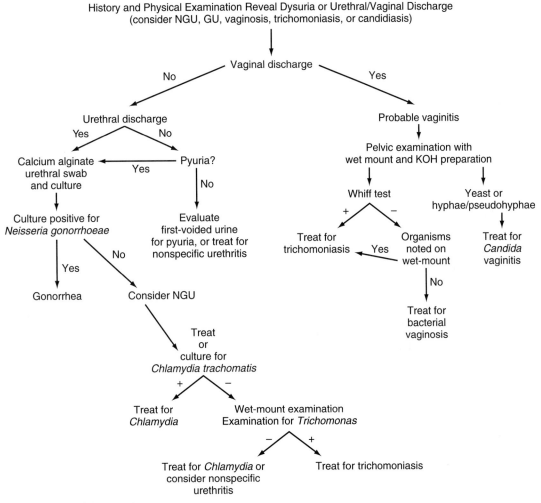

Figure 9-2
Evaluation of patients with dysuria and/or urethral/vaginal discharge. NGU, nongonococcal urethritis; GU, gonococcal urethritis; KOH, potassium hydroxide.

Infants and children may also be infected by *N. gonorrhoeae*. Infection among neonates usually results from peripartum exposure to infected endocervical exudates. It presents as an acute illness 2 to 5 days postpartum. Clinical manifestations range from rhinitis, vaginitis, urethritis, and inflammation at sites of intrauterine fetal monitoring to arthritis, meningitis, sepsis, or blindness from ophthalmia neonatorum. After the neonatal period, sexual abuse is the most common cause of gonococcal infection among children. Vaginitis, PID, anorectal, and pharyngeal infections may be seen. Any child suspected of having gonorrhea should be evaluated for sexual abuse.

Diagnosis

Diagnosis of gonorrhea is primarily based on examination and culture of urethral or endocervical swab specimens. Urethral specimens should be obtained at least 1 hour and preferably at 4 hours after the patient has voided. A calcium alginate swab should be inserted 2 to 4 cm into the urethra and rotated gently. Cotton swabs are not used owing to a bactericidal effect. Endocervical rather than urethral swabs are obtained from women. Rectal swabs should be obtained from homosexual men and all women. If there is a history of oral-genital contact, pharyngeal specimens are also obtained. Swabs are directly plated on culture media, and the same swab may be used for Gram staining. A slide is prepared by rolling the swab onto the slide to prevent damaging white blood cells. The presence of intracellular, gram-negative diplococci is diagnostic. Culture of *N. gonorrhoeae* requires special media, such as modified Thayer-Martin or New York City Transport Media, may be used when direct plating of specimens cannot be done.

Treatment

The CDC recommendations for treatment of gonorrhea in adults are outlined in Table 9–3.

Single-dose regimens are encouraged to enhance compliance. Resistance of *N. gonorrhoeae* to ceftriaxone has not yet been reported. Patients suspected of having disseminated gonococcal infections should be hospitalized and initially treated with parenteral therapy. Careful evaluation for endocarditis and meningitis should be performed. Twenty-four to 48 hours after clinical improvement is noted, therapy is switched to an oral regimen to complete 7 days of treatment (see Table 9–3). If meningitis is detected, parenteral therapy is continued for 10 to 14 days. Four weeks of intravenous therapy is required to treat gonococcal endocarditis.

Prevention of Transmission

As with all STDs, patients should be instructed to refer sex partners for evaluation and treatment. Persons with a history of sexual contact with an infected patient within 30 days of onset of symptoms should be evaluated and treated for gonorrhea and nongonococcal urethritis (NGU). If the infected patient is asymptomatic, all persons having sexual contact with the patient within the past 60 days should be evaluated and treated.

Use of a latex condom has been shown to prevent the spread of gonorrhea. Sexual activity should be avoided until treatment has been completed and all symptoms have resolved.

NONGONOCOCCAL URETHRITIS

Background and Incidence

As the name implies, NGU is an inflammation of the urethra not caused by infection with *N. gonorrhoeae*. The incidence of NGU has increased nearly as fast as HSV infection. A number of agents have been found to cause NGU. *C. trachomatis* is the most frequent cause, being identified in 25% to 55% percent of cases. It is also the most important pathogen because as outlined in the next section, *Chlamydia* can cause significant morbidity among infected men and women. *U. urealyticum* is the next most commonly identified organism, being found in 20% to 40% of cases. HSV, *T. vaginalis,* and cytomegalovirus (CMV) have also been identified as less common causes. Noninfectious agents such as caffeinated beverages, alcohol, and cigarette smoking have also been proposed as causes of urethritis.

NGU occurs most commonly among teenage and young adult males. It occurs more commonly among men of higher socioeconomic status than does gonorrhea. Conversely, it is a less common cause of urethritis among homosexual men. Up to one third of patients found to have gonorrhea also have NGU, most commonly due to *C. trachomatis* coinfection.

Symptoms of NGU generally develop 1 to 5 weeks after sexual contact with an infected host. The usual symptoms include dysuria and a thin urethral discharge. Discharge and dysuria may be absent, and the patient may note only a sensation of urethral itching. Asymptomatic infection is common among both men and women.

Diagnosis

As with gonorrhea, diagnosis is based on examination of an intraurethral swab specimen. One to 4 hours after the patient last voided, a calcium alginate swab is inserted 2 to 4 cm into the urethra and gently rotated. Cultures for *N. gonorrhoeae* and *Chlamydia* are obtained and a slide is prepared. NGU may be diagnosed by the presence of 5 or more polymorphonuclear leukocytes per oil immersion field. Alternatively, identification of 15 or more polymorphonuclear leukocytes in five random high-power fields of the spun sediment of the first-voided urine or a positive urine leukocyte esterase test can be used to screen for urethritis.

Treatment

Treatment for NGU is directed at treating *Chlamydia*. Alternate treatment with erythromycin or azithromycin may also be used. The CDC recommendations for the treatment of NGU are outlined in Table 9–3.

Sex partners should be identified and treated because they may harbor asymptomatic infection and act as a source for reinfection.

Recurrent or persistent symptoms may occur despite appropriate therapy. It is likely that the patient has a nonspecific urethritis that, although symptomatic, generally does not result in complications to the patient or his or her sex partners. Urologic examination with urethroscopy and uroflowmetry may be performed to evaluate for intraurethral lesions.

Prevention of Transmission

Sexual contacts of an affected patient should be identified, evaluated, and treated. Sex partners of symptomatic patients should be presumptively treated if they had sexual contact with the patient within 30 days of the onset of symptoms. Partners having sexual activity with an asymptomatic patient within 60 days of diagnosis should also be evaluated and treated.

CHLAMYDIAL INFECTION

Background and Incidence

In the United States, chlamydial genital infection is common among adolescents and young adults. As stated earlier, *C. trachomatis* is the most common cause of NGU. *Chlamydia* is an important pathogen not only because of its role as a venereal cause of urethritis but also because it is a potential cause of significant morbidity to men, women, and neonates. Although rarely a cause of serious problems in men, *C. trachomatis* infection has been shown to cause acute epididymitis and Reiter's syndrome (urethritis, arthritis, and conjunctivitis). Women, on the other hand, are much more likely to have important sequelae. PID, infertility, ectopic pregnancy, and chronic pelvic pain all have been linked to *Chlamydia* infection. PID may result in scarring of the fallopian tubes and ovaries. This scarring is believed to be a cause of infertility, ectopic pregnancies, and pain. The risk of becoming infertile increases with each occurrence of PID and has been shown to be more likely to occur in patients with nongonococcal rather than gonococcal PID.

Neonatal infection with *C. trachomatis* results from perinatal exposure to the mother's infected cervix. The initial infection involves the mucous membranes of the eye, oropharynx, urogenital tract, and rectum. *Chlamydia* has also been shown to be a cause of infant pneumonia. Infection most commonly presents 5 to 12 days after birth as conjunctivitis. As with neonatal *N. gonorrhoeae* infection, ophthalmia neonatorum may result. Asymptomatic infections of the oropharynx, genital tract, and rectum have also been noted. Prenatal screening of pregnant women is the best way to prevent chlamydial infection among neonates. Unlike gonococcal conjunctivitis, topical ocular prophylaxis does not prevent chlamydial conjunctivitis or its complications. Systemic therapy is required.

Chlamydial infection among preadolescent children almost exclusively results from sexual abuse. Perinatally transmitted infection of the nasopharynx, urogenital tract, and rectum may occasionally persist longer than 1 year. The suspicion or diagnosis of chlamydial infection in a child mandates investigation for sexual abuse.

Diagnosis

Because of the high prevalence of asymptomatic infection with *C. trachomatis*, routine testing of sexually active adolescent girls and young women is recommended and should be part of routine gynecologic examinations. A cervical swab specimen should be obtained, cultures for *Chlamydia* and *N. gonorrhoeae* prepared, and a slide should be made. In men, a urethral swab specimen is obtained as outlined in the section on NGU. Identification of polymorphonuclear leukocytes on Gram stain is an indication of infection, but culture results confirm that infection is due to *C. trachomatis*. Serologic or immunofluorescence tests are also available but less accurately confirm the diagnosis.

Obtaining a culture for *C. trachomatis*

among children suspected of having chlamydial infection is particularly important because of the potential for a criminal investigation of sexual abuse. Nonculture chlamydia tests should not be used because of the possibility for cross-reaction of the test reagents with *Chlamydia pneumoniae* or fecal flora. Nonculture tests are helpful in infants, however, when evaluating for *Chlamydia* conjunctivitis, ophthalmia neonatorum, and pneumonia.

Treatment

Prompt treatment of patients suspected of having chlamydial infections relieves symptoms, minimizes the chance of transmission, reduces the likelihood of developing serious sequelae, and prevents transmission of infection to neonates. The CDC recommendations for treatment of chlamydial infection in adults and adolescents are summarized in Table 9–3.

Prevention of Transmission

Recommendations for treatment of sex partners of a patient infected with *C. trachomatis* are the same as those for NGU. Sex partners of symptomatic patients should be presumptively treated if they had sexual contact with the patient within 30 days of the onset of symptoms. Patients having sexual activity with an asymptomatic patient within 60 days of diagnosis should also be evaluated and treated.

TRICHOMONIASIS

Background and Incidence

Trichomonal vaginitis is an STD caused by the protozoan *T. vaginalis*. Vaginal infection is usually symptomatic, resulting in vaginal itching, dysuria, frequency, and a malodorous vaginal discharge. Infection in men is generally asymptomatic but rarely causes urethritis. Men are often carriers of *T. vaginalis* responsible for reinfection of treated women. *Trichomonas* has not been reported to cause congenital infections or malformations but has been implicated as a cause of preterm delivery and premature rupture of the membranes.

Diagnosis

On vaginal examination, vulvar and vaginal erythema are often present. Spotty reddening of the cervix, "strawberry cervix," may be noted. The vaginal discharge is generally diffuse, malodorous, and yellow-green in color. The pH of the vaginal discharge is greater than 4.5. The Whiff test is positive (a fishy odor is noted after adding 10% KOH). One or 2 drops of normal saline is added to the discharge and placed on a slide to prepare a wet mount. Motile, pear-shaped organisms with three to five flagella are diagnostic for *Trichomonas*. Culture for *T. vaginalis* can be performed and is the most sensitive method of diagnosis.

Treatment

Metronidazole 2 g orally in a single dose is the recommended treatment. Alternatively, metronidazole 500 mg twice daily for 7 days may be given. Effective treatment results in relief of symptoms and prevents further transmission. If symptoms fail to improve, repeat treatment with metronidazole 500 mg twice daily for 7 days should be given. Pregnant women should not be treated until after the first trimester of pregnancy.

Prevention of Transmission

All sex partners should be treated to eradicate asymptomatic carriers. Sexual activity should be avoided until treatment is complete and patient and partners are asymptomatic.

Genital Warts

Background and Incidence

Genital warts occur commonly among men and women. They are caused by the DNA virus HPV. Infection occurs through contact with infected tissues. It is believed that exophytic warts are more infectious than subclinically infected tissues. Once infection occurs, rapid cell division may occur, producing replication of viral particles and exophytic warts. These lesions may occur singly or in groups. Adjacent tissues are subclinically infected.

Left untreated, the warts may grow, remain unchanged, or resolve spontaneously.

Causative Agents

Most genital warts are caused by HPV Types 6 or 11. Lesions occurring in the anogenital region are more commonly due to Types 16, 18, and 31. These three types are particularly important because they have been strongly associated with the development of cervical dysplasia in women and with genital dysplasia and carcinoma in both sexes. HPV Types 16, 18, and 31 often result in subclinical infection rather than exophytic warts.

Congenital infection of a fetus can rarely occur, but the mode of transmission is unknown.

Diagnosis

Genital warts are usually asymptomatic. Patients seek treatment because of the cosmetic appearance of the lesions. Diagnosis is based on physical examination. The lesions are easily recognized as 1- to 5-mm exophytic growths. They may be present on the glans penis, penile shaft, or urethral meatus, or in the intraurethral area. Lesions on the scrotum or perigenital skin may also be found. Lesions in women may be less noticeable to the patient and clinician. They may occur on the labia or inner thighs. Identification of lesions of the vagina and cervix requires careful vaginal examination or colposcopy. Perineal and perianal lesions are also seen. Occasionally, lesions are found on the oral and rectal mucosa.

Application of dilute (5%) acetic acid to the genitals or cervix may aid in the diagnosis of small or subclinical warts. These lesions may take on a white appearance after several minutes of exposure to acetic acid. This "aceto-white" testing is used as a more sensitive way of finding subclinical infection, especially in sexual contacts of an infected patient. The usefulness of aceto-white testing is somewhat limited, however, because normal tissues may become aceto-whitened whereas other infected tissues may not. Identification of urethral meatal warts may be assisted through the use of a nasal speculum. Occasionally, urethroscopy is required. Because of the risk of developing dysplasia or carcinoma with several subtypes of HPV, any atypically pigmented or persistent warts should be biopsied. Women being evaluated for genital warts should have a Papanicolaou smear to screen for cervical dysplasia or malignancy.

Treatment

Like genital herpes, no therapy has been shown to eradicate HPV. The goal of treatment is cosmetic improvement by removal of exophytic warts. Treatment of external genital warts has not been shown to decrease the development of cervical cancer, and although it is believed that exophytic lesions are more prone to transmit virus to sex partners, treatment has not been shown to decrease transmission rates. Currently available treatments have been shown to be 22% to 94% effective in clearing external exophytic genital warts. Recurrences are common (25% within 3 months) with all modalities of treatment. Small lesions present for less than 1 year are most successfully treated. Recurrence most commonly results from reactivation of subclinical infection than by reinfection by a sex partner.

Medical and surgical therapies are available (Table 9–4). The specific regimen is chosen based on the size and number of warts, anatomic site, convenience, expense, potential for scarring, and patient preference. Topical therapies are generally used for limited external disease, whereas surgical treatments with carbon dioxide laser, electrodesiccation, or excision are useful for more extensive or internal warts.

Several treatments require particular caution. Use of a cryoprobe on mucous membranes is not recommended because of the risk of perforation and fistula formation. Podophyllin and podofilox are contraindicated during pregnancy. To limit systemic absorption and toxicity, podophyllin should be washed off after 1 to 4 hours, less than 0.5 mL should be used per treatment, and it should not be applied to more than 10 cm^2 of surface area. Podophyllin should also not be applied intraurethrally and must be completely dry prior to removing the speculum if used to treat vaginal or urethral meatal warts. 5-Fluorouracil cream has been used to treat

Table 9–4
Treatment of Genital Warts

Site	Cryotherapy*	Podofilox† 0.5%	Podophyllin‡ 10–28%	Trichloroacetic Acid§ 80–90%	Electrocautery	Laser Therapy	Others
External genitalia and perianal	X	X	X	X	X	X	
Vaginal	X		X	X		X	
Urethral meatus	X		X			X	
Urethra						X	5-FU cream
Cervical							Consult gynecologist
Anal	X			X		X	Excision
Oral	X				X		Excision

*With liquid nitrogen or cryoprobe.
†Solution applied twice daily for 3 days; repeat for 4 cycles. Use <0.5 mg per session and wash off in 1–4 hours. Contraindicated in pregnancy.
‡In tincture of benzoin.
§May repeat weekly for 7 weeks. Powder with talc or sodium bicarbonate to remove excess acid.
5-FU, 5% 5-fluorouracil cream.

intraurethral warts, but its efficacy has not been well documented and it frequently causes local irritation. Interferon therapy is not recommended because of its cost and association with a high frequency of side effects. Finally, dysplasia must be excluded before treatment of women with cervical warts is initiated.

Human Immunodeficiency Virus Infection

Background and Incidence

AIDS was first reported in 1978. It was recognized as an STD before the causative agent was identified. AIDS is now known to be caused by infection with HIV. This disease was initially most prevalent among homosexual men and intravenous drug abusers. The spread of this illness has occurred at epidemic rates and is now a significant illness among heterosexuals. The virus has been isolated from body fluids including blood, tears, saliva, cerebrospinal fluid, pre-ejaculate, semen, vaginal secretions, and breast milk. Thus, transmission can occur through exposure to body fluids or blood and tissue transfusions.

This places sexual partners, patients receiving blood transfusions or organ transplants, and health care workers at risk. Congenital infection of a fetus by an infected mother also occurs.

Urologic Manifestations of HIV Infections and AIDS

Table 9–5 summarizes the most common genitourinary manifestations of HIV infection and AIDS. Adenocarcinoma of the prostate appears to have a more rapid progression among HIV-infected patients. Because of baseline hypogonadism often resulting from HIV infection of the testes, these cancers are often less responsive to androgen ablation therapy.

The prostate is often the site of opportunistic infections. The infecting agents may be those typically associated with prostatitis such as *Escherichia coli*, *Klebsiella pneumoniae*, or *Pseudomonas aeruginosa*. More opportunistic agents such as *Mycobacterium avium-intracellulare*, *Mycobacterium tuberculosis*, *Cryptococcus neoformans*, *Histoplasma capsulatum*, or CMV are often involved. Primary HIV infection of the prostate resulting in prostatitis has also been reported. Patients present with symp-

Table 9-5
Genitourinary Tract Manifestations of HIV Infection and AIDS

1. Renal
    a. Proteinuria 38–82%
    b. Nephrotic syndrome 7%
    c. Renal insufficiency 27%
       Focal and segmental glomerulosclerosis 5–10%
    d. Abscess 3%
2. Pyuria 52%
3. Hematuria 25%: asymptomatic, idiopathic microscopic hematuria in a majority of the patients
4. Urinary tract infection 20%: *Escherichia coli* (25%), *Pseudomonas aeruginosa* (33%), nosocomial with high fatality rates
5. Bladder: areflexic/hyporeflexic neurogenic bladder with urinary retention
6. Prostatitis—typical and atypical bacteria: 3–14%
    a. *Haemophilus parainfluenzae*, cytomegalovirus
    b. *Cryptococcus neoformans* and *Histoplasma capsulatum*
    c. *E. coli*, *Staphylococcus aureus*, *S. marcescens*, *Klebsiella pneumoniae*, *Salmonella typhi*, *Mycobacterium tuberculosis*, *Mycobacterium avium-intracellulare*
7. Prostatic abscess: most common causative agents are cytomegalovirus and Enterobacteriaceae
8. Cytomegalovirus cystitis
9. Epididymo-orchitis
10. Testicular atrophy (21%); also, abnormal hypothalamic-pituitary-testicular axis (28–38%)
11. Papillary necrosis and fungal balls
12. Urethral condyloma acuminata
13. Testicular malignancies: incidence is 0.2% (vs. 0.004% in general population), lymphoma (5%), and Kaposi's sarcoma (30%)
14. Impotence: erectile and ejaculatory dysfunction—neurogenic and hormonal

toms typical of prostatitis—fever, dysuria, frequency, urgency, hesitancy, and urinary retention. Prostatic abscesses occur more commonly among HIV-infected patients. Long-term antibiotic therapy or surgical drainage of prostatic abscesses may be required to alleviate symptoms and eradicate the infection.

Urinary retention is the most common presentation of AIDS-related complications involving the urinary bladder. Urodynamic testing of AIDS patients has revealed detrusor areflexia, hyperreflexia, hyporeflexia, and bladder outlet obstruction. These findings are believed to be most commonly due to AIDS involvement of the CNS and peripheral nervous system, most often due to CNS toxoplasmosis. Cystitis due to CMV, HIV, and toxoplasmosis can occur. As in other genitourinary locations, opportunistic malignancies such as Kaposi's sarcoma have been found in the bladder. Enterovesical fistulas have been reported to occur due to non-Hodgkin's lymphoma of the bowel causing erosion into the bladder.

Epididymitis

Background and Incidence

Epididymitis is inflammation of the epididymis; acute and chronic forms exist. Chronic epididymitis differs from the acute form in that the symptoms are present for more than 6 weeks and it is often believed not to be directly related to an infectious etiology. Acute epididymitis presents as a gradual or sudden onset of unilateral scrotal pain and swelling of the epididymis, testicle, and spermatic cord. Fever, dysuria, and scrotal erythema may be present. The acute inflammation may be due to reflux of sterile urine down the vas deferens. This reflux is believed to be due to straining against a closed external urethral sphincter. Most cases of acute epididymitis, however, are believed to be due to spread of bacteria from the urethra down the vas deferens. In children and older men, the causative organisms are not sexually transmitted. Commonly, gram-negative urinary pathogens are involved. In sexually active men younger than 35 years of age, how-

ever, sexually transmitted organisms are often the cause. Sexually transmitted epididymitis is most often due to *N. gonorrhoeae* and *C. trachomatis*. In these patients, an asymptomatic urethritis due to the same organisms also is present. Men who practice unprotected insertive anal intercourse may also acquire sexually transmitted epididymitis due to *E. coli*. *Haemophilus influenzae*, tuberculosis, *Cryptococcus*, and *Brucella* have also been noted to cause acute epididymitis.

The inflammation and swelling usually begin in the tail of the epididymis. The remainder of the epididymis, the distal spermatic cord, and the testicle may also become involved. In advanced cases, orchitis, epididymal or testicular abscesses, or infertility may result. Chronic pain may rarely occur after the acute inflammation resolves.

Diagnosis

Diagnosis of acute epididymitis is based on history, physical examination, urinalysis, urine culture, urethral swab specimens, and occasionally sonographic evaluation of the scrotum. Testicular torsion must be considered and ruled out in all cases of acute hemiscrotal pain. Distinguishing epididymitis from torsion may be difficult. Generally, epididymitis presents with gradual but progressive scrotal pain and swelling. Early on, the tail, body, or head of the epididymis is palpable, swollen, and tender. The testicle may also be tender, but less so. As the inflammation progresses, the testicle may also become exquisitely tender and indurated. Testicular torsion is most common among adolescents and presents with sudden onset of scrotal pain. Both the testicle and epididymis are tender. Pyuria, bacteriuria, and a positive urine culture are found with epididymitis but not with torsion. If *N. gonorrhoeae* or *C. trachomatis* is suspected, urethral swab specimens should be obtained.

Scrotal ultrasonography may be required to differentiate torsion from inflammation. Epididymitis causes the epididymis to appear swollen, with increased echogenicity. Doppler examination often shows increased blood flow to the epididymis and testicle. Absence of blood flow within the epididymis or testicle is diagnostic of testicular torsion. If any doubt about the presence of torsion exists, the patient should be referred for urologic evaluation and possible surgical exploration.

Treatment

Treatment should be initiated as soon as possible. If sexually transmitted epididymitis is suspected, antimicrobials effective against *N. gonorrhoeae* and *C. trachomatis* should be used. Treatment of epididymitis is summarized in Table 9–3.

Improvement should be seen within 3 days. If fever or symptoms persist, parenteral therapy may be required. Sonographic evaluation for testicular abscess, torsion, or cancer should be considered.

SUGGESTED READINGS

1. Berger RE: Sexually transmitted diseases: The classic diseases. *In* Walsh PC, Retik AB, Vaughan ED Jr, Wein AJ (eds): Campbell's Urology, 7th ed. Philadelphia, WB Saunders, 1998, pp 663–684.
2. Centers for Disease Control and Prevention: 1993 Revised classification system for HIV infection and expanded surveillance case definition for AIDS among adolescents and adults. MMWR Morbid Mortal Wkly Rep 41:RR–17, 1992.
3. Centers for Disease Control and Prevention: 1993 sexually transmitted diseases: Treatment guidelines. MMWR Morbid Mortal Wkly Rep 42:RR–14, 1993.
4. Krieger JN: Acquired immunodeficiency syndrome and related conditions. *In* Walsh PC, Retik AB, Vaughan ED Jr, Wein AJ (eds): Campbell's Urology, 7th ed. Philadelphia, WB Saunders, 1998, pp 685–706.
5. Kwon DJ, Lowe FC: Genitourinary manifestations of the acquired immunodeficiency syndrome. Urology 45:13, 1995.

10

Upper Urinary Tract Infections

Melanie Fisher

Upper urinary tract infections involve the kidney and/or the surrounding tissues. Acute pyelonephritis is an infection of the kidney characterized by fever, flank pain, and/or tenderness in the flank. Significant bacteriuria (>10⁵ bacteria per mL) and pyuria (>10 white blood cells [WBCs] per high-power field [hpf] on urinalysis) are usually present. Acute pyelonephritis is a common, serious infection that can result in bacteremia and septic shock, even in otherwise healthy people. Pyelonephritis may occur as a first infection in the urinary tract or may be due to a recurrent infection. Recurrences may be either relapses due to persistence of the same organism or may be new infections due to different organisms.

Pathogenesis

Upper urinary tract infections occur mainly through two different routes, ascending or hematogenous. The ascending route is most common and begins with the urethra becoming colonized with bacteria. In women the urethra is short and contamination occurs readily. The longer urethra in men is usually protective against colonization, and another factor is usually needed to predispose to cystitis followed by pyelonephritis. Once bacteria are present in the bladder, they multiply and then ascend the ureter to infect the renal pelvis and parenchyma. The ascending route is the most common pathogenic mechanism for gram-negative rods and enterococci to infect the upper urinary tract.

In the hematogenous route, the seeding of the renal parenchyma occurs from organisms in the blood stream. This most often occurs with *Staphylococcus aureus* bacteremia and candidemia.

Epidemiology

Both microbial and host factors influence the occurrence of upper urinary tract infections.

MICROBIOLOGY

Gram-negative bacilli are the most common bacteria that cause upper urinary tract infections. As in simple uncomplicated cystitis, *Escherichia coli* is the most common species causing upper urinary tract infections in the community-acquired setting. Host factors have been identified that enhance adherence and colonization by the gram-negative rods and subsequent invasion of the urinary tract. Additional host factors such as prolonged untreated cystitis, pregnancy, and urinary tract obstruction further predispose to the establishment of upper tract urinary infection by the ascending route.

The medulla of the kidney has a greater susceptibility to infection than the cortex. Only a few organisms are needed to infect the medulla. In contrast, 10,000 times as many bacteria are needed to infect the renal cortex. Several factors have been postulated that increase the susceptibility of medulla to infection: (1) impaired chemotaxis of neutrophils into the medullary environment of high osmolality, low pH, and low blood flow; (2) a high concentration of ammonia that may interfere with complement activation.

In an initial episode of urinary tract infection, *E. coli* is the pathogen in 90% of community-acquired cases. In recurrent upper tract infections, especially those with structural abnormalities, other bacteria are seen more frequently (just as in cystitis) including *Proteus* species, *Pseudomonas aeruginosa*, *Klebsiella* species, *Enterobacter* species, enterococci, and staphylococci. Multiple organisms may cause an infection in some cases. More antimicrobial resistance is likely also in this setting. In healthy young women, upper urinary tract infections would be most commonly caused by *E. coli*. *Staphylococcus saprophyticus*, a common cause of cystitis, is less commonly a cause of upper tract infection.

Nosocomial upper urinary tract infections share a similar microbiology with nosocomial cystitis. Important bacterial species include *Enterobacter*, *E. coli*, *Proteus*, *Klebsiella*, *P. aeruginosa*, and enterococci. *Candida* infections of the upper urinary tract may occur as well and are usually associated with indwelling catheters or obstruction of the urinary tract. Coagulase-negative staphylococci such as *S. epidermidis* occur as pathogens in lower urinary tract infections involving indwelling catheters and rarely may cause upper tract infections as well.

HOST FACTORS

Certain characteristics of patients predispose to the development of upper tract urinary infections. The predisposing factors for cystitis also predispose to upper tract disease. These factors include female gender, sexual activity in women, use of a diaphragm, pregnancy, indwelling urinary catheters, nephrolithiasis, and obstruction of the urinary tract, either mechanical or functional. Mechanical obstruction to urinary flow may be extrarenal or intrarenal. Causes of extrarenal obstruction include prostatic enlargement, congenital abnormalities, ureteral obstruction from stones, malignancy, fibrosis, and scarring. Intrarenal obstruction may result from nephrocalcinosis, polycystic kidney disease, or sickle cell trait or disease.

Vesicoureteral reflux (reflux of urine from the bladder to the ureters) predisposes to upper tract infection. The reflux may be due to congenital abnormalities or bladder overdis-

tention due to infection itself, such as that occurring in small children with lower tract infection. Reflux perpetuates infection by maintaining a pool of infected urine in the bladder. Patients with incomplete emptying of the bladder due to neurologic dysfunction are also at increased risk of upper tract disease. Patient-related predisposing factors to upper tract urinary infection are summarized in Table 10–1.

Clinical Manifestations

The classic presentation of acute pyelonephritis in adults consists of fever, flank pain, lower urinary tract symptoms, and pyuria with bacteriuria. The fever may be accompanied by chills and even frank rigors, which suggest bacteremia. Notably, fever is absent if only lower urinary tract infection (cystitis) is present. With pyelonephritis, fever may be absent in elderly patients, the subclinical pyelonephritis of young, otherwise healthy women who have early kidney infection that has ascended from the bladder, and patients on antipyretics or corticosteroids.

Flank pain may be reported by the patient or may be manifested as tenderness on physical examination over the costovertebral angle. Some adults with acute pyelonephritis report urinary frequency, urgency, and/or dysuria with the symptoms and signs of pyelonephritis occurring several days later. Table 10–2 compares the common features of cystitis and pyelonephritis in adults.

The clinical manifestations of pyelonephritis may vary considerably and may delay or confuse the diagnosis. For example, the pain may occur not only in the flank but anywhere in the abdomen and may mimic many intra-

Table 10–1
Patient-Related Predisposing Factors to Upper Urinary Tract Infection (UTI)

Lower UTI, delay in treatment
Obstruction to urinary flow
Indwelling catheter or instrumentation of bladder
Nephrolithiasis
Vesicoureteral reflux
Incomplete emptying of bladder due to mechanical or neurologic dysfunction
Diabetes mellitus

Table 10-2
Comparison Between Cystitis and Pyelonephritis in Adults

Signs and Symptoms	Cystitis	Pyelonephritis
Fever	Absent	Usually present
Urgency, frequency	Present	Sometimes present
Flank pain	Absent	Sometimes present
Vomiting	Absent	Often present
Pyuria	Always present*	Always present*
Bacteriuria	Always present	Always present
Positive blood cultures	Absent	Often present

*Except in neutropenic patients.

abdominal or pelvic conditions. If the pain is severe and radiates to the groin, a kidney stone may be suspected. In women, acute pyelonephritis can mimic pelvic inflammatory disease or atopic pregnancy, as well as other intrapelvic and intra-abdominal processes. In nosocomial upper urinary tract infections, flank pain is much less common even though bacteremia may be present. Patients with indwelling urinary catheters often have no lower tract symptoms at all. Fever, however, is still common in this situation, whereas flank pain is highly variable. The symptoms and signs of urinary tract infection in children are often nonspecific, particularly in infants. Failure to thrive, vomiting, and fever are common, especially in young children. A thorough discussion of urinary tract infections in children is presented in Chapter 11.

In elderly patients, symptoms of upper urinary tract infection are highly variable. Patients may experience dysuria and frequency or may have no lower tract symptoms. Although typical fever, flank, and/or abdominal pain may occur, elderly patients often lack one or all of these symptoms, or they have nonspecific symptoms such as a decrease in mental status mimicking a central nervous system infection and/or generalized weakness.

Diagnosis

Upper urinary tract infection should be suspected first by the typical symptoms and signs (e.g., fever, dysuria, flank pain, the sepsis syndrome). Certain clinical settings increase the likelihood, such as young women who are sexually active or who have had previous bladder infections and patients with indwelling urinary catheters, stone disease, or any of the risk factors as mentioned in the previous section. A high index of suspicion is needed to diagnose these infections when the symptoms and signs are atypical. The most important laboratory tests for making the diagnosis include urinalysis and urine culture.

A routine urinalysis performed on a clean-catch midstream specimen of urine or catheterized specimen is an extremely important diagnostic tool (in infants and small children, a suprapubic tap to obtain urine may be indicated) (see Chapter 11). Normal uninfected urine should have fewer than 10 WBCs per hpf in the sediment after centrifugation. The presence of more than 10 WBCs per hpf in the sediment is abnormal and represents 100 cells/mm^3. This amount defines pyuria. More specifically, in men five or more WBCs per hpf is abnormal and in women more than 10 WBCs per hpf is considered abnormal, defines pyuria, and should be worked up further. Infection of the urinary tract is one of the most common reasons for pyuria but is nonspecific. Other reasons for pyuria in the absence of infection include interstitial nephritis (e.g., drug-induced), other infections of the urinary tract such as tuberculosis, and urethritis from *Chlamydia* or other pathogens that do not grow in routine urine culture.

Most patients with symptomatic urinary tract infections, including those of the upper urinary tract, have significant pyuria. In the absence of pyuria, the diagnosis of urinary tract infection should be in doubt except in the case of the neutropenic patient. Another exception would include patients who have a renal abscess or perinephric abscess and may or may not have pyuria.

Microscopic or gross hematuria is occasionally seen in lower urinary tract infections; this finding is less commonly seen in upper tract infections. Hematuria is a nonspecific finding and may be from other causes that need to be ruled out such as malignancy, renal calculi, glomerulonephritis, vasculitis, or trauma. WBC casts may be seen occasionally in acute pyelonephritis. The absence of WBC casts, however, does not rule out upper tract infection. WBC casts on microscopic urinalysis can also be seen in other intrinsic renal diseases.

Gram's stain of the urine is also a helpful, simple laboratory test for supporting the diagnosis of upper urinary tract infection. In this test, the urine is left uncentrifuged and then examined microscopically for the presence of bacteria after Gram's stain has been performed. The presence of one bacterium per oil immersion field in a midstream clean-catch specimen correlates with the presence of more than 10^5 bacteria per mL of urine. This large quantity of bacteria would be evidence for urinary tract infection in the presence of significant pyuria. As in the diagnosis of lower urinary tract infections, rapid indirect methods to detect bacteriuria for a presumptive diagnosis have been studied. For example, the presence of nitrites in the urine can be suggestive of urinary tract infection if pyuria is also present. With many of the rapid indirect methods, however, false-negative tests are common and occasionally false-positive results also occur. Therefore, these methods should not be relied on to diagnose upper urinary tract infections.

The urine culture is a valuable tool for confirming the diagnosis of upper urinary tract infection. Urine in the bladder, ureters, and kidneys is normally sterile. Patients with infection usually have more than 10^5 bacteria per mL of urine. Voided urine carefully collected usually contains fewer than 10^4 bacteria per mL. About one third of young women, however, with symptomatic lower urinary tract infection may have fewer than 10^5 bacteria per mL; occasionally, patients with other conditions may also have this result. In upper urinary tract infection, reasons for lower colony counts in the presence of infection may include prior use of antimicrobials, antibacterial substances from the preparation falling into the urine sample, total obstruction below

the infection, infections with fastidious organisms, and renal tuberculosis. The criterion of more than 10^5 bacteria per mL applies only to the Enterobacteriaceae such as *E. coli* and *Klebsiella*. The criteria are less clear for gram-positive organisms and for fungi that may not reach such high titers in the urine and yet cause true infections. These limitations of the culture must be kept in mind when interpreting culture results. False-positive urine cultures occur most likely from contamination when the patient gives a sample. Samples obtained from catheterization of uninfected patients are less likely to become contaminated enough to demonstrate more than 10^5 bacteria per mL. Obtaining a sample through catheterization of the bladder with the catheter removed promptly after the sample is obtained may be a useful method to obtain the best sample of the bladder urine.

When the diagnosis of acute pyelonephritis is considered in women, in general, a pelvic examination should be performed to help rule out other pathology. Cultures should be obtained from the cervix for *Chlamydia* and *Neisseria gonorrhoeae*. Other sexually transmitted diseases should be considered as well. A bimanual examination is helpful in ruling out adnexal and cervical motion tenderness and other pelvic findings. A pregnancy test should be considered in all women who could be sexually active.

Blood cultures should be obtained, two separate sets drawn peripherally if possible, in any patient who is admitted to the hospital with presumed acute pyelonephritis. The bacteremia of acute pyelonephritis is intermittent, and negative blood cultures do not rule out the diagnosis. A positive blood culture, however, would help confirm the diagnosis as well as help in the treatment plan. Bacteremic patients should be treated longer with intravenous antimicrobials.

Localizing the site of the urinary tract infection, namely distinguishing cystitis from pyelonephritis, is sometimes difficult clinically. Patients who present with recurrences or relapses of cystitis may actually have subclinical upper tract infection and may be reinfecting the lower tract. Laboratory tests such as measuring the presence of antibody-coated bacteria have been disappointing. This technique is not widely available and has proved to be unreliable. It is mainly a clinical decision determining whether the patient has upper or lower urinary tract infection. The presence of fever would indicate upper tract infection as would the presence of flank pain. Subclinical pyelonephritis should be considered if a patient with clinically mild disease suggestive of cystitis relapses after reasonable therapy for cystitis. Making the diagnosis of upper tract disease influences the type and duration of treatment and also the need for observing the patient for possible complications. A positive blood culture would also indicate upper tract infection as well. The differential diagnosis of acute pyelonephritis is listed in Table 10–3.

Complications of Upper Urinary Tract Infection

Upper urinary tract infections may result in a serious complication including septic shock and/or abscess formation. Either the suspicion or diagnosis of a focal collection of pus such as intrarenal or perinephric abscess should always prompt consultation with the urologist. In addition, whenever urinary tract obstruction is suspected or proved, urologic consultation would also be warranted. The urologist would help identify patients who require surgical drainage or other procedures.

INTRARENAL ABSCESSES

Intrarenal abscesses may occur secondary to acute pyelonephritis. Gram-negative bacilli would be the most common etiologic organisms in this case. The intrarenal abscess can result from a coalescence of microabscesses that are frequently present in pyelonephritis. Intrarenal abscesses may also be a result of

Table 10-3
Differential Diagnosis of Acute Pyelonephritis

Appendicitis
Intra-abdominal abscess
Pelvic inflammatory disease
Diverticulitis
Acute cholecystitis
Other intra-abdominal processes

bacteremia particularly from *S. aureus*. *Candida* abscesses in the kidney may result from candidemia (see later section on renal candidiasis). In either case, if the abscesses are quite small, the patient may respond to prolonged antimicrobial therapy alone. If an abscess is large, percutaneous drainage in addition to antimicrobial therapy may be required. Surgical drainage may be necessary if percutaneous tube drainage is ineffective.

Perinephric abscess is an uncommon but serious complication of upper urinary tract infection. The most common predisposing factors for perinephric abscess are obstruction of the infected kidney or calyx (e.g., from nephrolithiasis) and diabetes mellitus. Gram-negative bacilli such as *E. coli* and *Klebsiella* are the most commonly cultured organisms if acquired as a result of ascending infection. Perinephric abscess may also occur secondary to bacteremia. In this case, *S. aureus* would be a likely pathogen.

The perinephric abscesses are confined by Gerota's fascia and may extend through the retroperitoneum to affect adjacent structures. The clinical presentation can be confusing. The patients may present with signs and symptoms suggestive of acute pyelonephritis and a few may have signs of lower urinary tract infection. Patients, however, may present nonspecifically with fever, weight loss, sometimes abdominal or flank pain, or the syndrome of fever of unknown origin.

The diagnosis should be considered in any patient with fever and abdominal or flank pain, particularly if they do not respond to treatment for presumed acute pyelonephritis and have pyuria. A palpable mass may or may not be present in the flank or abdomen.

Half of these patients have an abnormal plain film of the abdomen showing loss of ipsilateral psoas outline, swollen ipsilateral kidney, and shift in abdominal gas pattern. Thirty percent have a normal urinalysis and up to 40% have sterile urine cultures. An ultrasonographic examination of the kidney may show a perinephric abscess if it is at least 2 to 3 cm in diameter, as well as rule out intrarenal obstruction. A computed tomographic (CT) scan with contrast agent is the most helpful radiologic test and usually shows the perinephric abscess (Fig. 10–1). An intravenous pyelogram (IVP) helps delineate

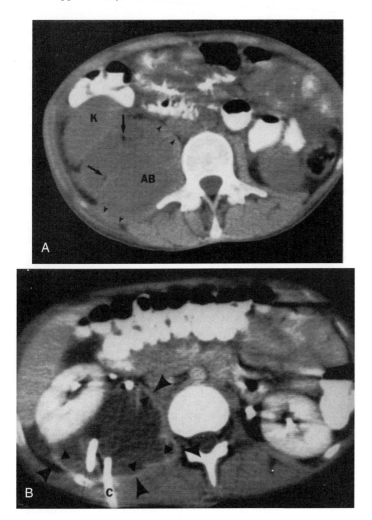

Figure 10-1
Perinephric abscess: a CT scan of the "rind sign." *A,* A large, septated perinephric abscess (AB) displaces the right kidney (K) anterolaterally and has a faint rind *(arrowheads)* of slightly increased attenuation. A few gas collections are seen *(arrows). B,* After administration of intravenous contrast material, there is enhancement of the wall ("rind sign") *(arrowheads).* A drainage catheter (C) has been placed percutaneously. (From Pollack HM [ed]: Clinical Urography: An Atlas and Textbook of Urological Imaging. Philadelphia, WB Saunders, 1990, p 876.)

the collecting system but is less useful for diagnosing perinephric abscess than the CT scan. The most common findings on CT scan include thickening of Gerota's fascia, enlargement of the kidney, and fluid and/or gas in or around the kidney.

To confirm the diagnosis of perinephric abscess, a diagnostic needle aspiration should be done with ultrasound or CT guidance. If it is confirmed, then percutaneous drainage with catheter placement can be tried along with appropriate antimicrobial therapy directed at the pathogen. A Gram's stain of the fluid obtained should be performed and cultures taken. The urologist should be involved in the evaluation of suspected or proven perinephric abscess from the start. Surgical intervention may be required if percutaneous drainage fails or if it is contraindicated. Also, percutaneous drainage has been

used for larger intrarenal abscesses and infected renal cysts. Tube drainage would need to be continued until the CT scan shows no further collection present. Antimicrobial therapy would need to be given initially intravenously (usually for several weeks) followed by an appropriate oral antimicrobial agent. Therapy would need to be continued until the CT scan shows no further collection. A high index of suspicion is essential for diagnosing perinephric abscess.

Management of Upper Urinary Tract Infection

Antimicrobial therapy should be given when there is reasonable evidence of infection in the urinary tract. Symptoms alone are not a reliable indication of infection. Properly collected urine specimens for urine culture (when there is pyuria), and other tests such as blood cultures when indicated should be obtained before starting antimicrobial therapy. Because acute pyelonephritis is a serious illness that can result in bacteremia and sepsis, once the cultures and studies are obtained and the diagnosis is suspected, therapy should be started promptly.

Most patients with acute pyelonephritis should be hospitalized and treated with intravenous therapy. This is particularly important in those patients who appear toxic or unable to keep liquids and medications down, those who are immunocompromised, and in children, pregnant women, and the elderly. Most oral antibiotics cannot achieve adequate serum levels that are above the minimum inhibitory concentration of most of the urinary pathogens, although renal levels may be higher. Although oral therapy is usually adequate for lower tract disease, in pyelonephritis intravenous therapy is the safest approach because of the possibility of bacteremia and sepsis. Also adequate blood levels of antibiotics may be important to cure patients who have renal parenchymal infection and who relapse.

If renal insufficiency is present, the dosages of some antimicrobials need to be modified. The major drugs in this category would include the aminoglycosides, ciprofloxacin, and trimethoprim-sulfamethoxazole (see Table 10–4 for modification of antimicrobial doses with renal insufficiency). The beta-lactam drugs, which include the penicillins and cephalosporins, are excellent choices even in renal insufficiency, but doses need to be altered with severe renal impairment.

Once the patient is begun on antimicrobial therapy for acute pyelonephritis, he or she must be observed carefully for symptoms and clinical signs of response. The patient may have a clinical cure, persistence of the infection, or relapse. Patients who do not improve clinically over the first 72 hours of therapy, including no decrease in fever after 72 hours, should be suspected of having complications such as abscess formation or a different diagnosis.

Microbiologic response to treatment means the bacteriuria has cleared, that is, follow-up Gram's stain and culture of the urine are negative. If the organism persists in the urine, a collection of pus or incorrect therapy should be suspected. Microbiologic relapse of acute pyelonephritis would be evident in a patient who has signs and symptoms again of lower tract or upper tract disease with the same organism 1 to 2 weeks after finishing appropriate antimicrobial therapy. This situation is usually associated with renal infection with structural abnormalities of the urinary tract or with chronic bacterial prostatitis. Further work-up and urologic evaluation would be indicated in these patients.

Choice of empiric antimicrobial therapy for acute pyelonephritis is crucial and should be

Table 10–4
Commonly Used IV Antimicrobials in Upper Urinary Tract Infection

		Doses in Adults		
		Creatinine Clearance (ml/min)		
Drug	Normal Renal Function	50–80	10–50	<10
Ampicillin	2 g q 4–6 h	Usual	1–2 g IV q 8 h	1–2 g IV q 12 h
Gentamicin, tobramycin*	1.7 mg/kg q 8 h (maintenance dose)‡	Use special nomograms to estimate doses of aminoglycosides with renal insufficiency		
Amikacin†	7.5 mg/kg q 8 h	Use special nomograms to estimate doses of aminoglycosides with renal insufficiency		
Piperacillin	3 g q 4 h	Usual	3 g q 8 h	3 g q 12 h
Ceftriaxone	1 g q 12–24 h	Usual	Usual	Usual
Ceftazidime	2 g q 8 h	Usual	1–2 g IV q 12–24 h	1 g q 24–48 h
Ciprofloxacin	400 mg q 12 h	Usual	400 mg q 18–24 h	400 mg q 24 h
Trimethoprim-sulfamethoxazole	3–5 mg/kg q 6–12 h	Usual	3–5 mg/kg q 12–24 h	Avoid

*First give loading dose of 2 mg/kg.
†First give loading dose of 7.5 mg/kg.
‡Check peak and trough levels around third dose.

based on clinical setting and Gram's stain of the urine, if available. An excellent choice for many cases of community-acquired pyelonephritis would be gentamicin plus ampicillin in patients who do not have a history of allergy to beta-lactam drugs such as ampicillin. Aminoglycosides such as gentamicin provide excellent coverage for most of the gram-negative rods. Ampicillin plus gentamicin gives good coverage for most of the enterococci. If the Gram's stain of the urine shows gram-negative rods only, then aminoglycosides alone can be considered. If the Gram's stain of the urine shows gram-positive cocci in chains, then enterococci should be suspected and the combination of ampicillin and gentamicin would be more appropriate. If *Staphylococcus* species are suspected (e.g., Gram's stain showing clusters of gram-positive cocci), then intravenous vancomycin may be indicated until cultures and sensitivities are available. In the hospital setting, more resistant gram-negative rods and even antimicrobial resistant enterococci may be possible. Antimicrobial therapy may need to be directed at more resistant pathogens (see section on nosocomial upper tract infections).

If gram-negative rods are growing from the culture, then gentamicin should be continued until sensitivities are available. If it is necessary to avoid gentamicin because of significant renal insufficiency, then use of a third-generation cephalosporin such as ceftriaxone or cefotaxime can be considered. A quinolone such as ciprofloxacin (intravenously at first) is another possibility. Norfloxacin should be avoided for pyelonephritis because adequate serum levels are not achieved. Once the culture results and sensitivities are known, it is often possible and prudent to switch therapy to a less toxic, narrower-spectrum agent. A drug should be picked that is the most effective by the sensitivities, the least toxic, and the most cost effective. In general it is best to keep patients on intravenous therapy until they have been completely afebrile for 72 hours before switching to an oral agent.

If there is no response in the fever and/or toxicity, then further work-up should be done. Ultrasonographic examination of the kidneys helps demonstrate obstruction and/or an abscess. The sonogram may be falsely negative, and if the patient still remains fe-

brile or not improving otherwise, then a CT scan with contrast agent is the more sensitive test and should be ordered. Finding urinary obstruction by any study should prompt urologic consultation immediately.

Most patients with uncomplicated acute pyelonephritis should be treated for 14 days' total therapy. In a patient who responds promptly the course may consist of 3 or 4 days of intravenous therapy followed by an appropriate oral agent for the rest of the course. In a patient who has had bacteremia or other complications, a longer course of intravenous antimicrobials may be necessary. For example, a patient with an abscess that complicates the pyelonephritis would need prolonged antibiotics in addition to percutaneous or surgical drainage. If patients relapse with their infection after 2 weeks of stopping therapy and no abscess or obstruction is found, then a longer course of therapy (4 to 6 weeks) should be considered. Compliance of the patient should be questioned as well. Again, urologic consultation would be important. The management of acute pyelonephritis is summarized in Figure 10–2.

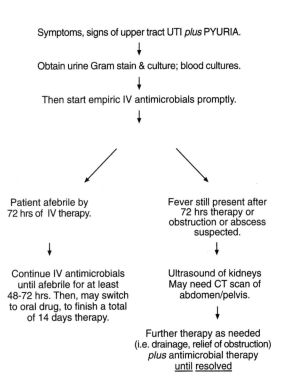

Figure 10–2
Management of suspected or proven pyelonephritis in adults.

Special Management Problems in Upper Urinary Tract Infections

RENAL CANDIDIASIS

Candida species are yeasts that are normal commensals from the female vagina and the skin (Fig. 10–3). *Candida* are capable of causing cystitis most often as a complication of indwelling urinary catheters, diabetes melli-tus, and/or patients receiving antibacterial drugs. Infection of either the upper or lower urinary tract with *Candida* generally manifests with pyuria plus a positive culture for *Candida* species, most often *Candida albicans*. Other species such as *Candida tropicalis* and *Candida glabrata* may cause infections as well. *Candida* renal infection is usually classified into two forms: primary which is presumably from the ascending route, and secondary, which occurs from hematogenous spread of

Figure 10-3

A, Candida albicans (yeast and my-celial forms) in urine sediment. (×400.) *B, Candida albicans* (yeast form) in urine sediment and en-gulfed by a polymorphonuclear leukocyte. The yeasts are the translucent oval bodies in the middle and right upper part of the cell. (*A* and *B* from Walsh PW, Gittes RF, Perlmutter AD, Stamey TA [eds]: Campbell's Urology, 5th ed. Philadelphia, WB Saunders, 1986, p 1031.)

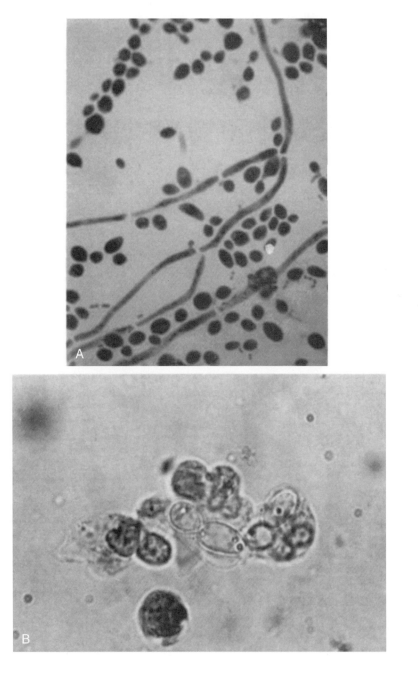

Candida, usually from a disseminated infection. Papillary necrosis, fungus balls, invasion of the renal calyces, and perinephric abscesses can result from ascending infection. These complications are most likely to occur in the presence of urinary tract obstruction, urinary diversion procedures, renal stones, or diabetes mellitus.

The hematogenous or secondary form of renal candidiasis is much more common. The kidneys are the most frequently involved organs in disseminated candidiasis. This condition occurs most often in patients with indwelling intravenous lines, those receiving chemotherapy, and postsurgical patients on intravenous antibacterial drugs. The pathologic changes in the kidney show multiple microabscesses, especially in the cortical areas.

The diagnosis of renal candidiasis is suggested by fever in a susceptible patient, pyuria, and a positive urine culture for *Candida.* The urine culture may occasionally be negative, especially if there is only a focal abscess present in the kidney that does not communicate with the collecting system. Patients often have leukocytosis as well. The most helpful imaging study is the CT scan with contrast agent that may demonstrate fungus balls. The presence of any but the tiniest abscesses and/or obstruction of the urinary tract from candidiasis should prompt urologic consultation. Fungus balls may need surgical drainage and removal. Abscesses generally require either percutaneous or surgical drainage.

The medical therapy of renal candidiasis includes an appropriate antifungal drug usually for several weeks and until abscesses are completely resolved by CT scan. Amphotericin B is the standard therapy. A test dose of amphotericin B must be given first of 1 mg in 50 mL of dextrose 5% in water over 2 hours while the patient is monitored closely. If the test dose is tolerated, then a daily dose of amphotericin 0.5 mg/kg/day is given, each dose given over 4 hours. Patients should be pretreated 30 minutes before the infusion with acetaminophen and diphenhydramine if this is feasible. Just prior to infusion and immediately afterward, if possible, patients should be given an intravenous saline infusion to help prevent the nephrotoxicity of amphotericin B. Side effects of the amphotericin B include anaphylaxis and hypotension, particularly during the test dose, nephrotoxicity, hypokalemia, hypomagnesemia, and renal tubular acidosis. Anemia may occur usually after several weeks of therapy. The total dose of amphotericin B for renal candidiasis is usually 1000 to 1500 mg, but the clinical situation must be monitored and patients treated until the infection has resolved. Newer formulations of amphotericin include liposomal amphotericin and lipid complex preparations, which appear to be associated with less nephrotoxicity.

The oral drug 5-flucytosine (5-FC) can be given along with the amphotericin B and may allow a lower dose of amphotericin B to be given. The dose of 5-FC is 50 to 150 mg/kg/day orally. Because of its frequent side effects of nausea, vomiting, diarrhea, skin rash, and even neutropenia, the drug is difficult for patients to take. In addition, the dose must be reduced significantly in the presence of renal failure. 5-FC should never be given alone for *Candida* infections because many *Candida* are de novo resistant to the drug, and *Candida* species may become resistant to the drug if used by itself.

Fluconazole is both an oral and intravenous antifungal agent that has excellent renal and urine levels when given by either route. It is a good alternative for renal candidiasis when the blood stream has not been involved and there is no evidence of disseminated candidiasis elsewhere. Most species of *Candida* are susceptible; however, *Candida krusei, C. tropicalis,* and some other species may be resistant. In seriously ill patients, the safest approach is beginning treatment with amphotericin B. The isolated *Candida* may then be checked for antifungal susceptibilities. If the isolate is susceptible to fluconazole, then this drug may be considered. Fluconazole is usually well tolerated. The dose in normal renal function is 200 mg orally once a day. The total duration of therapy would generally be several weeks. The patient would need to be treated until the infection clears clinically and abscesses have resolved by CT scan. Side effects of fluconazole include elevation of the liver transaminases, rash, nausea, vomiting, and diarrhea.

ELDERLY PATIENTS

Upper urinary tract infections in the elderly occur most often in the setting of indwelling urinary catheters, obstruction, and diabetes mellitus and in patients who have functional bladder obstructions such as urinary retention from autonomic neuropathy. The clinical presentation may be similar to that in younger adults but often is nonspecific. Patients may present with weakness, low-grade fever or even normal temperature, and sometimes decreased mental status. The risk of bacteremia and associated complications is great in the elderly.

Certain aspects of treatment need to be emphasized in the elderly. Risk factors such as obstruction and urinary retention need to be sought and corrected with the aid of the urologist. Antimicrobial therapy should be given for at least 14 days total in uncomplicated upper tract disease and longer if indicated.

The age-related decline in renal function should always be considered in dosing of antimicrobials, especially the aminoglycosides. The creatinine clearance of an elderly patient should always be estimated before dosing aminoglycosides.

In a patient whose renal function is worsening or improving, aminoglycosides need to be given cautiously, and peak and trough levels should be checked around the third dose. In the elderly patient, if the culture and sensitivities are available and a less toxic drug is effective to treat the patient's infection, then the aminoglycosides should be avoided. The doses for normal and impaired renal function are available in Table 10–3. If an aminoglycoside must be used in an elderly patient, it is best to give the drug no more often than every 12 to 24 hours.

The ability to empty the bladder completely may be impaired in elderly patients from a variety of causes including prostatic enlargement in men, bladder prolapse in women, and neurogenic bladder in either sex from diabetes mellitus or other conditions. Elderly patients who develop an upper urinary tract infection should be assessed for their ability to empty the bladder completely. A postvoid residual urine should be obtained by asking a patient who can cooperate to fully empty his or her bladder first. Then a catheter should be placed in the bladder using proper technique and the urinary volume that is left measured. If it is greater than 50 mL, incomplete emptying of the bladder is suspected and may be the cause of the urinary tract infection. Patients with this kind of impairment may need to be placed on intermittent bladder catheterization (e.g., every 6 hours with a straight catheterization) and have further work-up by a urologist.

PREGNANCY

Pyelonephritis in pregnancy carries an increased risk of bacteremia and sepsis in the mother as well as premature delivery of the fetus. Bacteriuria in the pregnant woman, whether asymptomatic and whether or not pyuria is present, must be managed properly with treatment with an antimicrobial to prevent the serious complication of pyelonephritis.

A pregnant woman who presents with signs and symptoms of pyelonephritis or even with an atypical syndrome such as fever, abdominal pain, and pyuria should be hospitalized because of the high morbidity and increased mortality. Blood and urine cultures should be obtained as well as urine Gram's stain. Both ampicillin and aminoglycosides such as gentamicin have been used extensively in pregnancy and are a commonly used initial regimen. Because of the potential toxicity to the kidneys and the auditory and vestibular toxicity, the aminoglycoside should be switched to a less toxic drug, if possible, once the culture results and sensitivities are known. In general the beta-lactam drugs such as the penicillins and cephalosporins are considered safe in pregnancy. Tetracyclines and fluoroquinolones should always be avoided in pregnancy. Trimethoprim-sulfamethoxazole should be avoided as well, particularly in the third trimester when it can be associated with kernicterus in the newborn.

The total duration of therapy for pyelonephritis in pregnancy is usually 14 days. Patients should then be followed closely after antimicrobials are stopped with clinical examination, urinalysis, and urine culture. A prophylactic oral antimicrobial (such as amoxicillin) should be given during the rest of pregnancy to help prevent recurrent bacteriuria.

If gentamicin or the other aminoglycosides are used in pregnant women, peak and trough levels should be obtained. The trough levels should be no higher than 1.5 to 2 mg/mL.

DIABETES MELLITUS

Involvement of the upper urinary tract is common in diabetic patients who develop cystitis. In addition, some of the pyogenic complications such as renal and perinephric abscesses are more common in diabetics as well. Diabetics frequently have incomplete emptying of the bladder due to autonomic neuropathy and must be assessed for this risk factor to help prevent future episodes of cystitis and pyelonephritis. These patients also need follow-up urinalysis and urine cultures after an adequate course of therapy is completed.

A serious form of upper tract involvement in diabetics is emphysematous pyelonephritis. This is most often seen in elderly women diabetics who have chronic urinary tract infections and renal vascular disease. The patients present very ill, often appear septic, and have abdominal and/or back pain. A flat and upright radiograph of the abdomen often reveals gas present in the kidney. Emphysematous pyelonephritis carries a high mortality in spite of appropriate antimicrobial therapy. Immediate urologic consultation is indicated and nephrectomy is usually necessary. Emphysematous pyelonephritis should be distinguished from a benign condition of emphysematous pyelitis, which is characterized by air in the collecting system only.

Another complication of pyelonephritis in diabetics is papillary necrosis. In this condition some of the calyces of the kidney are sloughed into the collecting system and obstruction can occur. Papillary necrosis may also occur in nondiabetic patients. This complication should be suspected in a patient with pyelonephritis who develops continued fever and an increase in flank pain and where renal ultrasonography may show obstruction. The management consists of appropriate antimicrobial therapy, relief of obstruction present under the consultation of the urologist, and adequate intravenous fluids.

NOSOCOMIAL UPPER URINARY TRACT INFECTIONS

Urinary tract infections are the most frequent nosocomial infections and a source of considerable morbidity and mortality. These infections are a frequent cause of bacteremia in the hospital also. The major risk factor for nosocomial urinary tract infection is exposure to an indwelling urinary catheter. Bacteriuria alone without either pyuria or symptoms in the hospitalized patient generally should not be treated, similar to the case of asymptomatic bacteruria in other settings.

Patients with true upper urinary tract infection that is nosocomially acquired often have fever. The illness may range from very mild to severe, even to septic shock. Flank pain and abdominal pain appear to be less frequent than in community-acquired pyelonephritis. A high index of suspicion for nosocomial pyelonephritis is necessary because many hospitalized patients are unable to manifest a febrile response or complain of symptoms.

To make the diagnosis, a urinalysis should be obtained as well as urine Gram's stain. If there is pyuria present, then a culture should be sent. When upper tract involvement is suspected (i.e., presence of fever and/or an ill patient), empiric intravenous antimicrobial therapy should be started after urine and blood cultures are obtained.

The choice of antimicrobial should be based, if possible, on the Gram's stain of the urine as well as the sensitivity patterns of bacteria in that particular hospital or long-term care setting. If the patient has been colonized with more resistant gram-negative rods, for example, this must be kept in mind in selecting empiric therapy. If the Gram's stain of the urine shows gram-negative rods, aminoglycosides such as gentamicin would be a reasonable first choice in addition to ampicillin if *Enterococcus* is a consideration. If *P. aeruginosa* is a strong consideration and/or if the patient is extremely ill, then piperacillin plus gentamicin would be appropriate, pending sensitivities. In patients who are allergic to beta-lactam drugs, gentamicin alone would be a consideration for gram-negative rods, pending cultures. In patients with renal insufficiency, other agents such as the third-generation cephalosporins or quinolones may be considered for initial therapy. Neither quinolones nor cephalosporins are effective against enterococci. When culture results are known, narrower-spectrum antibiotics would be appropriate.

The isolation of vancomycin-resistant enterococci presents a difficult problem. Patients should be placed in contact isolation. If they have no pyuria and are asymptomatic, then colonization alone is present. These patients may be observed only without antimicrobial therapy. If they are symptomatic, however, then therapy is difficult and investigational agents such as quinupristin and dalfopristin (Synercid) may be considered, but the results are variable.

The total duration of therapy for nosocomial urinary tract infections generally is 10 to 14 days in uncomplicated infections. As in community-acquired infections, once the patient is stable and has been afebrile for 72 hours, therapy may be switched to oral if the patient can tolerate oral drugs and the organism is susceptible. Whenever possible, indwelling urinary catheters should be removed to help prevent recurrent infections.

PATIENTS WITH NEPHROSTOMIES

Patients with nephrostomy tubes are at high risk for symptomatic pyelonephritis. The diagnosis is often confusing because many of the patients have some WBCs as well as bacteria present in the nephrostomy urine due to the indwelling tube. If the patients are completely asymptomatic without fever, particularly if the cultures show mixed organisms, then it may be reasonable simply to observe the patient. If the patient has fever or other signs or symptoms of systemic infection, such as an elevated total WBC count, then they should be treated for acute pyelonephritis according to regimens discussed previously.

RENAL TRANSPLANTATION PATIENTS

Patients who have received renal transplants have an increased risk of bacteriuria and urinary tract infections both of the lower and upper tracts. These patients need a prophylactic antimicrobial for the first 3 months after the transplant. Trimethoprim-sulfamethoxazole is the drug frequently used for this purpose. In general, lower tract infections in renal transplant patients should be treated even if they are asymptomatic to help prevent the serious complication of pyelonephritis. If they do develop pyelonephritis, it should be treated aggressively and the diagnosis confirmed with urinalysis, urine culture, and blood cultures. Follow-up urine cultures after therapy is finished are important as well. The aminoglycosides should be avoided, if possible, to help prevent renal toxicity. In a patient in whom *P. aeruginosa* is not a strong consideration, a third-generation cephalosporin such as ceftriaxone may be a useful intravenous drug to begin empirically until sensitivities are known and if the urine Gram's stain shows gram-negative rods. If an aminoglycoside is needed for synergy for the *Enterococcus* or because of *Pseudomonas*, then the dose should be calculated carefully according to the renal function and conservative dosing should be used (e.g., peak level < 4 to 5 μg/mL and trough levels < 1.5 μg/mL). The dosing interval needs to be appropriately lengthened, such as every 24 hours.

ILLUSTRATIVE CASES

Case Study No. 1

A 25-year-old woman complained of mild dysuria for 5 days. She then presented with fever, chills, right flank pain, and vomiting. She had been previously well with no history of urinary tract infections, renal calculi, or diabetes. She was sexually active.

On physical examination, her temperature was 39.5° C. Heart rate was 120 beats per minute and her other vital signs were normal. She appeared flushed and toxic. Her examination was notable for right costovertebral angle tenderness. Her abdominal and pelvic examinations were normal. Urinalysis revealed 20 to 50 WBCs and no red blood cells and was nitrite positive. Gram's stain of the urine showed gram-negative rods. Blood cultures and urine culture were obtained. The patient was hospitalized and begun promptly on intravenous gentamicin and ampicillin. On the second day she felt somewhat better. Her temperature remained elevated for 24 hours, then began to gradually decrease, and by day 3 of therapy she was afebrile. Her urine culture grew *E. coli*, colony count >100,000 bacteria per mL, while her blood cultures were negative. The isolate was sensitive to trimethoprim-sulfamethoxazole, aminoglycosides, and cefazolin and was resistant to ampicillin. The intravenous antimicrobials were continued until she was completely afebrile for 72 hours and sensitivities of the *E. coli* were known. The therapy was then switched to oral trimethoprim-sulfamethoxazole and she completed a total of 14 days therapy.

Comment

Case No. 1 demonstrates a typical case of acute uncomplicated pyelonephritis in an otherwise healthy young woman. She first developed cystitis, which then ascended into the kidneys. Appropriately, she was hospitalized and treated with intravenous antibiotics after cultures were obtained. She responded well to the intravenous therapy, which was then changed to a less toxic drug, trimethoprim-sulfamethoxazole, when culture and sensitivities were known. Outpatient follow-up after discharge would be important. If she develops further episodes of urinary tract infections, urologic evaluation would be indicated.

Case Study No. 2

A 35-year-old woman with Type I diabetes mellitus on insulin presented with a 2-week history of low-grade fevers, malaise, and vague abdominal pain. She also had a history of recurrent urinary tract infections treated as an outpatient.

On physical examination her temperature was 38.3° C. She appeared weak and moderately ill. Her examination was noted both for mild back pain in the left lower back and mild abdominal tenderness, particularly in the left upper quadrant. There was no rebound tenderness. Pelvic and rectal examinations were normal. Urinalysis revealed 10 to 20 WBCs per hpf; Gram's stain showed no bacteria. Blood and urine cultures were obtained. The patient's renal function was normal. Intravenous gentamicin and ampicillin were begun. A sonogram of the kidneys demonstrated 3+ hydronephrosis on the left and a possible fluid collection. CT scan of the abdomen and pelvis demonstrated fluid collection in and around the left kidney. Percutaneous drainage of the collection yielded puru-

lent material. Gram's stain showed many WBCs and gram-negative rods. The culture of the pus grew *Klebsiella pneumoniae* sensitive to cefazolin, gentamicin, and trimethoprim-sulfamethoxazole and resistant to ampicillin. The patient was allergic to sulfa drugs. The therapy was switched to cefazolin intravenously. Blood cultures were sterile. The catheter was left in place in the perinephric space and drained pus over the next 7 days. Repeat CT scan demonstrated no further collection. After 14 days of intravenous antimicrobial, therapy was then switched to cephalexin to complete a total of 6 weeks of treatment. Follow-up urine culture and urinalysis were normal. The CT scan at the end of therapy showed resolution of the perinephric abscess.

Comment

Case No. 2 demonstrates a patient with a perinephric abscess who had typical risk factors, namely prior urinary tract infections, diabetes mellitus, and obstruction of the urinary tract. The presentation was nonspecific, which is common for this condition. The high index of suspicion in a patient with these findings as well as pyuria prompted radiologic evaluation, including the CT scan, which demonstrated the perinephric abscess. Prompt antimicrobial therapy as well as urologic evaluation and drainage of the abscess were necessary to treat this patient's serious infection.

SUGGESTED READINGS

1. Andriole VT, Patterson TF: Epidemiology, natural history, and management of urinary tract infections in pregnancy. Med Clin North Am 75:359–373, 1991.
2. Edelstein H, McCabe RE: Perinephric abscess: Modern diagnosis and treatment in 47 cases. Medicine 67:118–131, 1988.
3. Evanoff G, Thompson CS, Foley R, Weinman EJ: The spectrum of gas within the kidney: Emphysematous pyelonephritis and emphysematous pyelitis. Am J Med 83:149–154, 1987.
4. Measley RE, Levison ME: Host defense mechanisms in the pathogenesis of urinary tract infection. Med Clin North Am 75:275–285, 1991.
5. Sobel JD, Kaye D: Urinary tract infections. *In* Mandell GL, Douglas RG, Bennett JE (eds): Mandell, Douglas, and Bennett's Principles and Practice of Infectious Diseases, 4th ed. New York, Churchill Livingstone, 1995, pp 662–690.
6. Stamm WE, Hooton TM: Management of urinary tract infections in adults. N Engl J Med 329:1328–1334, 1993.
7. Wood CA, Abrutyn E: Optimal treatment of urinary tract infections in elderly patients. Drugs Aging 9:352–362, 1996.

11 Urinary Tract Infections in Children

Melanie Fisher
William F. Tarry

Epidemiology

Urinary tract infections (UTIs) may affect children of all ages. The frequency of UTI in infants is about 1% to 2%. It is much more common in boys during the first 3 months of life but occurs later more often in girls. When UTIs occur in newborn boys, bacteremia is common.

Preschool girls are more likely to have UTIs than boys. When preschool boys do develop UTIs, they are usually associated with congenital abnormalities. Significant bacteriuria occurs in 4% to 5% of girls and in about 0.5% of boys in this age group. Infections during this period are often symptomatic. Several studies have indicated that much of the renal damage that occurs from UTIs takes place at this time. The presence of bacteriuria in childhood is a strong risk factor for the development of bacteriuria in adulthood.

Pathogenesis and Etiology

Most UTIs in children are acquired through the ascending route with bacteria originating in the periurethral area. In neonates, however, bacteria may enter the urinary tract via the hematogenous route as well. Several recent studies have shown that uncircumcised infant boys have a higher rate of UTI than circumcised infant boys possibly because of bacterial colonization of the prepuce followed by ascending infection.

After the neonatal period, the most important factor in the pathogenesis of UTIs is bacterial colonization in the periurethral area. *Escherichia coli* accounts for up to 90% of bacterial isolates in UTI in children, as in adults. Other species include *Klebsiella/Enterobacter*, *Proteus*, and *Staphylococcus saprophyticus*. Nosocomial pathogens tend to be more antimicrobial resistant and often include *Enterococcus* species and *Pseudomonas aeruginosa*. Pathogenic mechanisms include virulence and adhesion of certain bacteria such as *E. coli* to uroepithelium. In addition, host factors such as the presence of P and other blood group antigens on the uroepithelial cell surface may increase the likelihood of UTIs.

Vesicoureteric reflux is a common abnormality associated with UTI in children. With reflux, bacteria may easily ascend from the bladder to the kidney. The reflux may also lead to residual urine in the bladder, which also predisposes to UTI.

After their first symptomatic UTI, about 5% of girls and 13% of boys develop a renal scar. The scarring of pyelonephritis in children is believed to be due to an inflammatory response involving polymorphonuclear leukocytes and their toxic metabolites. The main determinants of renal damage are the presence of obstruction, the presence of reflux, the development of pyelonephritis in the first year of life, delayed antimicrobial therapy, bacterial virulence factors, and individual susceptibility of the host.

Predisposing Factors

Risk factors for UTI in children include neurogenic bladder and any anatomic abnormalities of the urinary tract that can interfere with host defense mechanisms. Any condition that impedes the unidirectional flow of urine through the urinary tract predisposes to UTI. Obstruction of the urinary tract may be anatomic or functional. Anatomic obstruction may occur because of posterior urethral valves, urethral strictures, ureteroceles, ureterovesical junction obstruction, stones, tumors, cysts, and other conditions (see Chapter 21). Vesicoureteric reflux, alone or in combination with dysfunctional voiding (enuresis, bladder instability), is a common predisposing factor. In addition, other medical conditions including diabetes mellitus, renal calculi, nephrocalcinosis, and immunodeficiencies increase the susceptibility of children to UTI.

Clinical Manifestations

The presenting symptoms of UTI depend on the age of the child. For example, the younger the child, the less likely are the symptoms to be localized to the urinary tract. In the neonatal period the signs are nonspecific and highly variable. A newborn may present severely ill with signs of sepsis including lethargy, irritability, apnea, metabolic acidosis, and/or temperature instability. A newborn may also present with vomiting, poor feeding, or paralytic ileus. A poor urinary stream may indicate urethral obstruction.

Up to the age of 2 years, the symptoms of UTI are usually nonspecific. In infancy fever is the most common presenting symptom of pyelonephritis. The physician should have a high index of suspicion for UTI when an infant is sick and no cause is readily apparent.

After children reach the age of 2 years, the symptoms of UTI are usually more specific and similar to those in adults. The symptoms of pyelonephritis may include fever, chills, flank or abdominal pain, and signs of toxicity. Lower tract symptoms may include suprapubic pain, dysuria, frequency, urinary urgency, and secondary enuresis in a child who was previously toilet trained.

Laboratory Diagnosis

As in adults, the diagnosis of UTI should be supported by a urinalysis and confirmed by a urine culture. The urinalysis should show pyuria defined as five or more white blood cells (WBCs) per high-power field of urine sediment. Pyuria is suggestive of UTI but may be secondary to other conditions as well. Pyuria is almost always present, however, with a UTI. Occasionally a second or third urinalysis is needed to show pyuria. A Gram's stain of an uncentrifuged urine specimen is also helpful in suggesting the diagnosis of UTI. The presence of one or more bacteria per oil immersion field correlates well with a bacterial colony count of 10^5 bacteria per mL of urine or higher.

Obtaining a proper urine specimen is of the utmost importance and is more difficult in children. The urine specimen must be collected in such a way to ensure that bacteria from the periurethral mucosa do not contaminate the sample. Bagged specimens obtained by attaching a sterile bag to the perineum of an infant have a high frequency of contamination and multiple organisms growing. The absence of bacterial growth from a bagged specimen collected over a short time would be helpful in ruling out a UTI in an infant. The optimal specimen from an infant would be obtained through suprapubic bladder aspiration. This technique can also be used in young children if it is performed by experienced personnel. It should not be performed on children with a coagulopathy or in children with abdominal wall defects. Most failures to obtain urine by this method are caused by absence of urine in the bladder. Suprapubic tap, therefore, should not be performed in an infant who has voided recently. The success rate is higher when ultrasonography is used to guide the aspiration. Complications include gross hematuria lasting less than 24 hours and the rare puncture of other abdominal organs.

In older children, a midstream urine specimen is obtained after antiseptic washing of the external genitalia. This technique may be used in children who can void on demand. Catheterization of the bladder to obtain a urine specimen for culture is not recommended in infants but may be used in toddlers who are too old to tap but too young to cooperate with the clean-catch technique. Unlike aspirations, catheterization is uncomfortable and stressful to the child and may introduce infection into the bladder. Whichever technique is chosen, the procedure should be performed by an experienced health care worker.

All urine specimens should be collected in a sterile container. The urine specimen should not be allowed to stand in room air and should be taken to the laboratory as soon as possible. The specimen may also be stored under refrigeration as long as 24 hours before plating on culture medium.

Work-Up of the Child with UTI

The diagnosis of a UTI in a child is often the first indication of a congenital or acquired structural abnormality of the urinary tract. Approximately 50% of children with UTI have an anatomic abnormality, and one third of all children with UTI have vesicoureteric reflux. Obstructive urinary problems should be diagnosed and treated at the earliest stage possible to minimize permanent renal damage (Fig. 11–1).

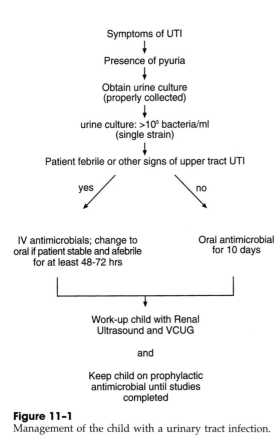

Figure 11–1
Management of the child with a urinary tract infection.

Every child in whom a diagnosis of UTI is made should have radiologic investigation. A renal ultrasound should first be done followed by a retrograde voiding cystourethrogram (VCUG). The renal ultrasound is noninvasive and can be done as soon as possible after the diagnosis of pyelonephritis is made so that urologic intervention may be carried out early. A plain radiograph of the abdomen should also be performed because it may detect renal calculi or skeletal abnormalities. An intravenous pyelogram should be done only if a more detailed anatomic visualization of the upper urinary tract is necessary.

A retrograde VCUG is needed to detect lower urinary tract abnormalities such as posterior urethral valves, ureteroceles, and diverticula. The VCUG is the only satisfactory method for the demonstration of vesicoureteric reflux. The VCUG should not be conducted during a period of acute infection. The VCUG may be difficult, and it should be explained carefully to help minimize apprehension and discomfort. A child who has abnormalities noted on either the ultrasound or the VCUG should be referred promptly to a urologist for further evaluation and management.

Other etiologic factors must be sought in children with UTI, including disturbance of bladder and bowel dysfunction. Unfortunately, these are difficult to evaluate by anatomic imaging studies. Their diagnosis requires an evaluation for infrequent voiding, urinary retention, other voiding disturbances, and constipation, which has also been known to be associated with UTI in children.

Treatment

Lower UTIs (cystitis) in a child can usually be treated with oral medication alone. Suggested daily doses of antimicrobials are listed in Table 11–1. The duration of treatment is controversial. Commonly recommended antimicrobials include trimethoprim-sulfamethoxazole, the cephalosporins, and nitrofurantoin. Up to 40% of community-acquired *E. coli* isolates are resistant to ampicillin and amoxicillin. These drugs, therefore, should not usually be used for initial treatment of UTI. If the sensitivities, however, show that the organ-

Table 11-1
Intravenous Antimicrobials for Urinary Tract Infections in Pediatric Patients Aged Beyond the Newborn Period*

Drug (Generic)	Dosage (per kg/day)†
Gentamicin	3–7.5 mg in 3 doses
Tobramycin	3–7.5 mg in 3 doses
Amikacin	15–22.5 mg in 3 doses
Ampicillin	200–300 mg in 4 doses
Trimethoprim-sulfamethoxazole (TMP-SXT)	8–12 mg TMP/40–60 mg SXT in 4 doses
Ceftriaxone	80–100 mg in 1 or 2 doses
Cefotaxime	150–300 mg in 3 or 4 doses
Ceftazidime	125–150 mg in 3 doses
Vancomycin	40–60 mg in 4 doses

*For further information, including dosing in newborns, consult the Red Book: Report of the Committee on Infectious Diseases, 24th ed. Elk Grove, IL, American Academy of Pediatrics, 1997.
†For normal renal function.

ism is sensitive to amoxicillin, therapy could be changed to this drug. The quinolones are not approved for use in children 16 years of age or younger.

Nitrofurantoin is a reasonable alternate drug for the treatment of UTI. It achieves a high urinary concentration, but it can be associated with nausea and vomiting. Hypersensitivity reactions such as pulmonary interstitial fibrosis and neurologic disorders have been rarely reported with this drug, and caution is advised.

Trimethoprim-sulfamethoxazole is a good, inexpensive antibiotic for initial therapy of lower tract UTI pending culture and sensitivity reports. Disadvantages include allergic side effects such as skin rashes (including Stevens-Johnson syndrome) and bone marrow suppression occurring in young children.

It is not recommended for children younger than the age of 2 months.

The cephalosporins are excellent alternatives if the other drugs cannot be given because of hypersensitivity or intolerance.

The optimal duration of treatment is controversial. Seven to 10 days of an appropriate antimicrobial agent are usually recommended for uncomplicated acute UTI in children.

For patients with pyelonephritis, the intravenous route should be used until the patient has been afebrile for at least 2 or 3 days. If the patient is stable, the therapy can be switched then to an appropriate oral drug based on the sensitivity tests. Suggested daily dose schedules for the intravenous antimicrobials for acute bacterial pyelonephritis are given in Table 11–2. A follow-up urinalysis and culture are important to assess the results of therapy. An aminoglycoside such as gentamicin plus ampicillin is an excellent combination to begin therapy in a child with acute pyelonephritis pending culture results. If a patient is allergic to the penicillins, then gentamicin plus vancomycin may be considered for pyelonephritis, particularly if the *Enterococcus* is suspected by Gram's stain of urine (gram-positive cocci in pairs or chains). If gram-negative rods only are apparent, then gentamicin alone pending further culture results would be a reasonable option. Vancomycin should only be used when a patient is allergic to penicillins and a gram-positive organism is the pathogen (e.g., *Enterococcus* or *Staphylococcus* species).

Prophylaxis

Patients who have demonstrated vesicoureteric reflux should be followed carefully until

Table 11-2
Oral Antimicrobials for UTIs in Pediatric Patients Aged Beyond the Newborn Period*

Drug (Generic)	Dosage (per kg/day)	Prophylaxis (single daily dose)
Trimethoprim-sulfamethoxazole (TMP-SXT)	8–12 mg TMP/40–60 mg SXT in 2 doses	1/4 mL/kg
Ampicillin	50–100 mg in 4 doses	—
Amoxicillin	25–50 mg in 3 doses	—
Cephalexin	25–50 mg in 4 doses	—
Nitrofurantoin	5–7 mg in 4 doses	1 mg/kg/day

*For further information, including dosing in newborns, consult the Red Book: Report of the Committee on Infectious Diseases, 24th ed. Elk Grove, IL, American Academy of Pediatrics, 1997.

it resolves or is corrected surgically. Any UTI should be treated to minimize the possible of renal damage from the reflux of infected urine. Optimally, the urine should be kept sterile at all times. Prophylaxis with either low-dose trimethoprim-sulfamethoxazole (1 to 2 mg/kg of trimethoprim and 5 to 10 mg/kg of sulfamethoxazole), or nitrofurantoin (1 to 2 mg/kg) at bedtime has been shown to be effective in the prevention of UTI. Breakthrough infections with bacteria resistant to the prophylactic drug may occur. In this case, prophylaxis should be changed to another drug if continued prophylaxis is necessary. In the absence of structural anomalies, for pediatric patients with frequent UTI, most experts advise prophylactic antimicrobials for a minimum of 3 to 6 months. Such patients will have reinfections throughout life.

ILLUSTRATIVE CASE

A two-year-old girl presented with a 2-day history of fever and poor appetite, followed by intermittent vomiting. Her past history was unremarkable. Physical examination was notable for a temperature of 38.5° C. A urinalysis obtained by suprapubic aspiration showed 50 to 100 per high-power field of WBCs and rare red blood cells, and was nitrite positive. Urine and blood cultures were obtained, and her peripheral WBC was 22,000/mm^3 with 85% neutrophils.

She was begun on intravenous ampicillin and gentamicin. The urine cultures grew more than 10^5 *E. coli* resistant to ampicillin but sensitive to all other drugs tested. She was completely afebrile by day 3 of therapy. An ultrasonographic examination was done that showed two normal kidneys without evidence of obstruction.

After she was afebrile for 48 hours, her therapy was switched to trimethoprim-sulfamethoxazole orally to complete a 2-week total course of antimicrobial therapy. Follow-up urinalysis and urine cultures were negative. Outpatient work-up then included a voiding cystoureterogram that showed Grade II reflux on the left side. She was continued on prophylactic trimethoprim-sulfamethoxazole, and follow-up VCUG was arranged at annual intervals. She remained free of infections, and at 5 years of age was found to have resolved her reflux.

Comment

This case is a fairly typical "success story." The radiologic evaluation would be the same if she had afebrile, lower tract infection because the goal is to identify reflux in children prone to infection before pyelonephritis scars the kidney. Some experts advocate nuclear renal scanning with dimercaptosuccinic acid in all patients with febrile infections to better delineate areas of focal scarring. Upper tract studies need not be repeated annually unless infection has occurred in the interim. Reflux with its surgical treatment is further detailed in Chapter 21. The most common reason for surgery in such cases is failure of antibiotic prophylaxis to prevent febrile UTI.

SELECTED READINGS

1. Koff SA: A practical approach to evaluating urinary tract infection in children. Pediatr Nephrol 5:398–400, 1991.
2. Leung AKC, Robson WLM: Urinary tract infection in infancy and childhood. Adv Pediatr 38:257–285, 1991.
3. Sherbotier JR, Cornfeld D: Management of urinary tract infections in children. Med Clin North Am 75:327–337, 1991.
4. Stull TL, LiPumar JJ: Epidemiology and natural history of urinary tract infections in children. Med Clin North Am 75:287–297, 1991.

12

Lower Urinary Tract Infections in Women

Raul C. Ordorica

The entire urinary tract of both men and women is susceptible to infection. Lower urinary tract infections (UTIs) in women comprise a significant part at an estimated cost of more than $1 billion annually required for their evaluation and therapy. With at least 7 million cases each year, these infections are probably seen more often by primary care physicians than by urologists. It is important, therefore, that the caregiver is able to recognize their presentation and prescribe appropriate therapy. Furthermore, it is essential to be able to differentiate it not only from more complicated UTIs, but also from other bladder, urethral, and vaginal pathology. This chapter deals primarily with the topics of bacterial cystitis and urethritis, their presentation, diagnoses, therapy, and prevention. In addition, consideration should be given to associated lower urinary tract pathology that may mimic these disorders or become apparent during evaluation.

Definition

Infections of the lower urinary tract are defined as involving either the bladder or urethra. This is in contrast to bacterial colonization, which is the presence of bacteria within the urine without actual tissue infection. The term *cystitis* implies the presence of an inflammatory condition of the bladder, such as that caused by a bacterial infection. The cause for cystitis in fact may be either infectious or noninfectious in nature. Infectious sources are primarily bacterial, with fungal or viral causes a much smaller portion. Examples of noninfectious cystitis would be those caused

by radiation or chemical irritants. The term *urethritis* likewise implies an inflammation of the urethra. Bacterial urethritis is often broadly classified as either gonococcal or nongonococcal.

An uncomplicated UTI is a lower UTI that superficially involves the bladder and urethra. Patients should be without symptoms of systemic infection and without upper tract involvement such as pyelonephritis. The implication of an uncomplicated UTI is that for those patients who present with their first infection, resolution can be expected with most antimicrobial therapy. For most women an uncomplicated UTI is an isolated occurrence, with approximately one fourth experiencing a repeat UTI within the next few years. To have an uncomplicated UTI, one must have a structurally and functionally normal urinary tract and immune system. The presence of any significant factors as those listed in Table 12–1 can result in what is termed a *complicated UTI*, which requires a more extensive course of antibiotic therapy, along with a substantial urologic evaluation.

Table 12-1
Factors Associated with Complicated Urinary Tract Infections

Anatomic or functional abnormality of the urinary tract
Foreign body
Obstructive uropathy
Vesicoureteral reflux
Azotemia
Diabetes mellitus
Advanced age
Pregnancy
Immunosuppression
Renal transplantation

For those patients who have recurrent infections, it becomes necessary to determine if this represents an otherwise benign process or one that is contributed to by significant underlying pathology. This is in part determined by the apparent source of the infections. Recurrent UTIs can be caused by bacteria either from within or without the urinary tract. If the recurrent infection is secondary to bacteria arising from outside of the urinary tract, this is classified as a reinfection and usually requires longer than 2 weeks to occur. With the source of reinfections being outside the urinary tract, the integrity of the urinary system is intact. Thus, extensive evaluations of these patients are often negative. Those that are caused by bacteria from within the urinary tract are described as a relapse, which usually occurs within a 2-week period. Patients with relapsing infections may have significant abnormalities of the urinary tract causing the inability for the antimicrobial therapy to clear the urinary tract of pathogens. It is for these people that urologic evaluation is warranted. To a significant degree apart from the history and physical examination of the patient, the need for extensive urologic investigations depends on the differentiation between reinfections and relapsing infections.

Pathophysiology

Lower UTIs typically arise in a retrograde fashion through the urethra. Therefore, it is understandable why lower UTIs are more common in women than men given the shorter length of the female urethra with the potential for contamination from the vagina and perineum. Those activities that encourage the passage of bacteria from these sites into the urethra and bladder, such as sexual activity, may predispose for infection. The normal bacterial colonization of the vagina is with nonpathogenic *Lactobacillus* species. With the harboring of these sites with fecal flora, the most common pathogen for lower UTIs is *Escherichia coli* at 80%, with *Staphylococcus saprophyticus* another typical organism causing 5% to 15% of infections. Other common pathogens include *Klebsiella* and *Proteus mirabilis*. These latter organisms are capable of

forming infectious urinary calculi, a potential source for relapsing infection and renal deterioration.

Once the bacteria have entered the bladder, they must find an environment in which they can multiply and overcome the host defense mechanisms of the bladder lining. If the bladder is emptied soon after bacterial contamination, then the pathogens are flushed from the system and infection is prevented. Likewise, if the bacteria are prevented from adhering to the bladder mucosa, infection is easily cleared. This is dependent on the interplay between bacterial adherence factors, most notably defined in *E. coli,* and specific characteristics of the vaginal and urothelial lining that is genetically determined. It is not uncommon to elicit a family history of UTIs in those patients with multiple reinfections. This should be contrasted with a family history of relapsing infections and pyelonephritis, such that could be caused by vesicoureteral reflux, a condition that also is more common in families.

Diagnoses

HISTORY

Most physicians are familiar with the presentation of lower UTIs, with symptoms of urinary frequency, urgency, and dysuria (Table 12–2). The onset of symptoms is typically acute, and patients usually seek medical attention within 24 hours. If there is a longer history, then prior antibiotic therapies and their clinical response should be recorded. This also includes whether the patient had been on antibiotic regimens for other infections, which may have altered colonic and vaginal flora, thus affecting the subsequent

Table 12–2
Signs and Symptoms of Urinary Tract Infections

Urgency
Frequency
Small-volume voids
Dysuria
Pelvic discomfort
Hematuria
Low-grade fever

UTI. Other factors that might affect vaginal flora such as the lack of estrogen in the postmenopausal state, or the use of a diaphragm for prophylaxis, may affect the eventual contamination of the urinary tract. Physiologic or anatomic alterations of the urinary tract, either temporary as in the case of pregnancy, or of a more permanent nature from surgical intervention, should be determined. Inciting events for the entrance of bacteria into the bladder should be elicited. These include instrumentation of the urinary tract, sexual intercourse, and frequent bathing.

Prior history of UTIs should be obtained, including those that may have occurred during childhood. A childhood history raises with it the suspicion for underlying urologic pathology. To be consistent with an uncomplicated UTI, the history should be negative for high fevers or bouts of pyelonephritis. These factors increase the risk that an upper UTI is present, which requires a more comprehensive evaluation and extensive course of therapy. Nor should there be a history of other urinary tract pathology such as vesicoureteral reflux, nephrolithiasis, or urinary tract malignancy. Their presence increases the risk of either more significant infection or an alternate disease process that would require therapy.

PHYSICAL EXAMINATION

The physical examination for those patients with a UTI should not only confirm the diagnoses but also rule out other pathology. There should be the absence of any high fever, which would be more consistent with systemic infection. There may be pain elicited with examination of the bladder, either with suprapubic palpation, or bimanual vaginal examination. Other urologic or gynecologic pathology that may be noted on physical examination is listed in Table 12–3.

URINALYSIS

The initial laboratory investigation in patients with symptoms consistent with a lower UTI is the urinalysis. In the case of lower UTI, clean-catch midstream urinalysis should demonstrate the presence of leukocytes and bacteria. This can be detected indirectly by dipstick method looking for the presence of nitrites (breakdown products by bacteria) or for leukocyte esterase (produced by neutrophils). Otherwise, these microbes and cells can be directly detected with microscopic analysis of the urine. Direct observation by microscopic examination brings with it additional benefit. Alternate sources for infection can be identified by the presence of white blood cell casts, which can provide evidence for pyelonephritis. Evidence for specimen contamination is signified by an abundance of epithelial cells and bacteria without pyuria. In women this most commonly represents vaginal contamination. For those women who have difficulty with collection secondary to vaginal contamination, urethral catheterization can be performed for specimen collection. The most accurate method of collection free of contamination is by suprapubic aspiration. However, because of its invasive nature, this procedure is rarely used outside of the pediatric population, where collection can be problematic.

The presence of red blood cells varies among cases, with some patients demonstrating none to those who experience gross hematuria. The presence of significant hematuria is rare in patients with urethritis or vaginitis, diagnoses often confused with UTI. These diagnoses should be differentiated from *painless* hematuria, which carries with it the suspicion for other causative pathology, with the onus on the caregiver to rule out the presence of malignancy. In addition, those patients with a documented infection who persist with hematuria should be assessed following therapy with a repeat urinalysis to exclude any underlying pathology. For patients who persist with hematuria despite the eradication of infection, evaluation for urothelial neoplasm is warranted.

URINE CULTURE

The diagnosis of a UTI is confirmed by urine culture. It is important that the specimen be obtained with a minimum of contamination to avoid false-positive results. The typical method is by use of a midstream clean-catch procedure. Contamination of the specimen is signified by growth of multiple organisms. If collection is problematic, a catheterized speci-

Table 12-3
Physical Exam for Urinary Tract Infection (UTI)

Examination	Finding	Pathology
Back	CVA tenderness	Renal infection, obstruction
Abdomen	Renal enlargement	Obstruction, mass
	Suprapubic fullness	Incomplete emptying of bladder
	Suprapubic tenderness	Cystitis
Vagina	Erythema, tenderness, discharge	Vaginitis
	Introital tenderness without erythema, discharge	Vulvar vestibulitis
	Levator spasm, tenderness	Pelvic floor dysfunction
	Atrophy	Facilitates recurrent UTI
	Other vaginal, uterine pathology	Herpes, cysts, Paget's disease, cervicitis, PID
Urethra	Tenderness, discharge	Urethritis
	Prolapse, swelling	Caruncle, diverticula, carcinoma
Bladder base	Tenderness	Cystitis
Neurologic	Decreased sensation, rectal tone, levator contraction, bulbocavernosus reflex	Neurogenic bladder

CVA, costovertebral angle; PID, pelvic inflammatory disease.

men can be obtained as in obtaining a urinalysis. The growth of 10^5 colony-forming units (cfu) per mL is used to define infection based on decades-old studies. However, significant infection may be missed with this standard, particularly early in the presentation. The Infectious Disease Society of America consensus definition of bacterial cystitis is the presence of 10^3 cfu per mL or more. The presence of significant growth is usually determined by 24 hours, with identification of exact organisms and their sensitivities to antibiotics by 48 hours.

Therapy

Symptomatic lower UTIs should be differentiated from bacterial colonization, which does not imply actual inflammation or infection of the lower urinary tract. Without tissue infection the bacteriuric patient may be asymptomatic, and there may or may not be the presence of pyuria. Although a UTI deserves therapy in practically all situations, the patient with asymptomatic bacteruria, or bacterial colonization, may or may not necessitate therapy, depending on the clinical situation (see sections on pregnancy, geriatric population, and patients with indwelling catheters).

Antibiotic therapy for UTIs can be by several modalities, as noted in Table 12–4. Antimicrobial therapy is optimally therapeutic, resulting in eradication of the offending bacteria from the infected tissue and urine during the acute infection. However, other uses include prophylaxis, in which reinfection is prevented by maintaining urine sterility despite periodic contamination with bacteria. In addition, there is suppressive therapy, implying the inability to eradicate the bacteria from the urinary source in the case of relapsing infections, for which the bacterial count is kept at a minimum to prevent acute infections.

UNCOMPLICATED URINARY TRACT INFECTION

Given the common scenario of uncomplicated UTIs in the female population, it is not unusual to treat patients who experience their first episode empirically based on history and urinalysis alone. For patients who present with a UTI for the first time, management typically consists of a course of antibiotics with reassessment following therapy. With the most common pathogen in 80% of cases being *E. coli*, therapy can be chosen from a range of antibiotics. Ideal characteristics for antimicrobials used for UTIs include those agents that are well absorbed from the gastrointestinal tract and are excreted at high concentrations in the urine. Although they should be effective against suspected pathogens, they should be relatively nontoxic to nonpathogenic flora of the lower gastrointestinal tract and vagina. The common antibiotics that meet most of these criteria include

Table 12-4
Antibiotic Regimens for Urinary Tract Infections (UTIs)

Modality	UTI Indication	Recommended Therapy
Therapeutic	Uncomplicated (short course)	TMP-SMX: 160–800 mg bid × 3 days TMP: 100 mg × 3 days Nitrofurantoin monohydrate/macrocrystals: 100 mg bid × 7 days Ciprofloxacin: 250 mg bid × 3 days Norfloxacin: 400 mg bid × 3 days Levofloxacin: 250 mg qd × 3 days Cefixime: 400 mg qd × 3 days Cefpodoxime proxetil 100 mg bid × 3 days
	Complicated (long course)	TMP-SMX: 160–800 mg bid × 7 days TMP: 100 mg × 7 days Ciprofloxacin: 250 mg bid × 7 days Norfloxacin: 400 mg bid × 7 days Levofloxacin: 250 mg qd × 7 days Cefixime: 400 mg qd × 7 days Cefpodoxime proxetil 100 mg bid × 7 days
Prophylactic	Reinfection: temporally related to inciting events (intermittent course)	Nitrofurantoin macrocrystals: 50 mg × 1 Nitrofurantoin monohydrate/macrocrystals: 100 mg × 1 TMP-SMX: 80–400 to 160–800 mg × 1 TMP: 100 mg × 1 Norfloxacin: 400 mg × 1
	Reinfection: no obvious inciting events (chronic course)	Nitrofurantoin macrocrystals: 50 mg qhs Nitrofurantoin monohydrate/macrocrystals: 100 mg qhs TMP-SMX: 80–400 to 160–800 mg qhs TMP: 100 mg qhs Norfloxacin: 400 mg qhs
Suppressive	Relapsing, persistence (chronic course)	Nitrofurantoin macrocrystals: 50 mg qhs Nitrofurantoin monohydrate/macrocrystals: 100 mg qhs TMP-SMX: 80–400 to 160–800 mg qhs TMP: 100 mg qhs Norfloxacin: 400 mg qhs

TMP-SMX, trimethoprim-sulfamethoxazole; bid, twice daily; qd, daily; qhs, nightly.

trimethoprim-sulfamethoxazole, trimethoprim, and nitrofurantoin.

The nitrofurantoins have the benefit of being rapidly excreted in the urine, which minimizes significant tissue levels. This results in the avoidance of altering the fecal and vaginal flora, which can result in the wiping out of normal vaginal colonization (*Lactobacillus* species), which can help suppress the overgrowth of potential pathogens. Alteration of nonpathogenic vaginal and fecal flora can lead to secondary vaginal fungal infections and colonization with antibiotic-resistant strains of bacteria. However, with the source of the UTI often being the vaginal reservoir, specific therapy against pathogens in this site may be beneficial to reduce the risk of reinfection. Nitrofurantoin tends to be less effective against *Proteus* than other agents. Resistance overall to community-acquired gram-negative pathogens has been noted to be at 15% to 20%. As a less potent systemic antibiotic, some studies have demonstrated that nitrofu-

rantoin is less effective in the treatment of uncomplicated UTI using a 3-day course in comparison to trimethoprim-sulfamethoxazole. Therefore, the usual course for nitrofurantoin is 7 days.

Trimethoprim or the combination of trimethoprim-sulfamethoxazole is an excellent choice for uncomplicated UTIs in which resistance to this form of therapy has not been demonstrated. Both medications achieve high concentration in the urine with a relatively long half-life. These antibiotics provide the benefit of eradicating the aerobic gram-negative pathogens not only from the urine but also from the lower gastrointestinal tract and vagina, which act as reservoirs for reinfection. However, normal anaerobic flora remain unaffected by these regimens, inhibiting further the overgrowth of pathogens. Duration of therapy should be from 3 to 7 days, with evidence that a 3-day course in using these antibiotics for uncomplicated UTIs is equally as effective as a 7-day course. Resistance of community acquired organisms has been noted at 5% to 15%.

The beta-lactam antibiotics have been found to be less effective in the treatment of UTIs in comparison with the aforementioned antibiotics. They have a relatively short half-life within the urinary tract. Their use can result in the rapid development of resistant strains, which has been noted in excess of 30%. In addition, there is a deleterious effect on normal vaginal and fecal flora, encouraging secondary infection and reinfection. However, their relatively benign side-effect profile and lack of teratogenicity make them ideal agents to use during pregnancy. Specifically, ampicillin is beneficial in the treatment of culture-proven *Enterococcus,* which may prove resistant to the usual empiric therapies.

Fluoroquinolones are markedly effective against the usual gram-negative pathogens found with UTIs. In addition, their long half-life allows for once- to twice-a-day dosing, depending on the specific antimicrobial. As that they are relatively broad-spectrum antibiotics, they may not be an ideal choice in the treatment of the first-time UTI, with concerns having been voiced regarding the potential development of resistant strains, which is currently at about 5%. Therefore, it may better be reserved for those cases in which organisms resistant to the other first-line agents are encountered or for the initial treatment of complex UTIs. Similar to trimethoprim or trimethoprim-sulfamethoxazole regimens, a 3-day course has been found to be as effective as a 7-day course. There is a clear decrease in efficacy when using single-day regimens with any of the antibiotics.

RECURRENT INFECTIONS

Several outcomes are possible with antibiotic therapy: complete response with resolution of symptoms and no further infections, initial response with recurrence of symptoms after 2 weeks (reinfection), initial response with recurrence within 2 weeks or a partial response (relapse), or no response at all. For those patients who have a complete response with symptom resolution, there is little left to do. The urinalysis can be rechecked in complete responders to ensure that there is no residual abnormality that deserves individual attention (e.g., pyuria, hematuria, and casts), and otherwise the follow-up may be on an as-needed basis.

Patients with a recurrence or continuation of their symptoms may benefit from the performance of a urine culture. Once a culture-specific organism is demonstrated, it allows for the direction of further therapy. UTIs are present when there are more than 10^3 cfu per mL present in a clean-catch midstream urine. Although antibiotics may be ineffective for various reasons in the in vivo setting, it may hinder bacterial growth in the laboratory setting. Therefore, the urine culture should be performed off all antibiotics. The culture alone may raise the suspicion for more significant urologic pathology, such as with urease-splitting organisms (e.g., *Klebsiella, Proteus*), which raise the possibility for infectious calculi.

Reinfection

Those infections that respond and recur outside of 2 weeks of therapy are considered to be occurrence of a reinfection. The anatomically normal urinary tract has been rendered sterile, and the source of the recurrent infection is from outside the system. This can result from conditions that promote the recurrence of infection in an otherwise healthy person. Typically, there is recontamination from outside the urinary tract such as from a vaginal reservoir. This is the most common form of recurrent UTI seen. This is secondary to the interaction between the reservoir of bacterial pathogens colonizing the perineum and vagina and the defense mechanisms against infection involving the urethra and bladder. Compromises of vaginal defense mechanisms, such as with vaginal atrophy in the postmenopausal state, can facilitate bacterial colonizations with pathogens. Alterations in urethral integrity as in the case of urethral dysfunction with stress urinary incontinence can result in the increased passage of bacteria into the bladder. The bladder itself, in the absence of anatomic abnormality, can have increased susceptibility to bacterial infection with various bacterial adherent factors. This increased susceptibility is genetically determined, and it is not unusual to identify patients' family histories of recurrent UTIs.

Relapsing Infection

Those patients who initially respond but recur within 2 weeks or only partially respond are considered to be incompletely treated, with the bacteria somehow protected from the antibiotic. This bacterial persistence is due either to a resistant strain or to the infected organism being isolated from the antibiotic. The bacterial resistance to the antimicrobial is either pre-existing or developed during therapy. Examples of bacterial foci that are not exposed to adequate concentrations of antibiotic include urinary stasis or other forms of pathogen sequestration (Table 12–5). In addition, low drug concentrations can be expected with poor excretion of the drug, such as with azotemia, or decreased patient compliance. Finally, there may be more than one species of bacterium within the urinary system, which is common with foreign bodies, such that as one type is eradicated, the other becomes the main pathogen. For those patients who partially respond, this provides evidence that the diagnosis of a UTI was at least partially correct.

NONRESPONDERS

Those infections that fail to respond altogether are either because the antimicrobial therapy is ineffective against the particular organism, or the patient does not have an infection as the cause of her symptoms. At this stage a thorough physical examination is repeated and a urine culture should be obtained. A list of alternative pathologies that should be considered when faced with lower urinary tract symptoms that do not respond

Table 12–5
Causes for a Relapsing Infection

Cause	Pathology
Urinary stasis	Poor emptying, vesicoureteral reflux, hydronephrosis, bladder or urethral diverticula
Sequestered organisms	Necrotic tissue (bladder cancer, papillary necrosis), foreign body (stones, stents, catheters), vesicoenteric fistula
Altered immune system	Diabetes, chemotherapy, steroid use
Altered antibiotic secretion	Azotemia, patient compliance

Table 12–6
Non-UTI Bladder Pathology

Interstitial cystitis	Ureteral calculus
Hemorrhagic cystitis	Bladder cancer
Radiation cystitis	Urethral syndrome
Herpes	Urethral cancer
Neurogenic bladder	Vaginitis
Bladder calculus	Vulvar-vestibulitis

to antibiotic therapy is included in Table 12–6. One should be aware that the presence of one of these disorders does not exclude the potential to suffer from UTIs also.

If an organism is cultured and found not to be sensitive to the initial antibiotic, then a 1-week course with the appropriate antibiotic is required. If the organism cultured is sensitive to the clinically ineffective antibiotic, then one must diagnose the cause for failed therapy. This may include problems with compliance, bioavailability, duration of therapy, or possible sequestering of bacteria, as in relapsing infections. If the evaluation for these factors is negative, including urologic examination, then a more prolonged course of the appropriate antibiotic may be attempted.

FOLLOW-UP AND PREVENTION

Patients with a history of recurrent infections should undergo urine culture following therapy and again at 1 month. If it is a relapsing infection, then the genitourinary pathology that is suspected based on the history and physical examination is worked up. Possible evaluations and their potential findings are listed in Table 12–7. If there is no evidence of underlying pathology, or one suspects that it is a reinfection, then deficiencies of host defenses can be addressed. An example of this is altering hygienic practice, such as with increasing fluid intake, voiding following potential bacterial contamination such as during intercourse, and minimizing perineal and vaginal colonization by wiping from anterior to posterior following voiding. Cranberry juice has been shown in vitro to inhibit the adherence of uropathogenic *E. coli* isolates to uroepithelial cells. Other causes of reinfection include the use of a vaginal diaphragm and spermicides for contraception. Alternatives to this form of contraception should be considered in patients with reinfection.

Table 12–7
Ancillary Tests for Relapsing Urinary Tract Infections

Test	Finding
KUB	Urolithiasis, renal mass, emphysematous pyelonephritis, emphysematous cystitis
IVP	Hydronephrosis, urolithiasis, emphysematous pyelonephritis, emphysematous cystitis, cortical thinning, renal scarring, calyceal diverticula, ureteral ectopia, renal mass, bladder trabeculation, urinary retention
US	Hydronephrosis, urolithiasis, cortical thinning, renal scarring, renal mass, bladder trabeculation, urinary retention
VCUG	Vesicoureteral reflux, bladder trabeculation, bladder diverticula, urethral diverticula, urinary retention
CT scan	Hydronephrosis, urolithiasis, renal mass, renal abscess, emphysematous pyelonephritis
Cystoscopy	Urethritis, urethral stenosis, urethral diverticula, ureteral ectopia, bladder tumors

KUB, kidney ureter, and bladder; IVP, intravenous pyelogram; US, ultrasound; VCUG, voiding cystourethrogram; CT, computed tomography.

The use of vaginal estrogen has been shown to reduce the rate of repeat UTI in postmenopausal patients. Application can be readily performed with an initial dose of 1 g of estrogen cream daily for 1 month followed by once- to twice-weekly applications for maintenance with minimal systemic effects. Other medications to improve host defenses include methenamine, which has an antiseptic effect by its conversion to formaldehyde in urine that has a pH of 6.0 or less.

If the findings are normal, and the prior measures of improving host defense mechanisms have been exhausted, then either the patient can treat the UTIs as they arise, or a prolonged course of prophylactic antibiotics can be used. If there is an obvious pattern to the infection (i.e., after intercourse), then prophylactic antibiotics are used during periods where infection is common. A common scenario is for the patient to take one or two doses of an effective antibiotic following intercourse to offset their occurrence. For those patients in whom reinfections are infrequent, self-initiated therapies of antibiotic regimens can be considered. If their symptoms do not resolve with 3-day regimens, or there is any

abnormality suspected, a more thorough urologic examination is performed.

For those patients who have more frequent reinfections than 2 per year, a 3- to 6-month course of prophylactic or suppressive antibiotics can be introduced. Nitrofurantoin, trimethoprim, trimethoprim-sulfamethoxazole, norfloxacin, or cephalexin can be used as a single nightly dose to maximize urinary concentrations. At some point this can be tapered to every other day and then discontinued, depending on the success of and the tolerance for the antibiotic. Caution should be exercised in the use of chronic nitrofurantoin use, with the potential development of a pulmonary reaction, signified by cough, dyspnea, and chest pain.

COMPLICATED URINARY TRACT INFECTION
Diabetes

Diabetes incurs a number of effects on the urogenital system that results in greater morbidity involving UTIs in women. There is an alteration in the vaginal flora, making recurrent vaginitis more common. This results in pathogenic colonization and subsequent contamination of the urinary system. Bladder dysfunction in the form of neurogenic bladder can be caused by diabetic neuropathy. Decreased bladder sensation and contractile function with resultant increases in postvoid residual volumes are most commonly cited. In addition, diabetes can have multiple effects on the upper urinary tract. This includes diabetic nephropathy, renal papillary necrosis, and renal artery stenosis. Finally, marked glucosuria has been shown to alter the phagocytic function of leukocytes.

These effects result in the complicated UTIs encountered, with bacteremia being two or three times more common in diabetic versus nondiabetic women with UTIs. This is secondary to the much higher rate of upper tract involvement in diabetics. This can be in the form of pyelonephritis, renal and perirenal abscess formation, emphysematous pyelonephritis, pyelitis and cystitis, fungal infections, and xanthogranulomatous pyelonephritis. Emphysematous pyelonephritis alone can result in a greater than 80% mortality if not surgically treated, despite aggressive medical management. This gas-forming, necrotizing infection of the renal parenchyma can be detected with a kidney, ureter, and bladder film, although computed tomographic (CT) scan is the image of choice for diagnoses.

The usual bacteria are encountered in the diabetic patient, with *E. coli* being the predominant organism, with a notable increase in the rate of *Klebsiella* pneumonia. *Enterobacter* species, *Enterococcus* species, and *Pseudomonas aeruginosa* can also be seen, particularly in patients who have been recently hospitalized, have undergone invasive urologic procedures, or have had recurrent UTIs. With all these elements for complicated UTIs, there is no role for short-course antibiotic therapy in the diabetic patient. A 7- to 14-day course should be used for those patients with lower UTIs, with culture documentation both of the pathogen and subsequent proof or eradication. Although in one study there was no benefit seen with a 6- versus a 2-week course in the therapy of female diabetic patients with lower UTIs, a more prolonged course is the standard with upper tract involvement.

Trimethoprim-sulfamethoxazole remains the first-line agent, although response to therapy must be monitored owing to the 5% to 15% resistance seen with community-acquired infections. It should be noted that high doses can potentiate the hypoglycemic effects of oral agents. Fluoroquinolones remain the second-line agent of choice, with only a 5% resistance rate. Nitrofurantoin is not recommended owing to its low tissue levels and subsequent lack of effect in treating upper tract involvement, although it still maintains a role as a prophylactic agent. Ampicillin and amoxicillin may be beneficial owing to the higher incidence of *Enterococcus* seen in this population, although this should be documented by culture.

By definition, UTIs in the diabetic patient are complicated. They have a higher rate of upper tract and systemic involvement, requiring aggressive management and follow-up. All infections should be documented by culturing of the organism with antibiotic sensitivity testing. Recurrent lower UTIs require evaluation of lower urinary tract function, and upper tract infections require prompt imaging and urologic attention. There is no role for short-course antibiotic therapy in the diabetic woman with lower UTI.

Pregnancy

The physiologic changes of pregnancy make many patients more susceptible for UTI, with greater potential to advance to pyelonephritis. Although asymptomatic bacteriuria may be tolerated in the elderly female population, this creates the risk in the pregnant patient for developing significant infection with the ramification of anemia, eclampsia, preterm labor, and low birth weight. Risk factors for the development of UTIs include functional or anatomic urinary tract abnormalities, history of recurrent UTIs, diabetes mellitus, low socioeconomic status, increased parity, sexual activity, and sickle cell trait. Initial urine screening is typically undertaken at 16 weeks' gestational age. If the initial screen is negative, it should be repeated in high-risk populations. If positive, confirmation should be obtained by quantitative culture with susceptibilities. Effectiveness of therapy should be evaluated with repeat testing 1 week following therapy. If bacteriuria is eliminated, screening should be repeated monthly. If there is persistence, retreatment with a longer course is necessary, with suppressive therapy used for further recurrence or persistence. **In the absence of noted risk factors, a 3-day course can be considered for either bacteriuria or isolated lower UTIs. Recurrent bacteriuria or infection requires longer 7-day courses. As in other UTIs, there is decreased efficacy with single-day regimens. Patients with persistent bacteriuria and recurrent UTIs require urologic evaluation. Patients with an episode of pyelonephritis should receive antibiotic suppressive therapy throughout the pregnancy. Those patients with pyelonephritis without a clear response to antibiotic therapy require upper tract evaluation and urologic evaluation.**

Antibiotics must be chosen that provide minimal risk to the developing fetus. Penicillin/cephalosporins and nitrofurantoin are Class B drugs, and trimethoprim-sulfamethoxazole and fluoroquinolones are Class C. Of all these, the penicillin/cephalosporins are the safest to use in terms of fetal safety. Commonly used agents are amoxicillin and cephalexin. Specific cautions include that for nitrofurantoin, which is contraindicated in patients with glucose-6-phosphate dehydrogenase deficiency, which might result in hemolytic anemia. Trimethoprim is teratogenic during the first trimester. Sulfamethoxazole can result in hyperbilirubinemia during the third trimester. Fluoroquinolones are contraindicated secondary to the resultant arrest of bone growth secondary to epiphyseal closure, and tetracycline secondary to dental alteration. For patients with recurrent bacterial colonization of UTIs, antibiotic prophylaxis during gestation can be considered during pregnancy. Sulfamethoxazole should be avoided at term owing to its effect on hepatic function.

Geriatric Population

With aging there are multiple changes that may promote entry of bacteria into the bladder and facilitate the persistence of infection. Other than the presence of actual anatomic pathology, voiding patterns may alter such that significant postvoid residual urine may be present, and vaginal and urethral atrophy may occur with alteration in defense mechanisms and flora. This brings with it treatment options such as estrogen replacement therapy.

A significant portion of this population of female patients may have bacteriuria and not benefit from antibiotic therapy. Whether the bacteriuria is the source of any symptoms may be difficult to discern. Elderly patients may have irritative voiding complaints of frequency, urgency, nocturia, and possibly incontinence, independent of any infection. In these patients, the determination that the bacteriuria is "asymptomatic" is made when the symptoms remain unchanged when the "infection" is successfully treated. The presence of infection can otherwise be defined by other indicators of host response, such as the constitutional signs of fever or failure to thrive, or the presence of pyuria. Attempts at treatment may bring a high recurrence rate despite long courses of antibiotics. Culture-specific therapy of even asymptomatic bacteriuria is warranted prior to urologic manipulation to avoid overt infection, including bacteremia and sepsis. Decreased renal function in the elderly should be considered during prescribing, with decreases in antibiotic dosage.

Catheterized Patient

The presence of an indwelling catheter for urinary drainage bypasses the defense mechanisms of the lower urinary tract to keep out bacteria. By definition we would expect that a urine culture from a patient with an indwelling catheter longer than 3 days would demonstrate significant numbers of bacteria. However, this often is indicative of colonization rather than actual tissue infection of the urethra and bladder. Moreover, attempts to treat the pathogen invariably results in the development of more resistant strains of bacteria. Therefore, therapy is reserved for patients who demonstrate actual tissue infection, typically signaled by the presence of leukocytosis and fever. The overall effectiveness of treating catheter-associated UTIs is the removal of the catheter itself. The chronic indwelling catheter results in microbial persistence with the development of resistant strains from repeated antibiotic therapy.

Manipulation of the catheter can result in the dissemination of the harbored organisms and the development of urosepsis. To minimize the potential for the development of significant infection, the bladder urine can be cultured prior to removal of the catheter or expected instrumentation, and therapy of the isolated organisms can be initiated based on the culture results. Often the microbiology laboratory will isolate multiple organisms, and laboratory personnel should be made aware of the presence of an indwelling catheter and that this is not a contaminated specimen that they would otherwise routinely discard.

URETHRITIS

Some patients may have lower urinary tract symptoms with negligible colony counts by urine cultures that respond to antibiotics. A potential source for this is urethritis. A bacterial urethral infection typically presents with urinary urgency, frequency, and dysuria, with a more gradual course in comparison to bacterial cystitis. Usual pathogens may include *Gonococcus* or *Chlamydia*, with a history significant for sexual activity. Because the nidus for infection is limited, the voided urine specimen may not demonstrate the pathogenic organism unless the bladder is also involved.

Physical examination may demonstrate tenderness in the area of the urethra with palpation. In addition, one may express purulent

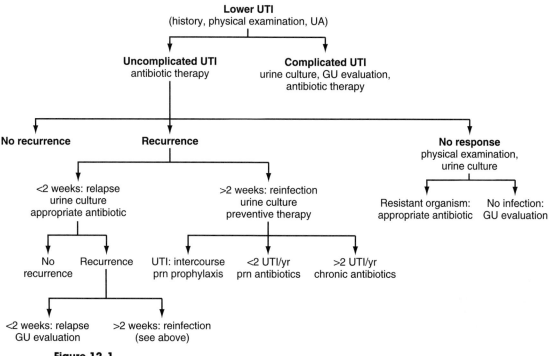

Figure 12-1
Algorithm for lower urinary tract infection (UTI) in women. UA, urinalysis; GU, genitourinary.

drainage that is evident either on physical examination or urethroscopy. Underlying pathology may include a urethral diverticulum. For many the culture is negative, with a partial response to short-course antibiotic therapy. Regimens for urethritis include the ruling out of sexually transmitted diseases. A subsequent course of doxycycline for 20 days will cover both gonococcal or nongonococcal sources. If this should fail, then additional antibiotics can be used to eradicate the potential infection of fastidious organisms (erythromycin, metronidazole, fluoroquinolones). Should these antibiotics also fail, urethral dilation is a potential therapy, although its routine use remains controversial.

Conclusion

Lower UTIs are commonly seen in the female population by the primary care physician. Their therapy is straightforward as guided by the history, physical examination, and laboratory data (Fig. 12–1). For those patients with recurrent infections, evaluation for more sig-

nificant urologic pathology is sometimes beneficial. Therapy for recurrent infections includes improving host defense mechanisms, prophylaxis, and suppressive therapy. For those patients with a significant history or examination, or who have a relapsing infection, a urologic evaluation is required. If the patient is consistently plagued by irritative voiding symptoms or hematuria with negative urine cultures, then the possibility of a non–infection-related inflammatory process of either the bladder, urethra, or vagina, including possible malignancy, should be considered. Although the myriad of maladies that can inflict the lower urinary tract can muddle the picture and cause difficulty in diagnosis and treatment, we can be thankful that the majority of illness that we treat in this area is the uncomplicated UTI.

SUGGESTED READINGS

1. Andriole VT: Urinary tract infections. Infect Dis Clin North Am 11:499, 1997.
2. Schaeffer AJ: Infections of the urinary tract. *In* Walsh PC, Retik AB, Vaughan ED Jr, Wein AJ (eds): Campbell's Urology, 7th ed. Philadelphia, WB Saunders, 1998, pp 533–614.

13 Lower Urinary Tract Infections in Men

Dennis R. La Rock
Grannum R. Sant

The lower urinary tract in men is a complex system that accommodates urine flow as well as the proper and timely emission of semen. Because these fluids use a final common pathway for egress, the problems associated with infection frequently affect both the genital and urinary systems. The continuity of the testicles with the prostatic urethra leaves a potential conduit through which ascending infection from the urethra can involve both the epididymis and the testicle. Infection occurs at every level of the male lower genitourinary tract. We review the common conditions that frequently come to the attention of the primary care provider.

Epididymitis

Epididymitis is an inflammation or infection of the male epididymis. It is often associated with orchitis and presents with persistent pain, edema, and a reactive hydrocele. Although it may be difficult to differentiate orchitis from epididymitis, a careful structured clinical examination of the external genitalia can usually make the distinction (Table 13–1).

ETIOLOGY AND CLASSIFICATIONS

Epididymitis is caused by infection from bladder urine, the prostate, or an ascending urethritis that spreads via the ejaculatory duct into the epididymis. The causes of epididymitis are bacterial, nonbacterial, or chemical. Bacterial epididymitis is most commonly caused by coliform bacteria via an ascending urethral route. This may be induced by direct

introduction of bacteria into the urethra during urethral instrumentation or catheterization. Other bacterial causes include sexually transmitted organisms. For instance, unprotected anal intercourse may permit direct introduction of bacteria into the urethra. Gonococcal epididymitis is another sexually transmitted type of epididymitis, and it is usually preceded by symptoms of urethritis and urethral discharge.

Nonbacterial epididymitis is usually associated with urethritis, the most common cause of which is *Chlamydia trachomatis* (Table 13–2). *Chlamydia* is a common cause of epididymitis in younger (<35 years of age), sexually active men. Other causes of nonspecific urethritis include *Ureaplasma urealyticum*. Although much less common, mycobacteria such as *Mycobacteria tuberculosis* can cause epididymitis. Tuberculous epididymitis may be on the increase in parallel with the increased prevalence of tuberculosis in North America. Tuberculosis should be considered in protracted cases of epididymitis when a bacterial pathogen cannot be isolated.

Noninfectious epididymitis is a surpris-

Table 13–1
"Structured" Physical Examination of the Scrotum

Cystic vs. solid
Tender vs. nontender
Confined to scrotum or extending into inguinal region
Anatomic position
  Testis, spermatic cord
  Epididymis
  Surrounding testis (hydrocele)
  Inguinoscrotal (hernias, hydroceles)

Table 13-2
Epididymitis

Types
Noninfectious
Infectious
    Bacteria such as coliforms
    Chlamydia

Physical Examination
    Tender, enlarged epididymis
    Associated orchitis (some cases)

Treatment Groups
>35 YEARS
    Signs and symptoms of cystitis/prostatitis
    Pyuria and bacteriuria
    Enterobacteria on urine culture
    Treat with TMP/SMX, fluoroquinolones
<35 YEARS
    Signs and symptoms of urethritis
    Pyuria
    Chlamydia
    Treat with tetracyclines or fluoroquinolones

TMP/SMX, trimethoprim-sulfamethoxazole.

ingly common entity and, as its name implies, is not caused by an infectious organism. It is a chemical inflammation caused by the reflux of sterile urine into the ejaculatory ducts. It occurs in settings of physical straining where increased abdominal pressure is transmitted to the bladder and in anatomic obstruction such as urethral strictures and congenital posterior urethral valves. This type of epididymitis is generally self-limited unless there is an anatomic anomaly. In such cases, urologic evaluation and treatment are warranted.

DIAGNOSIS

Epididymitis generally presents with "heaviness" and pain in the affected hemiscrotum.

If infectious, there can be fever, chills, dysuria, and marked edema and erythema. The differential diagnosis includes most other intratesticular pathologies. The distinction between epididymitis and testicular torsion is critical, especially in young and adolescent boys (Table 13–3). Other causes of scrotal pain and swelling include tumors (malignant and benign), hernias, hydroceles, and spermatoceles. Evaluation of the male patient with acute scrotal pain requires a careful and thorough examination of the scrotum, with particular attention to the epididymis. Urinalysis is essential, as is a rectal examination. Scrotal ultrasonographic study is an important adjunct to the physical examination in patients in whom the diagnosis is in doubt. Ultrasonography provides careful anatomic localization, and the Doppler mode can assess regional blood flow in cases of suspected testicular torsion.

TREATMENT

Epididymitis is usually treated on an outpatient basis with scrotal elevation, bedrest, and appropriate oral antibiotics. Patients with fever and leukocytosis may require hospitalization for intravenous antibiotics and close monitoring. Nonsteroidal anti-inflammatory drugs reduce scrotal discomfort and pain. Severe pain may require a spermatic cord block with a local anesthetic.

Because most infectious epididymitis is due to coliforms, oral quinolones generally provide the bacteriologic coverage and tissue levels needed for outpatient treatment. In a younger man where *Chlamydia* is suspected,

Table 13-3
Common Intrascrotal Conditions

	Testicular Torsion	Epididymitis	Testis Tumor
Symptoms			
Age	Neonate–early 20s	Childhood–old age	15–35 yr
Pain			
Nature	Sudden	Progressive	Absent or gradual
Degree	Severe	Variable	Absent or mild
Nausea/vomiting	Yes	No	No
Physical Examination			
Testis	Swollen, tender	May be swollen	Hard mass
Epididymis	Swollen, tender	Swollen, tender	Normal
Spermatic cord	Shortened	Thickened, may be tender	
Urinalysis	Normal	Pyuria, bacteriuria	Normal

doxycycline or ofloxacin provides the needed coverage. Ten days of coverage are generally sufficient for uncomplicated cases, but if bacterial prostatitis is suspected, a full 4 weeks of therapy is indicated (see later section on Prostatitis).

Most patients feel better within 48 to 72 hours, but swelling and discomfort may persist for weeks or months following bacteriologic eradication of the infecting organism. Persistent enlargement and/or induration frequently leads to a diagnosis of "chronic" epididymitis. Persistent fever in spite of adequate antimicrobial therapy suggests abscess formation and is an indication for sonographic evaluation. Surgical drainage of epididymo-orchiectomy may be required. Testicular necrosis, testicular atrophy, or infertility may complicate epididymitis. Chronic inflammation and fibrosis can block the ductal system and impair sperm production, especially in cases of severe bilateral epididymitis. Swelling and edema may compromise blood flow and lead to testicular atrophy.

Urethritis

Urethritis refers to the clinical symptoms and signs associated with urethral inflammation. It is one of the oldest urologic conditions, with references to it found in the earliest literature of antiquity. The classic symptoms include a urethral discharge, urethral burning, or itching and occasionally hematuria. Urethritis represents the end result of many causes: bacterial or nonbacterial, viral, or noninfectious immunologic causes.

ETIOLOGY AND CLASSIFICATION

The classic bacterial cause of urethritis is *Neisseria gonorrhoeae*. *N. gonorrhoeae* is a gram-negative diplococcus that may be seen on a Gram's stain of a urethral discharge. Gonococcal urethritis presents after a short incubation period of approximately 2 to 5 days as a purulent, mucoid discharge from the external urinary meatus. Occasionally the discharge initially is slight and clear but becomes purulent after about 24 hours. Patients also complain of dysuria. Untreated, the discharge subsides in about 8 weeks, and patients become completely asymptomatic in about 8 months.

Causes of nongonococcal urethritis include *C. trachomatis, U. urealyticum,* and other less common mycobacteria. They all produce irritative voiding symptoms but generally have a much less purulent urethral discharge compared with gonococcal urethritis. The discharge is generally thin, clear, and much less in amount. A significant proportion of patients have no discharge. This is important because as many as 10% of men infected with *Chlamydia* are asymptomatic. This has implications for their women partners, since *Chlamydia* is an important cause of pelvic inflammatory disease.

Less common causes of urethritis include parasitic infestations and viral infections. The most common parasite is *Trichomonas vaginalis,* a flagellated protozoa that is easily recognized by light microscopy and is transferred from an infected individual via intercourse. Viruses such as genital herpes and human papillomavirus also cause urethritis. A careful sexual history and inspection of the genitalia are therefore important in the assessment of men with urethritis.

DIAGNOSIS

When a patient with symptoms of urethritis presents for evaluation and treatment, the etiologic causes discussed earlier need to be considered (Table 13–4). To further complicate the issue, a number of noninfectious conditions, such as Reiter's syndrome, Wegener's granulomatosis, Stevens-Johnson syndrome,

Table 13–4
Urethritis

Symptoms
Urethral discharge
Irritative voiding symptoms
Associated symptoms of prostatitis/epididymitis
History of sexually transmitted diseases

Diagnosis
Urinalysis showing pyuria
Urethral swab (microscopy, cultures)

Treatment
Broad-spectrum fluoroquinolones
Tetracyclines
Metronidazole

and various chemical allergies, may manifest with urethritis.

The evaluation of a patient with urethritis includes a careful and complete medical and sexual history. In the physical examination, careful inspection of the genitalia and perineum must be performed. Because there may be perianal lesions, visual inspection and rectal examination are necessary. The external meatus must be closely inspected for the type and quality of urethral discharge, and the urethra must be swabbed for gonococcal cultures and *Chlamydia* identification (specific monoclonal antibody or an enzyme immunoassay). The swab specimen may be directly examined microscopically. In general more than four polymorphonuclear leukocytes seen in a 400-power field is enough to diagnose nongonococcal urethritis.

TREATMENT

Treatment of urethritis is aimed at complete eradication of the infection, particularly if it is gonococcal. Because of the high incidence of associated nongonococcal infection (e.g., *Chlamydia*), chlamydial coverage is advisable. Oral regimens for uncomplicated gonococcal urethritis include either a single dose of cefixime or ofloxacin plus 7 days of doxycycline. Posttreatment cultures to document cure are generally obtained about 4 to 7 days after treatment to ensure eradication, particularly if the person remains asymptomatic. In cases of human papillomavirus, therapy is aimed at eradication of the distinct lesion, and if it is noted to be within the meatus, cystoscopy is warranted to exclude urethral lesions. Treatment of warts, particularly in the urethra, can be troublesome. Trichomonal urethritis is treated with metronidazole.

Cystitis

The symptoms of cystitis are variable but include dysuria, frequency, urgency, suprapubic pain and pressure, and occasionally foul-smelling urine. In men, the additional symptoms of a narrowed urinary stream and urinary retention suggest involvement of the prostate. The incidence of simple cystitis is vanishingly small in men. The most common times of life for males to have a simple urinary tract infection (UTI) are as an uncircumcised neonate and as an elderly person, when either instrumentation or symptomatic prostate disease increases the risk of UTIs.

ETIOLOGY AND CLASSIFICATION

Cystitis is common in women and is due to a biologic predisposition manifest by adherence of pathogenetic bacteria to the vaginal mucosa and introitus. No such innate susceptibility occurs in men. In men, all UTIs should be treated as potentially complicated (see Table 13–3). Infected urine may be forced through patent ejaculatory ducts causing intraprostatic reflux of urine and prostatitis or epididymitis. Bacteriuria in young men is relatively uncommon, except in instances of anatomic anomalies and anal intercourse or with urethral instrumentation. As men age and the prostate begins to enlarge, the incidence of bacteriuria increases beginning in the fifth decade of life. With stasis of urine, cystitis with or without prostatitis becomes more common. Stasis eliminates one of the main defenses against infection; frequent and efficient bladder emptying. Neurogenic diseases such as spinal cord injury, multiple sclerosis, and diabetes mellitus also lead to impaired bladder emptying and an increased incidence of cystitis. Other anatomic factors that predispose men to cystitis include bladder outlet obstruction due to stricture disease, benign prostatic hyperplasia, and prostate cancer (Table 13–5).

Table 13–5
Cystitis

Prevalence

Uncommon in men
Associated with bacterial prostatitis, anal intercourse, uncircumcised neonates, outlet obstruction
Complicated infection

Work-up

Urologic evaluation
Radiologic imaging such as ultrasonography and intravenous pyelogram

Treatment

Specific underlying cause
Long courses of antibiotics
Need for surgical intervention such as transurethral resection of the prostate

CLINICAL EVALUATION AND DIAGNOSIS

When a patient is evaluated, confounding medical conditions need to be identified. For instance, a diabetic patient may have a poorly emptying bladder due to a subtle peripheral neuropathy, thereby increasing postvoid residuals. Patients with a past history of abdominal surgery, diverticulitis, or radiation should be queried for a history of pneumaturia that would suggest a vesicoenteric fistula. Careful attention is paid to the patient's voiding symptoms, such as dysuria, incomplete emptying, suprapubic pain, and frequency. Urinalysis reveals pyuria and possible bacteriuria. Urine cultures usually are positive and accurate in making the correct bacteriologic diagnosis. Offending organisms are generally aerobic, gram-negative bacteria, such as *Escherichia coli, Klebsiella,* or even *Pseudomonas* species. On physical examination there may be mild suprapubic tenderness on palpation, and a prostatic examination is important to help decide if there is prostatic involvement.

TREATMENT

Uncomplicated cystitis is best treated with antibacterial agents that achieve high urinary concentrations. Conventional 7- to 10-day treatment with trimethoprim-sulfamethoxazole (TMP-SMX), amoxicillin, and nitrofurantoin is safe and effective. **In enterococcal UTIs, in vitro TMP-SMX sensitivities are misleading, since in vivo the organisms can incorporate exogenous folates and escape the antibacterial action of TMP-SMX. Although uncomplicated UTIs in women are frequently treated with short courses of therapy (3 to 5 days), single-dose and short-course treatments are not recommended in men.**

All men with bacteriologically confirmed cystitis should be suspected of having a complicated UTI such as prostatitis and outlet obstruction. They deserve careful clinical and radiologic evaluation and a urologic assessment.

Prostatitis

Prostatitis is a condition of prostatic inflammation that can lead to a myriad of symptoms. It specifically refers to inflammation of the prostate but, in reality, has come to encompass any combination of irritative voiding symptoms and pain (such as perineal, pelvic, and scrotal). It has been estimated that 20% of patients presenting to a urology office have symptoms of prostatitis.

ETIOLOGY AND CLASSIFICATION

Acute bacterial prostatitis presents with symptoms of an acute cystitis and/or pyelonephritis with the sudden onset of malaise, low back and perineal pain, fever, and chills. Occasionally, patients complain of dysuria and even urinary retention. They may say that the "urine stream is narrowed." This situation may be a medical emergency. On physical examination these men are acutely ill and may appear toxic. The prostate itself may be anything from normal feeling to "boggy," but in all patients it is exquisitely tender and painful to palpation. Vigorous prostate examination is to be avoided because it can lead to bacteremia. Acute bacterial prostatitis may require hospital admission and parenteral antibiotic treatment.

The more common form of prostatitis is chronic prostatitis (Table 13–6). **About 5% to 10% of men with symptoms of chronic prostatitis have chronic bacterial prostatitis char-**

Table 13–6
Prostatitis

Types
Acute bacterial (rare)
Chronic bacterial (uncommon; 5–10%)
Chronic nonbacterial (extremely common)
　Possible infection, such as *Chlamydia*
　Prostatodynia

Diagnosis
Localization cultures
Post massage urine culture

Treatment
Antibiotics
　Acute bacterial
　Chronic bacterial
　Presumed chlamydial
Alpha blockers
　Prostatodynia
　Chronic nonbacterial
Others
　Skeletal muscle relaxants
　Biofeedback
　Exclude interstitial cystitis

acterized by the identification of bacteria (usually gram negative) in the prostatic fluid or ejaculate. This is a more prolonged, relapsing, and less severe form of prostatitis with intermittent low back and perineal pain, occasional dysuria, sexual dysfunction, and bacteriuria.

Prostate localization cultures are helpful and important in confirming the diagnosis of chronic bacterial prostatitis. This is done by collecting fractionated urine specimens as follows: the first 5 to 10 mL of urine (the voided bladder 1 [VB-1] specimen) detects urethral organisms; the next collection is the midstream urine referred to as the voided bladder 2 (VB-2) specimen that detects bladder organisms. Prostatic fluid is obtained by performing a vigorous massage of the prostate and is examined by culture and microscopically; this is referred to as the *expressed prostatic secretion* (EPS) and detects prostatic organisms. A final void called the voided bladder 3 (VB-3) specimen is a small amount of urine obtained after the prostatic massage and detects urethral and prostatic organisms. A simpler method of diagnosis is the postmassage test in which the urine obtained after prostatic massage is cultured. This approximates the EPS and/or VB-3 cultures and can be done in the primary care setting.

The pathogens causing prostatitis are the same as those that cause simple cystitis, including *E. coli, Enterobacter, Klebsiella, Pseudomonas*, or enterococcus. The problem with chronic bacterial prostatitis is that the infection is either recurrent or not completely eradicated with the first course of therapy. These patients require multiple courses of antibiotics or even chronic suppressive therapy. One potential cause of chronic bacterial prostatitis is the presence of prostatic calculi that harbor bacteria within the stone interstices.

Most prostatic calculi are clinically silent and insignificant. In fact as many as 50% of men have calculi on transrectal ultrasound examinations. Infected prostatic calculi can serve as a source of bacterial persistence and relapsing urinary infections. Such calculi harbor bacterial pathogens within the stone interstices, and consequently they cannot be sterilized with antibiotics. Permanent cure of infection can only be achieved by the success-

ful surgical removal of all infected calculi or temporized with chronic suppressive antibiotics.

Chronic nonbacterial prostatitis is a common condition in men. The symptoms generally tend to be somewhat milder than bacterial prostatitis but are nonetheless troublesome and persistent. A distinction must be made between noninfectious and infectious causes. Noninfectious prostatitis or prostatodynia is presumably caused by reflux of sterile urine into the ejaculatory ducts due to high pressure voiding. This may be caused by either internal or external sphincter spasm, and therefore therapy must be tailored to each situation. Infectious prostatitis that is nonbacterial may be due to *Chlamydia* or *Ureaplasma*. Therapy needs to be directed at these organisms. The patient's clinical presentation, past medical history, and physical examination play an important role in deciding initial therapy.

TREATMENT

The treatment of bacterial prostatitis is aimed at eradicating the offending bacteria. In acute bacterial prostatitis parenteral antibiotics may be indicated, especially if the patient is in urinary retention necessitating a suprapubic or urethral catheter. The most common agents are ampicillin and gentamicin, and further therapy may be directed by culture data. In less severe forms, outpatient therapy with oral quinolones has proven invaluable. The quinolones' high bioavailability and their penetrance into prostatic tissues make them ideal agents for treatment. They, however, must be used for at least 3 to 4 weeks for complete treatment. For patients who do not resolve on this therapy, other organisms must be considered and covered with the appropriate antibiotics, such as tetracycline for *Chlamydia*.

In men with chronic bacterial prostatitis, a number of possible treatment options exist. Oral antibiotic therapy, especially with the fluoroquinolones, effects clinical and bacteriologic cure in 60% to 70% of patients. Treatment failure after an appropriate course of antimicrobial therapy (usually 4 to 6 weeks) should alert the clinician to the possibility of infected calculi. For such patients who fail standard therapy, chronic antimicrobial suppression with TMP-SMX or nitrofurantoin is particularly useful in young men who want to avoid transurethral or open prostatectomy. Long-term administration of these antibiotics prevents the development of bladder infections and symptoms.

In older patients or patients in whom infected calculi are problematic, a transurethral resection of the prostate (TURP) can be considered. TURP can be curative if all infected calculi are removed. To achieve the latter, the resection needs to extend beyond the false, "surgical" capsule to the "true" capsule to remove the infected calculi and tissue from the posterior prostate lobes. Such a "radical TURP" for infected prostatic calculi requires an aggressive resection to remove as many infected stones as possible.

For patients with chronic noninfectious prostatitis (nonbacterial, prostatodynia), therapy is varied and empirical. Alpha blockers such as terazosin, doxazosin, and tamsulosin are used to combat the pelvic floor and prostatic muscle spasm believed to be present. These should be titrated to the maximal dose to achieve the greatest treatment effect with the least side effects. Most patients with noninfectious prostatitis (prostatodynia) have some response to this therapy. Unfortunately, most patients who stop taking medication relapse, making this a chronic problem with long-term therapy. Other treatments include skeletal muscle relaxants such as diazepam, pelvic floor education with biofeedback, and prostatic thermotherapy. Some patients with noninfectious prostatitis may actually have interstitial cystitis, and they respond to definitive treatment of that condition.

SUGGESTED READINGS

1. Berger RE: Urethritis and epididymitis. Semin Urol 1:38–45, 1983.
2. Krieger JN: Epididymitis, orchitis, and related conditions. Sex Trans Dis 11:173–182, 1984.
3. Meares EM Jr: Nonspecific infections of the genitourinary tract. *In* Tanagho EA, McAninch JW (eds): Smith's General Urology. Norwalk, CT, Appleton & Lange, 1992, pp 195–239.
4. Nickel JC: Rational management of nonbacterial prostatitis and prostatodynia. Curr Opin Urol 6:53–58, 1996.
5. Roberts RO, Lieber MM, Bostwick DG, Jacobsen SJ: A review of clinical and pathological prostatitis syndromes. Urology 49:809–821, 1997.

14 Uncommon Infections of the Genitourinary Tract

John Battin
Unyime O. Nseyo

This chapter discusses primarily the uncommon infections of the genitourinary tract, including tuberculosis and parasitic infections. However, tuberculosis can no longer be regarded as an uncommon infection in the United States. The concern is that the incidence of tuberculosis is increasing, and tuberculosis is becoming endemic in many parts of the world, including inner cities of the United States. The primary physician knows that this resurgence in tuberculosis is a major public health concern. Although the parasitic infections are rare, they are important from a public health standpoint.

Tuberculosis

Epidemiology

Since 1985 the incidence of tuberculosis has been increasing. One reason for this increase is the growing population of immunocompromised people secondary to an increased incidence of human immunodeficiency virus (HIV) infection and a larger number of people who have received organ transplantation. Immigration from countries where tuberculosis is more common is also an important source. In the United States the estimated incidence of tuberculosis is approximately 13 in 100,000 people. *Mycobacterium tuberculosis* commonly infects people between 25 and 44 years of age.

Pathogenesis

Most tuberculosis cases in the United States are caused by the aerobic organism *M. tuber-*culosis. This organism is an extremely slow-growing bacteria, which leads to its relative resistance to antibiotics. Tuberculosis is spread by small-particle aerosols generated by coughing and sneezing in infected people. After establishing infection in the lungs, *M. tuberculosis* spreads hematogenously to the kidney. This is usually the primary site of genitourinary involvement, although the prostate or epididymis can occasionally be the site of introduction to this system. All other genitourinary organs become involved via descent or ascent of bacteria. A low-grade inflammatory response develops in the small vessels near the glomeruli. This leads to granuloma formation consisting of giant cells surrounded by lymphocytes and fibroblasts. If bacteria continue to multiply, larger tubercles form, with caseating necrosis of renal tissue. Small abscesses can occur. Lesions may eventually slough into the renal collecting system, leading to bacilluria and spread to the lower genitourinary tract. With healing, calcium salts may be deposited, producing calcified lesions (Fig. 14–1). By impairing perfusion to a portion of renal parenchyma, hypertension may develop.

Ureteral tuberculosis is almost always an extension of renal infection. Because it usually occurs at the ureterovesical junction, distal ureteral obstruction may occur. This process usually occurs insidiously with the patient most often being asymptomatic. This slow, progressive narrowing and obstruction of the ureter can lead to hydronephrosis and autonephrectomy.

Bladder involvement usually occurs sec-

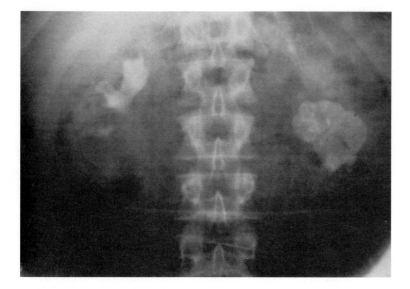

Figure 14-1
Calcification from tuberculosis in a kidney. (From Walsh PC, Retik AB, Vaughan ED Jr, Wein AJ [eds]: Campbell's Urology, 7th ed. Philadelphia, WB Saunders, 1998, p 814.)

ondarily from descent of bacteria from the kidneys. Most lesions start around the ureteral orifices. Late in the infection, ulcers may develop from tubercle breakdown. These patients can have sterile pyuria.

Prostatic tuberculosis is usually found incidentally at transurethral resection of the prostate (TURP). Spread to the prostate is either hematogenous or from descent of infection from the kidneys or bladder. Chronic infection of the prostate may lead to the creation of large calcified lesions. In advanced disease, perianal sinuses can develop.

Because the epididymis is well vascularized, spread of tuberculosis to this organ occurs hematogenously, as well as by direct extension of disease. Epididymitis may result as the primary and only presenting symptoms of genitourinary tuberculosis. With advanced disease, the vas deferens may develop nodularity. The testicle may become involved by direct extension. If a palpable nodule remains after full antibiotic treatment, testicular exploration is necessary to rule out malignancy.

Clinical Features

Genitourinary tuberculosis can present with a wide range of signs and symptoms. Early bladder complaints may include frequency starting at night and eventually occurring during the day. Women and children may complain of this symptom earlier in the course of the disease. Urgency usually occurs

with more advanced disease progression. Ureteral colic rarely occurs given the insidious nature of the obstruction caused by this infection. Renal and suprapubic pain are also late signs of disease. In advanced disease of the epididymis or testicle, a chronically draining sinus of the scrotum can occur. Clinical features of tuberculosis such as anorexia, loss of weight, and lassitude are late signs of this disease. The vas may feel "beaded" and thickened on examination. One or both epididymides can be thickened as well. On rectal examination, the prostate can feel nodular or indurated if involved. Flank pain to percussion is usually a late sign. Men often present with a swollen and tender scrotum as a result of epididymitis. Patients are often treated for urinary tract infections, but symptoms continue in spite of antibiotic therapy. About 20% of patients with bladder tuberculosis have superimposed *Escherichia coli* cystitis. Although urine cultures are usually negative, up to 80% of patients have more than 20 white blood cells per high-power field (hpf) on microscopy. Up to 50% of patients with this disease have microhematuria. Gross hematuria occurs in approximately 10% of patients with genitourinary tuberculosis. Hematospermia is also a rare finding, although tuberculosis should be ruled out if this is a recurrent problem.

Diagnosis

If genitourinary tuberculosis is suspected, urinalysis and three early-morning urine cultures should be obtained. Urine specimens should be as fresh as possible. Acid-fast staining of urine sediment may be positive in some cases. A subdermal tuberculin test using a protein-purified derivative of tuberculosis (PPD) should be performed. Maximum inflammatory response to this test occurs at 48 to 72 hours. A wheal more than 10 mm in diameter at the site of injection is usually considered positive. A 5-mm reaction is considered positive in those people who have had close contact with tuberculosis patients, in those with radiographic findings consistent with old healed tuberculosis, and in HIV-infected patients.

Laboratory studies should include a complete blood count, sedimentation rate, electrolytes, and blood urea nitrogen (BUN) and creatinine. Plain radiographs of the abdomen and pelvis should also be performed looking for calcified lesions in the kidneys, ureters, bladder, prostate, or scrotum. If genitourinary tuberculosis is suspected, an intravenous urogram can be helpful. Calyceal distortion or deformities may be apparent. Some describe the kidney as appearing "moth-eaten" (Fig. 14–2). Ureteral strictures or other lesions may also be defined. Renal scans are not usually necessary but may be helpful in determining the degree of function of an involved kidney. Computed tomographic (CT) scanning is also of little use in the evaluation of these patients but may be useful if malignancy is suspected. When the bladder is involved, cystoscopy may demonstrate erythematous lesions or ulcers. Cystoscopy is usually of low yield but plays an important role in ruling out malignancy when biopsies are performed.

Treatment

Culture and sensitivity studies should be performed prior to instituting any antibacterial therapy. For initial empiric treatment, a four-drug regimen, including isoniazid, rifampin, pyrazinamide, and either ethambutol or streptomycin for the first 8 weeks is recommended (Table 14–1). Isoniazid and rifampin are then used for the next 4 months, for a total of 6 months of therapy. The doses are as follows: isoniazid 300 mg orally; rifampin 600 mg orally daily; pyrazinamide 1.5 to 2 gm orally daily; streptomycin 1 g intramuscularly

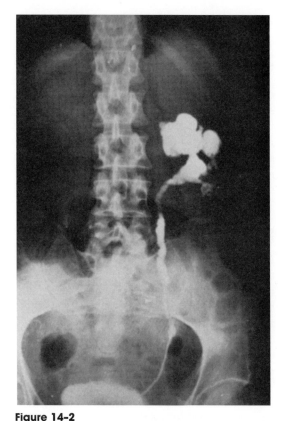

Figure 14-2
Severe calyceal and parenchymal destruction. (From Walsh PC, Retik AB, Vaughan ED Jr, Wein AJ [eds]: Campbell's Urology, 7th ed. Philadelphia, WB Saunders, 1998, p 821.)

daily; and ethambutol 25 mg/kg orally daily. Because of the increasing incidence of resistant organisms, this drug therapy may have to be tailored to the sensitivities of the organism.

Table 14-1
Classification of Antituberculosis Drugs

Classification	Agent	Activity
Primary agents	Rifampicin Isoniazid Pyrazinamide Streptomycin	Bacteriocidal
Secondary agents	Ethambutol Ethionamide Cycloserine	Bacteriostatic
Minor agents	Kanamycin Thiocetazone	Bacteriostatic

From Walsh PC, Retik AB, Vaughan ED Jr, Wein AJ (eds): Campbell's Urology, 7th ed. Philadelphia, WB Saunders, 1998, p 824.

Prognosis

The prognosis varies with the extent of disease; however, the overall control rate at 5 years is approximately 98%. It is important to check urine cultures every 3 to 6 months after starting therapy and then once a year for up to 10 years. Nephrectomy is almost never needed if the disease is caught in its early stages. Most long-term morbidity is due to secondary complications such as ureteral stricture and vesical contracture.

SECONDARY TUBERCULOSIS

Many patients with bladder cancer each year are treated intravesically with bacille Calmette-Guérin (BCG), an attenuated tuberculin bacterium (*Mycobacterium bovis*). This effective treatment for superficial transitional cell carcinoma of the bladder can cause many side effects. Most adverse reactions are limited to dysuria, hematuria, and low-grade fever. These mild symptoms can be treated with acetaminophen, diphenhydramine, and phenazopyridine (Pyridium). If these symptoms persist or become more severe, an immediate urology consultation is warranted. On rare occasions a potentially lethal secondary infection can lead to BCG sepsis. The diagnosis of BCG sepsis is generally not difficult. Patients typically, but not invariably, develop high fever, shaking chills, and then hypotension. Mental confusion, disseminated intravascular coagulopathy, respiratory failure, jaundice, and leukopenia may occur. While these reactions cannot be differentiated from gram-negative sepsis that occurs following instrumentation of the genitourinary tract, the temporal association with BCG administration makes coverage for BCG sepsis mandatory. Cultures of blood, urine, and bone marrow are typically negative in BCG sepsis, so treatment must be initiated on the basis of clinical suspicion.

When BCG sepsis does occur, consult with a urologist and start isoniazid 300 mg, rifampin 600 mg, and prednisone 40 mg daily. Prednisone is continued until sepsis abates and is then tapered for an additional 1 to 2 weeks. Isoniazid and rifampin are continued for 3 to 6 months, depending on the severity and duration of the reaction. It is important to proceed with antibiotic treatment when systemic BCG infection is suspected without waiting for culture results. Cultures are typically negative even with progressive infection.

HIGHLIGHTS

- Tuberculosis spreads hematogenously to the kidney from the lungs.
- Renal destruction can occur in the asymptomatic patient.
- Consider in patients with recurrent sterile pyuria.
- Kidney may appear classically "moth-eaten" in an intravenous urogram.
- A total of 6 months of antituberculosis therapy is required.
- The prognosis is excellent if treatment is instituted early in the course of this disease.
- Nephrectomy is usually not required.
- BCG sepsis is a potentially lethal disease that warrants an immediate treatment and urology consultation.

Schistosomiasis

Epidemiology

Schistosomiasis is caused by the parasitic blood fluke *Schistosoma haematobium*. It is endemic in the Middle East and throughout Africa, especially Egypt. Conservative estimates are that more than 200 million people worldwide are infected by this organism. Eighty to 90 million of those infected have genitourinary involvement. Furthermore, up to 60% of these patients demonstrate some degree of urinary obstruction. In endemic regions, schistosomiasis is a common cause of squamous cell carcinoma of the bladder and bladder calculi.

Pathogenesis

S. haematobium is the species most responsible for schistosomiasis involving the genitourinary tract. Larvae are found in infested fresh waters. Freshwater snails serve as intermediate hosts. Worms can penetrate the unbroken skin of humans and enter the blood stream. At 4 to 7 days, worms congregate in the lungs, and then invade the liver at 2 weeks. Adult worms then disseminate to the vesico-prostatic plexus of veins. Adult worms, which are approximately 1.5 cm long, can live here for 3 to 4 years before they die. They can produce 200 to 500 eggs per day. About 20% of ova penetrate the bladder wall and are released into the urine (Fig. 14–3). The remainder of eggs may become entrapped, initiating an inflammatory response that infiltrates the bladder wall, which is responsible for many of the symptoms and sequelae of this disease. T-cell-dependent granulomas and tubercles develop in the affected viscera, causing fibrosis and contracture of the bladder or stricture of the ureter. Chronic bilharzial ulcerations may develop in the bladder. Epithelial metaplasia and squamous cell carcinoma are frequent sequelae. Secondary bacterial infections are common. Extensive calcification of the bladder, lower ureters, and seminal vesicles can occur resulting from calcium salt deposition around dead ova. Ure-

teral obstruction can occur insidiously with progression of disease often resulting in severe hydronephrosis. In up to 25% of advance cases, ureteral reflux occurs.

Clinical Features

Within 4 to 7 days of onset of acute schistosomiasis, patients can develop a cutaneous hyperemia and a pruritic reaction. Patients also experience fatigue, malaise, and low-grade fevers. Up to 60% of patients complain of dysuria. As the disease progresses, painless gross hematuria can occur in about 30% of those infected. Irritative bladder symptoms such as frequency and urgency worsen as the patient develops secondary infections, bladder ulcerations, and malignancy. Patients may complain of incontinence or dribbling of urine. Flank pain is almost always a late complaint and is secondary to ureteral obstruction and hydronephrosis. These signs and symptoms are the most common with this disease. How-

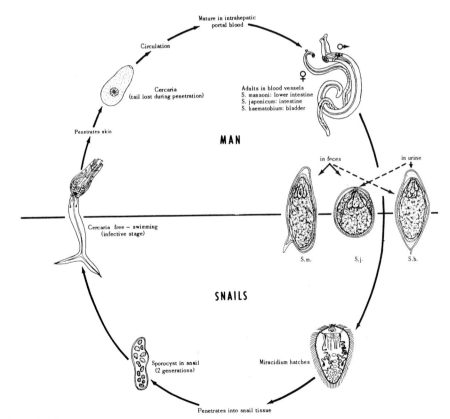

Figure 14-3
Life cycle of a schistosome. (From U.S. Department of Health and Human Services, Public Health Service Publications. Washington, DC, U.S. Government Printing Office, 1964.)

ever, most patients with chronic schistosomiasis exhibit few symptoms. On examination, lymphadenopathy and splenomegaly may be detected. Late in the course of the disease, patients may have a palpable suprapubic mass due to bladder carcinoma. Rectal examination may demonstrate an asymmetric firm prostate, enlarged seminal vesicles, or thickened bladder base. In older patients with advanced disease, perineal urinary fistulas can occur.

Diagnosis

Any time schistosomiasis is suspected, one must rule out malignancy and genitourinary tuberculosis. Definitive diagnosis of genitourinary schistosomiasis is dependent on the microscopic recognition of the ova in the urine sediment. These eggs have a characteristic terminal spine (Fig. 14–4). These eggs are almost always present in moderate and severe infections. Since egg laying is diurnal, urine is optimally obtained at mid-day. Viable eggs in the urine represent active infection. Secondary bacterial infection of the bladder is commonly detected. A complete blood count shows eosinophilia and hypochromic normocytic anemia in many cases. Detection of schistosome antigens in the blood and urine is now possible. They are detected by immunoassay and have about 100% specificity and

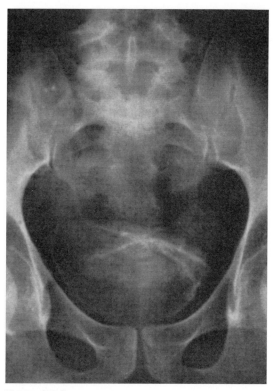

Figure 14–5
Bladder calcification of patient infected with *Schistosoma haematobium*. (From Walsh PC, Retik AB, Vaughan ED Jr, Wein AJ [eds]: Campbell's Urology, 7th ed. Philadelphia, WB Saunders, 1998, p 740.)

a high sensitivity. Most of these assays are expensive and are not in widespread use. Antibody detection methods exist but have not been particularly useful to the practicing clinician. On plain abdominal radiograph, bladder calcification is practically pathognomonic for chronic schistosomiasis (Fig. 14–5). An intravenous urogram can identify hydronephrosis, ureteral strictures, and a small contracted, irregular bladder. Ultrasonography can be helpful in making the diagnosis of schistosomiasis by demonstrating hydronephrosis, renal or ureteral calculi, or calcification of the bladder. Compared with other methods, ultrasonography is relatively sensitive and specific. Because it is portable, it is useful in rural endemic regions. All patients should undergo cystoscopy and biopsy to rule out malignancy.

Management

Two drugs are important in the medical management of *S. haematobium*. Praziquantel is the

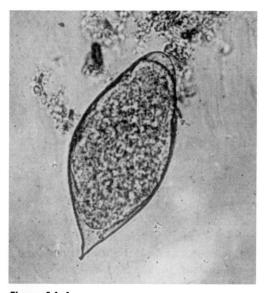

Figure 14–4
Egg of *Schistosoma haematobium*. (Courtesy of WTIM.)

drug of choice and is effective in all species of schistosome that infect humans. A single oral dose of 40 mg/kg is usually sufficient. Side effects include headache, dizziness, fever, fatigue, pruritus, and skin eruptions. None of these are usually long lasting and most resolve spontaneously. Metriphonate is an organophosphorus compound also commonly used in the treatment of *S. haematobium*. Standard dosing is 7.5 to 10 mg/kg given orally in three doses at an interval of 14 days. Side effects are usually minor and are similar to those caused by other acetylcholinesterase inhibitors. Surgical intervention may be necessary in patients with chronic schistosomiasis and its resultant sequelae. Ureteral strictures may require excision and neo-ureterocystostomy. In cases of squamous cell carcinoma of the bladder, a radical cystectomy with urinary diversion may be necessary.

Prognosis

The prognosis of these patients is related directly to the extent of their disease as lesion reversibility declines with progressive stages. It is important to check the urine for clearance of ova every 3 to 6 months for the first year, then at least annually for 10 years. The overall control rate is about 98% at 5 years. Medical cure occurs in more than 80% of those patients adequately treated.

HIGHLIGHTS

- Genitourinary schistosomiasis is most commonly caused by the blood fluke *S. haematobium*.
- Schistosomiasis is a common cause of squamous cell carcinoma of the bladder in endemic regions.
- Radiographically, extensive calcification of the bladder can be seen.
- Painless gross hematuria occurs in about 30% of infected patients.
- Eggs of *S. haematobium* found in urinary sediment have characteristic terminal spines.
- Praziquantel is the drug of choice for treatment of all *Schistosoma* species.

Aspergillosis

Epidemiology

Aspergillus fumigatus, *Aspergillus flavus*, and *Aspergillus niger* are responsible for most cases of aspergillosis in humans. These organisms are ubiquitous in soil, garbage, and bird excreta. Aspergillosis is an important opportunistic infection that afflicts debilitated patients with malignancy, diabetes mellitus, or those otherwise immunosuppressed. Those patients with severe neutropenia are particularly at risk for this infection. In one large study, of patients diagnosed with primary aspergillosis, 94% had pulmonary involvement and 13% had renal involvement.

Pathogenesis

Aspergillosis is usually acquired through the inhalation of airborne conidia by a susceptible host. In the kidney, aspergillosis can result in the development of multiple small abscesses with vascular occlusion and multiple small renal infarcts. "Fungus balls" can occur in the renal collecting system, causing obstruction of the renal pelvis or ureter. Prostatic involvement has been reported.

Clinical Features

Patients may present with fever and flank pain. Most patients with renal aspergillosis also have some degree of pulmonary involvement and may present with hemoptysis, wheezing, and dyspnea. Pleuritic symptoms can occur.

Diagnosis

Blood cultures in systemic disease usually are negative. Definitive diagnosis can be determined by tissue biopsy and periodic acid–Schiff or methenamine silver staining (Fig. 14–6). Tissue can be cultured on Sabouraud's medium. The complete blood count often demonstrates eosinophilia. Serum precipitating antibodies to *Aspergillus* antigens are present in 70% to 100% of cases. Fluffy pulmonary infiltrates can often be seen on chest radiograph. Intravenous urogram can demonstrate filling defects or deformities in the collecting

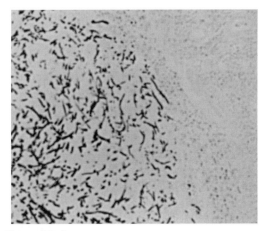

Figure 14–6
Photomicrograph of aspergillar mycelium in renal collecting system. (Hematoxylin & eosin with silver stain.) (From Irby PB, Stoller ML, McAninch JW: Fungal bezoars of the upper urinary tract. J Urol 143:447, 1990.)

system. Sites of urinary obstruction may also be identified.

Management

Currently, amphotericin B is viewed as the drug of choice for aspergillosis. The recommended dose is 0.8 to 1 mg/kg daily. The optimal length of treatment has yet to be determined. However, total doses of more than 1.3 g for up to 2 months with flucytosine (8 g daily) have been used effectively for the treatment of recalcitrant pulmonary infections. Recently, itraconazole has been approved by the U.S. Food and Drug Administration for the treatment of invasive aspergillosis refractory to amphotericin B. The loading dose is 600 mg daily orally for 4 days, then 200 mg twice daily. For aspergillosis of the urinary collecting system, amphotericin B irrigation via a nephrostomy tube has been used effectively as an adjunct to systemic therapy. When urinary obstruction occurs, nephrostomy tube or ureteral stent placement may be necessary until resolution of the disease. Occasionally, nephrectomy may be required in advanced disease.

Prognosis

The prognosis for these patients is improved with remission of the underlying disease and early diagnosis with aggressive treatment.

HIGHLIGHTS

- Aspergillosis is an important opportunistic infection that afflicts debilitated patients with malignancy, diabetes mellitus, or those otherwise immunosuppressed.
- Aspergillosis is usually acquired through the inhalation of airborne conidia by a susceptible host.
- Fungus balls can occur in the renal collecting system causing obstruction of the renal pelvis or ureter.
- Definitive diagnosis can be determined by tissue biopsy and periodic acid–Schiff or methenamine silver staining.
- Amphotericin B is viewed as the drug of choice.
- The prognosis for these patients is improved with remission of the underlying disease and early diagnosis with aggressive treatment.
- For aspergillosis of the urinary collecting system, amphotericin B irrigation via a nephrostomy tube has been used effectively as an adjunct to systemic therapy.

Filariasis

Epidemiology

Filariasis is endemic in countries bordering the Mediterranean, south China, and Japan. It is estimated that at least 79 million people are currently infected. It is usually caused by the filarial worm, *Wuchereria bancrofti*, which is responsible for about 90% of lymphatic filariasis. This threadlike worm is transmitted from person to person via mosquito. Most patients infected with this organism do not demonstrate clinical sequelae.

Pathogenesis

Filariasis is spread by transfer of the larvae from person to person via mosquitoes. After a minimum of 8 months, microfilariae appear in the blood of the host. Microfilariae are then ingested by the vector female mosquitoes during a meal. Larvae develop in the mosquito over a period of 10 to 12 days. Larvae migrate to the mouth parts of the mosquito and can enter humans during feeding. Larvae then migrate to human lymphatics, with a predilection for periaortic, iliac, inguinal, and intrascrotal nodes. Here they develop into mature worms and can live for many years (Fig. 14–7). Most related clinical sequelae are a result of the obstruction of these lymphatics. Acute bouts of lymphangitis and lymphadenitis become recurrent, occurring several times a year. Lymph vessels harboring worms become dilated with mild inflammation (Fig. 14–8). Chyluria from ruptured lymphatic varices around the collecting system may develop early in the course of the disease. Eventually, the lymph nodes become enlarged and matted. As the lymphatics of the genitalia become obstructed, lymphedema involving the scrotum and penis develops. Early in the course of this disease, the edema resolves spontaneously. However, in chronic disease, a nonpitting edema occurs, with skin thickening and loss of elasticity. It is not uncommon for adjacent veins to become inflamed and thrombosed. Funiculitis or epididymoorchitis can occur. Lymphangitis can lead to hydrocele formation. Sterile abscesses can develop beneath the rectus fascia of the lower abdomen. Lymphatic fistulas can develop near the calyces, leading to hypoalbuminemia and anasarca.

Clinical Features

Many patients develop an abrupt onset of fever, acute groin pain with swollen, tender lymph glands, and edema in the lower extremities during an acute attack of filariasis. **Funiculitis with acute pain and swelling of the spermatic cord may exist at presentation.** Patients may complain of milky colored urine secondary to chyluria. On examination, signs of acute inflammation such as local heat and redness may not be present. A painless lymphadenovarix of the inguinal regions can exist. As mentioned earlier, lymph nodes may feel matted and rubbery on palpation. Large hydroceles develop. The spermatic cord and epididymis can feel thickened and boggy when inflamed. Abscesses can be detected in the lower abdomen or inguinal region. Elephantiasis of the lower extremities, penis, and scrotum is not uncommon (Fig. 14–9). Early in the course of the disease, the edema is pitting in nature. However, later this massive edema becomes nonpitting as the skin becomes thickened.

Diagnosis

The presence of the aforementioned signs and symptoms should raise strong suspicion for

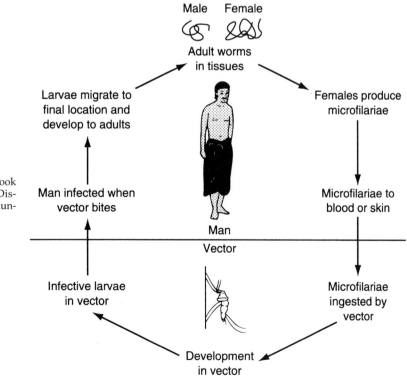

Figure 14–7
Life cycle of filariae. (From Cook G [ed]: Manson's Tropical Diseases, 20th ed. London, WB Saunders, 1996.)

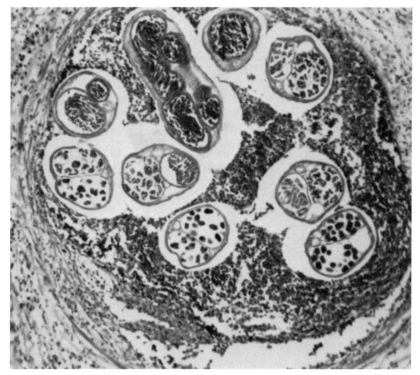

Figure 14-8
Photomicrograph of adult *Wuchereria bancrofti* in lymphatics of epididymis. (From Walsh PC, Retik AB, Vaughan ED Jr, Wein AJ [eds]: Campbell's Urology, 7th ed. Philadelphia, WB Saunders, 1998, p 759.)

filariasis, especially in endemic regions. Serum laboratory studies often demonstrate hypoproteinuria, eosinophilia, and sometimes microfilariae. An indirect hemagglutination titer of 1/128 is considered diagnostic. Demonstration of microfilariae in chylous urine or hydrocele fluid is also diagnostic. Chyluria can be detected on urinalysis with layering of the urine. Histologic discovery of adult worms in tissue is definitive. Monoclonal antibody–based tests for circulating antigens are available and appear to be quite specific for the detection of *W. bancrofti* antigen.

Management

The most common drug used for treatment of *W. bancrofti* is diethylcarbamazine citrate (DEC). This form of chemotherapy kills adult worms and eliminates microfilariae. Systemic reactions include joint and body pain, dizziness, headache, anorexia, vomiting, and malaise. Fever may also occur and appears to be related to the severity of the infection. Local reactions such as swelling and pain over the

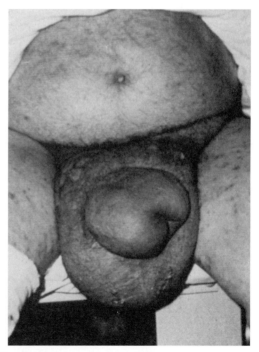

Figure 14-9
Elephantiasis of penis and scrotum. (Courtesy of Dr. M. Wittner. Reproduced from Zaiman H: A Pictorial Presentation of Parasites. Available from H. Zaiman, MD, PO Box 543, Valley City, ND 58072.)

lymph nodes are not uncommon. Another drug used in the treatment of this disease is ivermectin. Given in a single oral dose of 150 µg/kg, ivermectin has proved to effectively remove microfilariae. The side effects from this drug are similar to DEC therapy.

Surgical treatment for lymphatic filariasis includes excision of chronic hydroceles and grossly elephantoid skin. Usually the penis and scrotal contents can be preserved. Chyluria can usually be initially treated conservatively with DEC and restriction of dietary fats. However, if this approach proves to be ineffective, surgery may be necessary. Disruption or disconnection of the renal hilar lymphatics can be performed.

Analgesics and antipyretics should be used in conjunction with DEC for the treatment of symptoms. Bedrest and elevation of the scrotum and involved limbs should also be instituted.

Mosquito control is a significant proven prophylactic measure in the prevention of filariasis.

Prognosis

Prognosis is dependent on the extent of exposure and disease in individuals. If exposure has been limited, most people experience spontaneous resolution of their disease and the prognosis is excellent. Once medication is started, the progression of this disease usually ceases.

HIGHLIGHTS

- Filariasis is usually caused by the filarial worm, *W. bancrofti,* which is responsible for about 90% of lymphatic filariasis.

- This threadlike worm is transmitted from person to person via mosquito.
- As the lymphatics of the genitalia become obstructed, lymphedema involving the scrotum and penis develops.
- Elephantiasis of the lower extremities, penis, and scrotum is not uncommon.
- The most common drug used for treatment of *W. bancrofti* is DEC.
- Chyluria can usually be initially treated conservatively with DEC and restriction of dietary fats.
- Mosquito control is a significant proven prophylactic measure in the prevention of filariasis.
- Once medication is started the progression of this disease usually ceases.

SUGGESTED READINGS

1. Cook GC (ed): Schistosomiasis. *In* Manson's Tropical Diseases, 20th ed. Philadelphia, WB Saunders, 1996, pp 971–1013.
2. Gow J: Genitourinary tuberculosis. *In* Walsh PC, Retik AB, Vaughan ED Jr, Wein AJ (eds): Campbell's Urology, 7th ed. Philadelphia, WB Saunders, 1998, pp 807–836.
3. Reese R, Betts R: Genitourinary tract infections. *In* A Practical Approach to Infectious Diseases, 4th ed. Boston, Little, Brown, 1996, pp 511–513.
4. Sant G: Inflammatory diseases of the bladder. *In* Gillenwater JY, Grayhack JT, Howards SS, et al (eds): Adult and Pediatric Urology, 3rd ed. St. Louis, Mosby-Year Book, 1996, pp 1334–1335.
5. Smith JH, von Lichtenberg F: Parasitic diseases of the genitourinary system. *In* Walsh PC, Retik AB, Vaughan ED Jr, Wein AJ (eds): Campbell's Urology, 7th ed. Philadelphia, WB Saunders, 1998, pp 733–778.
6. Tanagho E (ed): Specific infections of the genitourinary tract. *In* Smith's General Urology, 14th ed. Norwalk, CT, Appleton & Lange, 1995, pp 245–259.
7. Wise GJ: Fungal infections of the urinary tract. *In* Walsh PC, Retik AB, Vaughan ED Jr, Wein AJ (eds): Campbell's Urology, 7th ed. Philadelphia, WB Saunders, 1998, pp 779–806.

15 Voiding Dysfunction and Urinary Incontinence in Women

Raul C. Ordorica

Urinary incontinence and voiding dysfunction can affect women of all ages. While the majority of these patients do not have a life-threatening disorder, the panorama of pelvic floor pathology can be significantly debilitating. Many patients do not tell their physician either due to embarrassment or the belief that reasonable treatments do not exist. Not only is it possible for the primary care physician to begin the initial diagnosis but often effective therapies can be initiated. While this is within the realm of the nonurologist, it should be emphasized that the best results are obtained by those clinicians who are appropriately equipped and committed to the care of women with pelvic floor pathology. This chapter defines bladder dysfunction in the female patient, its evaluation, and the various therapies available. The intent is not for the primary care provider to become the sole expert in caring for these disorders but rather to develop a basis for cooperative care strategies with other professionals. Thus, true continuity of care can be developed from the initial interview to even the most complex intervention.

Overview of Lower Urinary Tract Anatomy and Physiology

The urinary bladder is made of overlapping layers of detrusor smooth muscle with an inner lining of transitional epithelium. It is controlled by both sympathetic and parasympathetic innervation. To act as a low-pressure reservoir during storage, sympathetic inhibition of parasympathetic efferent nerve fibers results in the accommodation of increasing volumes of urine with minimal increases in intravesical pressure. Sensory nerve terminals within the bladder signal when the bladder is full and voiding is initiated if socially appropriate. During the voiding phase the sympathetic inhibition ceases and parasympathetic stimulation results in a coordinated and sustained contraction of the detrusor fibers with a resultant increase in bladder pressure.

The bladder outlet and urethra consist of multiple components that are interdependent for proper function. The bladder neck is formed by coalescing muscle and collagen fibers that open the bladder neck on voiding. The midportion of the female urethra is surrounded by striated slow-twitch nonfatiguing muscle fibers that form the external sphincter. It remains contracted during storage and relaxes during voiding in a coordinated pattern with the bladder as regulated by the sacral reflex arc. The epithelium of the urethra is able to form a seal against leakage due to the pliant, spongy characteristics of the underlying support tissue. The elastic characteristics of this support tissue are in part due to its vascular nature, which along with the remainder of the bladder outlet, is influenced by estrogen. The bladder neck and urethra are supported in position by the vagina and the endopelvic fascia, surrounded by the levator musculature.

The function of the bladder is to allow for low-pressure accommodation of urine during the storage phase and to contract to produce a sustained increase in intravesical pressure during the voiding phase. The purpose of the urethra is to maintain a pressure greater than that of the bladder during storage and to relax during emptying to permit low-pressure, efficient voiding. Therefore any dysfunction can be separated into those that involve failures in either storage or emptying as a result of an imbalance between the components of the lower urinary tract (Table 15–1). Storage failures result in urinary frequency, urgency, and incontinence, and for emptying failures there are varying degrees of voiding dysfunction culminating in urinary retention.

ALTERATIONS IN BLADDER ACTIVITY

Increased Bladder Activity

Increased activity of the bladder can result in increases in intravesical pressure. The patient may sense the need to void resulting in urinary urgency and frequency. If the vesical pressure exceeds outlet resistance, there is resultant urinary incontinence. Because the patient can often sense this increase in pressure, it is termed *urge incontinence.* This form of incontinence can often be more troubling to the patient in comparison to stress urinary incontinence (see decreased bladder outlet resistance). This is because not only can the volume of urine leaked be greater, with the patient spontaneously emptying her entire bladder, but it can occur with little if any warning.

Many patients can develop detrusor hyperactivity without any detectable neuropathy. It can be found with increasing prevalence in older populations. A particular form of increased bladder activity resulting in frequency and urge incontinence has been characterized in the geriatric population. In addition, the patient is unable to maintain a sustained detrusor contraction to efficiently empty her bladder. These combined effects of

Table 15–1
Classification of Lower Urinary Tract Dysfunction

> #### Failure to Store
> Increased bladder activity
> Increased bladder sensation
> Decreased outlet resistance
>
> #### Failure to Empty
> Decreased bladder activity
> Decreased bladder sensation
> Increased outlet resistance

Table 15–2
Causes of Neurogenic Bladder

> #### Supratentorial
> CVA
> Parkinson's disease
> Alzheimer's disease
> Cerebral palsy
>
> #### Spinal cord
> Spinal cord injury
> Spinal stenosis
> Central cord syndrome
> ALS
> Multiple sclerosis
> Myelodysplasia
>
> #### Peripheral Neuropathy
> Diabetes
> Alcohol
> Shingles
> Syphilis

CVA, cerebrovascular accident; ALS, amyotrophic lateral sclerosis.

urge incontinence with incomplete emptying have been termed *detrusor hyperactivity, incomplete contractility.*

A multitude of neuropathologic conditions can result in increased bladder activity (Table 15–2). Those that are supratentorial result in the coordinated release of urine given an intact sacral reflex arc, however, at socially inappropriate times. **Lesions of the spinal cord can result in dyssynergic voiding, along with alterations in bladder compliance with elevated bladder pressures and the potential for hydronephrosis and renal injury. Indeed, it is important for patients with neurogenic bladder to have lifelong monitoring for the development of hydronephrosis to prevent irreversible upper tract damage.**

Decreased Bladder Activity

The inability for the bladder to contract results in an elevation in residual urine following voiding. If the patient is unable to void at all, retention with overflow incontinence may result. Decreased bladder activity may result from either neuropathic or myopathic conditions. Neuropathic conditions may be temporary in nature, as with increases in sympathetic tone caused by pain following operative procedures, or during the acute phase of spinal cord injury. Permanent neuropathic conditions can result from both central and peripheral lesions (see Table 15–2). Myopathy can result from stretch injury of the detrusor fibers as with an episode of marked retention or the chronic delaying of voiding.

ALTERATIONS IN BLADDER SENSATION

Increased Bladder Sensation

Hypersensitivity of the bladder is manifested as the increased urge to void at low volumes. This can result from inflammatory conditions of the bladder such as urinary tract infection, radiation cystitis, or interstitial cystitis. Any irritative focus such as a foreign body, infiltrating tumor, or transitional cell carcinoma in situ can contribute to this. This situation typically presents with urinary frequency and urgency. Although incontinence rarely ensues in the individual with otherwise normal bladder dynamics, the compromised individual such as an elderly patient or one with a concomitant neuropathic condition may experience urinary leakage that otherwise would not normally be present.

Interstitial cystitis is a chronic idiopathic inflammatory condition of the bladder with potentially crippling results. Patients with interstitial cystitis typically complain of pelvic pain along with their irritative voiding symptoms. Although their symptoms include severe frequency and urgency, their detrusor is not hyperactive and any incontinence is incidental. Most patients have relatively normal compliance, with isolated cases of marked fibrosis and contracture of the bladder.

Decreased Bladder Sensation

A loss in bladder sensation can result in the inability to sense bladder fullness. With this, either spontaneous voiding may ensue, with perceived incontinence, or there is continued stretch injury of the detrusor muscle. A prolonged stretch injury with muscle hypoxia can lead to permanent loss of the contractile ability of the detrusor. This condition is outlined in the aforementioned description (see section on decreased bladder activity).

ALTERATIONS IN OUTLET FUNCTION

Increased Outlet Resistance

Increased outlet resistance can result from either neuropathic, behavioral, or anatomic conditions. Sustained or increased sympathetic tone, as outlined in conditions of decreased bladder activity, can result in failure of the bladder outlet and urethra to relax. In addition it has been found that there are those individuals who since early development do not sufficiently relax their outlet for coordinated voiding in the absence of any detectable neuropathology. This "pseudodyssynergia" may be associated with active contraction of the levator muscles with increased outlet resistance as the patient strains to void. This has been described as *nonneurogenic neurogenic bladder,* and it can lead to severe alterations in bladder dynamics and resultant renal deterioration.

Actual congenital anatomic abnormalities of the female urethra that result in increased bladder outlet resistance are rare. While acquired urethral strictures and stenosis are also uncommon, iatrogenic alterations of the bladder outlet secondary to bladder neck surgery for urinary incontinence are not. Performance of operative procedures to correct stress urinary incontinence and pelvic prolapse with overcorrection can result in pathologic increases in urethral resistance. Less common sources of outlet resistance are conditions such as urethral prolapse or urethral carcinoma, both of which should be evident on physical examination.

Increases in urethral resistance can result in difficulties with voiding with symptoms of decreased force of stream, straining, incomplete emptying, frequency, and double voiding. Possible outcomes include retention and overflow incontinence. In addition, the increased urethral resistance and elevated voiding pressures can result in detrusor irritability and hyperactivity, resulting in urgency and urge incontinence.

Decreased Outlet Resistance

This condition of decreased outlet resistance is the most emphasized of all female bladder dysfunctions. This is due not only to the prevalence of the condition but also to the fact

Table 15–3
Activities Associated with Leakage

Decreased Outlet Resistance
Coughing
Laughing
Sneezing
Lifting
Exercise
Running
Increased Bladder Activity
Running water
Hand washing
Change in position
Cold temperatures

that of all the bladder pathologies, it is the most amenable to surgical correction. Any condition that compromises the normal bladder outlet, including pelvic floor relaxation, decreases in sphincter function, or loss of mucosal coaptation, can contribute to decreased outlet resistance. This results in urinary stress incontinence. It has been attempted to separate this condition into either "genuine" stress incontinence characterized by bladder neck and urethral malposition versus intrinsic sphincter deficiency (ISD), implying defects in urethral muscle and mucosal integrity. However, it has been increasingly recognized that varying degrees of ISD are potentially involved in most, if not all, forms of decreased outlet resistance.

Patients with decreased bladder outlet resistance present with urinary leakage during those maneuvers that increase intra-abdominal pressure (Table 15–3). Because patients tend to leak when their bladder is full, they may tend to void at lower volumes to minimize the potential for "accidents," thereby resulting in urinary frequency. The leakage of urine and resultant skin breakdown may cause an increase in bacterial colonization of the perineum and vagina with more pathologic organisms, resulting in an increased rate of urinary tract infections.

Diagnosis

HISTORY AND PHYSICAL EXAMINATION

The history should qualify the pattern of voiding and any leakage and detect possible bladder or pelvic pathology (Table 15–4). The inciting events that result in leakage may give insight as to the underlying pathology (see Table 15–3). Specific questions should be posed, for patients may not realize that although the urgency, frequency, and nocturia is "normal" for them, it may characterize an underlying and treatable condition. Fluid intake, including type and volume, should be elicited. A voiding diary in which the patient records her volume intake, time and volume of voids, presence of any symptoms, and episodes of leakage can be helpful not only to clarify history but to monitor therapy. Pertinent past medical history would include any therapies that have previously been tried and their results. Past surgical and obstetrical history should be sought. Factors that might exacerbate difficulties with bladder control or impact on therapy, such as strenuous activity, obesity, or chronic obstructive pulmonary disease, should be considered.

Physical examination should include the back, lower abdomen, and pelvis (Table 15–5). The presence of any scars might signify prior surgery. Lower abdominal examination can check for any masses, bladder fullness, or areas of tenderness. The perineum may show evidence of chronic urinary leakage with skin excoriation. The vagina and introitus should be examined for atrophy. The urethra can be palpated for any tenderness or fullness that might detect the presence of urethritis, urethral diverticulum, or a urethral carcinoma.

Table 15–4
History

Voiding Symptom Checklist
Voided volume
Frequency
Urgency
Nocturia
Quality of stream
Double void
Sense of complete emptying
Straining
Leakage
Pelvic Pathology Checklist
Sense of dropping (prolapse)
Constipation
Fecal incontinence
Difficulty with stool evacuation
Dyspareunia
Pelvic pain
Vaginal bleeding

Table 15–5
Physical Examination

Back: CVA tenderness, spinal deformity/tenderness
Abdomen: suprapubic tenderness/fullness
Introitus: skin integrity, urethral meatus, prolapse
Vagina: atrophy, urethra, cystocele, enterocele, rectocele
Maneuvers: leak with cough/strain
Neurologic examination: T12–L1, S2–4
Laboratory studies: UA, creatinine

CVA, costovertebral angle; UA, urinalysis.

Pelvic examination should include observation of bladder position, the detection of any descensus, and the presence of any leakage with stress maneuvers. While the demonstration of leakage is of assistance, the inability to demonstrate it during the office examination does not rule out its presence. The presence of cystocele, enterocele, or rectocele, uterine size and position, presence of any pelvic masses, or areas of tenderness should be identified. The entire examination can be performed efficiently and with minimal patient discomfort using a single-speculum blade.

Sympathetic enervation to the bladder is through the T-12, L-1 roots, whereas parasympathetic enervation is through S-2, S-3, and S-4. Therefore, a focused neurologic examination is performed looking at the correlating dermatomes along the perineum and anus. **An intact sacral reflex arc can be detected by eliciting the bulbocavernosus reflex, in which the anal sphincter contracts with squeezing of the clitoris. Motor ability can be tested by voluntary contraction of the anal sphincter, contraction of the levator musculature of the pelvis, or dorsiflexion of the big toe.**

LABORATORY TESTS

Urinalysis is to be performed to rule out the presence of urinary tract infection or hematuria. Other findings such as proteinuria, crystalluria, or casts may signify the presence of upper tract diseases but would be incidental findings. **The chronic findings of low specific gravity may lend support to polyuria either from diabetes insipidus or polydipsia. Glucosuria may be the presenting finding for those patients with diabetes mellitus.** Urine culture and sensitivity should be performed for those patients with evidence of a urinary

tract infection by urinalysis. The presence of sterile acid pyuria may signify the presence of urinary tuberculosis.

Urine cytology is reserved for those patients in whom it is suspected that a neoplastic process involving the bladder is present (Table 15–6). This includes patients with hematuria in the absence of urinary tract infection, sensory urgency, or a prior history of bladder cancer. It is known that cigarette smoke and aniline dyes can contribute to the development of transitional cell carcinoma of the bladder. Chronic urinary tract infection and foreign bodies such as that found with indwelling catheters or untreated bladder calculi can contribute to the formation of squamous cell carcinoma of the bladder.

Serum creatinine measurement should be performed in those patients with urinary retention to rule out obstructive uropathy. This is a rare finding in women. Patients with a neuropathic cause for their voiding dysfunction with the potential for detrusor sphincter dyssynergia with chronically elevated bladder pressures, such as in spinal cord injury, myelodysplasia, or multiple sclerosis, should also be evaluated. The measurement of serum creatinine in these individuals can give only a rough estimate of renal deterioration following significant progression and should not be solely relied on (see diagnostic procedures). In addition, patients with severe sensory urgency either from interstitial cystitis or pelvic radiation can have fibrotic contracted bladders with decreased compliance. Elevated bladder pressures in these individuals or associated lower ureteral pathology can result in upper tract deterioration.

DIAGNOSTIC PROCEDURES

The initial evaluation of voiding dysfunction and incontinence can be performed in the

Table 15–6
In Whom Should We Suspect Cancer?

Isolated sensory urgency
Hematuria without UTI
Prior history of cancer
Cigarette smoke exposure
Aniline dye exposure
Chronic indwelling catheter
Chronic UTI
Schistosomiasis

UTI, urinary tract infection.

majority of patients without complex diagnostic procedures. The history is the most important element and should suggest if the patient is having a dysfunction of either bladder storage or emptying. The role of additional diagnostic procedures depends on the specific questions one is attempting to answer.

To determine if a patient is emptying completely, a postvoid residual should be measured. This can be performed with intermittent catheterization following voiding. Ultrasound provides a noninvasive modality, and low-cost specialized units are available. Therapy may not always need to be based on a single result, as wide variation may exist for a single individual. If multiple measurements are required either to confirm this finding or to alleviate the condition, then patients can be taught to perform this on their own. An elevation of postvoid residual marks either decreased bladder activity or increased outlet resistance. Elucidation of this requires urodynamic evaluation.

Urodynamic evaluations are typically performed by the urologist in an office setting. This may include a cystometrogram, which tests the storage phase of the bladder. A multilumen catheter is placed within the bladder. Pressure is continuously monitored as the bladder is filled, and notation is made of the patient's sensation during the study. The capacity and compliance of the bladder are determined, along with presence of any involuntary bladder contractions. This can be helpful in evaluating patients with urgency, frequency, nocturia, and urge incontinence (increased bladder activity). The patient may be asked to strain or cough, and the pressure at which leakage occurs is determined. These maneuvers are helpful in evaluating patients with stress incontinence (decreased outlet resistance).

The voiding phase can also be evaluated by measuring bladder pressure during emptying and in this way determine if there is an appropriately sustained detrusor contraction with coordinated relaxation of the urethral sphincters for efficient emptying. This can give insight into underlying neuropathology that might affect this coordination versus acquired dysfunctional voiding, decreased bladder activity, or fixed anatomic increases in

outlet resistance. In addition these studies can be performed with a radiographic contrast agent used as the medium, allowing fluoroscopic observation of the bladder and outlet during the study. All studies are performed on an outpatient basis without the requirement for anesthesia with little if any discomfort. No preparation is required.

Cystoscopy can be performed to evaluate the anatomy of the urethra and bladder. This is helpful in confirming the diagnosis of cystocele, for making evaluations following prior surgery, and in ruling out additional bladder pathology. The requirement to rule out bladder pathology is especially significant when one suspects the presence of bladder carcinoma, as in the case of microscopic hematuria or with sensory urgency without demonstrated urinary tract infection.

The initial evaluation of many patients with mild forms of urge or stress incontinence does not necessarily have to include endoscopic or urodynamic testing. However, if there is a history of failed therapies or complicating factors, then a urologic referral is advised.

Therapy

Therapies range from noninvasive to surgical. While the former can be easily instituted from the office setting, it does not follow that it should be used in all patients. An example for appropriate noninvasive therapy is the motivated compliant patient with mild stress incontinence (decreased outlet resistance). In contrast, there are those patients that are poor candidates for success by conservative measures, and the best initial therapy may in fact be surgical. This would include the patient with continuous leakage who had failed a surgical therapy with marked *decreased outlet resistance* (ISD). Table 15–7 provides a list of potential therapies for each of the bladder and outlet dysfunctions. Rather than adhering to strict guidelines for each given diagnosis, therapy should be tailored for the individual patient.

BEHAVIORAL THERAPY (increased bladder activity, increased bladder sensation, decreased bladder sensation)

There is usually some potential benefit with the use of behavior modification. There may

Table 15-7
Therapy Options for Bladder or Outlet Dysfunction

Presentation	Dysfunction	Therapy	Comment
Failure to store	Increased bladder activity	Behavior therapy Physical therapy Medical therapy Pessary Electrical neuromodulation Surgical augmentation	Conservative, nonsurgical therapies should be exhausted prior to surgical therapy
Failure to store	Increased bladder sensation	Behavior therapy Physical therapy Medical therapy Electrical neuromodulation Surgical replacement	Conservative, nonsurgical therapies should be exhausted prior to surgical therapy
Failure to store	Decreased outlet resistance	Physical therapy Medical therapy Surgical repair	Surgical therapy tends to be more successful than other methods; medical therapy is least effective
Failure to empty	Decreased bladder activity	Behavior therapy Medical therapy Intermittent catheterization Indwelling catheter Electrical neuromodulation	Other therapies should be exhausted prior to resorting to indwelling catheter; myogenic failure will not respond to electrical neuromodulation
Failure to empty	Decreased bladder sensation	Behavior therapy	Chronic bladder overdistention can lead to myogenic failure (decreased bladder activity)
Failure to empty	Increased outlet resistance	Physical therapy Medical therapy Intermittent catheterization Valves Electrical neuromodulation Surgical repair	Must define if due to functional (physical therapy, medical therapy, electrical neuromodulation) or anatomic causes (surgical repair); intermittent catheterization or valve can be used for either form

not be complete cure with some of the more conservative therapies but rather measures of improvement with the patient better able to cope with her condition. Behavior modification is based on the concept that the bladder dysfunction is dependent on bladder volume, and steps are taken to control this. Fluid intake can be reduced and the patient can void at more frequent intervals. In addition, the types of fluids can be modified, such as reducing caffeinated beverages that might stimulate detrusor activity, thus increasing urinary frequency and urgency. This form of therapy can be beneficial in initial treatment of urge incontinence (*increased bladder activity*), or sensory urgency (*increased bladder sensation*). It is not unusual that many patients have made these adjustments in their lifestyle by the time they seek treatment, and there may be little room for maneuvering if they have already restricted their volume intake and are voiding frequently to prevent incontinent episodes.

Another form of behavior modification can be used for decreased bladder sensation. The patient is unable to detect when the bladder is full, and capacities more than 500 mL can

result in decompensation of the detrusor muscle (decreased bladder activity). By increasing the frequency of voiding the final volume is decreased and a more normal bladder function can be achieved. To determine the appropriate interval for voiding, the patient must monitor her fluid intake and urinary output. This can be performed by rough estimation and voiding by the clock. To achieve more accurate results, personal ultrasound bladder volume monitors are available. These monitors can be applied intermittently, or they can be worn continuously with alarms set at specific volumes to alert the patient to empty her bladder.

Finally, for those patients with *increased bladder sensation*, in which they void at markedly low intervals, their bladder can be trained to hold more. A voiding diary is kept to establish their "normal" voiding interval. They are then asked to incrementally increase this on a weekly basis until an interval is reached that is more compatible with a normal lifestyle. An example of this is to go from voiding every 45 minutes to every 2 hours, achieved over several months. Key to all these forms of therapy is the motivated patient who is able to keep an accurate diary with aggressive follow-up and encouragement.

PHYSICAL THERAPY (increased bladder activity, decreased outlet resistance, increased outlet resistance)

Physical therapy is used to recondition the pelvic floor musculature and influence function of both the urethra and the bladder. Contraction of the pelvic floor results in the closing of the bladder outlet and shutting off the urinary flow. There is also indirect stimulation of the urethral rhabdosphincter. Both of these mechanisms are beneficial in treating stress urinary incontinence *(decreased outlet resistance)*. They appear to be more effective in lesser degrees of incontinence and do not cure gross anatomic defects such as pelvic prolapse or significant scarring. The closing of the bladder outlet has an indirect effect on bladder behavior with inhibition of detrusor contractions, thus reducing urgency and urge incontinence as well *(increased bladder activity)*. Therefore, they are often the first-line therapy for the appropriately chosen patient with either or both forms of incontinence.

Exercises of the pelvic floor are begun with voluntary contractions of the levator musculature. The evaluation for pelvic floor exercises begins with the initial physical examination when the patient contracts the pelvic floor on command. Patients with a strong contraction who have been performing pelvic floor exercises consistently may not benefit from continued use. However, those patients who either have not reliably performed the exercises or are unable to maintain an adequate contraction may benefit from proper training. The ability to properly contract the pelvic floor requires a hands-on approach by both the staff and patient. A finger placed in the vagina can sense the strength and duration of the contraction. Additional information can be achieved if the patient is able to interrupt her stream while voiding. Once the techniques are mastered, the exercise can be performed anywhere and anytime. A typical routine would be to perform three series per day of a dozen pelvic floor contractions, each sustained for 5 seconds. Given the compliance required to achieve good results, it often requires much more than a one-time cursory

instruction that is afforded by many simple patient handouts.

If the exercises are not reliably performed, then they can be verified by the use of biofeedback either in the office setting or at home. This can be done using a mechanical method, as in the use of Femina Cones, in which vaginal cones of increasing weight must be held in place, thus requiring the patient to accurately contract the pelvic floor. More sophisticated biofeedback monitors are available that can sense the pelvic contraction along with other musculature. This is to ensure adequate contraction and isolation of the targeted muscle. Finally, electrical stimulation can be directly applied by the use of a vaginal probe to provide the stimulus for muscle contraction. The more "invasive" methods typically rely on specifically trained nursing staff and physiotherapists for their use. Similar to behavioral therapy, the performance of physical therapy requires time, commitment, and ability by both the physician and the patient.

Physical therapy also can play a role in other forms of pelvic floor dysfunction, such as that responsible for *increased outlet resistance*. Some patients are unable to adequately relax their pelvic floor to allow for voiding. Therefore, they are taught relaxation techniques allowing them to voluntarily relax their pelvic floor. The degree of pelvic floor hyperactivity can result in spasm of the pelvic floor muscles and resultant marked discomfort. This can be identified with physical examination with the localization of affected areas. The use of trigger point therapy to relieve the spasm can result in marked improvement in symptoms, particularly in patients with *increased bladder sensation*. These methods require a knowledgeable physical therapist familiar with complete pelvic floor rehabilitation.

PHARMACOLOGIC THERAPY

Increased Bladder Activity

For those patients who are not good candidates for behavioral or physical therapy, or who have achieved maximal benefit from their use, medical therapy is often the next line used for *increased bladder activity* (Table 15–8). There is marked variation in the re-

Table 15-8
Medical Therapy for Increased Bladder Activity

Medication	Effect	Side Effects	Dose	Comment
Oxybutinin (Ditropan)	Antispasmodic, musculotropic	Xerostomia Dry skin Blurred vision Constipation Nausea	2.5–5 mg two or three times daily	Dry mouth most troubling; avoid with narrow-angle glaucoma; decrease dose in elderly patients
Tolterodine (Detrol)	Antispasmodic, musculotropic	Xerostomia Blurred vision Constipation	2 mg twice daily	Decreased side effects in comparison to oxybutinin
Dicyclomine (Bentyl)	Antispasmodic, antimuscarinic	Xerostomia Dry skin Blurred vision Constipation Nausea	20 mg two or three times daily	Similar profile to oxybutinin
Propantheline (ProBanthine)	Antimuscarinic	Xerostomia Dry skin Blurred vision Constipation Nausea	15–30 mg every 4–6 hours	Similar profile to oxybutinin
Hyoscyamine (Levsin, Levsinex, Cystospaz, Cystospaz M)	Antimuscarinic	Xerostomia Dry skin Blurred vision Constipation Nausea	0.125 mg four times daily 0.375 mg twice daily	Better tolerated than oxybutinin
Flavoxate (Urispas)	Antispasmodic	Xerostomia Dry skin Blurred vision Constipation Nausea	100–200 mg three or four times daily	Less effective, better tolerated than oxybutinin
Imipramine (Tofranil)	Tricyclic antidepressant	Weakness, fatigue, parkinsonian effect	25 mg nightly to four times daily	Avoid with MAO inhibitors; potential cardiotoxicity

MAO, monoamine oxidase.

Table 15-9
Medical Therapy for Increased Bladder Sensation

Medication	Effect	Side Effects	Dose	Comment
Phenazopyri-dine (Pyridium)	Topical urethelial analgesic	Orange staining Headache Rash Pruritus Nausea	200 mg three times daily	Caution with impaired renal function: methemoglobinemia
Pentosan polysulphate sodium (Elmiron)	Replenish mucopoly-saccharide lining of bladder	Anticoagulant Alopecia Diarrhea Nausea	100 mg three times daily	For interstitial cystitis
Amitriptyline (Elavil)	Tricyclic antidepressant	Sedative Anticholinergic effects	50–150 mg daily	For interstitial cystitis; avoid prompt withdrawal; potential cardiotoxicity
Dimethyl sulfoxide (Rimso-50)	Histamine release	Bladder irritation Garlic odor on breath	50 mL every 2 weeks for 3–6 doses	For interstitial cystitis; intravesical administration

sponse by patients to a given medication, such that some patients achieve marked results from medical therapy, whereas others derive no apparent benefit. One needs to pay close attention to the side effect profile, for which most of the therapies are typically started at a fraction of the available doses and titrated for the patient's ability to tolerate. For patients who require maximal medical therapy, combinations of medications can be used, such as adding oxybutynin and imipramine together.

Increased Bladder Sensation

The primary therapy in the treatment of increased bladder sensation is to treat the un-derlying cause for the problem. An example would be the antibiotic therapy of a lower urinary tract infection, rather than relying on phenazopyridine. Other than phenazopyridine, the agents listed in Table 15–9 are used for interstitial cystitis. Prior to starting what could be prolonged therapy for this debilitating disease, it is important to rule out the presence of infection or malignancy, which includes the requirement for a cystoscopic examination.

Decreased Outlet Resistance

While medical therapy is available to theoretically increase bladder outlet resistance (Table 15–10), and thus benefit patients with de-

Table 15-10
Medical Therapy for Decreased Outlet Resistance

Medication	Effect	Side Effects	Dose	Comment
Estradiol cream (Estrace)	Hormone	Breakthrough uterine bleeding Breast tenderness	2–4 g daily for 2 weeks, followed by 1–2 g daily for 2 weeks, followed by 1 g three times a week thereafter	Increased risk of endometrial cancer; avoid with breast cancer or thromboembolic disorder
Phenylpropanolamine	Alpha agonist	Elevated blood pressure	50 mg four times daily	Minimally effective; found in combination with multiple cold remedies
Pseudoephedrine (Sudafed)	Alpha agonist	Elevated blood pressure	30–60 mg four times daily	Minimally effective

Table 15-11
Medical Therapy for Decreased Bladder Activity

Medication	Effect	Side Effects	Dose	Comment
Bethanechol (Urecholine)	Muscarinic	Abdominal cramps Nausea	10–50 mg three or four times daily	Anecdotal benefit; use with alpha blockers
Metoclopramide (Reglan)	Increase acetylcholine activity	CNS effects Extrapyramidal reactions Galactorrhea	5–10 mg three or four times daily	Anecdotal benefit; use with alpha blockers

creased outlet resistance, there is little evidence of their effectiveness as individual treatment. The benefits of estrogen to improve mucosal integrity and prevent urinary tract infection may substantiate its use, particularly prior to surgical therapy. The limited effectiveness and side effect profile of alpha-agonist therapy typically prohibits its chronic use.

Decreased Bladder Activity

Despite its long history of use, there is not strong evidence to support the use of bethanechol for decreased bladder activity (Table 15–11). This is due to the findings that the increase in detrusor tone that results from its use not only does not translate into a sustained and coordinated bladder contraction but also is consistently opposed by a simultaneous increase in outlet resistance. Be that as it may, there are anecdotal reports of its effectiveness, particularly when combined with an alpha blocker to reduce bladder outlet resistance. Similar statements can be made of metoclopramide, which is used in an anal-

ogous fashion for diabetic gastroparesis in which gastric emptying is encouraged by increasing gastric motility and decreased pyloric sphincter contraction. It also has had anecdotal success either when used alone or in conjunction with alpha blockers.

Increased Outlet Resistance

The bulk of success involving alpha blockers remains in the treatment of male patients with benign prostatic hypertrophy (Table 15–12). For those women with fixed anatomic obstruction, surgical correction is best sought. For those patients with functional obstruction, a trial of these medications is reasonable, although none has clear superiority over another in terms of effectiveness. Therefore, if a patient is able to tolerate a maximal dose of one of these medications without success, then additional courses of the other forms is not warranted. In the absence of surgically corrected disease, physical therapy, intermittent catheterization, and perhaps electrical neuromodulation are strongly encouraged.

Table 15-12
Medical Therapy for Increased Outlet Resistance

Medication	Effect	Side Effects	Dose	Comment
Prazosin (Minipress)	Nonselective $alpha_1$ blocker	Orthostatic hypotension	1–4 mg two or three times daily	Least expensive form, titration required, tolerated by normotensive patients
Doxazosin (Cardura)	Nonselective $alpha_1$ blocker	Orthostatic hypotension	1–10 mg nightly	Titration required, tolerated by normotensive patients, scored tablets
Terazosin (Hytrin)	Nonselective $alpha_1$ blocker	Orthostatic hypotension	1–10 mg nightly	Titration required, tolerated by normotensive patients
Tamsulosin (Flomax)	Selective $alpha_{1a}$ blocker		0.4–0.8 mg daily	Titration not required

INTERMITTENT CATHETERIZATION
(decreased bladder activity, increased outlet resistance)

Of all the technologic breakthroughs regarding bladder pathophysiology and its management, none has had as profound an effect as the adoption of intermittent self-catheterization as a reliable, safe, and effective means for bladder management. For any given cause of a patient's failure to empty *(decreased bladder activity, decreased bladder sensation, increased outlet resistance)*, intermittent catheterization can be used to manage the condition. By using clean intermittent catheterization, voluntary urinary control is maintained with an infection and complication rate far less than that with an indwelling catheter. The hurdle that must be overcome is the patient's acceptance of the procedure. This can be achieved with proper teaching, encouragement, and support. Teaching is begun in the office, with training pamphlets and videos available. The patient must be followed closely, or else it is often discontinued. Subsequent measurement of her postvoid residual volumes provides feedback regarding the necessity of continuing this course.

INDWELLING CATHETER (increased
bladder activity, decreased outlet resistance, decreased bladder activity, decreased bladder sensation, increased outlet resistance)

A chronic indwelling Foley catheter provides continuous low-pressure bladder drainage. While it can be used to treat practically all failures of storage or emptying (except *increased bladder sensation*), there are some significant drawbacks to this form of therapy. Despite sterile methods of insertion and closed-drainage systems, the prolonged presence of a foreign body is a source of chronic bacterial colonization, increasing the risk of infection and stone formation. Catheters can be coated or impregnated with materials to reduce the degree of bacterial entrance along the catheter, but the risk for infection cannot be eradicated. Long-term indwelling catheter use can lead to bladder and urethral irritation, increasing the risk of squamous cell carcinoma. Patients who require chronic indwelling catheters for many years should be monitored for bladder malignancy, a task that currently requires cystoscopy. The use of non-latex catheters can result in less irritation than standard latex catheters and has been shown to be beneficial in reducing urethritis in the male population. The female urethra tends to dilate around the indwelling catheter, resulting in incontinence. Exchanging the catheter with a larger size is a temporary and limited solution, with subsequent further dilation and eventual leakage. A suprapubic tube can be inserted to bypass the urethra, but if performed to treat a markedly incompetent urethra, it should be accompanied with surgical correction or closure of the bladder neck. Thus, in most cases, an indwelling catheter is used only after exhausting other methods of therapy.

PESSARIES, SEALS, PLUGS, AND
VALVES (increased bladder activity, decreased outlet resistance, decreased bladder activity, increased outlet resistance)

Pessaries have classically been used to maintain the proper position of pelvic organs. Recent designs have been developed to support the bladder neck and thus treat *decreased outlet resistance* that is associated with bladder neck descensus (Introl device). Precise fitting is required as performed in the physician's office.

While the pessary may support and perhaps compress the urethra, a seal directly applied over the meatus has been designed to also treat *decreased outlet resistance* (Rejuvinate meatal cap). It has a cap in place to permit voiding. It requires fitting to provide an effective seal, and not all pelvic anatomy is conducive for its use. As another form of a urethral seal, a disposable urethral plug has been developed that is placed into the urethra with a small retention balloon inflated within the bladder (Reliance). It is deflated when the patient desires to void. While most often used for *decreased outlet resistance*, it also has some utility for *increased bladder activity,* because its presence within the urethra results in inhibition of bladder activity in some patients. As a variation on this, a urethral plug has also been designed with a valve mechanism that allows for the device to remain in place as the patient voids (Autocath 100). This makes the device applicable for *increased bladder activity, decreased outlet resistance, decreased bladder activity,* and *increased outlet resistance.*

While attractive in principle, these occlusive devices are invasive and require a high degree of patient ability and compliance. It is unusual for patients to fall within this category and not also be good surgical candidates with excellent results. In addition, these devices are prone to result in bacterial colonization and infection. Thus they usually are best reserved as either a temporary measure or resorted to for those patients who are not surgical candidates.

ELECTRICAL NEUROMODULATION
(increased bladder activity, increased bladder sensation, decreased bladder activity, increased outlet resistance)

As mentioned in the section on physical therapy, electrical stimulation can be directly applied to the pelvic floor musculature to cause contraction. Electrical stimulation can be applied using other modalities to alter bladder function. Direct stimulation or neuromodulation of the S-3 nerve roots accessed through the sacral foramina results in a decrease in detrusor activity and resultant urge incontinence *(increased bladder activity).* There may also be benefit in regards to voiding and pelvic floor dysfunction *(increased bladder sensation, decreased bladder activity, increased outlet resistance).* Following an initial percutaneous test stimulation, a permanent pacemaker can be implanted. Even though the U.S. Food and Drug Administration granted approval in 1997, experience is limited and this mode of therapy is currently reserved for patients who do not respond to more conservative measures such as behavioral, physical, or medical therapy.

SURGICAL THERAPY (increased
bladder activity, increased bladder sensation, decreased outlet resistance, increased outlet resistance)

While a full description of all the surgical options is beyond the scope and intent of this chapter, some insight into the urologist's armamentarium may be helpful. The majority of attention has been given to *decreased outlet*

resistance or stress urinary incontinence. Therapies include urethral injections of bulking agents that are performed under local anesthesia as ambulatory procedures, vaginal approaches with overnight stays, laparoscopic procedures, and open abdominal procedures. Success rates are high, complications low, and voiding is preserved. Additional pelvic pathology can be addressed simultaneously. Ideally, the proper therapy is chosen based on the clinical situation, the patient's desire, and the surgeon's ability. Given the myriad of therapies available and their success, many patients appropriately choose surgery for decreased outlet resistance as their initial therapy, bypassing other more conservative approaches.

Surgery for *increased outlet resistance* is best performed for patients with fixed anatomic obstruction that can be technically addressed. Examples of this are urethral prolapse, carcinoma, stenosis, and iatrogenic overcorrection. Given these examples, medical or physical therapy rarely plays a role, as compared to functional obstruction. Isolated urethral surgery and reconstruction is typically performed using a vaginal approach with minor hospital stays.

Surgery for *increased bladder activity* is usually resorted to when conservative therapies have failed. This may involve denervation procedures, bladder augmentation with intestine, or urinary diversion. Given the need often for extensive open surgery with the requirement for ongoing management, it is expected that the less invasive therapies are first exhausted. However it can be stated that with the urologist's complete surgical armamentarium, the motivated and able surgical candidate can achieve urinary control with the preservation of renal tissue, in practically all cases.

Conclusion

Voiding dysfunction and incontinence covers a wide range of bladder and urethral pathology. A comprehensive approach is to categorize the dysfunction into those alterations of bladder and urethral function as noted in Table 15–1. A systematic approach to their diagnoses can be initiated by the primary care physician, with specialized evaluations performed as required. Patients should be referred to those specializing in the care of these patients if there are implications of underlying pathology that is of significance or conservative therapies are unsuccessful. In many cases therapy can be instituted by the primary care physician in a stepwise fashion, with marked benefit for the patient. Given the motivated patient and the capabilities of both the primary physician and the specialist, excellent results can be expected for women with either voiding dysfunction or urinary incontinence.

SUGGESTED READINGS

1. Blaivas JG, Romanzi LJ, Heritz DM: Urinary incontinence: Pathophysiology, evaluation, treatment overview, and nonsurgical management. *In* Walsh PC, Retik AB, Vaughan ED Jr, Wein AJ (eds): Campbell's Urology, 7th ed. Philadelphia, WB Saunders, 1998, pp 1007–1043.
2. Klutz CG, Raz S: Evaluation and treatment of the incontinent female patient. Urol Clin North Am 22:481, 1995.
3. Leach GE, Dmochowski RR, Appell RA, et al: Female Stress Urinary Incontinence Clinical Guidelines Panel summary report on surgical management of female stress urinary incontinence. J Urol 158:875, 1997.
4. Resnick NM, Yalla SV: Geriatric incontinence and voiding dysfunction. *In* Walsh PC, Retik AB, Vaughan ED Jr, Wein AJ (eds): Campbell's Urology, 7th ed. Philadelphia, WB Saunders, 1998, pp 1044–1058.
5. Urinary Incontinence Guideline Panel. Urinary Incontinence in Adults: Clinical Practice Guideline. AHCPR Publication No. 92-0038. Rockville, MD, Agency for Health Care Policy and Research, Public Health Service, U.S. Department of Health and Human Services, March 1992.
6. Webster GD, Kreder KJ: The neurourologic evaluation. *In* Walsh PC, Retik AB, Vaughan ED Jr, Wein AJ (eds): Campbell's Urology, 7th ed. Philadelphia, WB Saunders, 1998, pp 927–952.
7. Wein AJ: Neuromuscular dysfunction of the lower urinary tract and its treatment. *In* Walsh PC, Retik AB, Vaughan ED Jr, Wein AJ (eds): Campbell's Urology, 7th ed. Philadelphia, WB Saunders, 1998, pp 953–1007.
8. Wein AJ: Pathophysiology and categorization of voiding dysfunction. *In* Walsh PC, Retik AB, Vaughan ED Jr, Wein AJ (eds): Campbell's Urology, 7th ed. Philadelphia, WB Saunders, 1998, pp 917–926.

SUPPORT GROUPS

1. Simon Foundation for Continence, P.O. Box 815, Wilmette, IL 60091.
2. National Association for Continence (NAFC), P.O. Box 8310, Spartanburg, SC 29305-8310.

16 Voiding Dysfunction in Men with Lower Urinary Tract Symptoms and Benign Prostatic Hyperplasia

Ashutosh Tewari
Perinchery Narayan

More than 15 million men in the United States are older than 50 years of age. This population group is expected to double in the next 50 years. Fifty percent of these men (17.2 million) will develop microscopic benign prostatic hyperplasia (BPH), of which half (8.6 million) will develop lower urinary tract symptoms (LUTS).

Lower Urinary Tract Symptoms

LUTS in men can occur as a result of several factors, including BPH, systemic illnesses, and medications.

Table 16–1 summarizes the various causes of LUTS. Several systemic and nervous system disorders can produce LUTS. These include cerebrovascular accidents (70% may have symptoms in the acute phase); parkinsonism (voiding dysfunction occurs in 25% to 75% of patients; 25% to 30% of patients with parkinsonism have associated BPH); multiple sclerosis (50% to 88% have voiding symptoms); diabetes mellitus (DM; DM occurs in 20% of men older than 65 years of age; 40% may have voiding symptoms); and alcoholism (third most common disorder in men 65 years of age or older). It is important to differentiate the predominant causes of LUTS to ensure proper management. When LUTS is secondary to extraprostatic causes, management of primary disease often results in a resolution of symptoms.

Table 16–2 summarizes commonly used medications that may result in urinary symptoms. Polypharmacy is a common problem in geriatric populations. Medications such as antihistaminics, diuretics, prostaglandin inhibitors, nicotine, clonidine, diazepam, calcium channel blockers, theophylline, isoniazid, amphetamine, lithium, and antidepressants all can cause various urologic symptoms.

BPH

BPH is the most common underlying etiologic factor in men with LUTS. The hyperplastic tissue is predominantly in the periurethral portion of the prostate gland. The relative proportion of adenoma versus supportive tissue and the composition of hyperplastic tissue in terms of glandular versus stromal elements vary significantly among patients with prostatic enlargement.

PATHOPHYSIOLOGY

BPH can interfere with normal voiding in several ways. The bulk of the enlarged prostate can become obstructive while the detrusor is contracting—this is known as *mechanical obstruction*. Obstruction secondary to spasm of smooth muscles of the bladder outlet (bladder neck, prostate, and prostatic urethra) is

Table 16-1
Factors Affecting Lower Urinary Tract Symptoms (LUTS)

Disease	Incidence/Symptoms	Effect	Mechanism
Neurologic			
Cerebrovascular disease and stroke	15-20% • Incontinence (following stroke)	Incontinence* due to: • Hyperreflexia • Decreased bladder sensation • Immobility • Stool impaction • Motor deficit • Mental impairment • Sleep disturbance • Emotional disturbance	• Bilateral mediofrontal cortical damage resulting in upper motor neuron–type lesion
Parkinson's disease	25-75%† • Urgency • Frequency • Nocturia • Urge incontinence	• Detrusor hyperreflexia • Sphincteric dysfunction • Drug induced and secondary to constipation and emotional dysfunctions	• Loss of normal inhibitory impulses from substantia nigra to pontine micturition center • Sphincteric bradykinesia secondary to overall skeletal dysfunction • Anticholenergics and associated side effects
Shy-Drager syndrome	67% • Urgency • Frequency • Nocturia • Urge incontinence	• Detrusor hyperreflexia • Sphincteric dysfunction	• Atrophy of areas of cerebellum, brain stem, and peripheral automomic ganglion • Overall diminished tone of muscles • Open bladder neck with denervation of sphincter
Dementia	25-75% have urge incontinence	• Detrusor instability	• Idiopathic • Secondary to medications • Fecal impaction • Restricted immobility • Poor cognitive function
Spinal spondylosis and stenosis	• Cervical or lumbar‡	• Detrusor hyperreflexia • Areflexia	• Compression on cervical or lumbar cord • Compression on lumbar cord
Normal-pressure hydrocephalus	• Urgency • Incontinence • Dementia • Gait abnormality	• Detrusor hyperreflexia	Paraventricular compression of frontal inhibitory centers causing; • Hyperreflexia • Lack of concern
Supra sacral spinal cord injury Above T6-7 (above sacral center and sympathetic outflow)	• Urinary incontinence§	• Acute spinal shock followed by detrusor hyperflexia • Synergic detrusor bladder neck • Dyssynergic detrusor external sphincter	May occur secondary to back injury or fall
Above L1 (above sacral center and sympathetic outflow)	• Retention§	• Acute spinal shock followed by detrusor areflexia • Dyssynergic detrusor bladder neck • External sphincter retains minimal tone—not under voluntary control	• Poor sensation • Normal to increased compliance
Sacral spinal cord injury	• Retention with overflow most common§	Initial increased compliance secondary to areflexic bladder followed by recurrent cystitis and fibrosis: • Fibrosis results in poor compliance and upper tract deterioration	• May occur secondary to fall or motor vehicle accident (most common)

Condition			
Vitamin B_{12} deficiency	Affects 15% of geriatric population	• Impaired bladder sensations • Detrusor areflexia • Retention with overflow	• Secondary to neuropathy • Urologic manifestations occur before megaloblastic anemia and serum cobalamin • Methylmalonic acid and homocystine levels may help in diagnosis—changes may be reversible
Multiple sclerosis	50–80% have bladder manifestations Range includes: • Frequency • Urgency • Retention	• Detrusor hyperflexia • Detrusor areflexia (1–40%) • Sphincteric dysfunction • Bladder neck dyssynergia	• Focal neural demyelination impairing nerve conduction • Posterior and lateral columns most common sites
Diabetic autonomic cystopathy	5–50% report voiding symptoms • Retention • Difficulty in voiding • Sometime urgency • Retention§	• Poor bladder sensations • Poorly contractile bladder	• Autonomic neuropathy is secondary to segmental demyelination
Disk disease		• Detrusor areflexia • Dyssynergic bladder neck–external sphincter may retain minimal tone or show signs of denervation	• Compression of sacral spinal roots due to disk protrusion
Pelvic surgery	15–20% develop voiding dysfunction	• Urinary retention • Obstruction due to residual sphincteric tone	• Poorly contractile bladder • Nonrelaxing sphincter • Sometimes poor compliance
Cardiovascular	Mainly indirect effects, including; • Frequency • Nocturia	• Fluid volume alterations • Sleep disturbances • Medication effects • Vascular diseases	• Congestive heart failure due to angina • Diuresis due to effects of antihypertensives and antianginal drugs • Anterior spinal artery syndrome in thoracic aortic aneurysm • Increased UTI due to disease and drugs
Musculoskeletal	• Urgency • Incontinence due to impairment in mobility/dexterity	• Impaired mobility • Rheumatoid arthritis	
Pulmonary	• Urgency	• Recurrent cough • Respiratory acidosis • Cor pulmonale	• Change in urinary pH • Congestive heart failure
Infectious Tuberculosis	• Urgency • Frequency • Sterile pyuria • Painless hematuria	• Tuberculosis of genitourinary tract • Chronic cystitis	• Mucosal irritation • Alteration of bladder capacity
Herpes zoster	• Retention • Frequency • Urgency	• Viral neuritis of sacral dermatomes • Viral prostatitis	• Poorly contractile bladder
Alcoholism	3rd leading health disorder in elderly men	• Urgency and retention	• Thiamine deficiency • Neuropathy • Detrusor hypocontractility • Sudden diuresis

*Results of TURP are unsatisfactory if stroke is recent (<12 mo).
†25–30% of men with parkinsonism may have associated BPH.
‡Common radiologic finding in 98% of old patients; urinary incidence unknown.
§Usually clinical picture is clear, and these patients are not part of differential diagnosis of LUTS.
TURP, transurethral resection of the prostate; BPH, benign prostatic hypertrophy; UTI, urinary tract infection.
From Bissada NK, Finkbeiner AE: Urologic manifestations of drug therapy. Urol Clin North Am 15:725–736, 1988.

Table 16-2
Drugs Affecting Bladder Function

Dysfunction	Site	Drug Group
• Urgency • Frequency • Incontinence	Bladder overactivity	**Alpha agonists** — **Anticholinesterase**: • Distigmine • Neostigmine — **Beta-adrenergic blockers** — **Smooth muscle stimulants**: • Angiotensin • Histamine • 5-Hydroxytryptamine • Oxytocin • Prostaglandins • Vasopressin — **Ganglion stimulants**: • Nicotine — **Opioid antagonists**: • Methadone — **Parasympathomimetics**: • Bethanechol • Carbachol — **Others**: • Digitalis • Furosemide • Metoclopramide • Metronidazole • Testosterone • Thioridazine • Valproic acid
• Urgency • Frequency • Incontinence	Outlet relaxation	**Alpha-adrenergic blockers**: • Alpha methyldopa • Clonidine • Guanethidine • Phenoxybenzamine • Phentolamine • Prazosin — **Beta-adrenergic agonists**: • Isoproterenol • Terbutaline — **Striated muscle relaxants**: • Baclofen • Dantrolene • Hydramitrazine — **Others**: • Bromocriptine • Levodopa • Lithium • Phenothiazines • Phenytoin • Progesterone
• Obstructive symptoms • Retention	By inhibiting brain's higher centers	**Antiepileptics**: • Carbamazepine • Clonazepam • Narcotic analgesics • Phenytoin — **Smooth muscle relaxants**: • Diazepam • Chlordiazepoxide • Methocarbamol
• Obstructive symptoms • Retention	Spinal cord level: polysynaptic inhibitors	Baclofen
• Obstructive symptoms • Retention	Bladder level by inhibition of detrusor	□ **Anticholinergics** — □ **Antihistaminics** — □ **Antiparkinsonism drugs**: • Benzotropine • Biperidine • Cycrimine • Levodopa • Procyclidine — □ **Beta-adrenergic blockers** — □ **Calcium channel blockers**: • Flunarizine • Nifedipine • Terodiline — □ **Diuretics** — □ **Ganglion blockers** — □ **Skeletal muscle relaxants**: • Diazepam • Diclomine • Flavoxate • Oxybutynin — □ **Prostaglandin inhibitors** — □ **Psychiatric drugs**: • Phenothiazines • Tricyclic antidepressants — □ **Others**: • Bromocriptine • Theophylline • Isoniazid • Hydralazine
• Obstructive symptoms • Retention	Bladder outlet level	**Alpha-adrenergic agonists** — **Beta-adrenergic blockers** — **Others**: • Amphetamines • Levodopa • Imipramine

termed *dynamic obstruction*. Sympathetic innervation of the prostate controls the closure of the bladder neck and contraction of the prostatic capsule, stromal smooth muscles, and seminal vesicle during normal ejaculation.

Approximately 30% of patients presenting with LUTS do not have urodynamically demonstrable bladder outlet obstruction. The source of LUTS in these patients could be primary bladder neck obstruction; chronic prostatitis; and other prostatic pathologies, including prostatic infarction, calculi, and possibly prostatic carcinoma.

Detrusor instability is a condition in which the bladder contracts involuntarily. Patients with BPH have obstruction in 38% of the cases, impaired contractility in 25%, and intrinsic sphincter deficiency in 8%. Involuntary bladder contractions may be detected in 30% to 50% of patients. The relief of BPH-induced obstruction often leads to resolution of the detrusor instability in two thirds of the cases.

Primary bladder neck obstruction results from dyssynergia between detrusor contraction and bladder neck relaxation in the absence of significant prostatic enlargement. This entity mainly affects younger men who have a component of psychological dysfunction. Diagnosis is confirmed by video-urodynamic evaluation that demonstrates a lack of bladder neck opening during voiding phase, trapping of contrast agent in the posterior urethra, high detrusor pressures, and poor urinary flow rates. These patients benefit from alpha-blocker therapy or endoscopic incision of the bladder neck.

EVALUATION

Since the process of BPH occurs over a chronic, prolonged period, changes within the urinary tract are slow and insidious. The pathophysiologic effects of BPH are a result of complex interactions between the resistance of the prostatic urethra (due to spastic as well as mechanical effects of BPH) and the intravesical pressure generated during voiding, the physical health and compensatory ability of the detrusor, the functional state of the neurologic system, and the general physical health of the patient (no conditions such as diabetes and alcoholism). After initial hy-

pertrophy to compensate for increased resistance, the detrusor muscle eventually decompensates, resulting in poor tone and ultimately in diverticula formation. Finally, poor intravesical muscular function and increasing volume from residual urine result in hydronephrosis and upper tract dysfunction.

SYMPTOMS

BPH symptoms may be obstructive or irritative in nature. The Boyarsky questionnaire designed to quantitate the severity of BPH consists of nine questions, five to assess obstructive symptoms and four to measure irritative symptoms. This scale has been modified as the International Prostate Symptom Score (IPSS). Although some limitations exist, this questionnaire is currently one of the most common measures used to quantitate symptoms of BPH.

Incontinence is not a common symptom with BPH, although with advanced disease, large residual urine results in a weak sphincter that opens to allow the escape of urine in small amounts corresponding to bladder filling in an already full, poorly compliant bladder. Dilation of the upper tract with urinary stasis in the ureters usually occurs with detrusor decompensation, although it may occasionally occur even earlier. Dilation of the ureter and pelvis eventually leads to functional renal damage, which may be amplified by ascending infection and pyelonephritis.

In the later stages of BPH, high residual urine, urinary stasis, and vesicoureteral reflux predispose to cystitis and pyelonephritis. Patients may therefore have more pronounced symptoms of urgency, frequency, dysuria, and flank pain. Urinary stasis may also predispose to bladder calculi, which result again in intermittent obstruction, frequency, and painful voiding. An enlarged prostate is also friable, and in the presence of infection or calculi it manifests gross and microscopic hematuria.

EXAMINATION

General physical examination of a patient with BPH may reveal signs of uremia if the disease is advanced and has resulted in renal failure. Signs of renal failure include elevated blood pressure, rapid pulse and respiration (manifestations of anemia and metabolic acidosis), uremic fetor, pericarditis, pallor of nailbeds, neurologic findings of asterixis, reduced mentation, and peripheral neuropathy.

Abdominal examination may reveal a palpable kidney or flank tenderness if there is hydronephrosis or pyelonephritis. A distended bladder may be noted on palpation and percussion. Examination of the penis and urethra is important to rule out other causes of outlet obstruction such as stricture, carcinoma, meatal stenosis, and phimosis. Rectal examination may reveal an enlarged prostate, cancer, rectal tone, and other rectal pathologic conditions.

In some patients one may have to perform detailed neurourologic examinations to identify the exact cause for LUTS.

INVESTIGATIONS

A urinalysis and microscopic examination are important to rule out the presence of white blood cells, bacteria, and infection. The presence of hematuria should also initiate a workup for causes other than BPH, such as upper urinary tract masses, calculi, and lower urinary tract pathology. Serum electrolyte, blood urea nitrogen, and creatinine determinations provide baseline information on renal function and metabolic status.

Uroflowmetery and Postvoid Residual Urine

Among the objective signs of BPH are a reduced urine flow rate, the documentation of prostate enlargement, and high residual urine. Rate of urine flow is governed by several factors, including detrusor contractile force, intravesical pressure, and urethral resistance. To obtain a representative urine flow, the patient must void at least 125 to 150 mL. The rate should be determined at least on two different occasions, and attempts must be made to provide a quiet environment, preferably with the patient alone, using an automated urine flow system. At very low volumes, the flow rate is inaccurate, because the bladder cannot generate adequate pressures. At least two determinations are necessary since there is some variation based on the patient's general state of health and emo-

tional well-being. Urine flow nomograms relating peak and average flow rates in relation to intravesical volumes suggest that at a volume of 125 to 150 mL, normal people have average flow rates of 12 mL/s and peak flow close to 20 mL/s. Mildly obstructed patients usually have flow rates 1 or 2 SDs below normal; their average flow rates range from 6 to 8 mL and the peak flow rates range from 11 to 15 mL. As the severity of obstruction increases, there is also an increase in frequency of voiding and a decrease in volume voided. **It has also been determined that approximately 7% of patients with symptomatic BPH have normal rates of urine flow. In such patients intravesical pressure determinations reveal detrusor voiding pressures in excess of 100 mm H_2O.**

Measurement of urinary flow rate is generally considered to be the most useful screening procedure for diagnosing bladder outlet obstruction. In fact, most men with bladder outlet obstruction have a diminished flow rate. **However, a decreased urine flow rate may also be secondary to impaired detrusor contractility.** There are no features of the flow curve that permit an accurate distinction to be made between obstruction and detrusor dysfunction.

Residual measurements may be made by catheterizations. Although there is no absolute volume of residual urine that is considered abnormal, residual urine volumes over 50 to 100 mL are considered significant.

Transrectal Ultrasonography

In the evaluation of the lower urinary tract in LUTS, ultrasonography (US) is most useful for measuring bladder and prostate volume as well as residual urine. US also detects bladder calculi, diverticula, large bladder tumors, and other obvious bladder pathology. Estimation of bladder and prostate volume with US is in the accuracy range of 80% to 87%. Estimation of prostatic size is important because most urologists prefer to perform transurethral resections for glands under 60 g, whereas open prostatectomy by the suprapubic or retropubic route is preferred for glands over 60 g. To estimate prostate volume by US, the suprapubic or transrectal route may be used. There is also a transurethral route, but this is more invasive and generally not popular. The suprapubic method is the simplest and gives a reasonably accurate estimation of prostatic volume. Transrectal ultrasonography (TRUS), in our experience, is more accurate. To assess the volume of the prostate accurately, precise measurements must be made in three dimensions.

URODYNAMICS IN THE EVALUATION OF LUTS

Based on our current understanding of BPH and its relationship to symptoms of prostatism and obstructive uropathy, the role of urodynamics as both a diagnostic tool and an instrument to assist in therapeutic management remains to be defined.

SYNCHRONOUS PRESSURE-FLOW STUDIES

From a hydrodynamic viewpoint, bladder outlet obstruction is defined as a low urine flow rate in the presence of a detrusor contraction of adequate force, duration, and speed. Impaired detrusor contractility is usually apparent from the characteristics of the detrusor pressure tracing. For an individual patient, however, it may be difficult to determine the relative contribution of the detrusor and the outlet with respect to the flow rate, and for this reason, many investigators have attempted to formulate a mathematical definition of bladder outlet obstruction.

Evaluation of detrusor pressure-urine flow rate dynamics has greatly enhanced our understanding of the mechanics of micturition and has narrowed the diagnostic "gray" zone. Nevertheless, it is not yet possible to define bladder outlet obstruction in a simple, quantitative way, and clinical judgment is essential in determining the potential efficacy of medical or surgical therapy in a particular case. Moreover, the pressure-flow data merely aid in the diagnosis of bladder outlet obstruction; the site of obstruction is best determined by videourodynamics.

VIDEOURODYNAMICS

Multichannel videourodynamic studies consist of the simultaneous measurement of urodynamic parameters with radiographic imaging of the lower urinary tract. The time, effort, and expense required to operate a videourodynamics facility are considerable; nevertheless, these studies offer unique advantages in select groups of patients and may be cost effective in distinguishing bladder outlet obstruction from poor detrusor contractility.

Other Investigations

In few rare cases patients may require specialized investigations such as magnetic resonanance imaging, computed tomography scanning, electromyography, and nerve conduction studies for establishing the causes and diagnosis of LUTS. In addition, some of the aforementioned diagnostic modalities, primarily synchronous pressure-flow studies and videourodynamics, are rarely used to evaluate patients with LUTS.

Management of BPH

MEDICAL THERAPY OF BPH

Medical treatment of BPH is the preferred first-line management by both physicians and patients. This is due to the reversibility of treatment, significant symptomatic improvement, established safety, and potential to prevent acute urinary retention and the need for surgery.

Alpha Blockers

Alpha blockers as a class are the most commonly used first-line drug in the management of symptomatic BPH. Approximately 80% of patients receiving medical management are prescribed alpha blockers by their primary care physician.

LONG-ACTING ALPHA$_1$-ADRENOCEPTOR ANTAGONIST

Terazosin. Terazosin, an antihypertensive drug, is a selective alpha$_1$-adrenoceptor antagonist that has been studied extensively. The half-life of this (treatment vs. placebo) agent is 12 hours, which allows for once-daily dosing. Benefits that have been reported include improvement in the American Urological Association (AUA) symptom score (20%) and peak urinary flow rate (1.5 mL/s) for terazosin. In this study the AUA Symptom Score improved from a baseline mean of 20.1 by 37.8% during terazosin therapy.

Treatment failure with this agent occurs in 10% to 12% of patients. The side effects include dizziness (11.7%), asthenia (7.5%), peripheral edema (4.0%), postural hypotension (1.9%), hypotension (1.3%), headaches (5.8%), and abnormal ejaculation (1.4%). These side effects are dose dependent.

Doxazosin. Doxazosin, a quinazoline derivative, is a highly selective alpha$_1$-adrenoceptor antagonist and binds with high affinity to all alpha$_1$-adrenoceptor subtypes. The long plasma half-life (22 hours) of doxazosin allows for once-daily dosing. The bladder outlet obstructive symptoms improve significantly with 8 mg of doxazosin.

The data on selective long-acting alpha-receptor antagonists reveal (1) sustained and consistent efficacy over placebo in men with symptomatic BPH at a dose of 10 mg daily of terazosin and 8 mg daily for doxazosin and (2) a significant lowering of blood pressure in men with hypertension (11 to 16 mm Hg). Overall, the side effects affect approximately 11% to 19% of patients. Treatment with the long-acting alpha-receptor antagonists should expect the most common side effects of dizziness, asthenia, somnolence, headache, postural symptoms, and nasal congestion. The incidence of retrograde ejaculation and impotence is relatively low (1% to 2%).

Tamsulosin. Tamsulosin is a sulfamoylphenethylamine derivative that possesses potent and selective alpha$_1$-adrenoceptor receptor antagonism. Tamsulosin has been shown to have 13 times more efficacy for prostatic smooth muscle as compared with urethral smooth muscles. Tamsulosin has a significantly lower degree of nonspecific binding as compared with other alpha-adrenoreceptor antagonists.

Tamsulosin was recently approved in the United States for treatment of patients with symptomatic BPH. The drug is available at a dosage of 0.4 mg given once daily, 30 minutes after breakfast.

The side effects include dizziness, headache, postural hypotension, syncope, asthenia, somnolence, and rhinitis. This drug, unlike other alpha blockers, does not appreciably affect blood pressure in hypertensive or normotensive patients with BPH.

Hormonal Manipulation

The fact that bilateral orchiectomy can cause improvement in BPH symptoms has been known for more than a century. Because of the accompanying psychological trauma, total loss of libido, impotence, and occurrence of hot flashes, this therapy has never gained popularity. Efforts at medical castration using drugs such as estrogens, progestational agents, and gonadotropin-releasing hormone analogues have also not found enthusiasm among patients. Most of these agents also cause total loss of libido and impotence. Additionally, estrogens have other side effects, including fluid retention and thromboembolism. Recently, agents that selectively blockade androgens at the prostate cellular level have been tested for treatment of BPH. These agents are termed *antiandrogens*. The prostate normally requires conversion of testosterone to dihydrotestosterone (DHT). The enzyme 5-alpha-reductase mediates the conversion to DHT. Finasteride is an antiandrogen that blocks this enzyme. Finasteride (5 mg daily) decreases prostatic size; improves urine flow rates; and, consequently, symptoms of BPH. Side effects of this drug are minimal and include impotence and decreased libido in fewer than 5% of patients. **One side effect of finasteride is that it lowers serum prostate-specific antigen levels by approximately 50% within 6 months of use. In clinical use this does not appear to have masked detection of prostate cancer.** Treatment with finasteride for up to 2 years more than halves the frequency of acute urinary retention and reduces surgical intervention. The implication is that long-term medical therapy can reduce the clinically significant incidence of acute urinary retention or surgery. Finasteride especially helps patients who have a larger prostate, and the duration of therapy must extend 6 months to expect clinical benefits in the favorable patients.

Minimally Invasive Therapy

Although TURP is considered the gold standard for surgical treatment of BPH, there is a small but significant incidence of impotence, incontinence, bleeding, fluid overload, and retrograde ejaculation associated with this procedure. Because of the moderate morbidity and costs associated with TURP, newer modalities such as transurethral needle ablation (TUNA), thermotherapy, lasers, VaporTrode, and stents have been developed; short-term results of these procedures are encouraging.

Generally, minimally invasive therapies use heat to destroy tissue. Heat destruction can be achieved by high-frequency current, radiofrequency (RF) current, laser beams, microwaves, or ultrasonic heating. When prostatic and most other tissues are treated, the lesions created depend on the intensity of heat delivered, the rapidity with which it is deposited in tissues, and the surface area in which it is deposited. In general, low-level heat applied to large volumes of tissue causes coagulation, whereas high-intensity heat deposited rapidly in small volumes of tissue causes vaporization. Minimally invasive procedures that cause vaporization achieve temperatures over several hundred degrees at the tissue. Minimally invasive procedures that cause coagulation reach temperatures between 45° and 100° C. The closer the temperatures are to 100° C, the higher the degree of coagulation and the better the tissue ablation achieved.

TRANSURETHRAL ELECTROVAPORIZATION OF THE PROSTATE

TURP and VaporTrode. Electric current between 100,000 and 4,000,000 Hz produces a variety of effects, depending on various tissue and technical factors. The various tissue effects of high-frequency current are due to conversion of electrical energy to thermal energy. Desiccation, coagulation, steaming, and vaporization all are important for transurethral electrovaporization (TVP) of the prostate. Clinical benefits with TVP have been similar to TURP.

The advantages of the VaporTrode over TURP are an excellent intraoperative hemostastis and a lack of bleeding and fluid absorption. There are less blood loss, fluid absorption, and cardiovascular instability with TVP because of this. Another advantage of the VaporTrode procedure is that patients are

allowed to go home on the same day, thereby contributing to significant cost savings. The potential long-term complication is impotence.

TRANSURETHRAL NEEDLE ABLATION

The TUNA procedure uses low-level RF energy to coagulate hyperplastic prostatic adenomas. Two needles are deployed at acute angles from the tip of the TUNA catheter and are strategically directed into the adenoma. Once deployed, these needles deliver low-level RF energy to the prostatic tissue. The fact that this procedure can be performed under local anesthesia with minimal sedation and morbidity makes this procedure one of the most promising advances in the treatment of BPH. TUNA results in short-term improvement in obstructive symptoms.

The most common acute side effects after TUNA are irritative voiding symptoms, which can last 24 hours to 3 weeks, and minimal hematuria. Transient urinary retention lasting between 2 and 7 days in some patients has been noted in most trials. There have been reports of late complications such as impotence, retrograde ejaculation, urethral stricture, or rectal injuries. Most procedures are performed in an ambulatory setting, either in the hospital or as an office procedure.

MICROWAVE THERMOTHERAPY

Another type of minimally invasive procedure for treatment of BPH uses microwaves to heat the prostate. Microwaves are transverse electromagnetic waves with frequencies in the 30- to 300-Hz range. These electromagnetic waves travel in a given medium and are reflected or scattered by media with differences in impedance. The first devices heated the prostate from 42° to 44° C using a transrectal probe.

The side effects of thermotherapy are retrograde ejaculation, diminished ejaculatory volume, hematuria, and transient irritative voiding symptoms, which usually resolve within 2 to 3 weeks after treatment. Major advantages include a procedure that can be done under local anesthesia on an outpatient basis or in an office with minimal bleeding. The major problem with thermotherapy is the cost of the machine, which—depending on the model—is around \$100,000 to \$300,000.

TRANSURETHRAL INCISION OF THE PROSTATE

Transurethral incision of the prostate (TUIP) is another minimally invasive procedure for the treatment of BPH. Outcome for TUIP is comparable to TURP. TUIP has been shown to have less perioperative complications and morbidity than TURP.

Advantages of TUIP include shorter operating times and fewer overall complications, resulting in lower overall costs. In the properly selected group of patients (prostate < 30 g), this procedure can be as efficacious as the standard TURP in relieving bladder outlet obstruction, with lower incidence of retrograde ejaculation.

LASERS

Because soft tissue is predominantly water, evaporation does not begin until sufficient heat accumulates in the tissue to cause water vaporization (2.5 J/mm^3 to reach 100° C and change from liquid to gas phase). For laser wavelengths that are strongly absorbed by water (>2100 nm), the depth in tissue at which evaporation occurs is essentially the depth of absorption of the beam in the tissue (<300 μm), thus creating a large zone of heat-denatured protein before vaporization begins. Vaporization begins when enough heat accumulates beneath the surface to raise the temperature of the tissue matrix fluid above 100° C, producing an abrupt change in phase to steam secondary to subsurface superheating and causing an explosion known as the "popcorn effect," thereby exposing a new layer of tissue.

The superheated tissue dehydrates, its thermal conductivity decreases, its temperature increases, and it starts to burn and carbonize at 300° C, forming a charred surface that is highly absorbent of light in the 400- to 2000-nm band of wavelengths. This photothermal process results in explosive evaporation, combustion of displaced tissue fragments, and exposure of fresh tissue. Heat that is not associated with steam production or tissue combustion is conducted to deeper layers, creat-

ing a subsurface zone of heat-coagulated tissue (the coagulation layer).

There are four basic methods of laser prostate ablation: (1) coagulation of the adenoma using a beam with a wide angle of divergence delivered by a sidefiring, slightly convex, metal reflector; (2) incision of the adenoma using a sapphire of fused-silica contact tips; (3) evaporation of the adenoma using a sidefiring, free-beam, internal-reflector fiber placed in contact with the adenoma; and (4) incision and vaporization of the adenoma by direct contact with the bare fiber tip. This last method could be considered a variant of the second method in the sense that the fiber tip itself is acting as a small fused silica tip.

Holmium laser ablation of the prostate (HoLAP) uses a sidefiring, dual-wavelength fiber to vaporize/ablate the prostate. A technique involving a Holmium laser creates a large cavity, exposing the surgical capsule. Of the three techniques, the HoLAP has the best results in relieving bladder outlet–obstructive symptoms at 6 months.

STENTS AND SPIRALS

Stents that have standing usage to maintain the patency of arteries have now been adapted to urologic conditions. Stents are used primarily to relieve prostatic obstruction in patients who have failed medical management and/or are not candidates for minimally invasive techniques or TURP. One of the drawbacks of the prostatic stents is encrustation with sediments from urine. The other complications of prostatic stent include displacement of the stent into the bladder or the urethra and obstruction due to epithelial overgrowth of openings in the stent.

Summary

Men with moderate symptoms of BPH are the best candidates for medical treatment, whereas surgery is usually indicated for patients with severe symptoms. Men with mild symptoms do not usually need treatment, but they might be re-evaluated annually if desirable. To be an effective treatment for BPH, the medical therapy must not only improve the patient's ability to urinate but also must have minimal side effects. Currently available medical therapies must be continued indefinitely to maintain a therapeutic response. Medical therapies must also be cost effective. A man who develops BPH at 50 years of age may need therapy for 20 to 40 years. The total cost of such treatment could be significant. As with any medication or treatment regimen, it is important to determine which patients are candidates for a trial of medical therapy for BPH. Any patient who is suffering from clinically significant symptoms of BPH and is not in urinary retention is a potential beneficiary from treatment with a 5-alpha-reductase inhibitor or an alpha$_1$-adrenergic antagonist. These therapies are not limited to the poor surgical candidate but can be useful for any patient with bothersome symptoms. Symptoms of a more severe nature and urinary retention, however, are relative contraindications to medical therapy.

SUGGESTED READINGS

1. Abrams P: Managing lower urinary tract symptoms in older men. BMJ 310:113, 1995.
2. Barry MJ, Cockett AT, Holtgrewe HL, et al: Relationship of symptoms of prostatism to commonly used physiological and anatomical measures of the severity of benign prostatic hyperplasia. J Urol 150:351, 1993.
3. Kabalin JN, Mackey MJ, Cresswell MD, et al: Holmium: YAG laser resection of prostate (HoLRP) for patients in urinary retention. J Endourol 11:291, 1997.
4. Lepor H: Long-term efficacy and safety of terazosin in patients with benign prostatic hyperplasia. Terazosin Research Group. Urology 45:406, 1995.
5. Lepor H: The treatment of benign prostatic hyperplasia: A glimpse into the future. Urol Clin North Am 22:455, 1995.
6. Lepor H, Henry D, Laddu AR: The efficacy and safety of terazosin for the treatment of symomatic BPH. Prostate 18:345, 1991.
7. Lepor H, Williford WO, Barry MJ, et al: The efficacy of terazosin, finasteride, or both in benign prostatic hyperplasia. Veterans Affairs Cooperative Studies Benign Prostatic Hyperplasia Study Group. N Engl J Med 335:533, 1996.
8. McConnell JD: The pathophysiology of benign prostatic hyperplasia. J Androl 12:356, 1991.
9. McConnell JD: Benign prostatic hyperplasia: Hormonal treatment. Urol Clin North Am 22:387, 1995.
10. Narayan P, Tewari A, Garzotto M, et al: Transurethral VaporTrode electrovaporization of the prostate: Physical principles, technique, and results. Urology 47:505, 1996.
11. Schulman CC, Cortvriend J, Jonas U, et al: Tamsulosin, the first prostate-selective alpha$_{1A}$-adrenoceptor antagonist: Analysis of a multinational, multicentre, open-label study assessing the long-term efficacy and safety in patients with benign prostatic obstruction (symptomatic BPH). European Tamsulosin Study Group. Eur Urol 29:145, 1996.

17

Benign Prostatic Hypertrophy

John L. Phillips
Kevin R. Anderson

Benign prostatic hypertrophy (BPH) affects 10 million males in the United States and costs $2 billion to treat annually. Approximately 50% of men aged 60 years and older have an enlarged prostate on rectal examination (> 30 g or 3 fingerbreadths). Half of these men have symptoms of urinary difficulty. BPH can cause a range of disease, from isolated, benign symptoms of poor voiding to irreparable bladder and kidney damage, renal failure, and death. Earlier diagnosis of disease and pharmacologic management make kidney damage an uncommon event. This improved morbidity of BPH remains one of the twentieth century's greatest medical achievements. Outlet obstruction from BPH is, however, an indolent process of gradual bladder damage. Therefore, the likelihood of maintaining good bladder and kidney function depends largely on early identification of at-risk patients for BPH by nonurologists and primary health care providers (Fig. 17–1 and Tables 17–1 and 17–2).

Underlying Defect: Failure of the Bladder to Empty

Failure of the bladder to empty is due to neurogenic causes (the bladder cannot raise enough coordinated pressure and fails to empty itself), bladder outlet obstruction (the bladder is normal but its outlet is blocked by an enlarged prostate or urethral stricture), or, not uncommonly, a mixture of both neurogenic (detrusor) and anatomic (BPH) etiology (Table 17–1). Because evaluations and treatments diverge greatly, neurogenic bladder (primary bladder failure) must be differentiated from a decompensated, chronically obstructive (secondary bladder failure) bladder. Often the delineation among primary, secondary, and mixed bladder failure is not always clear.

The process of voiding is a highly coordinated series of actions that requires a normally contractile bladder, intact spinal cord reflexes, and the ability to volitionally initiate and terminate the voiding response. When the bladder fills, afferent impulses to the spinal cord initiate a voiding reflex via efferent pelvic nerves that are volitionally inhibitable in the adult. When voiding is desired, external sphincter relaxation immediately precedes a coordinated bladder contraction mediated by pontine, cerebellar, and sacral cord pathways. Voiding is, therefore, highly controlled and there are numerous areas where neurologic defects can occur that produce poor voiding. Obstructive voiding is different in that there is an actual physical impediment to urine flow while the bladder, theoretically, is neurologically intact.

With age, governed by as-of-yet unknown growth factors, the prostate in most men enlarges and grows in mass and volume. With hypertrophy, the prostatic urethra becomes less compliant, more difficult to distend, and requires a higher pressure to open. The bladder's response to outlet obstruction is, like the myocardium in hypertension, concentric hypertrophy. The hypertrophic bladder can be smaller and its muscular wall appear trabeculated, named after a type of criss-cross-

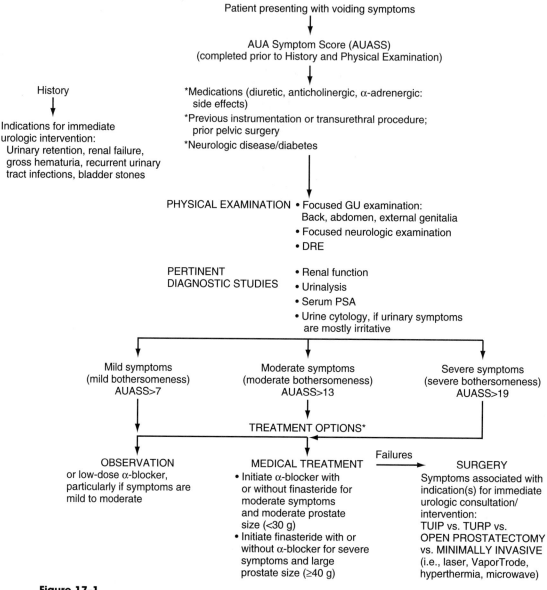

Figure 17-1

Critical pathway for patients with benign prostatic hypertrophy. GU, genitourinary; DRE, digital rectal examination; PSA, prostate-specific antigen; TURP, transurethral resection of the prostate; AUA, American Urological Association; TUIP, transurethral incision of the prostate.

*Treatment options in the absence of (1) indications for immediate urologic consultation/intervention and/or (2) abnormal DRE or PSA.

ing Italian latticework called *trabecula*. The bladder wall becomes thicker and less compliant. Such bladders do not conduct neurotransmission well and may interfere with the neurologic control of the bladder. This can cause the bladder to become irritated and spastic and can lead to symptoms even when a patient is not voiding. Gradually, the bladder begins to fail, the amount of urine it is able to void decreases, and residual volumes

increase. **Sustained residuals intermittently induce uninhibitable bladder contractions. Despite an intact sphincteric mechanism, a sense of urinary urgency can lead to leaking or frank voiding of urine at inappropriate and embarrassing times. Chronic residual urine can act as a nidus for infection and stone formation, and such processes can cause further neurologic damage.** With time, in unrelieved obstruction, bladder storage pressure gradually increases. **When storage pressures exceed 40 cm H_2O, kidney drainage can be impaired leading to chronic hydronephrosis and ischemic nephron damage.** Classically, patients in obstructive renal failure usually have decreased filtration from glomerular compromise and present with uremia, high blood urea nitrogen (BUN) and creatinine levels, hyperkalemic metabolic acidosis, and volume overload. Computed tomography almost always reveals severe bilateral hydroureteronephrosis and an enlarged bladder with a thickened wall. If a catheter can be placed in the bladder and it is ade-

Table 17–1
Causes of the Poorly Functioning Bladder

A. Neurologic disorders (neurogenic bladder)
  1. Central diseases
    a. Parkinson's syndrome
    b. Dementia
    c. Multiple sclerosis
    d. Stroke
  2. Peripheral diseases
    a. Cord injury
    b. Spinal dysraphism
  3. Diabetes mellitus
  4. Myasthenia gravis
  5. Guillain-Barré syndrome
B. Pelvic surgery, especially abdominoperineal resection
C. Infectious disorders
  1. Pathogens with neurologic sequelae
    a. Varicella/herpes zoster
    b. Syphilis
    c. Poliomyelitis
  2. Pathogens with obstructive sequelae
    a. *Neisseria gonorrhoeae*
D. Medications
  1. Agents that increase outlet resistance
    a. Alpha-agonists, especially nasal Neo-Synephrine
    b. Tricyclic antidepressants, especially imipramine
  2. Agents that decrease bladder contractility (negative cystotropes)
    a. Anticholinergics
      i. Sedatives, especially diphenhydramine (Benadryl)
      ii. Antispasmodics, especially dicyclomine HCl (Bentyl)
      iii. Tricyclic antidepressants, especially imipramine
    b. Other neurotropic drugs
  3. Calcium channel blockers, especially diltiazem
  4. Beta blockers, especially propranolol
  5. Dietary agents that can increase bladder irritability
    a. Caffeine (substituted xanthines)
    b. Ethanol
    c. Nicotine
    d. Food coloring (F.D. & C. Red #40, amaranth, tartrazine)
    e. Food additives (paprika, oleoresin, capsaicin)

Table 17–2
Signs and Symptoms of Difficult Urination

Signs

Enlarged prostate on digital rectal examination (> 3 fingerbreadths or 30 g)
Distended bladder
Postvoid residual > 100–125 mL in adult male
Hematuria, microscopic
Urinary tract infection, especially in male
Bladder calculus
Hydronephrosis, bilateral

Symptoms

IRRITATIVE VOIDING

Nocturia: being wakened by the need to urinate
Urgency: a sudden need to urinate quickly
Dysuria: pain with urination, i.e., initial, midstream, or terminal
Frequency: the perceived need to urinate often (e.g., cystitis)

OBSTRUCTIVE VOIDING

Hesitancy: a slowness in initiating the urinary stream
Dribbling: passage of urine after voiding has ceased
Decreased force of stream: a lessening in force, caliber, or pattern
Double voiding: multiple, incomplete attempts to empty the bladder
Splayed stream: turbulent or bifid flow
Strangury: a need to bear down to obtain urine flow
Incomplete voiding: sensation of residual urine after voiding

PERINEAL/SUPRAPUBIC PAIN
INCONTINENCE
HEMATURIA, GROSS

Obviously, none of these signs or symptoms are diagnostic of benign prostatic hypertrophy (BPH), and some, e.g., hematuria, may be indications of non–BPH-related disease.

quately drained, renal failure can often recover completely. Creatinine levels of even 20 mg/dL have been seen to correct themselves in several days. The postobstructive diuresis associated with the care of these patients is well documented and illustrates the acute medical management required for end-stage renal failure due to obstruction.

BPH is associated with, therefore, a tremendous range of uropathy, and it is the astute clinician who can preclude irreversible bladder and kidney damage by early recognition and treatment. This requires a well-organized urocentric office history and physical examination.

Assessment in the Office

HISTORY AND SUBJECTIVE DATA

A history of the patient must first be obtained especially since other diseases, infections, and conditions can have a marked effect on urinary control. Questions should first be directed toward identifying the neurogenic bladder, any underlying systemic neuropathology, use of neurotropic or vasculotropic medications, recent surgical history, and dietary intake (see Table 17–1). **Figure 17–1 outlines the critical pathway for evaluating, managing, and/or triaging patients with symptomatic BPH in the office or emergency department.**

When focusing on the voiding history a structured format is invaluable. Patients with voiding difficulties generally have two main groups of complaints: irritative and obstructive symptoms (see Table 17–2). Irritative symptoms arise from neurogenic changes to the bladder and may be among some of the earliest complaints of significant pathology. Obstructive symptoms are due, in part, to the physical impediment of a noncompliant prostatic urethra. The appearance of irritative and/or obstructive symptoms often mirrors the development, chronicity, and subjective severity of disease and allows identification of patients requiring further evaluation.

The major categories of symptoms have been conveniently outlined by the American Urological Association (AUA) into a patient-focused list of categories. One outline, known as the *AUA symptom score* (AUA-SS), allows the practitioner to qualitatively grade a complex array of complaints (Table 17–3). The AUA-SS is completely subjective and not definitive. In fact, some women with cystitis have as bad an AUA-SS as men with symptomatic BPH. Combined with the objective data described in the following section, however, the AUA-SS is exceedingly helpful with patient stratification. The symptom score can also be used as a gross assessment of a patient's improvement or worsening over time.

OBJECTIVE DATA

After the identification of patients with voiding disorders is made, regardless of severity, quantitative information should be obtained. A physical examination helps identify important features of bladder pathology. Digital rectal examination should elucidate prostate size, symmetry, tenderness, or nodularity.

Table 17–3
AUA Symptom Score and Index

Over the past month . . .	Never	20%	<50%	About 50%	>50%	100%
1. How often have you had a sensation of not emptying your bladder completely after you finished urinating?	0	1	2	3	4	5
2. How often have you had to urinate again in less than 2 hours after you finished urinating?	0	1	2	3	4	5
3. How often have you found you stopped and started again several times when you urinated?	0	1	2	3	4	5
4. How often have you found it difficult to postpone urination?	0	1	2	3	4	5
5. How often have you had a weak urinary stream?	0	1	2	3	4	5
6. How often have you had to push or strain to begin urination?	0	1	2	3	4	5
7. How many times did you most typically get up to urinate from the time you went to bed at night until the time you got up in the morning?	0	1	2	3	4	5

Additive symptom score:
Degree of severity: 0–7 Mild;   8–19 Moderate;   20–35 Severe

AUA, American Urological Association.

Baseline BUN and creatinine levels should probably be checked to confirm residual renal function, especially if one has not been obtained in a year and the patient has had voiding difficulties for 6 months or longer. Measuring the postvoid residual (PVR) remains the single most helpful objective measure of global bladder function: the ability to empty. A useful office tool in this regard is a commercially available bladder ultrasound device. By deriving the volume from multiple axial two-dimensional echo images, such bladder scanners have been found to have an accuracy greater than 90% when compared with catheterized controls. Catheterization remains, however, the gold standard for assessment of a PVR. PVRs greater than 100 to 125 mL in the setting of significant symptoms points to serious failure of the bladder to empty and requires urologic follow-up. What must thereafter be determined is if the elevated PVR is due to outlet obstruction or a weak, neurogenic bladder or both. Inability to pass a catheter through the penile urethra could suggest strictural disease. Urologic consultation should be obtained before a retrograde urethrogram is obtained.

A useful method of assessing bladder function when the PVR is elevated is urodynamic evaluation. This may be especially important in evaluating the male with voiding difficulties in the setting of significant neurologic disease, such as multiple sclerosis, or after recovery from extensive neuroablative surgery, such as an abdominoperineal resection. Formal urodynamics require videofluoroscopic evaluation, real-time flow manometry, and even electromyography and is best performed by a trained urologist.

Interpreting a Lot of Information

It is not the primary responsibility of the non-urologist to definitively diagnose and treat BPH, neurogenic bladder, or any of the sequelae of obstructive uropathy. Armed with a good history and physical examination and perhaps a PVR, the practitioner can identify those patients at higher risk for severe disease to be more quickly referred for urologic assessment.

No single test or finding is diagnostic of BPH, although symptoms continue to be the most important diagnostic and prognostic entity. There is no cutoff on symptoms or PVR for patients with and without BPH. AUA-SSs higher than 20 are certainly suggestive of significant obstructive disease, but the patient whose only problem is getting up at night two or three times to urinate may be as equally miserable. Likewise, the patient with a PVR of only 100 but an AUA-SS score of 15 may have as significant BPH as the patient with a PVR of 300 and an AUA-SS lower than 10.

Generally, all patients who present with frank urinary retention should be seen by a urologist. Patients with AUA-SSs higher than 20, PVRs higher than 150, and an abnormal creatinine level should be seen by a urologist soon after the initial interview. AUA-SSs of 8 to 20, PVRs less than 125, and an enlarged prostate on digital rectal examination in an otherwise healthy patient probably indicate BPH that may benefit from initiation of treatment before the patient is seen by a urologist (see Fig. 17–1). AUA-SSs of less than 7, minimal PVRs, and a normal examination may not indicate BPH, but the patient should still be seen by a urologist since his main problem is symptoms of difficult urination. The patient with symptoms of BPH (including lower AUASS of ≤ 7) and enlarged prostate (≥ 40 g) should be treated medically to prevent potential complications, including urinary retention. **No patient can ever be unnecessarily referred to a urologist if an abnormality of urologic concern is detected by the practitioner on physical examination or symptom interview. This tenet should be kept in mind when deciding when a referral should be made** (see Fig. 17–1).

Treatment and Options

The various treatments for BPH may have perhaps the widest range of any disease process in medicine. The goal of therapy in BPH is not only to relieve symptoms but to improve urinary tract drainage and prevent potential complications, such as urinary retention, as well as delay or prevent prostatectomy. Since the etiology of obstructive uropathy due to BPH is an obstructive prostatic urethra, all therapies are aimed at pharmacologically or surgically facilitating the passage of urine through this part of the urinary tract. Generally, patients with mild to moderate symptoms or those who will not be surgical candidates can be treated medically. Patients with severe symptoms and those who fail or cannot tolerate medical therapy may be candidates for surgical treatment. As with any disease treatment, however, efficacy, cost, risk-benefit ratios, and quality of life concerns all need to be assessed before any treatment for BPH can be initiated (see Fig. 17–1).

MEDICAL THERAPY

Alpha Blockers

The prostatic ductal epithelium is devoid of any smooth or skeletal musculature, but the endodermally derived prostatic capsule has a significant smooth muscle component. Innervated by sympathetic fibers, the capsule relaxes when exposed to alpha blockade. Capsular relaxation allows the hypertrophic prostate to expand; the prostatic urethra dilates and becomes more compliant. Additionally, there are alpha receptors scattered among smooth muscle cells of the bladder neck. Relaxation of the bladder neck and prostatic urethra serves as the basis for the use of alpha blockers in BPH. A randomized trial showed a 32% to 44% improvement in symptoms in patients treated with terazosin compared with a 23% improvement in the control group. Alpha blockers were originally used for the control of hypertension because of their vasodilatory effect on arteriolar smooth muscle. Symptoms related to low blood pressure occur in 10% to 15% of users and include weakness, postural hypotension, dizziness, or syncope. Such side effects can be dangerous and may thus severely limit alpha-blocker therapy. **Patients with significant peripheral vascular disease, a history of stroke, or who are concurrently taking calcium channel and/or beta blockers may not, therefore, be candidates for alpha blockade.** There is evidence that tamsulosin, an alpha blocker specific for the alpha$_1$ receptors of the prostate, has no to little vasodilatory effects and that it is well tolerated by patients maintained on multiple antihypertensives.

Finasteride

BPH occurs because of the stimulation of epithelial cells by growth factors derived from stromal cells. Prostatic stromal cells are stimulated, in turn, not primarily by testosterone (T) but by its metabolite, dihydrotestosterone (DHT), made predominantly in the prostate and male sexual glands. The hormone responsible for the conversion of T to DHT is DHT reductase and can be inhibited by the agent finasteride. The use of finasteride (Proscar) in BPH was initially believed to be a "magic bullet" since it would affect only hypertrophic prostate cells and thus actually treat the source of the disease. However, initial results were disappointing in that although 50% of men had a reduction in prostate volume by 6 months, only half of these men had symptomatic improvement. Patients generally responded earlier and subjectively did better on alpha-blocker therapy than finasteride. However, whereas alpha blockers enhance urethral compliance, finasteride may reverse the disease process itself. It may, therefore, ultimately be of best use for patients with larger prostate glands (> 40 g). **Finasteride has few or no side effects, except occasional report of erectile and/or ejaculatory dysfunction. It is well tolerated and can be used by patients with significant cardiovascular disease. Finasteride causes a 50% reduction in PSA after 6 months; however, finasteride therapy does not mask the diagnosis of prostate cancer.**

INTERMITTENT CATHETERIZATION

The goal of all therapies in BPH management is to optimize bladder emptying. No agent including surgery does this as effectively and as safely as a rubber catheter. Intermittent self-catheterization (ISC) is a highly efficacious regimen which is well tolerated by many patients, especially those who have been dissatisfied with other options or who are not candidates for pharmacologic therapy. ISC can be learned by almost anyone who can understand medical instructions and has good use of the fingers and hands. It is a treatment of choice for the nursing home patient with chronic urinary retention and who is not a candidate for pharmacologic or surgical intervention. The risk of infection in the male is low and is certainly lower than the risk in males who have chronic bladder residuals. ISC obviates the need for any other medications except topical iodine and surgical lubricant. In the urologic community, ISC is among the most recommended forms of treatment for BPH as well as for any other disease that leads to poor bladder drainage. Unfortunately, some patients do not accept ISC, especially those who believe it may interfere with lifestyle or who do not wish to include it in their activities of daily living.

SURGERY

Few other fields in surgery have become so advanced yet remain so controversial as transurethral surgery on the prostate. Originally, surgeons attempted to open the prostatic urethra with a cystoscope with a kind of coring device that had little visualization and a poor ability to achieve hemostasis. Morbidity was high. Endoscopy and continuous flow irrigation, developed in the 1970s, has made transurethral surgery of the prostate highly effective, and it continues to evolve. Transurethral resection of the prostate (TURP) is the classic approach toward opening up the prostatic urethra and is the gold standard for surgical intervention in terms of improving patients' quality of life, voiding parameters, and renal function. Because of the rich blood supply to the prostate and the intricate connection of the prostate to the urinary sphincters, postoperative bleeding and incontinence continue to be areas of concern. Retrograde ejaculation occurs after TURP, and the procedure is therefore not indicated for men desiring children. The desire for even safer methods of prostate resection has yielded a host of other approaches, none of which yet have superior success to TURP. Laser ablation, cryotherapy, vaporization, and microwave needle ablation (TUNA) all have their proponents and are theoretically safer procedures, but none have yet to replace the classic TURP.

For patients with very large prostates for whom TURP may not be adequate, the obstructing adenomas of the prostate can be removed from within the capsule via a suprapubic incision, known as a simple prostatectomy. Radical prostatectomies are performed for prostate adenocarcinoma and are never indicated for BPH.

Regardless of surgical procedure, there are few to no absolute contraindications to transurethral or open surgery. Patient selection for surgery is a urologic decision and is generally based on BPH severity, the presence of comorbid disease, and the patient's likelihood to tolerate blood loss and general anesthesia. Most patients selected for surgery do well. The bladder in BPH, as discussed earlier, can be abnormal due to long-standing obstruction. In such patients, symptoms may not improve for several weeks following surgery. Despite optimal prostatic resection and a "wide-open" prostatic urethra, patients may continue to have irritative voiding symptoms until the hypertrophic detrusor myothelium begins to normalize.

Outcomes and Cost Analysis

Few other fields in medicine are as rapidly growing and as potentially significant as clinical outcome data analysis. For the management of patients with BPH, such information is exceedingly useful to the physician as well as to the patient who is expected to make an informed decision about the various treatment modalities available to him. Independent of cost are patients' lifestyle decisions as well, and this may be the single most important issue to address in the management of BPH.

A direct comparison of watchful waiting, medical therapy, and surgery has been difficult. Many patients who undergo surgery have completed a lengthy course of medical therapy. Age differences, comorbidities, and disease severity significantly affect overall options. Improvements in technique have decreased hospital stays and costs in recent years following surgery. Furthermore, short-term costs, such as hospital stays or nursing, need to be carefully compared to overall long-term costs as well. In one large cohort study, watchful waiting, surgery alone, medical therapy alone (both alpha blocker and finasteride) and mixed medical and surgical therapies were compared for age groups 45 to 85 years of age (Table 17–4). Generally, transurethral surgery tends to have the best overall outcome, regardless of disease severity, in terms of subjective improvement, especially in younger men (45 to 55 years of age). Its

Table 17-4
Comparison of Different Benign Prostatic Hypertrophy Therapies

	Watchful Waiting	Medical Therapy	Surgical Therapy
Improvement in symptom score (AUA) (%)	31–55	33–86	75–96
Complication rate (%)	1–5	1–10	5.2–30.7
Need for retreatment within 5 years (%)	15.3–65.2	Continued therapy	9.4–10.6
Cost/case over lifetime ($)	3339	9087	9516

AUA, American Urological Association; NA, not available.

Adapted from Chirikos TN, Sanford E: Cost consequences of surveillance, medical management, or surgery for benign prostatic hyperplasia. J Urol 155: 1311–1316, 1996.

costs have recently approached that of life-long medical therapy in selected patients. Because the life span is shorter in older patients, their overall costs for all therapies tend to be lower.

When to Refer

Urologists are responsible for evaluating all patients referred to them for any voiding complaint or finding. Most men with voiding difficulties and who even have BPH probably do not need immediate attention by a urologist but can be greatly helped by their primary care provider following the outline of this text. In the managed care environment, the initial evaluation of a patient with voiding difficulties more frequently occurs in the primary care setting. Most often, patients present to their primary care provider with a mixture of often confusing symptoms, and it is unclear when a urologist should be seen. To aid in this regard, this chapter discussed how the most important features of obstructive uropathy and BPH can be assessed by the nonurologist and how treatments can be started. It requires years of disease before

BPH manifests itself as a voiding disorder and so the treatment may not have overnight improvements. It therefore becomes more important that the primary care provider and the patient have a long-term relationship regarding the treatment of this disease. Early input by a urologist can help the practitioner with the subtle decisions that we all face when assessing the patient with BPH.

SUGGESTED READINGS

1. Barry MJ, Fowler HJ Jr, O'Leary MP, et al: The American Urological Association symptom index for benign prostatic hyperplasia. J Urol 148:1549, 1992.
2. Chirikos TN, Sanford E: Cost consequences of surveillance, medical management, or surgery for benign prostatic hyperplasia. J Urol 155:1211–1216, 1996.
3. Coroneos E, Assouad M, Krishnan B, Truong LD: Urinary obstruction causes irreversible renal failure by inducing chronic tubulointerstitial nephritis. Clin Nephrol 48:125–128, 1997.
4. Duffy LM, Cleary J, Ahern S, et al: Clean intermittent catheterization: Safe, cost-effective bladder management for male residents of VA nursing homes. J Am Geriatr Soc 43:865, 1995.
5. Lepor H, Williford WO, Barry MJ, et al: The efficacy of terazosin, finasteride, or both in benign prostatic hyperplasia. Veterans Affairs Cooperative Studies Benign Prostatic Hyperplasia Study. N Engl J Med 335:533–539, 1996.
6. Tammela T: Benign prostatic hyperplasia: Practical treatment guidelines. Drugs Aging 10:349–366, 1997.

18

Urologic Problems in Pregnancy

David M. Hall
Unyime O. Nseyo

The genitourinary tract undergoes physiologic and pathologic changes during pregnancy. The increase in cardiac output and decrease in renal vascular resistance results in a 30% to 50% increase in the renal plasma flow (RPF) as well as the glomerular filtration rate (GFR). The heightened hormonal milieu of pregnancy, particularly placental progesterone, causes relaxation of the ureters and renal pelvis partly contributing to gestational hydronephrosis. Pregnancy-induced high levels of progesterone, aldosterone, deoxycorticosterone, placental lactogen, and chorionic gonadotropin help mediate these hemodynamic changes. Increases in urinary excretion of amino acids, glucose, and even therapeutic medications are a consequence of increases in the RPF and GFR. Increases in RPF and GFR increase calcium filtration and calcium absorption secondary to high serum levels of calcitriol. Consequently, pregnancy is associated with hypercalciuria; however, there is no net increase in the incidence of nephrolithiasis because there is a similar increase in stone-inhibiting factors such as citrate, magnesium, and glycosaminoglycans in the urine. The gravid uterus undergoes dextrorotation with resultant mechanical compression of the right ureter as well as of the urinary bladder. The consequences are predispositions to upper and lower urinary tract dysfunction. This chapter discusses the clinical implications of these pregnancy-induced physiologic and pathologic changes of the urinary tract.

Asymptomatic Bacteriuria and Urinary Tract Infections

Pregnant women are particularly prone to acquire acute urinary tract infections; however, asymptomatic bacteriuria is a significant problem of pregnancy. Pregnancy causes ureteropyelocaliectasis resulting from either abnormal physiologic changes or mechanical obstruction by the gravid uterus. Consequently, pregnant women are at increased risk for pyelonephritis when bacteriuria is present. It is for this reason that all pregnant women should be screened for asymptomatic bacteriuria and treated if it is present. Frequently, cystitis occurs first and may then lead to ascending bacteriuria with resultant renal parenchymal infection or pyelonephritis.

INCIDENCE

Approximately 20% to 40% of pregnant patients with asymptomatic bacteriuria during the first trimester develop pyelonephritis in the third trimester. About 20% to 30% of cases of pyelonephritis in pregnancy occur in patients who had sterile urine cultures on their initial prenatal visit. However, 14% to 63% of patients with bacteriuria develop acute antepartum urinary tract infection. Three percent of pregnant women with severe pyelonephritis can develop endotoxic shock. Importantly, 60% to 70% of cases of severe urinary tract infections during pregnancy can be prevented if intensive screening and treating of bacteriuria of pregnancy occurs. Such an intensive surveillance and treatment can prevent neonatal complications of prematurity, growth retardation, and low birth weight.

PREDISPOSING FACTORS TO BACTERIURIA OF PREGNANCY

The prevalence of significant bacteriuria of pregnancy ranges from 2% to 10%. Predisposing factors to significant bacteriuria during pregnancy include socioeconomic status (2% to 3% of nonindigent vs. 6% to 10% of indigent), age and parity, race, sickle cell trait (twice as common in black women with sickle cell trait), bladder distention and urethral trauma associated with normal delivery, as well as underlying disease (e.g., diabetes mellitus).

DIAGNOSIS

By definition "significant" bacteriuria of pregnancy occurs with a bacterial colony count of 100,000 or more organisms per mL from two or three consecutive clean-voided urine specimens. Routine urethral catheterization should be discouraged because bacteria may be introduced into the bladder that is sterile.

A rapid, simple screening procedure is to examine a drop of uncentrifuged urine under the microscope ($43\times$ microscopic objective). Presence of any bacteria denotes a colony count of 10^5/mL of urine.

BACTERIOLOGY

The bacteriology of asymptomatic bacteriuria as well as urinary tract infections of pregnancy involves gram-negative rods, namely *Escherichia coli, Klebsiella, Enterobacter,* and *Proteus.* Gram-positive cocci and enterococci also have been reported. Group B streptococcus is often found colonized in diabetics, without increased incidence of group B urinary tract infection. Diagnosis of a chlamydial infection should be regarded as serious and should be treated to prevent neonatal complications such as pneumonia, nasopharyngitis, and conjunctivitis.

TREATMENT

Approximately 25% of untreated patients with bacteriuria of pregnancy develop clinical disease compared with 4.2% of treated patients. A short course of 10 to 14 days of nonteratogenic antimicrobial therapy with continued surveillance is the recommended management of pregnant patients with significant bacteriuria. About 5% to 10% of pregnant patients demonstrate persistent or recurrent bacteriuria after adequate therapy. Treatment of bacteriuria of pregnancy involves eradication of the pathogen followed by uroprophylaxis using the same drug as a single bedtime dose throughout pregnancy. Urinary bacteriologic cultures should be performed regularly, probably every month throughout the pregnancy. Table 18–1 lists an-

Table 18-1
Antibiotics in Pregnancy

Drug	Toxicity	Pregnancy Class*
Penicillin	No known fetal toxicity	B
Cephalosporins	No known fetal toxicity	B
Erythromycin	No known fetal toxicity	C
Aminoglycosides	CNS toxicity, ototoxicity	C
Nitrofurantoin	Hemolysis in G6PD	B
Sulfonamides	Kernicterus, hemolysis in G6PD	B (D at term)
Trimethoprim	Folate antagonism	C
Tetracycline	Tooth dysplasia, inhibition of bone growth	D
Metronidazole	Inhibits nucleic acid synthesis	B (avoid in first trimester)
Clindamycin		C
Quinolones	Abnormality of bone growth	C

*B, Animal studies have not shown an adverse effect on the fetus, but there are no adequate clinical studies in pregnant women. C, Animal studies have shown an effect on the fetus, but there are no adequate studies in humans; the drug may be useful in pregnant women despite its potential risks. D, There is evidence of risk to the human fetus, but the potential benefits of use in pregnant women may be acceptable despite potential risks.
CNS, central nervous system; G6PD, glucose-6-phosphate dehydrogenase.

tibiotics that are considered safe during pregnancy.

Urolithiasis of Pregnancy

INCIDENCE

Acute urolithiasis in pregnancy is rare with an incidence ranging from 0.35% (1 in 286) to 0.03% (1 in 3000). The incidence is quite low; however, clinicians must be alert to the possibility. Early diagnosis and treatment can eliminate complications of urinary tract obstruction with the resultant infection and impairment of renal function, as well as potential loss of pregnancy. The rate of urolithiasis varies during pregnancy, with 12% of cases being diagnosed in the first trimester and 88% of cases diagnosed in the second and third trimester.

ETIOLOGIC FACTORS

Generally, pregnancy induces decreased ureteral peristalsis, hydronephrosis, infection, and calcium supersaturation. However, these predisposing factors are counterbalanced by increased excretion of stone inhibitors and neutralizing effectors, including citrate, magnesium, and glycosaminoglycans. However, other etiologic principles include

1. Pregnancy-induced hydronephrosis: Pregnancy induces hydronephrosis. However, this phenomenon, with the resultant stasis and urinary tract infection, has not really been proven to be an important etiologic factor in urolithiasis of pregnancy. The incidence of urolithiasis in pregnancy is no greater than in nonpregnant female patients. There is no evidence of right-sided preponderance in incidence of upper urinary tract stones.

2. Parity and trimester of pregnancy: The incidence of kidney stones appears to be relatively higher in multiparous women; however, this finding may reflect the propensity of the incidence of urolithiasis to increase with age. There is no evidence to indicate that either parity or trimester is directly related to etiology of urinary stones in pregnancy. However, the basis for the reported higher incidence of calcium-based stones in women

who suffer spontaneous abortions has not been elucidated.

3. Underlying disease: As with the nonpregnant stone former, the underlying disease must be sought with the same intensity in the pregnant stone former.

CLINICAL EVALUATION

Signs and Symptoms

Microscopic hematuria, lateralizing abdominal and/or flank pain, and other signs and symptoms may suggest urolithiasis. Hematuria may be indicative of other urinary pathologic conditions. Therefore, hematuria of pregnancy warrants urologic consultation. Often urinary infection may be the obvious presenting sign.

Most causes of abdominal pain during pregnancy are obstetric in nature, such as ectopic pregnancy (1:300) and placental disruption (1:100). Other causes of pain include appendicitis, intestinal obstruction, and cholecystitis. The urologic causes of acute pain in the pregnant patient include acute cystitis, pyelonephritis, hydronephrosis, and urolithiasis (Table 18–2). In rare cases rupture of the renal collecting system or parenchyma have been reported. At 5 to 8 months of gestation, pain is atypical for urolithiasis.

Diagnosis

History of kidney stones, recurrent urinary tract infections, and family history of urinary stones in the presence of suggestive symptoms and signs in a pregnant women must alert the treating clinician to the diagnosis of urolithiasis (Table 18–3). Obstructive uropa-

Table 18–2
Differential Diagnosis of Abdominal/Flank Pain in Pregnancy

Urinary tract	Urolithiasis
	Blood clots
	Sloughed tissue
Gastrointestinal	Appendicitis
	Cholecystitis
	Colitis/ileitis
Gynecologic	Ectopic pregnancy
	Ovarian cyst
	Pelvic inflammatory disease

Table 18-3
Evaluation of Urolithiasis of Pregnancy

	Sign/Symptom	Recommended Evaluation
History	Flank pain, history of stones, family history of stones, dehydration	*Ultrasonography:* hydronephrosis, calculus *Intravenous urogram:* delayed visualization; ureteral columnization *KUB:* radiopaque calculus *Laboratory tests:* urinalysis: hematuria, pyuria, bacteriuria
Physical examination	Focal, unilateral tenderness, including costovertebral angle tenderness, suprapubic tenderness, fever, chills, hypotension (with septic shock)	Urine culture is warranted if urinalysis suggests infection; serum calcium, phosphorus, alkaline phosphate, parathyroid hormone levels needed with history of recurrent stones or oxalate stone

KUB, kidney, ureter, and bladder.

thy, including obstructing stones, must be suspected in a pregnant patient with acute pyelonephritis or urinary tract infection responding poorly to appropriate antibiotic therapy.

Imaging Studies

The diagnosis of urolithiasis usually involves use of an ultrasound first. However, because of the physiologic hydronephrosis of pregnancy, its diagnostic value is severely limited. Renal pelvis stones can usually be easily seen on ultrasound, but these do not cause pain as often as ureteral stones. Although often difficult, a ureteral stone can sometimes be located with an ultrasound in the hands of an experienced ultrasonographer. Using a renal Doppler duplex ultrasound, internal vascular resistivity indices can be determined. This can aid in determining whether hydronephrosis is physiologic or is caused by obstruction. The next step would be a limited intravenous urogram, which would aid in locating the stone and in determining the degree of obstruction, if present.

Significant doses of radiation to the pelvis (5 to 15 rads) during the first trimester increase the risk of fetal abnormalities from 1% to 3%. A standard intravenous urogram delivers a total of 1.5 rads. A limited study, employing only two or three films can reduce the level of radiation to relatively "safe" levels. In general, each abdominal film delivers 0.2 rads to the fetus.

TREATMENT

In general, the spontaneous passage of upper tract stones is size dependent. Most (70%) upper tract stones pass spontaneously. Stones 5 to 6 mm in diameter have a greater than 50% chance of spontaneous passage. The spontaneous passage rate is 45%, 20%, and 12% for proximal, mid, and distal ureteral stones, respectively. Pregnancy is likely to adversely modify the above predictions and reduce spontaneous passage to 50%, particularly in cases of stones in the right upper urinary tract.

Since most stones pass on their own, management is conservative. The patient's pain is often controlled with oral analgesics on an outpatient basis (Table 18–4). If the patient remains symptomatic or admission is indicated (Table 18–5), urologic consultation is warranted urgently. Irrespective of the patient's disposition in the emergency department, urologic consultation must follow. Other urologic management options include ureteral stent placement, ureteroscopy with

Table 18-4
Pain Relief in Pregnancy

Drug	Toxicity	Pregnancy Class*
Narcotics	None in proper doses	C
Tylenol	None in proper doses	B
Aspirin	Fetal cerebral hemorrhage	D

*See Table 18–1 for legend.

Table 18-5
Indications for Hospitalization

Obstructed solitary kidney
Urinary tract infection
Diabetes mellitus
Stone of large size (>1 cm), which is unlikely to pass
  spontaneously
Nausea and vomiting
Uncontrollable pain in the emergency department

stone extraction, placement of a nephrostomy tube, or open lithotomy. Extracorporeal shock-wave lithotripsy is relatively contraindicated during pregnancy because of the unknown effects on the fetus and the excess radiation exposure during fluoroscopy.

Management of urolithiasis in pregnancy must be individualized based on the location of the stone, its size, degree of obstruction, the presence of infection, and the patients' overall condition and stage of pregnancy.

HIGHLIGHTS

- Most causes of abdominal pain in pregnant women are obstetric in nature.
- Acute cystitis and pyelonephritis can be diagnosed with urinalysis.
- Urolithiasis can be diagnosed with an ultrasound or a limited intravenous urogram.
- Small stones can be treated conservatively with hydration and oral analgesics.
- Larger and persistent stones require more invasive procedures.
- The normal physiologic hydronephrosis of pregnancy can lead to severe flank pain and, rarely, renal pelvis rupture.

Lower Urinary Tract Dysfunction

As a consequence of the pregnancy-induced physiologic and pathologic changes in the kidneys and the urinary bladder, the pregnant patient often complains of urinary frequency, stress urinary incontinence, urinary urgency, urge incontinence, incomplete bladder emptying, and slow urinary stream.

Urinary frequency is a common problem seen in up to 60% of pregnant women. This clinical presentation is mainly due to increased GFR and the resulting increased urinary output. The gravid uterus impressing on the bladder is an important contributing factor in this symptom. It is important to rule out significant gestational diabetes mellitus in the pregnant patient with dysfunction of micturition. No further work-up is indicated unless dysuria is present and a urinary tract infection needs to be ruled out. Patients can similarly complain of nocturia. Treatment is aimed at patient education and reassurance. Both of these symptoms can be expected to resolve post partum as urine output returns to normal.

Urinary incontinence, primarily stress, occurs in 30% to 50% of pregnant women. Again, the significant etiologic factor is the gravid uterus impressing the bladder. Both stress incontinence and urge incontinence often coexist in the same patient. Pregnancy-induced intrinsic dysfunction in the urethral smooth muscle has been proposed as another etiologic factor of stress urinary incontinence of pregnancy. Incontinence tends to become progressively worse during the pregnancy; however, 60% to 80% of the cases regress after delivery. Treatment is aimed at patient education and reassurance. If symptoms persist post partum, conservative measures such as Kegel exercises can be employed or a urologic consult can be obtained for severe cases.

HIGHLIGHTS

- Dysfunction of micturition, primarily urinary frequency and nocturia, during pregnancy resolve postpartum in most patients.
- Most cases of stress urinary incontinence of pregnancy resolve postpartum.

SUGGESTED READINGS

1. Cunningham FG, Whalley PJ: Asymptomatic bacteriuria during pregnancy. *In* Buchsbaum HJ, Schmidt JD (eds): Gynecologic and Obstetric Urology. Philadelphia, WB Saunders, 1982, pp 519–537.
2. Lipsky H: Dilatation of the urinary tract during pregnancy and its management. Eur Urol 10:372–376, 1984.
3. Loughlin KR: Management of urologic problems during pregnancy. Urology 44:159–169, 1994.
4. Marchant DJ: Effects of pregnancy and progestational agents on the urinary tract. Am J Obstet Gynecol 112:487–501, 1972.

5. Meares EM: Urologic surgery during pregnancy. Clin Obstet Gynecol 21:907–920, 1978.
6. Mikhail MS, Anyaegbunam A: Lower urinary tract dysfunction in pregnancy: A review. Obstet Gynecol Surv 50:675–683, 1995.
7. Nathan L, Huddleston JF: Acute abdominal pain in pregnancy. Obstet Gynecol Clin North Am 22:55–68, 1995.
8. Schmidt JD: Urinary calculi in pregnancy. *In* Buchsbaum HJ, Schmidt JD (eds): Gynecologic and Obstetric Urology. Philadelphia, WB Saunders, 1982, pp 562–572.
9. Weiss JP: Distinguishing normal from pathologic urologic changes during pregnancy. Infect Urol 10:111–117, 1997.
10. Weiss JP, Gillenwater J: Management of urologic problems in pregnancy. *In* Gillenwater JY, Grayhack JT, Howards SS, et al (eds): Adult and Pediatric Urology, 3rd ed. St. Louis, Mosby-Year Book, 1996, pp 353–367.

19 Renal Function in Pregnancy

Karen MacKay
Ossama Hozayen

Physiologic Changes in Normal Pregnancy

Pregnancy induces a number of alterations in systemic hemodynamics, renal function, and electrolytes (Table 19–1). Cardiac output increases early in pregnancy and reaches a plateau, at 30% to 50% above prepregnancy values, by the 16th week of gestation. This increase occurs as a consequence of a decrease in afterload and an increase in preload. Systemic vasodilation and the low-resistance circuit in the uterus combine to lower afterload. Vasodilation results in a fall in systemic blood pressure to a mean of 105/60 mm Hg during the second trimester. Preload increases by virtue of a 6- to 8-L expansion of extracellular fluid volume. The combination of increased plasma renin activity and slightly reduced atrial natriuretic peptide levels suggest that

the volume expansion occurs secondary to the increase in vascular capacitance. Volume expansion appears to be important for the fetus, as demonstrated by the positive relationship that exists between volume expansion and fetal growth.

Renal blood flow and glomerular filtration rate (GFR) also increase markedly during pregnancy. The GFR begins to increase approximately 6 weeks following conception and continues to rise until 12 to 20 weeks, when it stabilizes at a level 50% above prepregnancy values. This increase in GFR is reflected in a decrease in the serum creatinine concentration. Serum creatinine falls from a mean of 0.8 mg/dL prepregnancy to approximately 0.5 mg/dL during the second and third trimesters. Thus, serum creatinine values considered normal for the nonpregnant woman may be indicative of underlying renal

Table 19–1
Physiologic and Anatomic Changes Associated with Normal Pregnancy

Alteration	Clinical Consequence
Increase in cardiac output secondary to decreased systemic vascular resistance and increased extracellular volume	Normal blood pressure falls to a mean of ~105/60 mm Hg during the second trimester; localized edema occurs in ≤83% of normal pregnancies
Glomerular filtration rate increases by ~50%	Serum creatinine level falls from mean of 0.8 mg/dL to 0.5 mg/dL during pregnancy
Decreased tubular reabsorption of glucose	Glycosuria is common and is not necessarily indicative of glucose intolerance
Decreased tubular reabsorption of uric acid	Reduction in plasma uric acid concentration Increased urinary uric acid excretion
Increase in renal length by ~1 cm	Decrease in renal size following pregnancy is normal
Urinary tract dilation	Hydroureter of pregnancy, typically greater on the right, occurs in 90% of pregnancies
Chronic respiratory alkalosis	Modest fall in P_{CO_2}
Reset osmostat	Serum sodium level decreases by ~5 mEq/L

disease if that same value is seen during pregnancy. The GFR and serum creatinine level return to prepregnancy levels within 3 months after delivery.

Alterations in renal tubular function during pregnancy include decreased glucose reabsorption and increased uric acid excretion. The clinical consequences of these altered tubular functions are glycosuria, which is not necessarily associated with impaired glucose tolerance, increased urinary concentrations of uric acid, and reduced plasma uric acid levels.

Substantial anatomic changes also occur in the kidney and urinary tract. Swelling of the kidney leads to an increase in kidney length of approximately 1 cm. Hydroureter of pregnancy occurs in 90% of gravid women. Dilation of the renal pelvis and ureters begins at 6 to 10 weeks, progresses until term, and resolves within 1 to 2 months of delivery. Hydronephrosis extends to the level of the pelvic brim and is typically more pronounced on the right than the left. The mechanisms responsible for ureteral and pelvicaliceal dilation are likely to be multifactorial. Dilation of the ureters early in pregnancy suggests that mechanisms other than mechanical obstruction cause hydroureter of pregnancy. Progesterone and prostaglandins are suspected mediators of this early ureteral dilation. Later in pregnancy the enlarging uterus causes compression of the ureters as they cross the pelvic brim. Changes in the bladder include a decrease in tone with an associated increase in capacity. The bladder may contain twice its usual volume without discomfort during the later stages of pregnancy.

Electrolyte changes associated with pregnancy include chronic respiratory alkalosis and a decrease in the serum sodium concentration. The respiratory alkalosis, reflected by a modest fall in P_{CO_2}, results from direct stimulation of the respiratory center by progesterone. The decrease in serum sodium begins as early as the fifth week of pregnancy, falls by 5 mEq/L by 10 weeks, then remains at this level throughout pregnancy. Normally the serum sodium concentration is tightly regulated by thirst and antidiuretic hormone (ADH)-directed renal free water retention or excretion. This same close regulation is in place during pregnancy; however, the set point for

cessation and stimulation of ADH secretion appears to be shifted. This reset osmostat allows the serum sodium concentration to be tightly maintained at the new lower level despite variable water and sodium intake. Attempts to correct serum sodium to levels normal for the nonpregnant woman are ineffective and unnecessary because the change is small and is not associated with symptoms. A role for human chorionic gonadotropin (hCG) is suggested by the temporal correlation between serum sodium decline and hCG increase, and by the finding that the administration of hCG to women during the luteal phase of the menstrual cycle can induce a similar resetting of the osmostat. Serum sodium returns to prepregnancy levels within 1 to 2 months following delivery.

Hypertension and Pregnancy

Hypertensive disorders in pregnancy occur in about 6% to 8% of pregnancies. These disorders are important because hypertension is among the leading causes of maternal and perinatal mortality. Recently, it has been suggested that the deprived intrauterine environment caused by maternal hypertension not only leads to small-for-gestational-age infants but also may increase the prevalence of essential hypertension in affected infants as they reach adulthood.

As described earlier, normal pregnancy is a low-blood-pressure state associated with marked vasodilation. Blood pressure falls during the first trimester to average values of 103 ± 11 mm Hg systolic and 56 ± 10 mm Hg diastolic. Blood pressure then begins to rise slightly after the 28th week of gestation. **A diastolic blood pressure above 75 mm Hg during the second trimester or above 85 mm Hg during the third trimester is therefore abnormal. Fetal mortality increases if diastolic blood pressure exceeds 85 mm Hg, particularly if associated with proteinuria.**

Preeclampsia is the most common cause of hypertension in pregnancy. Women with preeclampsia have a reversal of the vasodilation characteristic of normal pregnancy. Clinically this disorder, whose onset is almost always after 20 weeks' gestation, is characterized by the combination of hyper-

Table 19-2
Risk Factors for Preeclampsia

Nulliparity
Multiple gestation
Age >40 yr
Family history of preeclampsia
Smoking
Diabetes
Hypertension
Renal disease
Obesity
Fetal hydrops
Antiphospholipid syndrome
Vascular disease

tension, proteinuria, and edema. An elevation in plasma uric acid concentration may also be a clue to the presence of preeclampsia. The vasoconstriction induced by preeclampsia decreases renal blood flow, lowers urate clearance, and leads to the elevated plasma levels. These elevated uric acid levels contrast with the low levels found during uncomplicated pregnancy. Risk factors for the development of preeclampsia are listed in Table 19–2. **Treatment balances the knowledge that sustained hypertension increases the risk of** prematurity, intrauterine growth retardation (IUGR), perinatal death, and maternal death with the concern that aggressive antihypertensive therapy may compromise uteroplacental blood flow. Induction of labor is indicated when the pregnancy is near term because preeclampsia resolves rapidly following delivery. **Pregnancy can be continued if the fetus is not mature and ominous signs are absent: severe hypertension persisting after 24 to 48 hours of treatment, thrombocytopenia, increasing hepatic transaminase levels, progressive renal insufficiency, premonitory signs of eclampsia (headache, hyperreflexia, epigastric pain), or fetal distress.**

Treatment of mild hypertension associated with preeclampsia (diastolic blood pressure < 95 mm Hg) typically involves bed rest. Pharmacologic treatment is employed in those with moderate hypertension (diastolic blood pressure ≥ 95 to 100 mm Hg). Suitable antihypertensive agents and some whose use should be avoided in pregnancy are listed in Table 19–3. Hydralazine and labetalol are the agents most frequently used to treat severe hypertension (diastolic blood pressure ≥ 100

Table 19-3
Antihypertensive Drugs and Pregnancy

Drug	Comments
Methyldopa	The drug of choice. Safety and efficacy supported by randomized trials and long-term follow-up of children born to mothers treated during pregnancy
Hydralazine	Appears to be safe and is often used along with methyldopa. May cause reflex tachycardia. It has been reported to induce neonatal thrombocytopenia
Atenolol and metoprolol	Appear to be safe and efficacious in late pregnancy. Fetal growth retardation has been noted when treatment was started in early or mid-gestation. Fetal bradycardia may occur
Labetalol	Appears to be as effective as methyldopa. There are no follow-up studies of children born to mothers treated with labetalol. May cause maternal hepatotoxicity. Fetal bradycardia was not detected in most studies.
Calcium channel blockers	Less experience than with the above-listed drugs. Role at present is uncertain. Nifedipine has been used without major problems. Not recommended as a first-line agent throughout pregnancy
Diuretics	Use is controversial. They may blunt the extracellular volume expansion that is important for fetal growth. These drugs may be continued in women for whom they were prescribed before pregnancy or if hypertension appears to be salt sensitive
Angiotensin-converting enzyme inhibitors	Absolutely contraindicated in pregnancy. Adverse fetal outcomes were seen in women treated during the second and/or third trimesters. No adverse fetal outcomes reported in those whose use was limited to the first trimester. If a woman taking these drugs becomes pregnant, she should be immediately switched to another agent
Angiotensin II receptor antagonists	Contraindicated based on the experience with the angiotensin-converting enzyme inhibitors

Table 19-4
Classification of Hypertension in Pregnancy

Type	Characteristics
Chronic hypertension	Elevated blood pressure >140/90 mm Hg presents before pregnancy or diagnosed before the 20th week of gestation or that persists beyond 6 weeks postpartum
Transient hypertension	Elevated blood pressure during pregnancy or in the first 24 hours postpartum with no other signs of preeclampsia or preexisting hypertension; this pattern, a manifestation of latent chronic hypertension, usually recurs in subsequent pregnancies and is responsible for most misdiagnoses of preeclampsia in multiparous women
Preeclampsia	Increased blood pressure appearing after 20 weeks' gestation usually accompanied by proteinuria and edema in a previously normotensive woman. The hypertension and proteinuria resolve following delivery
Preeclampsia superimposed on chronic hypertension	In women with chronic hypertension, increase of blood pressure of 30 mm Hg systolic or 15 mm Hg diastolic in addition to proteinuria or edema
Eclampsia	Seizures with preeclampsia

to 110 mm Hg). The risk of fetal cyanide toxicity limits the use of sodium nitroprusside to only a few hours.

Preeclampsia and the other types of hypertension associated with pregnancy are listed in Table 19–4. For many women, pregnancy may represent their first sustained contact with health care providers. Because of this, problems whose onset predated pregnancy, such as hypertension or underlying renal disease, may be first identified during pregnancy. **The presence of renal insufficiency, proteinuria, and/or hypertension prior to the 20th week of gestation strongly suggests an underlying renal disease or hypertension rather than preeclampsia. Factors that may assist in differentiating those with preexisting hypertension from those with preeclampsia are outlined in Table 19–5.**

Treatment recommendations for mild non-preeclamptic hypertension are not clear. Studies demonstrate increased fetal mortality with diastolic pressures higher than 85 to 90 mm

Hg; however, clinical trials have not consistently demonstrated a fetal or maternal benefit of treatment of hypertension of this severity. Treatment is clearly indicated for those with diastolic pressures higher than 100 mm Hg. Alpha methyldopa remains the drug of choice because of its extensive record of use and safety. Other drugs are listed in Table 19–3.

Pregnancy in Women with Underlying Renal Disease

The two central issues when a person with underlying renal disease considers pregnancy are what the effects of pregnancy are on the kidney disease, and what the effects of kidney disease are on the pregnancy. In people with primary renal diseases, the answer to these questions is largely dependent not on the specific type of histology, but rather on the severity of the underlying renal disease.

Table 19-5
Characteristics that May Aid in Differentiating Preeclampsia and Chronic Hypertension

Characteristic	Preeclampsia	Chronic Hypertension
Age	Extremes	Older
Parity	Nulliparous	Multiparous
Onset of hypertension	Third trimester	Earlier, often <20 wk
Funduscopic examination	Retinal edema; arteriolar spasm	Hypertensive retinopathy
Cardiac status	Normal	Left ventricular hypertrophy
Deep tendon reflex	Hyperactive	Normal
Proteinuria	>300 mg/d	Absent or minimal
Serum uric acid	Often elevated	Normal or low

The outlook is quite good for both fetal and maternal outcome in those with normal or only mildly reduced renal function (serum creatinine < 1.4 to 1.5 mg/dL). Fetal survival is only moderately reduced and a pregnancy-induced permanent decline in renal function is seen in up to 10% of pregnancies. A recent comparison of renal survival between 360 women with primary glomerulonephritis (serum creatinine ≤ 1.25 mg/dL) who did (171 women) or did not (189 women) become pregnant revealed no significant difference in renal survival during a mean follow-up of 15 years. Increases in the severity of proteinuria, edema, and hypertension occur frequently during pregnancy but generally resolve after delivery. Two additional factors to consider in women with normal or mildly reduced renal function are high levels of proteinuria and hypertension. **Women with nephrotic-range proteinuria with marked hypoalbuminemia present prior to conception or during the first trimester have a higher rate of spontaneous abortion, IUGR, and prematurity.** As is the case with women without underlying renal disease, hypertension present at conception or developing early in pregnancy is associated with an adverse effect on fetal outcome.

The picture is different in women with more severe underlying renal disease. Advances in care have led to a marked improvement in fetal survival when compared with that seen in earlier decades. A recent report of 82 pregnancies that continued beyond the first trimester in women with a serum level of 1.4 mg/dL or higher revealed an infant survival rate of 93%. However, these infants had a high rate of preterm delivery (59%) and IUGR (37%). The effect on maternal renal function is more grim. Forty percent of women with a creatinine level between 1.4 and 1.9 mg/dL had a pregnancy-related loss of renal function. This loss of function reversed following delivery in only half of the affected women. An even worse outcome was seen in those with an initial creatinine level of 2.0 mg/dL or higher. Nearly two thirds of these women had a rise in serum creatinine level during the third trimester. This decline in renal function persisted in nearly all the women and was associated with a rapid progression to end-stage renal disease in more

than half of those affected. The number of fetal complications were also high when baseline serum creatinine was at least 2.5 mg/dL. The frequency of preterm deliveries was found to be 73%, with IUGR in 57%. Prospective parents should be clearly informed of the risks associated with pregnancy undertaken in the face of moderate or severe renal insufficiency. If they elect to proceed, they should have access to high-risk obstetric care with an attendant neonatal intensive care unit.

Pregnancy is uncommon in those with severe renal dysfunction (serum creatinine ≥ 3 mg/dL) because of the frequency of amenorrhea or anovulatory menstrual cycles. If pregnancy does occur in this situation, patients should be cautioned to expect a high rate of obstetric complications and permanent loss of renal function. Fertility is even less common in those on dialysis. Not surprisingly, fetal outcome is poor with a high rate of fetal loss and prematurity. Women on dialysis should be encouraged to delay pregnancy until 1 or 2 years following successful transplantation. In transplanted women, 93% of pregnancies that continued beyond the 20th week ended successfully, albeit with high rates of preterm delivery (50%) and IUGR (40%). Pregnancy does not appear to have an adverse effect on allograft survival if the grafted kidney is functioning well at the onset of pregnancy.

Diabetic nephropathy and reflux nephropathy warrant comment because they are common in women of childbearing age. Pregnancy does not appear to accelerate the onset of diabetic nephropathy. Diabetics with proteinuria and normal or near-normal renal function have a consistent, but reversible, increase in proteinuria and hypertension during pregnancy. Worsening of renal function does not appear to be a concern in this population. By contrast, women with diabetic nephropathy with impaired renal function tend to have more difficulty. A study of diabetic women with baseline serum creatinine values of 1.4 to 1.7 mg/dL revealed that 45% experienced an accelerated progression of renal failure during pregnancy.

Pregnancy does not affect renal function in those with reflux nephropathy except in those with preexisting renal failure. As is the case for women with other causes of renal disease, some of these women with chronic renal insufficiency due to reflux nephropathy may suffer an irreversible accelerated loss of renal function with pregnancy. **A recent study of pregnancy in women with reflux nephropathy found that urinary tract infections complicated 22% of pregnancies. Forty percent of these infections involved pyelonephritis. Upper urinary tract infections were more common in those with previous episodes of pyelonephritis and in those with persistent vesicoureteral reflux.** Antibiotic chemoprophylaxis should be considered in those young pregnant patients with recurrent urinary tract infections or bacteriuria.

Acute Renal Failure in Pregnancy

Acute renal failure is an uncommon complication of pregnancy. The differential diagnosis of acute renal failure during pregnancy includes any of the disorders capable of inducing acute renal failure in nonpregnant persons. Early in pregnancy prerenal azotemia may occur as a consequence of hyperemesis gravidarum or hemorrhage. History and associated laboratory findings typical of persistent vomiting (hypokalemic metabolic alkalosis and low urinary chloride concentration) point easily to these diagnostic possibilities.

Renal cortical necrosis may occur secondary to severe complications of pregnancy such as septic abortions, placenta previa, amniotic fluid embolus, and prolonged intrauterine fetal death. In women suffering from severe complications of pregnancy, renal cortical necrosis presents with the abrupt development of oliguria or anuria, at times accompanied by gross hematuria and flank pain. Ultrasonography or computed tomographic (CT) scanning may help establish the diagnosis by demonstrating hypoechoic or hypodense regions of the renal cortex. Renal biopsy or arteriography, which demonstrates either absent or a nonhomogeneous cortical flow, is usually not required for diagnosis. Irreversible end-stage renal disease is the most common outcome of this severe disorder. However, with supportive therapy, 20% to 40% of patients have partial recovery of renal function, with creatinine clearances between 15 and 50 mL/min.

The differential diagnosis of acute renal failure late in pregnancy associated with evidence of microangiopathic hemolytic anemia and thrombocytopenia includes severe preeclampsia, hemolytic-uremic syndrome, and thrombotic thrombocytopenic purpura (TTP). Severe preeclampsia is usually preceded by the hypertension, proteinuria, and edema characteristic of preeclampsia. Patients may also have evidence of the HELLP syndrome (*h*emolysis, *e*levated *l*iver enzymes, *l*ow *p*latelet count). Acute renal failure is uncommon, even with severe preeclampsia, unless complications of severe bleeding, hemodynamic instability, or marked disseminated intravascular coagulation are superimposed. The abnormalities resulting from the severe preeclampsia resolve spontaneously within the first 2 weeks following delivery.

Hemolytic-uremic syndrome and TTP, which are likely different spectra of the same disease process, may occur during or in the weeks following pregnancy. The clinical picture of microangiopathic hemolytic anemia, thrombocytopenia, and renal insufficiency should raise concern about this diagnosis. Fever and neurologic abnormalities may be present in those with the clinical picture more characteristic of TTP. Unlike severe preeclampsia, this disease does not spontaneously resolve following delivery. The use of plasma infusion or plasma exchange has markedly improved the prognosis in this disease, which was formerly associated with a 90% mortality.

Acute renal failure secondary to obstruction is a rare finding during pregnancy. As indicated earlier, functional hydronephrosis is a common finding in normal pregnancy and is not associated with renal dysfunction. The diagnosis of obstruction secondary to the gravid uterus may be established by the demonstration of normalization of renal function with the patient in the lateral recumbent position and its recurrence when supine. Urinary tract obstruction secondary to stones is discussed later.

Urinary Tract Infection During Pregnancy

Bacterial infections of the urinary tract are the most commonly encountered infections during pregnancy. Although asymptomatic bacteriuria is more common, symptomatic infection may affect the lower urinary tract, causing cystitis, or the upper urinary tract, causing pyelonephritis. The prevalence of bacteriuria during pregnancy is similar to that in nonpregnant women ranging, in most studies, from 4% to 7%. The prevalence of bacteriuria rises with parity, age, sexual activity, lower socioeconomic status, and sickle cell trait. Women with an antepartum history of urinary tract infections have a higher prevalence of bacteriuria during pregnancy than do women without such a history. Most women with bacteriuria at delivery had bacteriuria at their first prenatal visit, and another 1% to 2% acquire bacteriuria later in pregnancy.

Physiologic and anatomic changes associated with pregnancy, which include dilation of the upper collecting system and reduction in ureteral peristalsis, may provide an opportunity for symptomatic urinary tract infections to develop. **Between 20% and 40% of women with untreated asymptomatic bacteriuria progress to acute pyelonephritis during pregnancy. By contrast, only 1% to 2% of those without bacteriuria early in pregnancy develop symptomatic urinary tract infection. Development of pyelonephritis is of concern not only because of the associated maternal morbidity but also because prematurity rates of 20% to 50% have been found in women with symptomatic urinary tract infection.** Fortunately, treatment of bacteriuric women lowers the incidence of symptomatic urinary tract infections by 80% to 90%. These concerns led to the recommendation that women be screened for the presence of bacteriuria during pregnancy.

Screening during the 16th gestational week may be the optimal time to screen to maximize bacteriuria-free gestational weeks. A midstream, clean-catch urine sample is the most common and practical method of collecting urine for screening. Catheterized urine specimens eliminate the problem of vaginal contamination, but the procedure should be avoided because it is associated with a 4% to 6% risk of introducing infection. Suprapubic aspirates are not practical for use in a screening program.

A midstream specimen containing more than 10^5 cfu/mL of a single pathogen per milliliter is the standard definition of a positive urine culture in an asymptomatic individual. There are several available methods for determining urinary bacterial counts. The presence of bacteria in an uncentrifuged drop of urine using the high-dry objective correlates well with the presence of at least 10^5 bacteria per milliliter. This technique is quick and inexpensive, but it lacks the sensitivity required of a good screening test. The semiquantitative dip inoculum method involves dipping an agar-coated slide in urine. After a 24-hour incubation, growth on the slide is compared with photographic standards. This method yields excellent results in screening for gram-negative bacteria and has been recommended as an initial screening procedure. A positive result on the dip inoculum test should be followed by a standard urine culture using a calibrated inoculum loop.

Some have challenged the cost effectiveness of screening populations with a low prevalence of bacteriuria. A suggested alternative in low-risk groups is to inform them to report immediately for care if they develop chills, fever, flank pain, or urinary symptoms. Advice regarding urinary symptoms may be problematic because irritative symptoms typically associated with urinary tract infections have such low predictive value for identifying those with bacteriuria during pregnancy.

Organisms involved in urinary tract infections during pregnancy are similar to those seen in nonpregnant women. Coliforms including *Escherichia coli*, the *Klebsiella-Enterobacter* group, and *Proteus mirabilis* are responsible for most infections. Gram-positive organisms, including *Staphylococcus saprophyticus*, other coagulase-negative staphylococci, and enterococci are responsible for a small percentage of urinary tract infections. *Streptococcus agalactiae* growth may represent contamination with vaginal flora rather than bacteriuria. It is unclear whether *Ureaplasma ureolyticus* and *Gardnerella vaginalis*, which may be cultured in 10% to 15% of pregnant women, play any significant pathogenic role.

Antibiotic choice in pregnancy is based on the need to use effective drugs while avoiding those drugs that have potential for fetal toxicity (Table 19–6). The optimal duration for treatment of asymptomatic bacteriuria is not

Table 19-6
Antibiotic Use During Pregnancy

Drug	Comments
Amoxicillin	Well tolerated; extensive clinical use during pregnancy
Nitrofurantoin	Those with G6PD deficiency may develop hemolytic anemia
Sulfisoxasole	Associated with hyperbilirubinemia near term
Cephalexin	May have lower cure rates than drugs listed above
Amoxcillin/clavulanic acid	Limited experience during pregnancy
Trimethoprim-sulfamethoxazole	Not recommended during pregnancy because of potential teratogenicity
Quinolones	Not recommended—may induce abnormalities of fetal bone growth

G6PD, glucose-6-phosphate dehydrogenase.

well defined. Single-dose treatments are effective but have cure rates of only 70%. A three-day treatment course may reflect a good balance between efficacy and side effects in those with asymptomatic bacteriuria. Others recommend the more standard 7- to 10-day course of therapy. Follow-up cultures should be done approximately 1 week after initial treatment. Women whose infections have cleared should be followed with monthly cultures until delivery. Those who fail their initial course of treatment should be treated again with a different antibiotic to which the organism is sensitive. The small number of women who fail to clear after two courses of antibiotics should be treated with a third course, followed immediately by suppressive therapy with 50 to 100 mg of nitrofurantoin nightly until delivery. These women should be recultured on a regular basis to detect infection with a resistant organism.

Presentation and treatment of pyelonephritis are similar to that of nonpregnant women. More than 95% of patients respond within 72 hours to appropriate intravenous antibiotics, usually ampicillin and an aminoglycoside. Treatment of pyelonephritis should be followed immediately with suppressive therapy and regular surveillance cultures until delivery.

Nephrolithiasis During Pregnancy

The pathogenesis of nephrolithiasis involves an imbalance between factors that favor stone formation and those that protect against stone formation. Several changes in normal pregnancy may predispose to stone development.

Dilation of the collecting system allows urinary stasis that provides an opportunity for crystal formation, aggregation, and stone growth. Circulating levels of 1,25-dihydroxyvitamin D increase during pregnancy and contribute to increased intestinal absorption of calcium and increased calcium mobilization from bone. As a result, urinary calcium excretion may increase by twofold to threefold. Uric acid excretion also increases substantially during pregnancy. These factors that favor stone formation are countered by increased excretion of substances that inhibit stone formation: citrate, magnesium, and glycoproteins.

The true incidence of nephrolithiasis during pregnancy is uncertain. Estimates vary and indicate that stones complicate 0.03% to 0.12% of pregnancies. The frequency of stone disease during pregnancy does not appear to be greater than that found in the general population. A study of 78 patients with a history of stone disease who later became pregnant found that pregnancy had no effect on the frequency of stone episodes. The types of stones formed during pregnancy mirror those seen in the general population with approximately 75% calcium, 10% to 20% uric acid, 10% struvite, and 1% cystine stones. When stones do complicate pregnancy, 80% to 90% of episodes occur during the second or third trimester.

Symptoms of nephrolithiasis during pregnancy are similar to those of the general population. Flank pain is present in 84% to 100% of patients. Hematuria, either microscopic or macroscopic, is present in 90% to 100% of patients. However, examination of the urine on two or three occasions may be necessary to demonstrate such a high prevalence of hematuria. Flank pain with accompanying abdominal pain is a common presentation, while abdominal pain alone was noted in only 6% of patients in one series. Frequency, urgency, and dysuria may also occur. These symptoms may be difficult to evaluate because they are seen with uncomplicated urinary tract infections and also are commonly experienced in pregnancy. Infection of the lower urinary tract or pyelonephritis was present in 9 of 15 patients reported in one series. Clues to the presence of nephrolithiasis in patients presenting with urinary tract infection may be the greater severity of pain in women with concomitant stone disease and persistent fever following administration of appropriate antibiotics. The time at which persistent fever should prompt a search for nephrolithiasis is uncertain. A recent study of nonpregnant individuals with pyelonephritis indicated that the median duration of fever was 34 hours. It seems reasonable to perform imaging studies in those whose fever persists longer than 48 or 72 hours.

The wide availability of ultrasonography and its lack of radiation exposure have made this the best initial study for evaluation of suspected nephrolithiasis in pregnancy. Unfortunately, ultrasonography has far from ideal sensitivity for detection of nephrolithiasis during pregnancy. In one series the diagnosis of urolithiasis was confirmed by ultrasonography in only 7 of 15 patients. A larger study found that only 20 of 75 patients with renal colic had a clearly abnormal renal ultrasound. Stones may be difficult to locate because most are located in the ureters in pregnancy and ureteral stones are difficult to identify, except when they are located in the most proximal and distal portions of the ureter. Transvaginal ultrasonography may be helpful in the detection of calculi in the lower portion of the ureter. Another challenge associated with interpretation of ultrasonography is that of differentiating the physiologic hydronephrosis seen in most pregnancies from pathologic dilation secondary to stone-induced obstruction. Measurements of the resistive indices of intrarenal vessels may allow better differentiation of these two processes. Ureteral obstruction causes an increase in intrarenal vascular resistance with consequent reduction in diastolic blood flow. **Resistive**

indices, which are normal in women with physiologic hydronephrosis of pregnancy, may be elevated in the acutely obstructed kidney. Color-flow Doppler ultrasonography may add further to the diagnostic usefulness of ultrasound in these patients. This study may be used to detect ureteric jets, which may be absent or show low continuous flow in the presence of a high-grade obstruction.

The intravenous pyelogram (IVP), the gold standard for imaging with nephrolithiasis, can be modified to decrease fetal radiation exposure. **Beam collimation, short exposure time, high-speed screens, and prone rather than supine positioning can be used to decrease fetal radiation dosage. Limiting the number of films, shielding the maternal pelvis, and filming only the involved side can also decrease radiation exposure.** Limited-stage IVP has been variously defined. A scout film, followed by a 15- to 20-minute kidney, ureter, and bladder and delayed films as necessary, has been recommended. In some studies delayed films consistently failed to identify calculi if none were evident on the 20-minute film. These authors recommended a plain abdominal film, followed by films at 30 seconds and 20 minutes.

Magnetic resonance (MR) urography using T2-weighted fast-spin, echo-type imaging can provide good-quality images that accurately determine the level of obstruction. Because stones do not elicit a characteristic MR signal, they are detected as a signal void superimposed on the high-contrast signal of urine. The effect of MR imaging on fetal development is unclear; thus, it is not recommended during the first trimester. The lack of wide availability and the expense of MR imaging further limit its usefulness. Unenhanced helical CT scanning is reportedly highly sensitive in the diagnosis of nephrolithiasis and has the ability to differentiate calculi from tumor or blood clot. However, the high delivered radiation dose, particularly to the pelvis, makes it unsuitable for routine use in pregnancy. Urologic consultation is warranted in every case of nephrolithiasis during pregnancy.

Conservative treatment with hydration, bed rest, and analgesia results in the spontaneous passage of 50% to 84% of stones. Codeine has been associated with fetal defects and is best avoided in the first trimester. Morphine is not known to cause any fetal problems. Nonsteroidal anti-inflammatory drugs have been associated with fetal pulmonary hypertension and carry the theoretical risk of premature closure of the ductus arteriosus when given close to term. Segmental epidural anesthesia has been used to treat severe renal colic during pregnancy. This technique may decrease ureteral spasm and facilitate the passage of calculi.

Indications for intervention in pregnant patients with stones include persistent fever with obstruction, anuria in a solitary kidney, worsening renal function with persistent obstruction, intractable pain, sepsis, failure of conservative therapy, and renal colic precipitating premature labor that is refractory to tocolysis. Ureteral stents placed under ultrasound guidance is a suitable therapy for many of these indications. Ultrasound-guided percutaneous nephrostomy is preferable for those in whom stents cannot be placed or in acutely ill or septic patients because it allows immediate drainage and culture. Encrustation, which may occur at an accelerated pace during pregnancy, may require frequent (every 3 to 8 weeks) tube replacement. Ureteroscopy has been used successfully, although some consider that it exposes the mother and the fetus to unnecessary risks. Extracorporeal shock-wave lithotripsy is contraindicated in pregnancy because of possible adverse effects on the fetus. The availability of these options for management of complicated stone disease allows for management of all but a few patients without the use of open surgical techniques.

Prevention is an important factor in managing patients with a history of stone disease who are pregnant or planning pregnancy, or in those with newly active stone disease. These women should be reminded of dietary measures that may decrease recurrence rates. Fluid intake should be sufficient to maintain a urine output of more than 2000 mL per 24 hours. Sodium intake should be limited to 2 g daily, because excess renal excretion of sodium increases renal calcium excretion. Excessive animal protein intake should be discouraged because high-protein diets serve to increase uric acid and calcium excretion and

decrease citrate excretion. **Dietary calcium restriction should not be advised. In the Nurses Health Study, low dietary calcium intake was associated with an increased frequency of calcium stone disease, possibly because it allows increased oxalate absorption.** Calcium supplementation was, by contrast, associated with an increased frequency of stone disease. If women with a history of stone disease choose to take calcium supplements, they should be advised to take them with meals.

Most drugs used to prevent stone formation are best avoided during pregnancy. Thiazide diuretics, which decrease urinary calcium excretion, may blunt the maternal volume expansion needed for normal fetal growth and possibly cause fetal thrombocytopenia. Allopurinol has not been associated with adverse effects on fetal animals; however, the lack of information regarding its effects in humans makes it also a drug whose use during pregnancy is not advised. Penicillamine, which is used to treat cystine stones, is not recommended for use because of its teratogenic effects in rats and reports of fetal defects in humans.

SUGGESTED READINGS

1. Andriole VT, Patterson TF: Epidemiology, natural history, and management of urinary tract infections in pregnancy. Med Clin North Am 75:359, 1991.
2. Brown MA, Whitworth JA: The kidney in hypertensive pregnancies—victim and villain. Am J Kidney Dis 22:427, 1998.
3. Epstein FH: Pregnancy and renal disease. N Engl J Med 335:277, 1996.
4. Gorton E, Whitfield HN: Renal calculi in pregnancy. Br J Urol 80(Suppl 1):4, 1997.
5. How SH: Pregnancy in women with chronic renal disease. N Engl J Med 312:836, 1985.
6. Jungers P, Chauveau D: Pregnancy in renal disease. Kidney Int 52:871, 1992.
7. Krane NK: Acute renal failure in pregnancy. Arch Intern Med 148:2347, 1988.
8. Loughlin KR: Management of urologic problems during pregnancy. Urology 44:159, 1994.
9. MacLean AB: Urinary tract infection in pregnancy. Br J Urol 80:10, 1997.
10. Maikranz P, Coe FL, Parks J, et al: Nephrolithiasis in pregnancy. Am J Kidney Dis 9:354, 1987.
11. Paller MS: Hypertension in pregnancy. J Am Soc Nephrol 9:314, 1998.
12. Swanson SK, Heilman RL, Eversman WG: Urinary tract stones in pregnancy. Surg Clin North Am 75:123, 1995.

20 Perinatal Urologic Consultation

William F. Tarry

Prenatal ultrasonography has greatly enhanced the early detection of many congenital anomalies, particularly those involving the genitourinary system. The kidneys are readily identifiable by 16 weeks' gestation in most fetuses. The incidence of genitourinary anomalies in populations where virtually all pregnancies undergo screening sonography is about 0.2%. However, since there is a significant diagnostic error rate (9% to 20%), many of these kidneys do not have a significant lesion and do not come to surgery. Perinatal urologic consultation is useful in sorting out which kidneys need further attention. While dilation of the kidneys is by far the most common genitourinary finding, dilation of the lower urinary tract is also readily identifiable. Conversely the absence of a detectable bladder is also always a significant finding, signaling the presence of either bladder extrophy or one of the cloacal malformations. As a general rule, a renal pelvic diameter of less than 1 cm in the fetus rarely signifies any significant obstructing lesions. Most experts recommend further evaluation of any kidney with the pelvis diameter wider than 8 mm in the immediate postnatal period.

The postnatal evaluation of patients exhibiting prenatal hydronephrosis consists of a repeat ultrasound examination of the entire urinary tract accompanied by a voiding cystourethrogram. Although there has been some debate about the timing of these studies, it appears reasonable to perform them prior to discharging a healthy newborn from the nursery on postnatal day 2. If the postnatal ultrasound shows no hydronephrosis, most experts believe that a follow-up sonogram at 3 or 4 months of age should be performed. It is unlikely, however, that such a patient has a significant anomaly. The voiding cystogram has two purposes: to look for vesicoureteral reflux or, in males, posterior urethral valves. In most instances the ureters as well as the renal collecting system will have been dilated prenatally. The management of reflux is discussed in Chapter 21. The management of valves is discussed in this chapter. **All patients with prenatal hydronephrosis should be maintained from birth on prophylactic antibiotics, usually a penicillin derivative; this prophylaxis should be continued at least until the diagnosis is clear and possibly as long as 3 months postnatally.**

Ureteropelvic Junction Obstruction

Ureteropelvic junction obstruction is the most common cause of hydronephrosis in the newborn. It is somewhat more common in boys and on the left side. In 15% of cases it is associated with vesicoureteral reflux that may be present on the same or the opposite side. The infant who has persistent significant hydronephrosis on postnatal sonography should be evaluated with a diuretic nuclear renal scan (usually done with either diethylenetriamine-penta-acetic acid [DTPA] or mercaptoacetyltriglycine [Mag 3]) labeled with ^{99m}technetium. This examination quantitates renal function in each kidney and defines obstruction by means of the washout curve after the furosemide (Lasix) administration. This study should be delayed until after 3 weeks of age because there is no rush to make the diagnosis, and the quality of the study is improved by maturation of the kidney. Patients with normal function in the affected kidney and a normal furosemide washout curve are usually followed for 1 or 2 years with sequential renal scans. Most of them resolve spontaneously, but a small percentage come to surgical correction either because of worsening function or drainage or the development of other symptoms such as urinary tract infection or failure to thrive. Patients who have markedly delayed excretion of the nuclide after furosemide administration or those who exhibit diminished function in the affected kidney need urologic referral and generally come to surgery promptly.

The surgical repair of this lesion in the newborn has become a routine, uncomplicated procedure. It is generally done through a relatively painless posterior lumbar incision, and the patients are discharged from the hospital within 48 hours. The failure rate or reoperation rate in most large series is about 2%. Surgical failures are usually asymptomatic and must be detected by follow-up nuclear studies that are done at 3 months and 1 year postoperatively. Reoperation is generally successful in preserving renal function and resolving the obstruction.

Posterior Urethral Valves

Posterior urethral valves is the most common cause of bladder outlet obstruction in the newborn. The valve appears as a diaphragm at the junction of the prostatic and membranous urethra near the verumontanum where the valve is inserted. The incidence is about 1 in 5000 to 8000 boys, and the spectrum of severity of symptoms and degree of obstruction with its effect on renal development is quite variable. **Currently the most common presentation is that of prenatal hydronephrosis involving both kidneys and ureters as well as the bladder. On fetal sonography the bladder is seen not to empty as it normally would.** Alternatively, the patient may present in the newborn nursery with poor urinary stream or failure to void and a palpable abdominal mass. Prior to the advent of fetal sonography the typical presentation consisted of an abdominal mass, failure to thrive,

and sepsis, occasionally accompanied by urinary ascites. In severe cases where the fetal urinary production is impaired, oligohydramnios may result in pulmonary hypoplasia and postnatal ventilatory difficulties.

In any baby with a lower abdominal mass, bladder catheterization is usually the definitive diagnostic maneuver, and disappearance of the mass with drainage of the bladder clarifies the situation. If these boys are observed to void, the urinary stream trickles down over the perineum and the diagnosis of bladder outlet obstruction is obvious. Once the catheter is in place and urine is draining, the definitive study is a voiding cystourethrogram (VCUG) to delineate the valve and to document the presence of vesicoureteral reflux that is present in about half the cases. Serum creatinine is usually equal to maternal creatinine level for the first 48 hours and after that time reflects the infant's own renal function. The presenting creatinine level is quite variable but usually a rapid drop is observed with decompression of the bladder. Occasionally catheterization is difficult and placement of a suprapubic catheter is required. In the absence of respiratory compromise, prematurity or other metabolic difficulties that preclude safe anesthesia, the patient can be taken to the operating room and have the valves ablated endoscopically within the first day or so of life, thus avoiding the period of catheter drainage with its attendant risk of infection. **Whether the obstruction is relieved by catheter drainage or valve ablation, the creatinine level should drop fairly promptly and a nadir below 0.8 mg/dL is believed to denote a good long-term prognosis.** Another prognostic factor is the sonographic appearance of the kidneys, with increased echogenicity suggesting an element of renal dysplasia and long-term poor function. The presence of reflux also correlates with poor renal function in the refluxing kidney(s). Nuclear renography after relief of the obstruction further defines renal function.

Several issues regarding management remain somewhat unclear. In the past proximal urinary diversions using cutaneous ureterostomies were done in patients whose creatinine level did not drop below 0.8 mL/dL. Such diversion does not improve renal function, is detrimental to bladder function, and therefore may compromise subsequent transplantation. Primary valve ablation to relieve the obstruction is almost invariably the appropriate course of action. Traditionally a great deal of attention has been paid to persistent reflux, and early reimplantation of refluxing ureters in valve patients was frequently done. The results in general were dismal, and some of the poor outcomes predicted by the presence of reflux may in fact have resulted from surgical complications. Rarely is reimplantation necessary; about half the time the reflux resolves spontaneously with relief of the obstruction. Reimplantation is usually carried out if recurrent pyelonephritis occurs, or prior to transplantation if that becomes necessary. There may be a few instances in which massive reflux of most of the bladder volume up the ureters precludes proper bladder cycling, and reimplantation facilitates development of normal bladder function.

When patients with posterior urethral valves are studied urodynamically early in infancy, they are found to void more frequently and at higher pressures compared with normal subjects. As they age some of them revert to a more normal pattern, whereas others progress to a situation in which they empty frequently in small amounts and do so with high voiding pressures; they develop either bladder instability or noncompliance. In such cases incontinence is typically present throughout the school years. In past years it was thought that no treatment for this incontinence was warranted and that the onset of continence at puberty was to be expected. Recent evidence suggests that those patients who experience the onset of continence at puberty in fact are about to undergo a rapid decline into renal failure and that the incontinence should be treated early with anticholinergic drugs to eliminate the bladder instability. The rare patient with significant residual urine should be worked up for residual obstruction and then treated as necessary with intermittent catheterization. In most instances if the obstruction has been adequately relieved, the bladder will empty well. Some of the poor results with valve bladders have been largely iatrogenic. **If the bladder is allowed to cycle normally, bladder instability is treated, and infection is prevented, further renal deterioration can be delayed as long as possible, and the success of a later renal transplant is improved.**

The children with reflux should be maintained on antibiotic prophylaxis until the reflux resolves. All the infants with posterior urethral valves should be on antibiotic prophylaxis for the first 3 months of life. Probably the only group of patients with a really good long-term outlook are those whose creatinine level returns to normal (0.4 mg/dL in the newborn). Those between 0.4 and 0.8 mg/dL probably represent patients who will come to end-stage renal disease in adult life, whereas those whose creatinine level never becomes lower than 0.8 mg/dL in the first year of life will progress much more rapidly and come to dialysis or transplantation during the childhood years. **Unless the renal function is completely normal, these patients need to be followed by pediatric nephrologists as well as urologists for optimum growth and prevention of metabolic derangements.** Many of them exhibit concentrating defects and difficulties with acid-base balance before they exhibit extreme decline in their glomerular filtration.

Duplication Anomalies: Duplex Ectopic Ureters and Ureteroceles

Duplication of the ureter is common, occurring in about 10% of the general population. In a small fraction of cases one of the duplex ureters terminates ectopically or in a ureterocele, which is a balloon-like dilation of the terminal ureter. This condition may cause unilateral or bilateral obstruction and is the third most common cause of newborn hydronephrosis. It is somewhat more common in females. A variety of sequelae are possible depending on bilaterality, degree of obstruction, and the association of reflux in the lower pole ureters. **Often the upper segment of kidney subtended by the ectopic ureter is dysplastic and has little or no appreciable function even after the obstruction is relieved. The lower pole ureter on the other hand often refluxes and is located somewhat** laterally in the bladder. **Large ureteroceles may obstruct the bladder outlet via a ball-valve mechanism and may even occasionally prolapse through the urethra in females, presenting at the introitus as a necrotic mass. Urinary tract infection and gram-negative sepsis are commonly associated with this entity and, in fact, sepsis was the most common presenting sign in the preultrasound era.** Thus, when these lesions are discovered prenatally or at birth, the patient must be placed on prophylactic antibiotics. **Should this lesion escape detection in the newborn, a frequent presentation in girls with ectopic ureters is constant dribbling incontinence due to the production of small amounts of urine by the upper pole segment whose ureter terminates outside the urethral sphincter mechanism; the most common locations for these ectopic ureters are adjacent to the urethral meatus or on the anterior vaginal wall.**

Whether the patient presents with prenatal hydronephrosis or with infection, the initial examination is usually an ultrasound. A good ultrasound should demonstrate all of the relevant anatomy, including the duplication of the collecting system, the dilated obstructed ureter, and the presence of the ureterocele within the bladder. If the lower pole ureters reflux they are usually dilated as well. The next appropriate study would be a VCUG to confirm the presence of the ureterocele in the bladder and to diagnose any associated reflux that may be contralateral, ipsilateral, or both. In rare instances duplex ectopic ureters may be bilateral. The work-up is completed by a functional upper urinary tract study. Both intravenous pyelography and nuclear renography have advantages and proponents. **The traditional pyelogram is better for demonstrating the location and course of ureters, remembering that the upper ureter associated with the ureterocele or the ectopic orifice generally does not visualize.** The nuclear study is better at measuring function. It is useful in that if there is function in the upper pole segment, one is more inclined to preserve that segment. In addition refluxing lower pole segments sometimes demonstrates diminished function, further complicating the management.

No standard management is appropriate

for all cases, and indeed there is not a general agreement about the details of managing these complex lesions. Removal of the upper pole segment associated with the ectopic ureter sacrifices little functioning tissue and allows the distal dilated ureter and ureterocele to decompress, thus obviating the bladder outlet problems. If there is no associated reflux and the ureterocele is not overly large, partial nephrectomy may be sufficient treatment. Alternatively, endoscopic incision of the ureterocele allows the obstructed system to drain and may be sufficient therapy in some cases, even if the upper pole segment fails to develop any function. On the other hand, the presence of a large ureterocele, which may continue to obstruct the bladder outlet or impair continence later in life, coupled with high-grade reflux into the lower pole system, precludes treatment with a single minor procedure.

While there have been advocates of total correction of these patients at the initial surgery, particularly when they presented with infection at 6 months to 2 years of age, this is rarely done in the asymptomatic newborn. Generally the initial procedure is one of the earlier discussed simple preliminary operations. If there are continued episodes of infection, voiding problems, or bladder outlet obstruction, or if the upper pole system remains persistently dilated in spite of the incision, a more definitive procedure at the bladder level becomes necessary. Refluxing ureters are reimplanted and the ureterocele or the distal dilated ectopic ureter is excised completely with reconstruction of the bladder neck muscle and epithelium to facilitate later development of urinary control. About 60% of patients with ectopic ureters and ureteroceles require this more extensive reconstruction. Follow-up consists of radiographs to document the absence of reflux or obstruction. Failure to resolve these problems with the initial surgery is uncommon but can be successfully corrected. Persistent incontinence has frequently been noted in the past. When reviewing older series it is not clear whether this incontinence results from overzealous dissection around the distal ureteral segment or distortion of the continence mechanism by the expanding ectopic ureter itself. Recent experience has been that normal urinary control is usual with careful dissection, and in general the entire abnormal segment should be removed.

Multicystic Dysplastic Kidney

The final lesion to be mentioned in the category of prenatal hydronephrosis is actually a misdiagnosis. **The multicystic dysplastic kidney is the second most common abdominal mass in the newborn and may be confused on sonography with a hydronephrotic kidney.** A careful postnatal examination, however, should be diagnostic since this lesion is characterized by randomly distributed noncommunicating cysts and a complete absence of any identifiable renal parenchyma. Rarely should a nuclear study be needed to confirm the complete absence of function in such kidneys. While they were historically removed due to the lack of good radiographic studies and the possibility of malignancy in an infant with a palpable mass, **most urologists today would follow these lesions and allow them to resolve spontaneously. Although the kidney cannot develop any function, it rarely produces any symptom or problem warranting surgical intervention.** There have been rare reports of hypertension, Wilms' tumor, or renal cell carcinoma associated with these kidneys later in life, but the incidence is so low as to make the risks of early nephrectomy exceed the benefits. Rarely in a small baby a large multicystic kidney produces symptoms such as poor feeding or respiratory compromise, prompting the nephrectomy in the neonatal period. **These patients should undergo a VCUG because there is a 15% to 20% incidence of ureteral reflux in the contralateral, solitary functioning kidney.** Refluxing patients should receive antibiotic prophylaxis and be managed like any other patient with reflux (see Chapter 21). In clinical practice this is invariably a unilateral lesion and is not associated with other anomalies. It should not be confused with polycystic kidney, which is bilateral and inevitably leads to chronic renal failure.

The genitourinary system is the most common site for developmental anomalies, and many of these malformations of the upper urinary tract are asymptomatic and not obvious from external examination. Thus it is worth noting that if anomalies are present in two systems, there is a 50% chance that a third anomaly exists and the urinary tract is the most likely place for it to be located. Another interesting association is that of hydronephrosis and cyanotic heart disease. **Newborns with cyanotic heart disease have a 20% incidence of a renal lesion such as those described earlier.** All such babies should be screened with sonography of the urinary tract. Early detection of such lesions prevents deterioration of renal function and the complications of infection. Efforts at such detection are generally worthwhile and cost effective.

Neurogenic Bladder and Myelomeningocele

Patients with neurogenic bladder and myelomeningocele require long-term urologic care, and there is a great deal more to be said about their management later in life. In the newborn it is sufficient to ensure that bladder emptying occurs and that they remain uninfected. Almost invariably the kidneys are normally functioning at birth, and interventions are designed to preserve that situation. An ultrasound of the kidneys and bladder at the earliest convenient time is a reasonable baseline study. Dilation of the kidneys at this early stage is rare but is a warning that bladder emptying is inadequate. Renal function may be monitored with the serum creatinine level. **Perhaps the most important thing one can do in the neonatal period is palpate the abdomen frequently, looking for a distended bladder.** In the infant the bladder is easy to palpate or percuss, and its persistence is diagnostic of poor bladder emptying due to the neurologic abnormality. Pressure on the bladder to empty it is almost never helpful and indeed may be harmful. The Credé maneuver should be employed only in the rare patient with a completely flaccid bladder and urethral sphincter. One may suspect this situation where the bladder is persistently distended but there is absence of perineal reflexes or anal sphincter activity and minimal pressure on the bladder expresses the urine from the urethra.

Most patients with spina bifida exhibit some degree of bladder hypertonicity or instability and variable but fixed outlet resistance. Urodynamic studies are useful in predicting which children will get into trouble later and should be done sometime within the first few months of life. **If the pressure at which fluid leaks from the bladder is higher than 40 cm H$_2$O, that patient needs to be managed with intermittent catheterization or, in the female infants, urethral overdilation.** Emptying the bladder at low pressure preserves storage capacity and facilitates later management as well as prevents infection and damage to the kidneys in infancy. Those who empty at pressures below 40 cm H$_2$O and do not exhibit significant residual urine can be left alone to void into the diaper. They should be monitored with periodic ultrasonography of the kidneys to detect any dilation of the upper urinary tract. It is not necessary to put all newborns with spina bifida on intermittent catheterization as a preventive measure. If the bladder is emptying well, they do not need routine prophylactic antibiotics.

Ambiguous Genitalia

The newborn with ambiguous external genitalia presents a most stressful situation for the physician and the parents. **The evaluation must be rapid, accurate, and as simple as possible; it must result in identification of an appropriate gender assignment and clarification of any serious metabolic abnormalities. Names of syndromes with gender connotations, such as female pseudohermaphrodite, should be avoided; at no time prior to the final gender assignment should the child be referred to as he or she. Inadvertent reference to the incorrect gender pronoun may have long-lasting effects on the parents' acceptance of the child and may alter the child's self-perception and sexual development. In determining the sex of rearing, important guiding principles include the following:**

Adequate sexual function as an adult is an important consideration, particularly for the reconstructive surgeons.

Preservation of fertility where feasible and hormone production by an existing gonad that is consistent with the gender assignment are desirable.

Neonatal imprinting by ambient hormones is a real phenomenon, and its impact should be taken into consideration.

The best approach to the work-up incorporates the attitude that the proper sex of the infant will be discovered and that poorly developed or inappropriately developed parts will be reconstructed surgically as indicated. Parents should never be left with the impression that their boy or girl could have been something other than what it is, or that it could become whichever sex they choose for it.

While the external genital appearance of individual patients varies considerably, and the detailed genital examination is important for planning management, the physical examination contributes relatively little to the diagnosis. Basically all intersex patients exhibit similar ambiguous features. **There are two salient features of the physical examination of the newborn with ambiguous genitalia. The labioscrotal folds and inguinal regions must be palpated extremely carefully for the presence of a gonad. A gonad that descends partially or completely toward a scrotal location is almost invariably a normal testis. If the normal testis is palpable, the patient is almost certainly either a normal male with hypospadias and an undescended contralateral testis or a true hermaphrodite, the former being much more likely. In this case the gender identification is male, although the hermaphrodite requires gonadal biopsies to prove the point. It is wise to keep in mind that 85% of babies with ambiguous genitalia are genetic females with congenital adrenal hyperplasia; some of the precursors of cholesterol synthesis have androgen activity and masculinize the fetus. These patients are always reconstructed as females and have normal fertility and sexual function. For this reason metabolic evaluation including electrolytes, cortisol levels, and measurement of urine and serum levels of precursors to identify the specific enzyme defect should be done promptly.** When those tests are completed, the evaluation is finished. All other patients require laparotomy or laparoscopy and possibly gonadal biopsies to establish the diagnosis and arrive at a correct gender identification. Obviously consultation on the first day of life with the pediatric endocrinologist and the pediatric urologist is mandatory. The adult specialist in these areas is of no use either in the initial evaluation or in the long-term management of these problems.

Laparoscopy has replaced laparotomy in most centers for the examination of the internal genital structures and the gonads. It should be done in the first few days of life, as soon as congenital adrenal hyperplasia has been ruled out as a diagnosis. It is not necessary to wait for the karyotype because this has relatively little bearing on either the sex of rearing or the surgical management of the infant. At the same time endoscopy of the perineal opening or urogenital sinus should be carried out because this contributes a great deal to planning of the external reconstruction. A radiograph in which contrast agent is injected in the urogenital sinus is often helpful and may be done under the same anesthetic or separately in the radiology department. Ultrasound examination of the pelvic organs is often done but usually is nonspecific and does not eliminate the need for direct examination of these organs. If the nature of the gonads is not obvious from their external appearance, a careful biopsy of each gonad must be done in such a way as to preserve gonadal tissue. Under no circumstances should unidentified gonads be removed completely prior to definitive diagnosis, gender identification, and management planning. The karyotype may aid in the decision regarding gonadal disposition. **In the presence of a Y chromosome dysgenetic gonads are prone to malignant degeneration.** On the other hand a gonad may provide endogenous hormone if not contribute to fertility in certain instances, such as a true hermaphrodite with a normal testis on one side reared as a male.

Congenital adrenal hyperplasia is the most common intersex problem, and 21-hydroxylase deficiency is the most common enzyme defect, accounting for about 80% of cases. The remainder have a deficiency of 11-hydroxylase with essentially the opposite metabolic effects. Of the former about 70% have salt wasting and hypotension, whereas of the latter about 30% have salt retention and severe hypertension. Usually these syndromes manifest themselves in the third or fourth week of life. The accumulation of precursors has an androgenic effect and results in variable masculinization ranging from mild labioscrotal fusion and severe hypospadias to a completely normal male phenotype. The gonads are never palpable because they are normal ovaries in the usual intra-abdominal location. There is a urogenital sinus with an opening somewhere on the perineum and a junction of the vagina with the urethra usually close to the perineal skin but occasionally up toward the bladder neck. The uterus and fallopian tubes are normal. Although some regression of the phallus is achieved with steroid treatment, it is insufficient to obviate surgery. Early reconstructive surgery produces psychological benefits by allowing the baby to go home looking like a normal female. In general the urogenital sinus is incised and a posterior flap is rotated up into the vagina to enlarge the introitus. The urethra then is seen to have a normal location. The clitoris is recessed or partially resected, and the excessive phallic skin and labioscrotal folds are fashioned into normal-appearing labia minora and majora. The cosmetic results are quite nice. The one drawback to early surgery is the potential for subsequent stenosis of the introitus, which can usually be managed with gentle dilation under anesthesia or a small surgical procedure at the time the patient is ready for sexual activity to begin. Unfortunately long-term psychological problems have arisen in these patients, presumably due to early androgen imprinting of the brain. A complete discussion of these aspects is beyond the scope of this chapter.

True hermaphroditism is defined by the presence of both ovarian and testicular tissue regardless of the karyotype, which may be XX, XY, or a mosaic. Most commonly they exhibit a 46XY karyotype. In general the gonadal development and that of the internal and external genital structures correlate. Each gonad may be pure testis, pure ovary, or a combination of the two. Fertility is occasionally documented in hermaphrodites. **Therefore, if a relatively well-developed uterus accompanies a gonad that looks like a normal ovary, that could be left in place and a**

female sex of rearing would be appropriate. On the other hand if the external genitalia are masculinized and a partially descended functioning testis is present on one side, a male sex of rearing would be preferable. Historically, most hermaphrodites have been raised as males (about 66% of the cases).

Mixed gonadal dysgenesis is the third most common intersex disorder and is defined again by the gonadal tissue that consists of a dysgenetic testis on one side and a streak gonad with no germinal epithelium on the other. These infants have a more female appearance externally and have only rudimentary development of both müllerian and wolffian duct derivatives. Generally there is a little more wolffian development on the side of the testis and müllerian maturation on the side of the streak gonad. Fertility and pregnancy are impossible given the nature of the internal structures. Most of these patients have been raised as females. The reconstruction is fairly similar to that described for the patients with congenital adrenal hyperplasia. **The gonads are always removed because they contribute nothing and do develop malignancies even in the first decade of life. The karyotype in this group is an XO/XY mosaic pattern.**

Finally, the male pseudohermaphrodite group consists of two lesions: (1) an androgen insensitivity syndrome due to a cytoplasmic receptor defect and (2) the 5-alpha-reductase deficiency whereby testosterone is not converted to dihydrotestosterone. **Those patients have normal male internal structures and female external genitalia.** They respond normally to androgen at puberty and masculinize considerably. Fertility is possible and generally reconstruction as males using standard hypospadias techniques is the rule; the testes if undescended are brought into the scrotum. The androgen insensitivity group, on the other hand, exhibits a much wider spectrum of phenotypes ranging from nearly normal female with slight clitoromegaly to near-normal male. The response to androgen at puberty is also variable depending on the degree of receptor deficiency. The more feminized patients need to be reared as females and reconstructed along the lines described for adrenogenital syndromes because the phallus will not develop at puberty. The gonads produce quite high levels of androgen, which of course has no effect on any of the tissues of the body, and they are usually removed because of the predisposition to malignancy. Fertility is not possible in these patients. The reconstruction and the sex of rearing depends almost entirely on the external genital development and the possibilities for future sexual function. Hormonal imprinting does not seem to be a factor in this group, since there is no androgen receptor in the brain anymore than there is in the genitalia.

Other External Genital Malformations

Hypospadias and cryptorchidism are two of the most common urologic genital anomalies. They are addressed in the chapter on congenital anomalies because they do not really require any diagnosis or management in the newborn, except to exclude an intersex state when they coexist. This chapter also addresses neonatal testicular torsion and the much more common hydrocele/hernia that is often identified in the newborn nursery or the neonatal intensive care unit.

TESTICULAR TORSION

Neonatal testicular torsion is a relatively rare event, and it almost invariably occurs in utero. There is no reported case of a salvageable testis resulting from early exploration of these patients. Therefore, neonatal transport and emergency surgery is not warranted because the risk outweighs the potential benefit. However, because subsequent contralateral torsion has been known to occur in rare instances, exploration with orchidectomy on the involved side and contralateral fixation of the testis in a dartos pouch is usually done to prevent anorchia. For some reason the patients often appear completely normal at birth, but within the first 24 hours of life the scrotum swells and a hard unilateral mass is palpated. Blue discoloration is common. Occasionally the problem is bilateral; such patients at exploration are invariably found to have bilateral infarcted testes and are referred to the endocrinologist for management at an appropriate age. In the past it was common to leave the infarcted testis in place; it is probably better to remove it to prevent any adverse effects on the contralateral testis. This has been documented to occur in older children with torsion and in animal models, although the mechanism remains a mystery. Fertility is affected in those instances. Removal seems to ameliorate subsequent infertility.

HERNIAS AND HYDROCELES

Hernias and hydroceles are both common in the newborn and are similar in the anatomic structure but different in their management. **The conventional definition is that a hydrocele sac contains only fluid, whereas a hernia sac contains intestine or omentum.** In general the hydrocele sac tends to narrow at the top and the scrotal portion gets quite large and may have a blue appearance when tensely distended. The amount of fluid tends to wax and wane, so that the hydrocele may come and go or be larger or smaller at various times. With a true hernia the bulk of the swelling is near the internal ring and not down in the scrotum. In these cases there is a 25% risk of incarceration and strangulation of the intestine that requires emergency surgical reduction and sometimes bowel resection. For this reason hernias are generally fixed within a week or so of being identified unless the defect is quite large and easily reducible. **Hydroceles, on the other hand, tend to resolve spontaneously with time; most of them disappear within the first 3 or 4 months of life.** Conventionally, if they are still present at 1 year of age, they are repaired to prevent enlargement over time and progression to a hernia, although there is little evidence in the literature that this actually occurs. There has never been a large series followed to document adequately the natural history of communicating hydrocele. In the infant bilateral hernia repair is generally done up to 1 year of age, whereas after that time only the symptomatic side is fixed if the contralateral side is normal on physical examination. Occasionally a hernia or hydrocele is associated with a cryptorchid testis. In that case the orchidopexy must be carried at the time of the hernia repair. If it is left until later the dissection is much more difficult with some risk of compromise to the testicular blood supply. Parenthetically it should be noted that inguinal hernias in phenotypic females or hernias in the absence of a palpable gonad on that side are frequently associated with some form of intersex state.

SUGGESTED READINGS

1. Josso N (ed): The Intersex Child. New York, S. Karger, 1981.
2. Kelalis PP, King LR, Belman AB: Clinical Pediatric Urology, 3rd ed. Philadelphia, WB Saunders, 1992.
3. Mandell T, Peters CA, Petik AB: Perinatal urology. *In* Walsh PC, Retik AB, Vaughan ED Jr, Wein AJ (eds): Campbell's Urology, 7th ed. Philadelphia, WB Saunders, 1998, pp 1601–1618.

21 Congenital Anomalies

Emmanuel M. Schenkman
William F. Tarry

The genitourinary system is the most common site for congenital anomalies. The evaluation and management of these urologic problems are dynamic. The purpose of this chapter is to discuss some common urologic congenital anomalies that are encountered by the primary care physician. These include cryptorchidism, vesicoureteral reflux (VUR), and hypospadias. The etiology, diagnosis, and management of these common congenital problems are presented.

Cryptorchidism

Cryptorchidism or the maldescended testicle is the most common disorder of the testicle. The incidence in full-term boys is 3% to 6%, and in premature males 20% to 30%. By 1 year of age the incidence is approximately 1%, which remains unchanged into adulthood. The right testicle is affected more often than the left (70% to 30%, respectively). Both testicles are affected one third of the time. Twenty percent of the time the testicle is nonpalpable, but up to 80% of these testicles are found at surgical exploration.

A basic understanding of normal testicular development is essential for determining different treatment options. At the seventh week of gestation, the Testis Determining Factor *(TDF)* gene located on the short arm of the Y chromosome provides a signal for differentiation of the gonadal stroma into the testicle. By the eighth week, the testis migrates to the internal ring but remains within the abdomen. The testicle remains in that position until the seventh month of gestation when the tunica vaginalis evaginates through the internal ring into the inguinal canal. From the seventh month of gestation to 1 year postnatally, the testes migrates through the inguinal canal to reside in the scrotum.

Testicular descent depends on mechanical, neural, and hormonal factors. Mechanical factors, which probably play a small role, involve the dilation of the inguinal canal by the gubernaculum. The normal groin anatomy and increases in abdominal pressure may aid in pushing the testes through the internal ring. Neural factors also play a small role in testicular descent. Hormonal factors are the major cause for testicular descent. Müllerian inhibiting substance produced by Sertoli's cells in the testis is important in abdominal descent, whereas inguinal descent is dependent on the interplay of the gonadotropins and androgens.

The clinical aspects of cryptorchidism, including diagnosis, pathology, treatment, and prognosis, vary depending on testes position. The physical examination should be performed in a warm room. The cross-legged position is optional. **The testis can be described as maldescended, ectopic, or retractile. A maldescended testicle may be either palpable or nonpalpable. An ectopic testicle descends normally but is located outside of the normal tract of descent. Ectopic testes may be found in the perineal, prepenile, contralateral scrotal, femoral, and superficial inguinal areas. The superficial inguinal pouch is the most common location for an ectopic testis. A retractile testis descends** normally but remains in the upper scrotum near the external ring. The retractile testis can be brought down into the scrotum during the physical examination. Almost half of all "undescended testes" seen by primary care physicians are retractile.

The most common urogenital anomaly associated with cryptorchidism are vasal or epididymal abnormalities, which occur in one third to two thirds of patients. Other anomalies include posterior urethral valves (<5%), upper tract abnormalities (<5%), and hypospadias (<6%). Hypospadias in association with maldescended testicle should raise the possibility of intersex (mixed gonadal dysgenesis).

The pathologic changes of undescended testes demonstrate a decreased number of Leydig's cells and germ cells, and peritubular fibrosis. Most histologic changes in cryptorchid testes are noted by 2 years. The more cranially placed testes exhibit more severe histologic changes. Abdominal testes are associated with a greater loss of germ cells than are prescrotal testes. Germ cell counts in contralateral testes are in the low-to-normal range, regardless of patient age at repair.

The most significant long-term sequelae of maldescended testes are infertility and malignancy. There are few long-term studies on fertility in patients with cryptorchidism. As mentioned previously, the germ cells are abnormal in both the undescended testicle and contralateral testis, despite surgical correction. Overall, sperm counts are low in this patient population but are not predictive of paternity.

The risk of testicular malignancy is markedly increased in cryptorchid testes. Up to 5% of these patients develop a testes tumor by age 45. Moreover, 10% of patients with testes tumor have a history of an undescended testicle. Seminoma is the most common tumor in cryptorchid testes, representing 60% of the cases. Testicles located higher along the path of normal descent have a greater risk of malignancy. Orchidopexy allows for self-examination but does not change the malignant potential of the testicle. Most urologists would perform orchiopexy until puberty. After puberty, undescended testes should be removed. After age 32, an undescended testicle may be observed because the risk of surgery is greater than the malignant potential of the testicle.

Surgical exploration, with placement of the testis in the scrotum if possible, is recommended at age 1 year (Fig. 21–1). The incidence of cryptorchidism is the same for a 1-year-old and adults, and histologic damage to the testis is marked by age 2. Overall, the success rate is 90% for orchidopexy. Complications include testicular atrophy (7%), retraction of testes (3%), and vas deferens injury (1% to 2%), and an orchiectomy is required in 5% of patients. Medical treatment uses hormone manipulation to cause the testes to descend into the scrotum. Luteinizing hormone–releasing hormone (LHRH) and human chorionic gonadotropin (hCG) are given

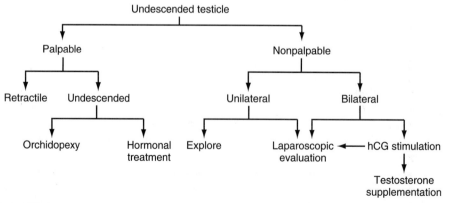

Figure 21–1
Algorithm for the evaluation and treatment of the undescended testicle in children. hCG, human chorionic gonadotropin.

sequentially with a 37% to 65% success rate. LHRH is given as a nasal spray in Europe and is the preferred treatment. Biopsy data suggest that it enhances germ cell counts even when it fails to produce descent. Unfortunately the spray is not available in the United States. No data exist regarding use of the injectable form for cryptorchidism, and appropriate doses are unknown.

Vesicoureteral Reflux

VUR is the abnormal flow of urine toward the kidney; it may occur during the voiding or filling phase. VUR is responsible for a significant portion of childhood urinary tract infections and subsequent complications of recurrent urinary tract infections in childhood.

INCIDENCE AND DEMOGRAPHICS

The incidence of VUR in healthy children is less than 1%. The peak age of incidence is 3 to 6 years; 85% of affected patients are girls in the United States, but European data reveal no gender difference. **VUR is an inherited disorder, and 33% of siblings have VUR.** The condition is most common among whites with blond hair and of northern European ancestry.

DIAGNOSIS

VUR may be diagnosed in newborns who have a postnatal renal ultrasound for follow-up of prenatal hydronephrosis and in siblings of known patients with reflux who are screened. These patients require a voiding cystourethrogram (VCUG) to diagnose reflux. Most often it is discovered during the evaluation of a urinary tract infection. **Two thirds of newborns and one third of older children with urinary tract infection will be found to reflux. The sequelae of untreated reflux and infection are focal renal scarring (30%), hypertension (20%), and end-stage renal disease (30%). Therefore, any child with a urinary tract infection should have a VCUG** (Fig. 21–2). The patient should have a sterile urine obtained prior to performing a VCUG. The study is performed on the unsedated child, and the importance of visualizing the

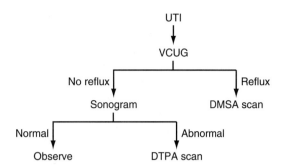

Figure 21–2
Algorithm for radiologic evaluation of children with urinary tract infection (UTI). VCUG, voiding cystourethrogram; DMSA, dimercaptosuccinic acid, technetium labeled; DTPA, diethylenetriamine penta-acetic acid, technetium labeled.

bladder during voiding cannot be overemphasized. The VCUG provides anatomic detail of the lower urinary tract and allows for classification of the severity of reflux. The nuclear cystogram is an alternative method for detecting reflux, but it does not allow for accurate grading. The advantages of a nuclear cystogram are that it is more sensitive than the standard VCUG and exposes the patient to less radiation. A nuclear cystogram is often recommended for sibling screening of patients with VUR. Renal ultrasound is performed to rule out hydronephrosis (obstruction), to assess renal size and growth, and, in experienced hands, to provide a reasonable assessment of focal renal scarring. Nuclear renal scans are useful, albeit expensive, to demonstrate renal function, obstruction, and renal scarring. **Technetium 99m diethylenetriamine penta-acetic acid (DTPA) assesses renal function and obstruction, whereas technetium 99m dimercaptosuccinate acid (DMSA) diagnoses acute pyelonephritis, visualizes renal scars in the cortical tissue, and measures function. No single test suffices to answer all the questions in a particular case.**

CLASSIFICATION AND GRADING OF REFLUX

Primary VUR secondary to an inherited malposition of the ureter into the bladder is the most common cause of reflux. Normally, the ureter enters obliquely into the bladder and is supported posteriorly by the detrusor muscle. As the bladder fills, the ureteral orifice closes through a passive mechanism. Funneling of the bladder neck during voiding results in active closure of the ureteral orifice by the ureterotrigonal muscle complex. **Refluxing ureteral orifices are noted to be laterally located on the trigone; this location shortens the submucosal tunnel formed by the ureter's oblique course through the bladder wall, which subsequently allows for reflux.**

The most widely used grading system is the International Reflux Classification (Fig. 21–3). Reflux is graded I through V. Grade I reflux demonstrates reflux of contrast medium into the ureter on a VCUG. Grade V reflux shows a severely dilated ureter and blunted calyces with effaced papillary impressions on a VCUG. The grading system has prognostic significance, which is discussed in subsequent sections.

SEQUELAE

Why should reflux be treated? VUR can facilitate bacterial pyelonephritis, which may result in focal renal scars. Renal scarring can be a cause of decreased renal and somatic growth, hypertension, and renal insufficiency.

The prevention of renal scarring is the goal of the treatment of reflux. The pathogenesis of renal scarring is multifactorial. The most widely accepted theory is that the combination of VUR and a urinary tract infection causes renal scars. There is little evidence to suggest that years of sterile reflux cause scarring. Bacterial virulence factors contribute to the development of pyelonephritis. **Patients with dysfunctional voiding, such as infrequent voiding, or bladders that store urine at high pressure, are more susceptible to renal scarring. The first infection is usually the most devastating in terms of renal scarring.** Thirty percent of patients have renal scars at diagnosis. Successful treatment of VUR may result in increased renal and somatic growth. VUR may also be secondary to an infectious or neuropathic mechanism. Transient reflux may occur during a urinary tract infection. This type of reflux usually resolves spontaneously after appropriate treatment of the infection. Voiding dysfunction can coexist in 15% to 60% cases. The peak age of occurrence is 3 to 5 years. Patients usually have uninhibited bladder contractions and complaints of urgency, frequency, and nocturnal enuresis. These patients are often treated effectively by managing the bladder with anticholinergic medications. This form of treatment allows for urine storage at a low pressure and facilitates resolution of reflux. VUR in these patients is treated similar to primary reflux, using antibiotic prophylaxis. **Note that VUR combined with high-vesical-pressure voiding dysfunction is bad for the kidney, and the child must undergo urologic evaluation and treatment.**

VUR in pregnancy may increase the risk of pyelonephritis. Asymptomatic bacteriuria occurs in 4% to 6% of pregnant women, and up to 4% of these women develop pyelonephritis. Any bacteriuria in pregnant women needs to be treated with a nonteratogenic antibiotic, usually a penicillin or cephalosporin. Nitrofurantoin is useful for long-term prophylaxis during pregnancy. The surgical correction of reflux in postpubertal females remains controversial; some evidence suggests a higher incidence of pyelonephritis during pregnancy in reimplanted women.

As previously mentioned, VUR is genetically transmitted, and there is an increased prevalence of VUR in siblings. Approximately 33% of siblings have reflux. It is recommended that all siblings younger than 10 years of age undergo either a VCUG or radionuclide VCUG to screen for reflux.

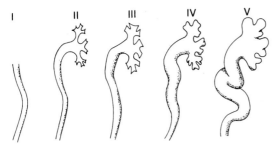

Figure 21–3
International classification of reflux. (From Walsh PC, Retik AB, Vaughan ED Jr, Wein AJ [eds]: Campbell's Urology, 6th ed. Philadelphia, WB Saunders, 1992.)

PROGNOSIS

Overall, if properly treated, low-grade (Grades I and II) reflux resolves. Reflux resolves in approximately 90% of Grade I, 80%

of Grade II, 50% of Grade III, and 10% of Grade IV, and rarely in Grade V. Overall, there is a 10% to 15% resolution rate per year.

Renal scarring has occurred in 30% to 50% of patients on initial evaluation, and fewer than 5% of patients treated either medically or surgically develop new renal scars. VUR is the most common disorder causing severe hypertension in children. There is a 10% to 20% incidence of hypertension in patients with VUR regardless of the grade of reflux. Hypertension is usually associated with the degree of renal scarring. VUR is responsible for 30% to 40% of the cases of renal failure in children. Proteinuria on routine examination in patients with focal renal scarring is an ominous sign; pregnancy often precipitates a decline in renal function.

TREATMENT

All children with VUR should be treated with prophylactic antibiotics. When reflux is discovered, antibiotic prophylaxis is calculated at one fourth to one eighth of the therapeutic dose. Trimethoprim-sulfamethoxazole or nitrofurantoin are good choices for initial prophylaxis. In children younger than 3 months of age, amoxicillin is the drug of choice.

Patients should be followed with a yearly VCUG to assess resolution of reflux. Any urine cultures should be obtained by a catheter or suprapubic aspirate to reduce the possibility of contamination. Once the VCUG shows resolution of reflux, antibiotic prophylaxis may be discontinued. Prophylaxis may also be stopped when the child reaches puberty, since renal growth is completed by puberty.

Surgical management of VUR is effective 95% of the time. Indications for surgery include pyelonephritis despite antibiotic prophylaxis, noncompliance, and Grade V reflux. Although surgery is effective in preventing pyelonephritis, these patients may still develop recurrent cystitis.

Hypospadias

Hypospadias is a congenital defect in the penis that results in incomplete development of the anterior urethra. The abnormal opening may occur any place along the course of the urethra. The more proximal meatus is associated with a ventral curvature of the penis. The incidence of hypospadias is about 1 in 300 male children. The defect is usually easily recognized at birth and is characterized by a prepuce with an excessive dorsal hood. There may be a genetic disposition, since 8% of fathers and 14% of siblings have hypospadias. The cause of hypospadias remains unknown.

The normal anatomy of the penis consists of paired corpora cavernosa and the urethra, which traverses the corpus spongiosum. The urethra is on the ventral side of the penis. Hypospadias results in a deficiency of the prepuce over the glans. Hypospadias can be classified or described by the position of the meatus. Distal hypospadias includes glanular, subcoronal, and distal shaft meatal loci and accounts for 50% of cases (Fig. 21–4). Middle hypospadias is found in 30% of cases and includes the middle third of the penile shaft. Proximal hypospadias includes the posterior third of the shaft, penoscrotal junction, scrotum, and perineum and accounts for 20% of cases (Fig. 21–5).

Chordee or ventral curvature of the penis is a poorly understood process often associated with hypospadias. Certain anomalies are not uncommon with hypospadias. Cryptorchidism or an inguinal hernia is found in 9% to 18% of these patients. Urinary tract anomalies are infrequent, and routine radiologic evaluations in these patients are not warranted. Intersex may be confused with severe hypospadias. Patients with normally descended testes and hypospadias do not require further investigation. However, patients with severe hypospadias and a nonpalpable testis should have a karyotype performed. Mixed gonadal dysgenesis is the most common form of intersex in patients with hypospadias. This state is characterized by a testis on one side and a streak gonad on the other side.

The treatment of hypospadias is surgical and is usually performed as a one-stage repair. The elements of the surgical repair include meatoplasty, glanuloplasty, urethroplasty, penile straightening, and proper skin cover. These patients do well with surgery between 6 months and 1 year of age. By 6 months of age, these infants are a lower anesthetic risk, and patients have no recall of such a trau-

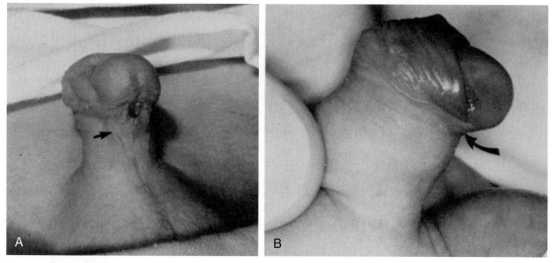

Figure 21-4

"Subglanular" or coronal hypospadias. *A,* The orifice is usually more stenotic than this; prepuce is "hooded" on the dorsal surface and deficient ventrally. The arrow points to the eccentric penile raphe and to a chordee deformity producing ventral curvature of the shaft proximal to the orifice. *B,* Ventral tilt of the glans on the shaft. (From Ashcraft KW [ed]: Pediatric Urology. Philadelphia, WB Saunders, 1990.)

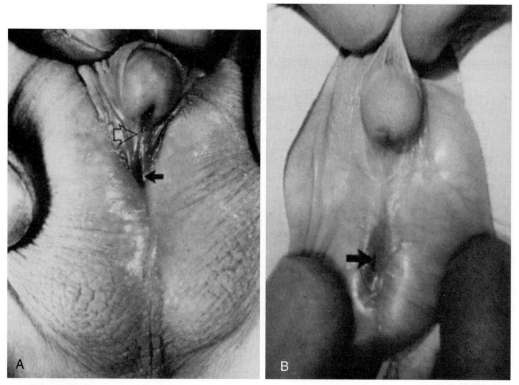

Figure 21-5

Two views of proximal hypospadias. *A,* Penoscrotal hypospadias (*black arrow* marks the orifice) and gross chordee deformity (*open arrow*). A blind pit is seen on the glans. *B,* Perineal hypospadias with the orifice at the base of the scrotum (*arrow*). Gross chordee and ventral angulation of penis. (From Ashcraft KW [ed]: Pediatric Urology. Philadelphia, WB Saunders, 1990.)

matic event. Hypospadias surgery is readily accomplished on an outpatient basis.

Early complications includes urinary tract infection, meatal stenosis, and loss of skin flaps. The most common late complication is a urethrocutaneous fistula, which occurs in fewer than 5% of distal repairs and about 12% of proximal cases. Other late complications include residual curvature, stricture, urethral diverticulum, inflammation, or a hairy urethra. Most of these complications occur in older patients and are associated with outmoded techniques. Long-term follow up on patients treated with one-stage repairs is lacking.

SUGGESTED READINGS

1. Atala A, Keating MA: Vesicoureteral reflux and megaureter. *In* Walsh PC, Retik AB, Vaughan ED Jr, Wein AJ (eds): Campbell's Urology, 7th ed. Philadelphia, WB Saunders, 1998, pp 1859–1916.
2. Duckett TW: Hypospadias. *In* Walsh PC, Retik AB, Vaughan ED Jr, Wein AJ (eds): Campbell's Urology, 7th ed. Philadelphia, WB Saunders, 1998, pp 2093–2119.
3. Rozanski T, Bloom DA, Colodny A: Surgery of the scrotum and testis in childhood. *In* Walsh PC, Retik AB, Vaughan ED Jr, Wein AJ (eds): Campbell's Urology, 7th ed. Philadelphia, WB Saunders, 1998, pp 2193–2209.
4. Smith DE: Hypospadias. *In* Ashcraft K (ed): Pediatric Urology. Philadelphia, WB Saunders, 1990, pp 353–396.

22

Pediatric Enuresis and Voiding Dysfunction

Emmanuel O. Abara
Margaret Moyo

Children achieve urinary continence when they develop the ability to store urine in the bladder until it is convenient and socially appropriate to void. Urinary incontinence or enuresis occurs when this ability has not been attained or there is a disease process. We define *enuresis* or *incontinence* as the involuntary elimination of urine and consider various forms of enuresis as problems within the larger context of voiding dysfunction. *Nocturnal enuresis (bedwetting)* refers to those children who have attained voluntary bladder control but wet their beds at night, whereas *diurnal enuresis* refers to daytime wetting. The first section of this chapter discusses the assessment and management of voiding problems and enuresis in children who do not have overt neurologic or anatomic abnormalities and may not require extensive investigations. Clinical features that set this group of children apart from the minority with clinically significant functional and anatomic abnormalities of the urinary tract are emphasized (Figs. 22–1 to 22–6).

It is hoped that at the end of the chapter, the primary care physician will be able, by history, physical examination, and simple urine tests, to separate a child with voiding dysfunction into one of the following treatment groups: (1) watchful waiting (no treatment); (2) medical and/or behavioral and conditioning treatment; or (3) referral to the urologist and/or other specialists for further investigations and treatment.

By 4 years of age, most children have acquired an adult pattern of urinary control. The typical trend for the development of bladder and bowel control has been described as follows: (1) nocturnal bowel control, (2) daytime bowel control, (3) daytime control of voiding, and (4) nocturnal control of voiding.

There are considerable individual and cultural variations in this flow of events. Most parents begin to worry if their child has not

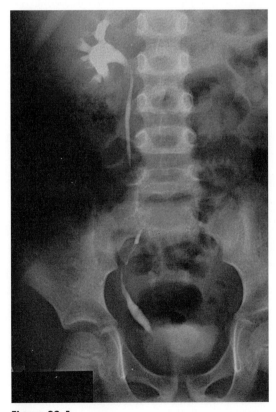

Figure 22-1
Intravenous pyelogram showing a nonfunctioning left kidney in a 4-year-old boy with hesitancy, slow stream, and daytime incontinence.

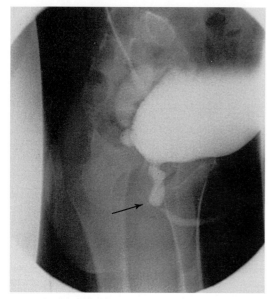

Figure 22-2
Voiding cystourethrogram showed posterior urethral valves *(arrow)* with Grade 5 reflux.

attained the fourth stage in continence development by 5 years of age, and this concern is heightened if this goal has not been attained by the seventh or eighth year of life. At this time, the parents and the child are quite anxious to have something done, because this is the age when peer pressure begins; the child gets involved in sports and other social events that may necessitate that the child sleep away from the home. By the time the parents bring the child to the primary care physician, a number of techniques must have been tried at home. Parents need to be reassured at all times that variation in developmental milestones may be normal within certain limits and no active therapy is necessary before the age of 5 years if there are no other abnormalities.

Nocturnal Enuresis

Epidemiology

Nocturnal enuresis, or nighttime incontinence, is common in children younger than 6 years of age, affecting at least 25% of children. It is self-limiting, with a spontaneous resolution rate of 15% each year, so that by the age of 15 years only 1% to 2% of adolescents

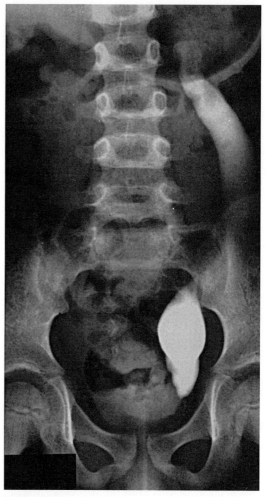

Figure 22-3
Posterior urethral valves with Grade 5 reflux shown in Figure 22-2 is best demonstrated in a postvoid film after successful transurethral resection valve ablation.

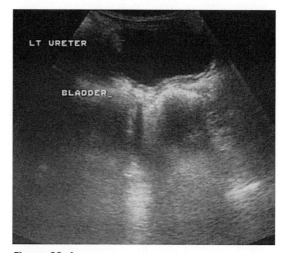

Figure 22-4
Prevalve ablation pelvic ultrasound showing large residual urine and dilated distal left ureter.

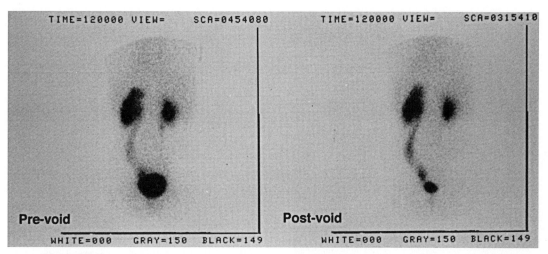

Figure 22-5
DTPA renal scan demonstrated some contrast medium in the left kidney and ureter (some function and refluxed urine).

remain incontinent. This small group remain enuretic through adult life.

About 15% to 20% of the children who are bedwetters also have daytime incontinence, a prevalence that decreases rapidly in children older than 5 years of age. This group of enuretic children need detailed investigation to rule out significant urinary tract abnormalities. Nocturnal enuresis is more common in boys, whereas daytime incontinence occurs more commonly in girls.

Positive Family History

Because nocturnal enuresis is prevalent in the general population, there is a well-documented familial incidence. In one survey of families in which both parents had a history of bedwetting, there was a 77% incidence of nocturnal enuresis in their children. Therefore, a good account of family history should be obtained except in cases of adopted children, for whom this information may not be readily available.

Etiology

There have been several studies in search of the possible causes of nocturnal enuresis. However, controversy still exists. This is not surprising because there may be more than one cause. More important, if enuresis is regarded as a symptom rather than a disease,

it is possible that it can be affected by several etiologic factors.

Attempts at determining specific causes in individuals with nocturnal enuresis have not been rewarding in the management of most patients. However, awareness of these etiologic factors is important because they form the basis of various treatment options currently available.

SLEEP DISORDERS

Most parents of enuretic children often volunteer the information that the affected child sleeps unusually deeply compared with the siblings. This had led to the studies that suggest a relationship between sleep patterns and enuresis; however, in later, more sophisticated sleep studies, investigators noted that enuretic events occurred randomly throughout the night in each sleep stage. No specific brain wave pattern or stage of sleep associated with bedwetting has been identified. The sleep patterns of enuretic children do not differ appreciably from those of normal children. Sleep patterns change during childhood; this may account for the high spontaneous resolution rate as well as the high success rate achieved with alarm systems that wake the patient during enuretic episodes.

MATURATIONAL LAG OR DEVELOPMENTAL DELAY

Delayed maturity theory, although not generally accepted, has been used to explain enure-

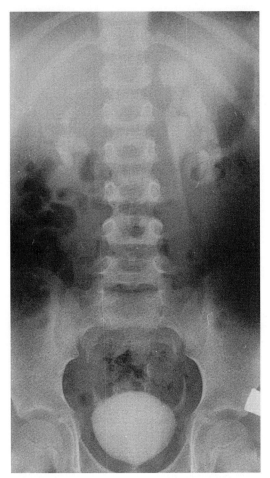

Figure 22-6
Intravenous pyelogram 6 weeks after a left tapered reimplant.

NOCTURNAL POLYURIA AND ANTIDIURETIC HORMONE

There are reports of extensive studies on the nocturnal secretion of antidiuretic hormone (ADH) in enuretic children. It has been suggested that a failure of the normal nocturnal rise of ADH leads to increased urine production beyond the bladder capacity. Once bladder capacity was exceeded, an enuretic episode occurred. This theory does not account for why enuretic children do not wake with a full bladder, as occurs in most children, but it does suggest that nocturnal polyuria with or without abnormal ADH secretion may be an important factor in some enuretic children; hence the use of desmopressin acetate (DDAVP) (see later).

Psychological Factors

The role of emotional disturbances and psychopathology in enuretic children has been studied by a number of investigators. The conclusion of several large reviews is that, although a higher proportion of enuretic children are maladjusted and exhibit measurable behavioral symptoms, only a few enuretic children actually have significant underlying psychopathology. However, several studies show that enuretic children tend to be more immature and less self-reliant than are nonenuretic children.

URINARY TRACT INFECTIONS

Although uncommon, urinary tract infection (UTI) is a clinically important cause of nocturnal enuresis. Enuretic girls tend to exhibit a higher incidence of bacteriuria (5.6%) than nonenuretic girls. Recurrent UTIs in girls with enuresis often resolve after successful treatment.

UTI may be more prevalent in children with daytime and nighttime incontinence or secondary enuresis and should be excluded.

Assessment

Although most enuretic children have the idiopathic variety of enuresis, a thorough clinical evaluation is necessary to diagnose and treat rare causes such as UTI, neuropathy, and congenital anomaly (Figs. 22–7 and 22–8).

sis and why, if left untreated, most enuretic children eventually develop complete control. Other studies suggest that enuresis represents a developmental delay due to deficient learning of a habit pattern and not a lag in neurophysiologic maturation. The developmental level at 1 and 3 years of age, in addition to a family history of enuresis, is predictive of the age of attainment of urinary control.

Successful response to conditioning therapy has been cited by behaviorists as evidence that control of nocturnal enuresis can be "learned" and therefore does not necessarily depend on maturation of the central nervous system.

However, neurophysiologic maturational delay may well play a greater role in children who also have associated daytime voiding dysfunction.

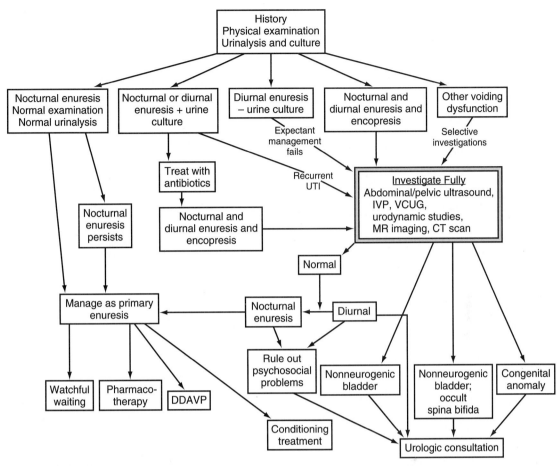

Figure 22-7
Algorithm of management of pediatric enuresis and voiding dysfunction. IVP, intravenous pyelogram; VCUG, voiding cystourethrogram; MR, magnetic resonance; CT, computed tomography; UTI, urinary tract infection; DDAVP, desmopressin acetate.

The initial evaluation should include the medical, social, and family histories. Information should be sought regarding the following:

1. Onset pattern—primary or secondary?
2. Pattern 7 days per week?
3. Severity of enuresis—volume voided and persistence?
4. Circumstances in which enuresis occurs?

Children who consistently wet their bed more than once per night may have nocturnal polyuria, especially those with a normal bladder capacity. Voiding history should ask specific questions to obtain valid voiding pattern, including daytime frequency and urgency, daytime enuresis, intermittent or weak stream, and urgency. Urinary frequency and urgency may suggest underlying small blad-

der capacity, bladder instability, or other types of acquired voiding dysfunction. A history of a weak or intermittent stream and associated hesitancy may suggest detrusor-sphincter dyssynergia, or, in boys, a stricture or posterior urethral valve. Constant dribbling of urine may suggest a fistula or ureteral ectopy.

VOIDING DIARY AND FUNCTIONAL BLADDER CAPACITY

For the enuretic child with daytime voiding dysfunction, a voiding diary and determination of the child's functional bladder capacity may help identify the type of voiding dysfunction.

Children who often void small amounts with urgency, urge incontinence, and squat-

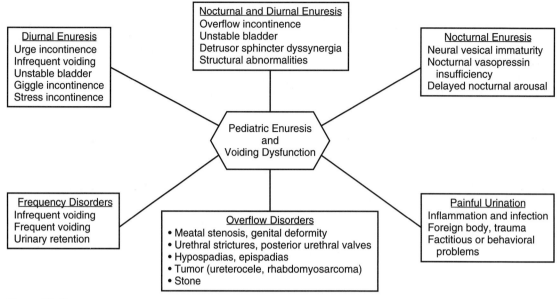

Figure 22-8
Model of the "cube" of pediatric enuresis and voiding dysfunction: six "faces" of the problem.

ting with posturing may have underlying bladder instability and a small functional bladder or UTI, whereas enuretic children who void infrequently have a large bladder capacity, void only two or three times a day, and may have paradoxic urgency and urge incontinence when their bladder reaches maximum capacity.

Enuretic children with diurnal voiding dysfunction often have associated chronic constipation and/or encopresis. A bowel-habit history should be obtained. Chronic constipation is present in two thirds of bed wetters and children with history of UTIs. For this information, the child should be interviewed directly because some children may reveal that they are not aware when they have to urinate. These children are often found to be sitting in a pool of urine when involved in some activity and truly may have a sensory neurologic deficit.

A psychological history may help identify factors that have precipitated involuntary voiding especially in secondary enuresis. Environmental factors such as socioeconomic status and stress play a role. It is important to determine if there is a family history of nocturnal enuresis and how the problem was managed, because this may influence the family's opinion about treatment options. Some parents want to be reassured that their child is physically normal and that the enuresis will likely resolve spontaneously.

The child's sleeping habits, any prior history of UTI, and other medical history should be ascertained.

An attempt should be made to evaluate the attitude of both child and parents toward the bedwetting because this may influence the decision to treat, and the timing and choice of treatment.

It is uncommon for a child younger than 6 years of age to be concerned enough about bedwetting to want to undergo any form of treatment. However, an 8-year-old child who participates in competitive swimming or hockey and has to go out of town will be pleased to have a dry weekend to play his or her sports without the embarrassment of bedwetting.

The physical examination should be complete. Abdominal and genital examination should be able to detect any physical abnormality such as a palpable distended bladder or a bifid clitoris in girls that may explain the child's voiding dysfunction. If the child is constantly wet, pooling of urine within the vaginal vault may be detected. When an underlying neurologic abnormality is suspected, peripheral reflexes, perineal sensation, and anal sphincter tone should be checked; the child's gait should be observed and the lower back visually inspected for evidence of sacral dimpling and cutaneous anomalies.

In most children with isolated nocturnal enuresis, however, the results of physical examination are normal. A urinalysis and urine culture should be done at least once during the course of evaluation.

UNCOMPLICATED VERSUS COMPLICATED NOCTURNAL ENURESIS

Children with isolated nocturnal enuresis, a normal physical examination, and a normal urinalysis and sterile urine culture have uncomplicated enuresis and form the majority of the enuretic group.

Some may have mild daytime frequency or enuresis, a positive family history of enuresis, and perhaps slightly delayed developmental milestones. In this group, the incidence of organic uropathology is not significantly higher than that of the normal population. Therefore, no further urologic imaging, urodynamic studies, or cystoscopic evaluation are necessary.

Patients with a positive urine culture, a history of UTI, an abnormal neurologic examination, and a history of significant daytime voiding dysfunction have complicated enuresis and merit further investigation. These patients constitute an important, although small, minority of the enuretic population.

Further assessment with abdominal and pelvic ultrasonography, voiding cystography, and lumbosacral spine radiographs is necessary to exclude secondary vesicoureteral reflux and/or hydronephrosis associated with trabeculated unstable bladder, or a urethral abnormality such as posterior urethral valve or stricture. A urethral duplication in boys, ureteral ectopy in girls, and ureteroceles in boys and girls can lead to daytime incontinence with associated nocturnal enuresis. These abnormal findings suggest the need for further urologic evaluation (such as urodynamics and/or cystoscopy).

Treatment

Most parents bring their enuretic child for evaluation when several home remedies have failed. Such remedies as withholding fluids in the evening, random awakening of child to void, rewards for staying dry, and punishment are ineffective and should be discouraged, especially the punishment, because the child does not have voluntary control of the enuretic episode.

Numerous techniques that may work include behavior modification treatment (conditioning therapy, motivational therapy, counseling) and pharmacotherapy (imipramine, desmopressin, and oxybutynin).

Treatment should be individualized and guided by the patient's age; the patient's and parental attitudes toward the problem; and socioeconomic status. Since the rate of spontaneous resolution is high, it is important that treatment is not worse than the condition. Some children will have lost considerable self-image and self-esteem because of their enuresis and are highly motivated to deal with the problem.

BEHAVIOR MODIFICATION

Motivational therapy promotes development of a positive relationship between parents and child and provides positive reinforcement ranging from words of praise to actual material rewards. It involves a series of counseling interviews during which the child is encouraged to assume responsibility for his or her enuresis and to become an active participant in the treatment program. This approach has been termed *responsibility-reinforcement therapy*. A record of the child's progress, such as a gold star or a sticker on a calendar for each dry night, is kept. As the child progresses stepwise toward the ultimate goal of dryness, the parents and physician provide positive reinforcement as a means of response shaping.

An estimated cure rate with motivational counseling is 25%; its main use is to lay the groundwork for a successful trial using conditioning therapy with a portable alarm system.

Conditioning therapy is based on the use of a signal alarm that is triggered by contact with urine when the child voids. A conditioned response of awakening and inhibition of urination is gradually evoked by the repetitive association of waking to the alarm and bladder distention. Since success depends on a cooperative and motivated child and family, conditioning therapy is generally reserved for children older than 7 years of age. This is the age when these children are involved in outdoor sports and may want to spend the weekends at their friends' homes—these are additional incentives to enlist the cooperation of the child.

The most effective alarm systems are battery operated with a small sensor attached to the child's underwear and a buzzer alarm on the shoulder.

This system has a cure rate averaging 82% if used for a minimum of 4 to 6 months. A relapse rate of 30% has been reported; however, a similar favorable outcome with re-treatment after relapse has been reported. It is the most effective therapy available for uncomplicated nocturnal enuresis. The device is safe and relatively inexpensive, and the only absolute contraindication is a patient who is deaf. Relative contraindications include emotional disturbances and patients whose siblings sleep in the same room, but this is often not a problem because these siblings understand the reason for the alarm.

The alarm often fails to wake the child; someone else (adult) has to awaken the child in response to the alarm for good results. Not understanding this and convincing the parents to assume this responsibility is the most common cause of alarm failure and dissatisfaction.

Relapse is said to be less likely to occur after a discontinuation of use of the alarm after a dry period of at least 4 weeks rather than a briefer dry period.

TRICYCLIC ANTIDEPRESSANT: IMIPRAMINE

Several tricyclic antidepressants, especially imipramine, have been employed in the treatment of nocturnal enuresis with variable results. The mechanism of action in enuresis is not well understood but may relate to (1) alterations in arousal and sleep patterns, (2) anticholinergic and antispasmodic effects, and (3) its antidepressant effect. A recent study suggests that imipramine may also work by increasing the secretion of ADH from the posterior pituitary.

Imipramine in a dose of 25 to 50 mg taken 1 to 2 hours before bedtime is usually pre-scribed in children over the age 6 years. Initial success rates have been reported to be as high as 40% to 50%; the maximum effect usually occurs within the first week of treatment. The treatment should be maintained for at least 6 months before trying to wean the child by reducing the dose and/or frequency. Should relapse occur, a second course of treatment for an additional 6 months can be resumed. Since the effect of imipramine is immediate, it can be used on an "as necessary" basis in situations when staying dry is important to the child (e.g., sleepovers, camp, sports).

Side effects are fairly common and include anxiety, insomnia, dry mouth, nausea, and personality changes.

Imipramine should be kept out of the reach of young children because overdose from excessive accidental ingestion can cause fatal toxicity with cardiac arrhythmias and conduction blocks, hypotension, and convulsion. Parents should be counseled regarding this danger and should monitor the drug carefully at home.

ANTICHOLINERGIC: OXYBUTYNIN

Anticholinergic drugs such as oxybutynin reduce or abolish uninhibited detrusor contractions and increase bladder capacity. It is useful in children who have bladder detrusor instability and/or small bladder capacity associated with daytime urgency and urge incontinence in addition to nocturnal enuresis. This medication is rarely beneficial in children who have only nocturnal enuresis.

Common side effects include dry mouth and facial flushing. Hyperpyrexia may occur, especially in hot weather. Blurring of vision and hallucination may occur with excessive dosage.

Oxybutynin, the most common anticholinergic, is often used empirically when there is clinical evidence of detrusor instability or urge incontinence associated with nocturnal enuresis.

DESMOPRESSIN ACETATE

The use of DDAVP for nocturnal enuresis gained popularity in the 1990s. DDAVP has an antidiuretic effect, a prolonged half-life, and long duration of action. When administered intranasally, it is said to reduce nocturnal urine output to a volume less than the functional bladder capacity. This assumes that the enuretic child wets the bed when the bladder capacity is exceeded. DDAVP may be useful in the subgroup of enuretic children who have a relative deficiency in the nocturnal ADH secretion. Currently, there is no reliable means to differentiate this subgroup from others.

DDAVP is commercially available as a nasal spray pump, which delivers a dose of 10 μg of desmopressin per spray. The recommended initial dose is 20 μg (10 μg per nostril) 1 hour before bedtime for at least 6 months. The response to DDAVP appears to be dose related. Repeated long-term cure rates range from 5% to 22%, and relapse rates after discontinuation of short-term treatment are high. Significant side effects with desmopressin are rare, although severe hyponatremia has been described.

This medication is expensive and is best reserved for a minority of children who really need it (e.g., the child who needs to stay dry for specific periods such as summer camp).

Response to pharmacotherapy can be rapid, but these agents do not cure nocturnal enuresis. Most patients require long-term treatment to remain dry. In double-blind studies, reported response rates for imipramine and DDAVP are similar. DDAVP is more expensive than imipramine, but has fewer side effects and is less toxic. Anticholinergic drugs such as oxybutynin, may benefit children with small bladder capacity and/or daytime frequency or incontinence, but it has not proved helpful for nocturnal enuretics. When four treatment groups are compared, (1) observation, (2) imipramine, (3) desmopressin acetate, and (4) alarm therapy, only the bedwetting alarm system demonstrated persistent effectiveness at 12 months.

Triage

Since spontaneous resolution is high, children younger than 6 years of age require reassurance and encouragement only. Older children, who are motivated, are best managed with a portable alarm system, because it is inexpensive and highly successful. Proper instruction regarding the operation of the device and use

for 4 to 6 months results in a success rate of over 60% to 80%.

Pharmacologic therapy is associated with immediate results but lower rate of achieving and maintaining dryness and should be used in selected cases. Urologic consultation should be reserved for patients with diurnal enuresis, abnormal physical findings, or those who have failed 1 year of standard therapy.

In some individuals with enuresis and no structural anatomic anomalies, response to standard therapy may not occur, and such children may have to go through adult life with periods of bedwetting. In such individuals, supportive therapy, behavioral modification, and wise application of new anti-incontinence devices such as urethral plugs may be worthwhile.

Complicated enuresis includes several functional voiding disorders seen in children who do not have any obvious abnormalities. These children often have nocturnal enuresis in addition to daytime urinary frequency, urgency, infrequent voiding, weak or intermittent stream, straining to void, and a history of UTI.

Assessment should be as described earlier for the child with noncomplicated nocturnal enuresis. It is necessary to assess the patient's voiding and bowel habits, in addition to the functional bladder capacity. Abdominal and pelvic ultrasound with prevoid and postvoid residual urine estimations should be done. Increased postvoid residual urine, trabeculated bladder, and lower ureteral dilation may point to significant urologic disease (see Figs. 22–1 to 22–4).

Girls who have continuous dribbling night and day may have renal upper tract duplication anomaly with or without hydronephrosis and ectopic ureter. The boy whose underwear is constantly wet may have urethral duplication, with the ectopic urethral meatus in the perineum.

In addition to the abdominal and pelvic ultrasonography, voiding cystourethrogram should be done in any child with a history of UTI, which would include all children with severe dysfunctional voiding, such as those with Hinman's syndrome.

Many pediatric urologists reserve spine radiographs for patients with some objective physical finding (sacral dimpling, gait change) or other neurologic signs. In selected cases, full urodynamic studies are necessary to define and treat the problem.

Organic Causes of Diurnal Enuresis

Approximately 5% of children with diurnal incontinence have the type with organic causes. UTIs are the most common. Dysuria, urinary frequency, urgency, suprapubic pain. and sudden onset of daytime wetting characterize this diagnosis. Older children with UTIs may present with urinary frequency and dysuria and no incontinence. Girls are more often afflicted with UTI than boys. In fact, some authors have suggested that girls who use bubble bath are prone to daytime incontinence as a result of chemical distal urethritis. Some of these children often have small-capacity, irritable bladders with detrusor instability and may benefit from a combination of anticholinergic and antibacterial therapy.

The UTI may be associated with other anomalies such as ectopy of the ureter and/or urethra. Mothers of children with ureteral ectopy almost always complain that the children are wet all the time. It may not be a "shower" of urine but a steady trickle of urine and dampness day and night, in spite of normal voided volumes at normal intervals.

Daytime Enuresis or Other Voiding Dysfunction

Daytime enuresis may be defined as lack of urinary control during waking hours in a child old enough to maintain bladder control. The age of 2½ years has become an arbitrary age cut-off for a child who has not responded to toilet training, if intelligence and motor development are normal. These children tend to empty the whole contents of their bladder, and their clothes are completely soaked. In some, it may occur several times a week and in others there is continuous wetting. This is often quite embarrassing to the child of school age.

Nocturnal enuresis is commonly associated with daytime incontinence in 50% to 60% of children who have this problem. It is gener-

ally accepted that most episodes of daytime incontinence are under voluntary control, whereas nocturnal incontinence is involuntary. Diurnal incontinence associated with urinary urgency, squatting, and constipation is caused by detrusor instability and responds to hydration, bowel and bladder training, and anticholinergics. Urologic referral and evaluation may be indicated in those who fail this initial management. The toilet-trained child who is too busy playing with a new Christmas toy and postpones voiding only to end up wetting himself or herself does not need investigation. Occasional leakage of a few drops of urine in a child of any age is so common that it should be considered normal.

Obstruction of the lower urinary tract may lead to poor bladder emptying, urinary retention, and overflow incontinence. A history of hesitancy, straining at urination, dribbling, or small stream should alert the clinician to the possibility of obstructive element. In boys, posterior urethral valves should be suspected. Other causes include ureteroceles, hydrocolpos, urethral cyst, urethral duplication, or tumors such as rhabdomyosarcoma. **Fecal impaction in a child with chronic constipation is associated with detrusor instability and sphincter pseudo-dyssynergy.** Diagnostic imaging studies are essential in defining the pathology that may dictate surgical therapy to resolve the incontinence associated with the condition.

Neurogenic bladder is a rare cause of diurnal incontinence alone. There are usually other associated conditions such as gait disturbances and inadequate bowel control. Recently, the study group at the Hospital for Sick Children, Toronto, has reported on a cohort of children with occult spinal dysraphism or tethered cord syndrome that appeared to improve following neurosurgical division of the filum terminale.

Vaginal reflux of urine is often seen in girls during urination. When such girls stand up and walk after normal voiding, urine leaks out of the vagina and may continue for some time, wetting the underwear. This problem is often seen in obese girls or those with anterior displacement of the posterior labial frenulum. Although not essential, voiding cystourethrogram may demonstrate this vaginal reflux of urine.

Ectopic ureter associated with incontinence occurs most frequently in girls and usually ends in the vagina. Such children are best referred to the urologist early for detection and treatment of this condition.

CASE REPORTS

Case 1

A 4½-year-old boy was referred by the family physician because of nocturnal enuresis. He had good daytime urinary control. His bowel movements were regular and normal. His growth and development were normal. There was a history that the father was a bedwetter till the age of 6 years. Physical examination did not show any abnormality. Urinalysis was normal. Based on the history and clinical findings, the parents were reassured that the problem would resolve spontaneously. At the follow-up evaluation 6 months later, the mother confirmed that the child had not wet the bed since the last visit.

Between the ages of 1 and 2 years, conscious sensation of bladder fullness develops, setting the stage for voluntary urinary voiding control. The ability to urinate or inhibit urination voluntarily at any degree of bladder filling develops usually in the second and third years of life.

Case 2

A 7-year-old boy was referred because of bedwetting 7 days a week. There were no other complaints. The parents confirmed that he was a deep sleeper, difficult to arouse from sleep, and occasionally walked in his sleep. Examination did not reveal any physical or emotional abnormalities. In particular, there were no neurologic deficits. The child's growth and development were normal. The mother and a maternal uncle wet the bed till they were 10½ and 10 years of age, respectively. The boy was a gifted child—an avid piano and violin player. Various treatment options were discussed, including watchful waiting, desmopressin (DDAVP), imipramine, and the bell. The child was not keen on any treatment. The parents were concerned about the side effects of DDAVP and the anticholin-

ergic effects of imipramine and were not willing to try the bell because the child would feel embarrassed. Two years later at the age of 9, he was still wetting the bed every day. He was now involved in competitive sports, highly motivated—and requested some treatment. The enuretic bell was recommended— because the child and the family were now well motivated. After 3 months, the child was dry, and with further use of the enuretic bell for another 3 months, the child has remained dry and happy.

Case 3

A 10-year-old girl was referred because of bedwetting and daytime urinary frequency and occasional incontinence. There was no dysuria, and she had no systemic symptoms. No family history was available because she was adopted. She had never been toilet trained. Physical examination showed no abnormalities. She had microscopic hematuria and bacteriuria. Urine culture, however, was sterile. Prior to referral, she had been treated with desmopressin (DDAVP) and imipramine at different times with good response for a short period.

Abdominal and pelvic ultrasound studies were normal. Cystoscopy under general anesthesia revealed cystitis cystica. She was therefore treated with a long-term low-dose antimicrobial agent for 6 weeks. The daytime incontinence and frequency stopped, but she still wet the bed three to five times a week.

DDAVP was again recommended, and this partially but not completely alleviated the problem. Small doses of imipramine starting from 12.5 mg and increasing to 25 mg were added to the regimen, and with this combination therapy, she was able to achieve daytime and nighttime continence with occasional bedwetting.

The girl is now 16 years old; she participates in all activities and takes her medication only when she has to sleep away from home or in a stressful situation (e.g., impending competition).

Case 4

A 12-year-old boy was referred because of daytime and nighttime incontinence. The child was adopted at 5 years of age; therefore, no family history was available. The growth and development were said to be normal since he was adopted. The mother complained that he did not appear to empty his bladder. On physical examination, he looked healthy with normally developed genitalia, but suprapubic fullness was noted. Ultrasonographic examination of the abdomen and pelvis revealed bilateral hydroureteronephrosis and trabeculated bladder with 400 mL of residual urine. The serum creatinine level was 285 μmol/L (normal, 90 to 130 μmol/L). Renal scan confirmed hydronephrosis with thinning of the cortices. Voiding cystourethrogram showed bilateral Grade 4/5 reflux and no posterior urethral valves and the presence of trabeculations. Lumbosacral spine radiographs, CT scan, and MR imaging of the spine showed no spina bifida occulta. Urodynamic studies showed he had detrusor sphincter dyssynergia and detrusor instability with high residual postvoid urine. He was managed by self-intermittent catheterization. Recent assessment after 6 years of this regimen showed normal creatinine values, a normal intravenous pyelogram with zero residual urine, and a stable bladder on urodynamics. He did not require surgery.

Comments

Cases 1 and 2

Toronto Children's Hospital also reported that chronic constipation, poor bowel evacuation, and abnormal manometric rectal pressures may occur in most children with primary nocturnal enuresis. Therefore, rigorous bowel regimens (tapering enema schedule for 3 months) should result in improved bowel evacuation, normal manometrics, and complete resolution of the enuresis.

Case 3

Evaluation and management in this case would have been satisfactory without cystoscopy.

Case 4

This case represents the classic Hinman-Allen syndrome, which may be associated with family and bowel dysfunction. Spinal radiographs are virtually always normal in the absence of neurologic findings; this is often called pseudo-dyssynergy because it lacks any neurologic cause.

SUGGESTED READINGS

1. Churchill BM, Abara EO, McLorie GA: Ureteral duplication, ectopy, and ureterocele. Pediatr Clin North Am 34:1273–1289, 1987.
2. Essen J, Peckham C: Nocturnal enuresis in childhood. Dev Med Child Neurol 18:577, 1976.
3. Fergusson DM, Hans BA, Horwood LJ, et al: Factors related to the age of attainment of nocturnal bladder control: An 8-year longitudinal study. Pediatrics 78:884, 1986.
4. Koff SA, Byard MA: The daytime urinary frequency syndrome of childhood. J Urol 140:1280–1281, 1988.
5. Marshall A, Marshall HH, Lyons RP: Enuresis: An analysis of various therapeutic approaches. Pediatrics 52:813, 1973.
6. Monda JM, Husmann DA: Primary nocturnal enuresis: A comparison among observation, imipramine, desmopressin acetate, and bedwetting alarm systems. J Urol 154:745–748, 1995.
7. Muellner SR: Development of urinary control in children: Some aspects of the cause and treatment of primary enuresis. JAMA 172:1256, 1960.
8. Yeates WK: Bladder function in normal micturition. In Kolvin I, MacKeith RC, Meadow SR (eds): Bladder Control and Enuresis. London, Heinemann, 1973, p 28.

23 Genitourinary Malignancies in Children

Farhad B. Nowzari
William F. Tarry

Wilms' Tumor

EPIDEMIOLOGY

Wilms' tumor, also known as *nephroblastoma,* was first described thoroughly by Max Wilms in 1899. It is the most common malignant neoplasm in the urinary tract of children, accounting for about 500 new cases annually in the United States, with an incidence of 1 in 10,000 children. This tumor represents 5% to 6% of childhood cancers in the United States. The incidence peaks at age 36.5 months for males and 42.5 months for females. The frequency is slightly higher in girls in the United States. There is some ethnic variation but no consistent environmental association in the incidence of Wilms' tumor. Synchronous bilateral disease occurs in about 5% and metachronous lesions in only 1% of patients.

GENETICS AND ASSOCIATED SYNDROMES

Wilms' tumor appears to occur in either heritable or nonheritable form. In children with the heritable form, the tumor develops at an earlier age and is more likely to be bilateral and multicentric. All bilateral cases and 15% to 20% of unilateral Wilms' tumors may be attributable to the heritable form of neoplasm.

The three chromosomal abnormalities found in Wilms' tumor are constitutional deletion at the short arm of chromosome 11 (11p13), loss of heterozygosity (LOH) in 11p15 region, and possibly LOH for the long arm of chromosome 16q.

Other significant anomalies associated with this tumor include aniridia, hemihypertrophy, congenital genitourinary anomalies, as well as syndromes such as Beckwith-Wiedemann, Denys-Drash, Perlman, and Wilms' tumor, *an*iridia, *g*enitourinary abnormalities, and mental *r*etardation (WAGR). The incidence of these anomalies in National Wilms' Tumor Study patients is summarized in Table 23–1.

CLINICAL PRESENTATION

Most children with Wilms' tumor present with an abdominal mass. The tumor is palpable on physical examination in more than 90% of patients. Gross hematuria occurs rarely, but microhematuria has been found in up to 50% of patients at the time of diagnosis. Hypertension is present in 25% to 50% of cases and has been attributed to either production of

Table 23–1
Incidence of Congenital Anomalies Associated with Wilms' Tumors*

Anomaly	Rate (per 1000)
Aniridia	7.6
Beckwith-Wiedemann syndrome	8.4
Hemihypertrophy	33.8
Genitourinary anomalies	
Hypospadias	13.4
Cryptorchidism	37.3
Hypospadias and cryptorchidism	12.0

*Patients reported to the National Wilms' Tumor Study.

renin due to ischemia produced by tumor compressing the renal parenchyma or renin secretion by the tumor itself. Other symptoms such as general malaise, abdominal pain, weight loss, and vomiting occur less frequently and may reflect advanced disease.

DIAGNOSIS

The usual laboratory studies include a complete blood count and differential, platelets, urinalysis, chemistries, and urinary catecholamines to rule out neuroblastoma. Chromosome studies are important in children with associated congenital anomalies.

Classically, intravenous pyelography shows distortion of the renal contour with splaying of the collecting system. A nonfunctioning kidney may occur in up to 10% of patients and suggests extensive disease. Curvilinear calcification may occur in 5% to 10% of patients and is usually located on the periphery.

Ultrasonography is the usual first study in children with abdominal masses. It can differentiate solid from cystic lesions, determine if the mass is of renal origin, and assess whether tumor thrombus extends into the renal vein, inferior vena cava, or right atrium. Wilms' tumors often have echo-free zones with scattered internal echoes that probably represent necrotic areas within the mass.

Computed tomography (CT) is the most sensitive examination for demonstrating the extent of the disease and involvement of contiguous structures as well as detecting unsuspected contralateral Wilms' tumor. The distinction between renal and adrenal or paravertebral masses (neuroblastoma) is usually clear on CT.

Inferior venacavography and arteriography are virtually never helpful in children.

DIFFERENTIAL DIAGNOSIS

Wilms' tumor accounts for more than 90% of renal tumors in children. Other diagnoses in the child with a renal mass include clear cell sarcoma, rhabdoid tumor, congenital mesoblastic nephroma, and renal cell carcinoma.

PATHOLOGY

Grossly, Wilms' tumor appears spherical and light gray or tan on cross-section. Cysts are common and may be a dominant feature. Microscopically, this tumor is variable, and the classic triphasic pattern includes blastemal, stromal, and epithelial cells. Additionally, patients can be separated on the basis of favorable and unfavorable histologic type. **Unfavorable histology includes anaplasia and monomorphic sarcomatous-appearing tumors. These unfavorable features occurred in only 10% to 12% but accounted for almost half of the tumor deaths in the first early National Wilms' Tumor Study.**

MANAGEMENT

Management of Wilms' tumor is rather complex and beyond the scope of this chapter. It includes surgery, chemotherapy, and radiation therapy, depending on stage and histology of the tumor.

Complete surgical removal of the tumor continues to be an essential part of management. Initial thorough exploration of the abdominal cavity and contralateral kidney is crucial to exclude local or regional tumor spread as well as involvement of the opposite kidney. Current chemotherapeutic agents used are doxorubicin, vincristine, actinomycin D, and cyclophosphamide.

STAGING AND SURVIVAL

The current staging system of Wilms' tumor reflects nodal involvement and local residual disease or tumor spillage. The following are the definitions of each stage:

Stage I: the tumor is limited to kidney with complete excision

Stage II: tumor extends beyond the kidney but is completely excised

Stage III: residual nonhematogenous tumor remains and is confined to the abdomen

Stage IV: tumor deposits are outside the abdomen

Stage V: bilateral renal involvement

The distribution by stage of favorable histology tumors was stage I, 47%; II, 22%; III, 22%; and IV, 9%. Patients with unfavorable histology are twice as likely to present with stage IV disease than those with favorable counterparts.

The present survival for children with

Wilms' tumor is excellent. Two-year relapse-free survival (which is comparable to more recent 4-year relapse-free survival data) is summarized in Table 23–2.

Neuroblastoma

EPIDEMIOLOGY

Neuroblastoma was first described by Virchow in 1864. It is the most common malignant tumor of infancy, and, after brain tumors is the most common solid tumor of childhood. It is also the most common intra-abdominal malignancy of childhood. This tumor accounts for 7% to 8% of all pediatric cancers, 15% of all pediatric cancer deaths, and 50% of all neonatal malignancies.

The peak age at presentation is 1½ years, with 50% of cases occurring in children younger than 2 years of age and 75% noted by the fourth year of life. This is younger than the peak age for Wilms' tumor by 18 months.

GENETICS

About 20% of neuroblastoma cases occur in patients with an inheritable mutation. The familial cases are believed to represent an autosomal dominant pattern of inheritance. The median age at diagnosis is significantly younger in familial cases versus in sporadic cases (9 vs. 21 months, respectively). The risk of this tumor developing in a sibling or offspring of an affected patient is less than 6%. Numerous karyotypic abnormalities have been found in neuroblastoma; however, dele-tion of the short arm of chromosome 1 is observed most frequently (in 70% to 80% of patients) and is believed to represent the loss of a neuroblastoma suppressor gene.

An association has been found between this tumor and neurofibromatosis, and there is increased risk of brain and skull defects.

PATHOLOGY

Neuroblastoma is known to arise from cells of neural crest origin that form the adrenal medulla and sympathetic ganglia. Tumors derived from the sympathetic nervous system are differentiated along two lines: the pheochromocytoma and the sympathoblastoma. The latter includes neuroblastoma (malignant and least differentiated), ganglioneuroblastoma (intermediate cellular differentiation), and ganglioneuroma (benign and most differentiated).

Microscopically, this tumor is the prototypical small "blue cell" tumor of childhood.

CLINICAL PRESENTATION

The clinical manifestations of this tumor vary depending on the site of primary tumor, the presence of metastases, and the secretion of catecholamines. More than half of neuroblastomas originate in the abdomen, and two thirds of these arise in the adrenal glands. **The most common presentation of this disease is an abdominal mass that is usually firm, fixed, and nodular, often extending beyond the midline. This is in contrast to Wilms' tumor, which usually occurs as a smooth flank mass that does not cross the midline. Pelvic neuroblastoma may cause urinary retention and constipation. Unilateral Horner's syndrome may develop in cervical or upper mediastinal tumors. Neuroblastoma is usually silent in its early stages, and up to 70% of patients have metastatic disease at the time of diagnosis. The first sign of illness may be caused by widespread disease, with weight loss, irritability, fever, anemia, and bone pain from bone or bone marrow metastases. Other presentations of metastatic disease include proptosis, periorbital ecchymosis, and subcutaneous nodules known as "blueberry muffins."**

Table 23–2
Survival Rates for Patients with Wilms' Tumor

Stage	Two-Year Survival (%)
I	95
II	90
III	84
IV	54
Nodal disease	
Negative	82
Positive	54
Histologic pattern	
Unfavorable	54
Favorable	90

DIAGNOSIS

Minimal criteria for establishing a diagnosis of neuroblastoma are an unequivocal pathologic diagnosis made from tissue by standard methods, or the bone marrow containing unequivocal tumor cells (pseudorosettes) and the urine with increased urinary catecholamine metabolites.

Complete work-up includes complete blood count (anemia may be the presenting sign especially in those with bone marrow involvement), coagulation parameters, liver function tests, chest radiograph (to evaluate posterior mediastinum), skeletal survey, CT scan of abdomen, bone marrow aspiration (at least 50% of patients have bone marrow involvement), and urinary level of catecholamine metabolites (elevated in 90% to 95% of cases), vanillylmandelic acid and homovanillic acid. Other laboratory markers include neuron-specific enolase, which is elevated in more than 90% of patients with metastases, and elevated serum ferritin levels, which are found in 40% to 50% of patients with advanced disease. A plain abdominal film shows speckled calcification in 50% of cases. CT scan with contrast agent shows inferolateral displacement of the ipsilateral kidney and ureter, creating a "drooping lily" appearance, when the tumor arises in the adrenal gland; the kidney may be displaced in other directions by tumors of paravertebral origin.

STAGING AND PROGNOSIS

Accurate staging of patients with neuroblastoma is important because it provides information regarding prognosis (Table 23–3) and dictates treatment. Of the different staging classifications, the one most widely used clinically was proposed by Evans, as follows:

Stage I: tumor is confined to organ of origin
Stage II: tumor has unilateral regional spread
Stage III: tumor extends across the midline
Stage IV: distant metastasis
Stage V: limited metastasis to skin, liver or bone marrow, without bony involvement

There are many variables that have an impact on the prognosis of neuroblastoma. However, the site of origin (non-adrenal primary tumors with better survival), the age at the diagnosis (<1 year of age with far better survival), and stage of disease are the most important, with Stages I, II, and IV-S all having a favorable outcome and Stages III and IV fairing poorly.

TREATMENT

Complete surgical removal of Stages I and II alone is an adequate treatment providing a 2-year disease-free survival of about 80%. The kidney is rarely invaded by tumor and can routinely be spared. In Stage IV-S tumors, resection of the primary is not mandatory and the likelihood of spontaneous remission is high; therefore, treatment may be directed toward complications. Radiation therapy and/or chemotherapy may be used for symptomatic infants with massive hepatic involvement. Advanced tumors as in Stages III and IV require multimodal management, which includes surgery, chemotherapy, radiation therapy, and autologous bone marrow transplantation. Aggressive attempts at resection, including spinal cord extension of tumor, are required.

METASTASIS

Metastases occur in 60% to 90% of patients at the time of presentation. Metastasis in retroperitoneal structures is via direct extension and to other tissues by lymphatic and hematogenous routes. Dissemination of this tumor develops early in the lymph nodes, liver, and bone and later in the lungs and brain. Most common skeletal metastases are skull and long bones. Neuroblastoma also exhibits a propensity to invade the spinal cord via the foramina.

Table 23–3
Number of Patients with Neuroblastoma Surviving 2 Years by Age and Stage at Diagnosis

Age (Years)	Stage					%
	I	II	III	IV	IV-S	
<1	12/14	10/11	5/8	5/15	14/21	67
1–2	4/4	3/5	4/7	2/33	0/0	26
>2	6/8	2/5	0/10	12/81	1/1	20
Total %	85	71	36	15	68	

Testicular Tumors

Testicular tumors in children are rare, constituting only 1% to 2% of all pediatric solid tumors. They are the seventh most common childhood tumor seen. The peak incidence of pediatric testicular tumors is at 2 years of age. The incidence decreases after the age of 4 years; however, it then begins to rise again at puberty. The incidence of germ cell tumors in children is not as high as in adults, constituting only 65% of prepubertal testicular tumors. A greater percentage of benign testicular lesions occurs in children. The etiology of testicular cancer is unknown, but there is a clear link between cryptorchidism and germ cell tumors of testis (Table 23–4).

CLINICAL PRESENTATION AND DIAGNOSIS

The most common presentation of testicular tumor is a painless scrotal mass. The mass is usually nontender and does not transilluminate. There is often a delay of about 7 months from first recognition of the scrotal swelling by the parents and initiation of treatment.

Abdominal CT is the most common tool used to examine the retroperitoneal spread of malignant tumors. Chest radiograph or chest CT is mandatory to exclude pulmonary metastases.

Alpha-fetoprotein (AFP) is produced by yolk sac tumor and also by fetal yolk sac, liver, and gastrointestinal tract. Its serum half-life is about 5 days; thus, the AFP level should return to normal within 25 days if there is no residual disease after resection of primary tumor. The beta subunit of human chorionic gonadotropin is produced by embryonal carcinoma and mixed teratomas, and its half-life is approximately 24 hours.

STAGING AND SURVIVAL

The current staging system for germ cell tumors comprises the following:

Stage I: tumor limited to testis
Stage II: local microscopic disease or nodal involvement ($\leq$ 2 cm) and/or persistent elevated tumor markers
Stage III: bulky retroperitoneal nodal disease
Stage IV: distant metastasis

Overall survival for patients with yolk sac tumors is excellent (99%) but less optimal for more advanced disease (Stages III and IV).

Yolk Sac Tumor

Yolk sac tumor is the most common prepubertal testicular tumor (followed by teratoma), and it accounts for about 60% of all testis tumors. **More than 75% of pediatric yolk sac tumors occur in the first 2 years of life, and they are believed to arise from the yolk sac elements. The characteristic histologic finding in this tumor is Schiller-Duval bodies.** Unlike its adult counterpart, spread of the childhood yolk sac tumor to the retroperitoneal lymph nodes is uncommon; routine retroperitoneal lymph node dissection is unnecessary. Distant metastases are most likely to be hematogenously disseminated to the lung (in 20% of patients).

TREATMENT

Treatment of germ cell tumors depends on the stage of disease. Clinical Stage I patients do not receive additional adjuvant treatment after radical orchiectomy. Stage II patients are given chemotherapy (bleomycin, cisplatin, and etoposide) in addition to surgery. Stages III and IV patients receive chemotherapy after initial retroperitoneal lymph node sampling. All of these patients need to be followed carefully after treatment.

Table 23–4
Pathology Categories for the Prepubertal Testicular Tumor Registry

Pathology	N	Percentage
Yolk sac	197	62
Teratoma	45	14
Gonadal stroma	18	6
Leydig's cell	4	1
Sertoli's cell	2	1
Other (e.g., rhabdomyosarcoma, leukemia, epidermoid cyst, gonadoblastoma)	51	16
Unknown	3	1

Table 23-5
Summary of Characteristics of Pediatric Tumors

Pearls	Wilms' Tumor	Neuroblastoma	Testicular Tumor	Rhabdomyosarcoma
Symptoms	Thriving with abdominal fullness	Depends mainly on site of origin Abdominal fullness or constitutional symptoms	Painless scrotal swelling	Depends mainly on site of origin Urinary retention Unilateral painless scrotal swelling
Signs	Flank mass that usually does not cross midline Hematuria, HTN	Mass usually cross midline "Blueberry muffin"	Scrotal mass that does not transilluminate	Abdominal mass Prolapse vaginal mass Scrotal mass distinct from testis
Associated factors/anomalies	Associated with aniridia, hemihypertrophy, Beckwith-Wiedemann, Denys-Drash, Perlman, and WAGR syndromes	Neurofibromatosis Brain and skull defect	Cryptorchidism	Li-Fraumani syndrome Neurofibromatosis Gorlin's basal cell nevus syndrome Fetal alcohol syndrome
Staging systems Pathology/genetics	I through V Deletion 11-13, 11-15, LOH 16q Triphasic pattern Favorable vs. unfavorable histology	I through IV and IV-S Familial cases autosomal dominant Deletion of 1p Neural crest cells	I through IV Yolk sac tumor 60% of testis tumor Yolk sac elements Schiller-Duval bodies	Depends on different centers Primitive mesenchymal cells Highly malignant Embryonal is most common subtype

Treatment	Surgery, chemotherapy, radiation therapy	Stage I—surgery only Stage II—surgery only Stage IV-S—treat complications	Stage I—surgery only Stage II—surgery and chemotherapy Stage III/IV—chemotherapy	Surgery, radiation therapy, chemotherapy
Prognosis/survival	Overall good (Table 23–3)	Stage I and II—75–80%. With surgery alone Stage III/IV—debulking (with BX), ± BMT—poor prognosis—30%; Stage IV-S—65–70% (Table 23–3)	Overall excellent	Better prognosis for vaginal and paratesticular Rhabdomyosarcoma > 90% survival rates for localized disease
Diagnostic pearls/tools	Older age than neuroblastoma Ultrasound and CT scan	Peak age 1½ to 2 years Tissue BX, pseudorosettes in bone marrow aspirates, elevated urinary VMA, HVA Speckled calcification of plain abdominal radiograph "Drooping lily" Deformity on contrast imaging	Peak at age 2 years Ultrasound of scrotum CT scan of abdomen Chest radiograph or CT AFP/β-HCG	Peak at age 2–6 and 15–19 years Male:female 3:1 Ultrasound and/or CT of abdomen Cystoscopy with BX

HTN, hypertension; WAGR, Wilms' tumor, aniridia, genitourinary abnormalities, mental retardation; LOH, loss of heterozygosity; CT, computed tomography; BX, biopsy; BMT, bone marrow transplant; VMA, vanillylmandelic acid; HVA, homovanillic acid; AFP, alpha-fetoprotein; β-HCG, beta human chorionic gonadotropin.

Rhabdomyosarcoma

EPIDEMIOLOGY AND INCIDENCE

Rhabdomyosarcoma is the most common soft tissue sarcoma in infants and children, and it accounts for about half of all pediatric soft tissue sarcomas. It is the fifth most common solid tumor in children and accounts for 15% of all pediatric solid tumors. Genitourinary rhabdomyosarcoma constitutes about 20% of these tumors and occurs at two age peaks: 2 to 6 years of age and 15 to 19 years. It has a male-to-female ratio of about 3:1. The most common genitourinary sites are the prostate, bladder, and vagina, with vaginal and paratesticular primaries having a better prognosis than bladder and prostate primaries.

ETIOLOGY AND PATHOLOGY

The etiology of rhabdomyosarcoma is unknown; however, familial aggregations of rhabdomyosarcoma with other sarcomas, breast cancers, and brain tumors (Li-Fraumeni syndrome) suggest a possible genetic factor. Other associated congenital anomalies include neurofibromatosis, Gorlin's basal cell nevus syndrome, and fetal alcohol syndrome.

Rhabdomyosarcoma arises from primitive mesenchymal cells and is highly malignant, spreading by local invasion as well as lymphatic and hematogenous routes. The three histologic subtypes are embryonal, alveolar, and pleomorphic, in descending order of frequency. All genitourinary rhabdomyosarcomas consist of the embryonal subtype.

DIAGNOSIS

Clinical presentation of patients with genitourinary rhabdomyosarcoma depends on the site of the primary tumor. **A common manifestation of rhabdomyosarcoma of the bladder and prostate is urinary retention due to bladder outlet obstruction.** On examination an abdominal mass from either tumor or a distended bladder is often present. Ultrasound or CT shows the extent of tumor and evaluates the involvement of the retroperitoneal and pelvic nodes. Finally, cystoscopy with biopsy establishes the diagnosis. Para-testicular rhabdomyosarcoma often presents as a unilateral painless scrotal swelling or mass usually distinct from the testis. Ultrasound can confirm the solid nature of the lesion, and CT imaging of the retroperitoneum identifies nodal metastases, as lymphatic spread is evident in up to 40% of patients. Patients with vaginal and vulvar rhabdomyosarcoma may present with prolapse of the mass from the vaginal introitus as well as vaginal bleeding or discharge. The diagnosis is made by vaginoscopy and biopsy of the lesion.

STAGING

The outcome of treatment of rhabdomyosarcoma is most dependent on the stage at diagnosis. Staging for RMS is dependent on the resectability of the primary tumor and nodal involvement. The intergroup Rhabdomyosarcoma Study Staging outlines the following:

Group I: completely detectable localized tumor
Group II: only microscopic residual after tumor resection
Group III: gross residual tumor after resection
Group IV: distant metastasis

These systems share conceptual similarities but contain important differences.

TREATMENT

Before the advent of combination chemotherapy and the realization that genitourinary rhabdomyosarcoma is radiosensitive, genitourinary rhabdomyosarcoma was treated with radical surgery (i.e., radical cystectomy or pelvic exenteration). Combined modality therapy, including extirpative surgery, local radiation, and 1- to 2-year multiagent chemotherapy with vincristine, actinomycin D, cyclophosphamide, doxorubicin, and cisplatin has produced survival rates of greater than 90% and maximal preservation of functional distal urinary tract in patients with localized disease.

Summary

The essential facts or clinical pearls concerning each of these tumors are summarized in convenient tabular form in Table 23–5. These items recur frequently in board examinations as well as in clinical practice, and constitute the principal similarities and differences among the genitourinary malignancies of childhood.

SUGGESTED READINGS

1. Broecker BH: Childhood genitourinary rhabdomyosarcoma. AUA Update Series 5(Lesson 16):2–7, 1986.

2. Coplen DE, Evans AE: Neuroblastoma update. AUA Update Series 12(Lesson 35):274–279, 1993.

3. Kay R, Kaplan GW: Testicular tumors in infants and children. AUA Update Series 2(Lesson 15):114–117, 1982.

4. Kramer SA: Pediatric urologic oncology. Urol Clin North Am 12:31–42, 1985.

5. Mesrobian HGJ, Kelalis PP: Wilms' tumor. AUA Update Series 10:146–151, 1991.

6. Ritchey ML, Andrassy RJ, Kelalis PP: Pediatric urologic oncology. *In* Gillenwater JY, Grayhack JT, Howards SS, et al (eds): Adult and Pediatric Urology, 3rd ed. St. Louis, Mosby-Year Book, 1996, pp 2675–2754.

7. Shapiro E, Strother D: Pediatric genitourinary rhabdomyosarcoma. J Urol 148:176–178, 1992.

24

Prostate-Specific Antigen

Michael Stifelman
Mitchell C. Benson

The widespread use of serum prostate-specific antigen (PSA) determinations was supposed to simplify the diagnosis and treatment of prostate cancer. Unfortunately, like many medical discoveries that at first appear straightforward, once the dust settles, controversy and confusion can remain. In every PSA application, as a screening tool, as a prognostic indicator, or as a determination of response to therapy, there has been at least some disagreement on how PSA should be used and interpreted. This chapter attempts to identify these issues and, when possible, clarify them. We review the physiologic function of PSA and factors that influence the production and release of PSA into the serum. The role PSA plays in prostate cancer screening is reviewed, with a discussion of the benefits and pitfalls of screening. The PSA derivatives that have been developed in the last decade (PSA density [PSAD], PSA velocity [PSAV], age-specific PSA, race-specific PSA, and free-to-total PSA) to improve the specificity of PSA-based prostate cancer screening are highlighted. Finally, how PSA may be used as a tumor marker for staging and prognosis is addressed.

What Is PSA?

PSA was first demonstrated in prostatic tissue in 1970 and in seminal fluid in 1971. In 1979 Wang and associates purified this antigen from prostatic tissue and tested an antibody against PSA in other tissue extracts. This antigen was not found in other tissues and hence was named *prostate-specific antigen*. We now know that PSA can be identified in other tissues, including periurethral glands (Skene's glands in women), breast cancer, and renal cell cancer. However, the highest concentration by more than 1000 to 1 is within the prostate gland and seminal fluid. PSA is a single-chained glycoprotein with 237 amino acids and a molecular weight of 28,430 daltons. The gene for PSA is located on the long arm of chromosome 19 and is androgen regulated. PSA is synthesized in the ductal epithelium of prostatic acini; it is a serine protease inhibitor, exhibiting proteolytic activity, and is a member of the kallikrein family. Its physiologic function is to liquefy the coagulum that forms at ejaculation. This liquefaction is accomplished through proteolysis of the gelforming proteins within the semen. The liquefaction allows for the release of the spermatozoa from the coagulum.

PSA, although found in greatest concentration in the seminal fluid, is also found in the serum. In preliminary studies conducted at Roswell Park Cancer Institute in the 1980s, observations regarding serum PSA were extended to the clinical setting. Using an assay approximately 200 times less sensitive than our current assays (capable of detecting only 0.5 µg of PSA per mL), Papsidero and colleagues examined serum PSA in patients with and without prostate cancer. They found that approximately 8% of 219 patients with advanced prostate cancer exhibited activity compared with 0% reactivity in 20 age-matched controls, and 0% reactivity in 175 patients with late-stage nonprostatic cancer.

These observations led to the development of a more sensitive enzyme immunoassay with a minimum detectable dose of 0.1 ng/mL. Using this assay they noted that 79% to 86% of patients with prostate cancer (Stages A through D) had serum PSA levels above the their upper limits of normal (1.8 ng/mL). It was these findings that triggered the explosion of research into the role of PSA as a tumor marker and possible screening tool for prostate cancer.

Factors Influencing Serum PSA Concentration

PSA is a prostate epithelial cell secretory product that is supposed to be secreted into the ejaculate. However, a quantum of PSA leaks into the serum from each prostate cell via "wrong way diffusion." Since each prostate cell is responsible for a quantum of this diffusion, serum PSA is a rough indicator of prostate cell number. Cancer is a growth process. Patients with prostate cancer will, on average, have more prostate cells than patients without prostate cancer. Therefore, PSA can be used to establish the risk of prostate cancer. Unfortunately, factors other than the development of prostate cancer can influence the amount of PSA in the serum. The "normal" total serum PSA level is currently defined as 4 ng/mL. Patients with a PSA above 4 ng/mL are deemed to have an abnormal level. One process that may cause an abnormal elevation in serum PSA is prostate cancer. Prostate cancer cells do not produce more PSA than their nonmalignant counterparts. Rather, more PSA reaches the serum either because of greater cellularity per unit volume of prostate tissue or the fact that the PSA produced by invasive malignant cells has no access to the lumina of the prostate, and all of the secreted PSA is eventually absorbed into the blood stream. In patients undergoing prostate resection for removal of benign hyperplastic prostatic tissue, researchers at Stanford University demonstrated that the serum PSA falls at a rate of 0.3 ng/mL per gram of resected tissue. Patients with prostate cancer experience a serum decrease of 3.5 ng/mL per gram of resected tissue.

Although PSA increases with prostate cancer, it is not prostate cancer specific. PSA is produced by all prostate cells and is an important component of seminal fluid. Thus, a patient with an enlarged benign prostate may also have an elevated serum PSA. Other factors that may lead to elevated serum PSA levels include infection, ejaculation, and prostate manipulation by vigorous digital rectal examination (DRE), instrumentation, or biopsy (Table 24–1). PSA elevations secondary to prostatitis have been frequently reported. It has been suggested that the inflammatory response and resultant hyperemia associated with acute and chronic prostatitis causes a disruption of the prostate interstitium allowing PSA to "leak out" into the blood stream, increasing the levels of serum PSA. Treatment of patients with acute bacterial prostatitis with 2 to 6 weeks of appropriate antibiotics results in a normalization of serum PSA, but this normalization may take 3 to 6 months to accomplish. There is another inflammatory entity, which can also be a source of PSA elevation, that is referred to as *subclinical prostatitis* or *chronic nonbacterial prostatitis.* Asymptomatic patients with a normal DRE, who on biopsy have pathologic features consistent with prostatitis, define this clinical syndrome. In this cohort of patients, about 6% have an elevated PSA level. Antibiotics do not have a significant effect on serum PSA concentrations in this group of patients, and thus a course of antibiotics for patients with a suspicion of subclinical prostatitis is not usually beneficial.

Table 24–1
Factors Affecting Serum Prostate-Specific Antigen (PSA)

Factors Affecting Serum PSA	Duration of Effect
Prostate cell number	Not applicable
Prostate size	Not applicable
Recent ejaculation	6–48 hours
Prostate manipulation	
Vigorous massage	1 week
Cystoscopy	1 week
Prostate biopsy	4–6 weeks
Prostatitis	
Acute	3–6 months
Chronic	Unknown
Prostate cancer	Not applicable
Drugs: finasteride (Proscar)*	3–6 months

*Lowers PSA for as long as patient is on the medication.

The relationship between ejaculation and transiently elevated serum PSA levels has been controversial. Some studies have shown that a transient elevation of PSA may be observed if ejaculation occurred within 6 to 48 hours of serum collection. One study demonstrated a modest elevation in 87% of patients older than 50 years of age following ejaculation. Of the patients who displayed an increase in PSA serum concentration, 92% returned to baseline within 24 hours, 97% returned to baseline in 48 hours, and 100% returned to baseline by 1 week. Based on these observations, some have recommended that men abstain from ejaculation for at least 48 hours prior to a serum PSA determination.

Prostate manipulation by routine DRE does not increase PSA levels enough to alter treatment decisions and thus is not clinically relevant. Prostate massage for evaluation of expressed prostatic secretions may increase PSA levels significantly and should not be performed prior to obtaining a serum PSA level. Transrectal ultrasound (TRUS) of the prostate causes a statistically significant rise in up to 20% of patients that can last for up to 7 days, and it is recommended that serum PSA determinations are done before a TRUS examination.

Prostate biopsy disrupts prostatic architecture and can result in a serum PSA elevation that lasts for 4 to 6 weeks. Changes in serum PSA secondary to vigorous rectal examination, TRUS, or cystoscopy should be short lived with returned to baseline within 1 week. Acute urinary retention has been shown to elevate serum PSA levels by as much as 6-fold to 10-fold, and thus PSA levels in patients in retention are unreliable.

These factors raise serum PSA levels and can result in false-positive test results. There is one agent that causes serum PSA to decrease. The drug finasteride (Proscar, Propecia) blocks the enzyme 5-alpha reductase. This enzyme is responsible for the prostatic intracellular conversion of testosterone to dihydrotestosterone (DHT). DHT is the most active moiety of testosterone, and, as a result, finasteride causes a selective partial castration of the prostate gland. This partial castration causes prostate cell death and, as a result, a decrease in prostate cell numbers. Prostate cells not dying may also decrease their indi-

vidual PSA production. As a result, patients taking finasteride 5 mg (Proscar) experience a 25% to 50% decrease in their serum PSA that occurs over a 3- to 6-month period after starting therapy. Recently, finasteride 1 mg (Propecia) has been released for the treatment of male-pattern baldness. The effect of finasteride 1 mg on serum PSA is less dramatic and more variable. **For patients on finasteride 5 mg, failure of the serum PSA to fall should be considered an indication for further evaluation and urologic referral.**

If finasteride is stopped, the patient's PSA will return to baseline. The time necessary for this return to baseline PSA is variable and to some extent a function of how long finasteride therapy had been maintained. Most patients return to baseline within 6 months.

It is the multitude of factors that affect serum PSA (see Table 24–1) that makes it so difficult to interpret the etiology of an elevated PSA. **Thus, an elevated PSA value (> 4.0 ng/mL) may be secondary to adenocarcinoma of the prostate, benign prostatic hyperplasia (BPH), prostatitis, recent ejaculation, or prostate manipulation.**

Prostate Cancer Screening

The American Cancer Society (ACS) and the American Urological Association (AUA) have recommended that all men 50 years of age or older undergo annual prostate cancer screening by DRE and serum PSA. Both organizations also recommend earlier screening for men at increased risk of prostate cancer (those with a family history or African Americans). The AUA recommends that this screening begin at the age of 40 years, and the ACS recommends age 45. All men with an abnormal DRE should be sent to a urologist for further work-up, regardless of the PSA level. When the serum PSA is abnormal, the clinician should search for factors that may cause a transiently elevated PSA (see Table 24–1). When appropriate, these causes should be treated and a repeat PSA performed. If no cause for a PSA elevation can be discovered or if the PSA does not return to normal after therapy, patients should be referred to a urologist for further work-up to determine if the patient's abnormal examination or PSA elevation is secondary to prostate cancer.

The only way one can exclude a diagnosis of prostate cancer with 100% certainty is to remove the entire prostate and to step-section the entire gland. This is clearly both impractical and overly invasive. However, anything short of total examination of the entire prostate has a reduced sensitivity; that is, some cancers will be missed owing to sampling error. The urologist's work-up begins with a careful evaluation of why the PSA may be spuriously elevated and a careful DRE. If the DRE is abnormal or the PSA is elevated, the next step is TRUS and TRUS-guided needle biopsy of the prostate and, when appropriate, digital-guided prostate biopsy (for an abnormal DRE only). This is an ambulatory procedure requiring a Fleet Enema the night prior to or the morning of the biopsy and 3 to 4 days of prophylactic antibiotics. At the time of TRUS the prostate volume may be measured and hypoechoic regions identified. When hypoechoic regions and/or palpable abnormalities are identified, preferential biopsies in addition to random biopsies are performed. Random prostate biopsy involves the direction of the biopsy needle into the various anatomic regions of the prostate. These include the apical portion, the midportion, and the base of the prostate posteriorly and possibly the transitional zone ventrally on both the right and left sides. Often, 6 to 12 cores of tissue are obtained. The number of biopsies often depends on the clinical setting, the magnitude of the PSA elevation, the size of the prostate, and whether or not the patient has undergone prior biopsies. Positive findings are beyond the scope of this chapter. Negative biopsies allow the patient to be placed on surveillance.

PSA-based prostate cancer screening has unquestionably increased the detection of prostate cancer and appears to increase the detection of curable disease. Most epidemiologists relate this dramatic increase to better screening techniques (i.e., PSA). Regarding PSA's ability to increase detection of curable disease, one may compare pathologic stage at time of diagnosis. **In the pre-PSA era (DRE-detected cancers), the incidence of pathologically organ-confined disease averaged only 33%. In contrast, in the post-PSA era, 60%** **to 70% of patients are found to have organ-confined disease and the lower the PSA, the higher the likelihood of prostate cancer confined to the prostate gland and surgical specimen.** Despite this obvious increase in early detection and strong suggestion of increase in the detection of curable disease, it still remains to be demonstrated that PSA-based prostate cancer screening has improved survival. As a result, PSA-based prostate cancer screening remains controversial owing to its cost to society both financially and in terms of morbidity secondary to prostate cancer therapies.

Several large studies have been designed throughout the world to determine if PSA screening improves patient survival. One study, the European Randomized Study of Screening for Prostate Carcinoma (ERSPC), enrolled 9200 men between 55 and 70 years of age to be randomized between PSA-based screening and no screening. Patients with a PSA level greater than 4 ng/mL, abnormal DRE, or abnormal TRUS underwent TRUS-guided sextant biopsies. The cancer detection rate in those patients screened was 174 (4%) in 4286. Of the 174 cancers detected, 41% were detected because of an elevated PSA alone and theoretically would have been unrecognized in the pre-PSA era. To determine the significance of these cancers, they were compared to incidentally found latent prostate cancers (pathologically insignificant) in radical cystoprostatectomy specimens removed for bladder cancer. These incidentally found latent prostate cancers had a mean cancer volume of 0.04 mL, with only 3% demonstrating extracapsular extension. **This is compared to the PSA-detected carcinomas where the average tumor volume was 50 times as large as the latent carcinoma's volume and extracapsular extension was detected in 30% to 40% of pathologic specimens. These findings suggest that PSA-detected prostate cancers are not latent incidental carcinomas but have a real potential for malignancy and death.**

Another study conducted in Austria enrolled 21,078 men, all without a history of prostate cancer or prostatitis. All volunteers were subjected to a serum PSA measurement. PSA cut-off levels were based on age-specific reference levels: 2.5 ng/mL in men aged 40 to 49 years, 3.5 ng/mL in men aged 50 to 59 years, 4.5 ng/mL in men aged 60 to 69 years, and 6.5 ng/mL in men aged 70 to 79 years. The concept behind age-specific PSA levels and other PSA derivatives is fully discussed later in this chapter. Age-specific PSA was developed to account for the rise in PSA that occurs in men as they age. In this study, all men with an elevated PSA according to age-specific reference ranges were invited to undergo a DRE to determine if a nodule was palpable and a TRUS-guided sextant biopsy. **The overall cancer detection rate was 1.2%, and of these lesions, 70% were missed by DRE and detected solely by PSA. Organ-confined prostate cancer was discovered in 70% of patients compared with historical rates of 30%.**

These two studies confirm the ability of PSA to increase the detection of seemingly curable prostate cancer and suggest that these cancers, when treated, may lead to increased survival and decreased cancer death. However, neither study has the longitudinal follow-up to prove this final and crucial point.

The pitfalls of PSA screening are largely secondary to its poor specificity. From the large screening studies described earlier, it is clear that the percentage of patients in the population who test positive (PSA > 4 ng/mL) is much higher then those with the disease. In other words, there is a high percentage of false-positive results, implying that PSA as a tumor marker for diagnosing prostate cancer has a low specificity. In terms of sensitivity, which is driven by the number of patients with false-negative results, PSA is considered very good. Although there are patients diagnosed with prostate cancer who have a "normal" PSA, this cohort is relatively small. Positive and negative predictive values improve with age secondary to the fact that the prevalence of prostate cancer increases with age. However, the benefit of detecting prostate cancer in some older patients diminishes.

PSA Derivatives

Although the effect of PSA screening on mortality has yet to be proven, there is consensus regarding its usefulness in diagnosing pros-

tate cancer and for many primary care physicians, general practitioners, and internists, it has become a standard part of the annual physical examination. Thus, although the debate continues, the reality is that most men are aware of PSA and are strongly desirous of its inclusion in their examination. The sensitivity of PSA has never been questioned. It is the test's lack of specificity (the number of false-positive results that lead to invasive evaluations) that has caused the most concern. In an attempt to improve specificity, several modifications in the interpretation of PSA have been proposed. These modifications are called *PSA derivatives*. Numerous PSA derivatives have been developed and are being tested clinically with the purpose of optimizing the use of PSA as a screening tool by improving the specificity while preserving its sensitivity.

PSA DENSITY

PSAD is one such variation and is defined mathematically as total serum PSA (in nanogram per milliliters) divided by the volume of the prostate gland (in cubic centimeters). The concept of PSAD is based on the assumption that PSAD calculation would standardize the amount of PSA produced per cubic centimeter of prostate tissue. It assumes that for a given volume of prostate tissue, a volume occupied by cancer results in a higher serum PSA than a volume occupied by benign tissue owing to increased cellularity and the inability of invasive cancer cells to secrete PSA into a glandular lumen. It was postulated that PSAD would be able to identify which patients had an elevated PSA secondary to benign enlargement, BPH, versus those with elevations secondary to prostate carcinoma.

The concept of PSAD was introduced at Columbia-Presbyterian Medical Center in New York by the authors in collaboration with Dr. William Cooner of Mobile, Alabama, as a means of decreasing the number of false-positive findings and thus decreasing the number of unnecessary biopsies. An analysis of 773 patients with a negative DRE and a PSA between 4 and 10 ng/mL who subsequently underwent prostate biopsy led to the proposal of a PSAD cut-off of 0.15 mg/mL. In this preliminary study, only patients with an abnormal TRUS (hypoechoity or asymmetry) underwent an initial biopsy. The positive prostate biopsy rate in this group was 6% for patients with a PSAD less than 0.15 and 18% for patients with a PSAD greater than 0.15. An initial study by Bazinet and coworkers from Montreal confirmed these findings. In a study of 142 patients with a negative DRE and a PSA between 4 and 10 ng/mL who underwent prostate biopsies, they noted only 2 patients had positive biopsies with a PSAD less than 0.15 compared with 20 patients with positive biopsies if they had a PSAD greater than 0.15.

Despite these encouraging results, other studies have failed to show improved cancer detection rates using PSAD compared with total serum PSA. Factors responsible for the conflicting results and conclusions may involve anatomic and technical difficulties in determining prostate volume (the "Achilles heel" of PSAD), lack of uniformity regarding the statistical analysis applied to the different studies, and the fact that the epithelium-to-stroma ratio differs considerably between patients. Differences in the amount of epithelium versus stroma in an individual's prostate allow for a wide range of PSA production in prostates of similar size. Because of these observations, PSAD as a means of increasing specificity is not universally accepted.

AGE-SPECIFIC PSA

Age-specific reference ranges for serum PSA is another variation of total PSA designed to increase specificity. The concept of age-specific reference ranges for serum PSA is similar to PSAD. Most men, as they get older, develop BPH (prostatic cellular proliferation) with a resultant increase in their prostate size, benign prostatic hyperplasia, and thus an increase in their serum PSA. In 1993, Oesterling and associates at the Mayo Clinic in Rochester, Minnesota, enrolled 537 men into a screening protocol that included serum PSA, DRE, and a TRUS. Of the 537 men, 471 had all three tests completed and showed no evidence of prostate cancer. Using this subset of patients, the researchers correlated serum PSA with age and prostate volume. The results indicated that serum PSA increased by 0.04 ng/mL (3.2%) per year. From these re-

sults and using the 95th percentile confidence limits, age-specific reference ranges for serum PSA were developed (Table 24–2).

Based on age-specific ratios, it was hypothesized that sensitivity would be increased by detecting more cases of organ-confined prostate cancer in younger men and specificity would be increased by decreasing the number of biopsies performed in older men. Several investigators have tested this hypothesis and examined its clinical usefulness in decreasing the normal value in younger men and raising the normal value in older men. It appears that lowering the normal range in younger men is valid and appropriate. Catalona and colleagues, in a multi-institutional study, used a patient population base consisting of 6630 men undergoing PSA and DRE screening followed by prostate biopsy for a positive result. They reported that a cut-off of 3.5 ng/mL in men aged 50 to 59 years resulted in a 15% increase in cancer detection rate. Partin and coworkers from Johns Hopkins Hospital in Baltimore used patients who had undergone a radical prostatectomy whose only indication was an elevated PSA. They concluded that in men younger than 60 years, a significant number of additional tumors would been detected using age-specific reference ranges. **Thus, it appears that the PSA cut-off of 4 ng/mL may be too high in younger men. However, it must be realized that decreasing the level of normal will result in more false-positive results (more patients will undergo biopsies).**

The validity of an increasing normal range in older men is less compelling. Catalona and associates showed that in men aged 60 to 69 years, 15% fewer biopsies would have been required but 8% of organ-confined tumors would have been missed. In men older than

Table 24–2
Age-Specific Reference Ranges for PSA

Age (yr)	Serum PSA (ng/mL)		
	Whites	**Japanese**	**African American**
40–49	0–2.5	0–2.0	0–2.0
50–59	0–3.5	0–3.0	0–4.0
60–69	0–4.5	0–4.0	0–4.5
70–79	0–6.5	0–5.0	0–5.5

PSA, prostate-specific antigen.

70 years of age, 44% fewer biopsies would be required but 47% of organ-confined cancers would be missed. Partin and colleagues also observed that the sensitivity of serum PSA would be decreased by raising the limit of normal in older men but raised the question of clinical significance and clinical consequence of the missed tumors.

In summary, investigators support the theory that the use of age-specific reference ranges would improve the sensitivity of PSA in younger men, allowing for the diagnosis of more organ-confined prostate cancer. For now, most investigators are unwilling to raise the upper limit of normal in older men. The question remains, however, about what percentage of these missed patients is clinically relevant.

RACE AND AGE-SPECIFIC PSA

The database that led to the development of age-specific reference ranges was composed of mainly white men. It has been known for a long time that Asian men, in general, have smaller prostates and a lower incidence of prostate cancer than whites or African American men do and that African American men have the highest incidence of prostate cancer in the United States. These facts led investigators to evaluate the effect of race on age-specific reference ranges. Oesterling performed a study similar to the one outlined earlier in an attempt to clarify age-specific reference ranges in Japanese men. The study results suggested that the age-specific reference ranges for Japanese men are 0 to 2 ng/mL for men aged 40 to 49 years, 0 to 3 ng/mL for men aged 50 to 59 years, 0 to 4 ng/mL for men aged 60 to 69 years, and 0 to 5 ng/mL for men aged 70 to 79 years (see Table 24–2). The difference between Japanese and white age-specific reference ranges was postulated to be secondary to the fact that Japanese men have smaller prostates than white men.

Morgan and coworkers completed a study examining age-specific reference ranges in African American men (see Table 24–2). This study confirmed that the PSA concentration correlates with age and that the upper limit of normal serum PSA should be also be age dependent in African Americans. Morgan de-

termined that if traditional age-specific reference ranges were used, as outlined by Oesterling for white men, 41% of cancers in their African American cohort would be missed. Therefore, the age-specific reference ranges for African Americans are 0 to 2 ng/mL for men aged 40 to 49 years, 0 to 4 ng/mL for men aged 50 to 59 years, 0 to 4.5 ng/mL for men aged 60 to 69 years, and 0 to 5.5 ng/mL for men aged 70 to 79 years. The differences appear minor but have tremendous clinical significance because it is in African American men that prostate cancer is more prevalent, occurs at an earlier age, and has a higher death rate.

PSA VELOCITY

Another derivative used to improve PSA screening, introduced by Carter and associates from Johns Hopkins in 1992, is known as PSAV. Carter and associates, using data and frozen serum from the Baltimore Longitudinal Study of Aging, were able to plot the PSA of 73 men, 60 years of age or older, over a 7-year period. They observed that men without prostate symptoms or prostate cancer had no change in their PSA over time. Patients with BPH had a linear slope of PSAV. Patients with prostate cancer had an initial linear component that became exponential. They calculated PSAV with an equation using at least three separate points and suggested that a PSAV higher than 0.75 ng/mL per year was indicative of prostate cancer.

The "normal" PSAV was examined by several studies, including one by Smith and Catalona, which prospectively enrolled 982 men to examine the efficacy and utility of PSAV. This study calculated that for patients with a PSA lower than 4.0 ng/mL, the cut-off point that predicts cancer is 0.75 ng/mL per year. However, they found that for patients with a PSA greater than 4.0 ng/mL, the cut-off point that predicts cancer is 0.4 ng/mL per year.

The major questions surrounding PSAV are how many serum measurements are required and how far they should be spaced. Carter and associates addressed these issues by retrospectively examining serial PSA measurements in 806 men, focusing on the number of PSA determinations, the time interval between PSA measurements, and the effect on the calculated PSAV. They concluded that three or more measurements are necessary and that longer intervals (> 6 months) between readings are more accurate in determining velocity than shorter intervals. This is the greatest shortcoming of PSAV.

The clinical utility of PSAV is limited since it is of greatest value retrospectively and of least value when the PSA determinations occur less than 1 year apart. Therefore, at a minimum, 2 years of PSA measurements are required to accurately stratify patients by PSAV, and most patients are far too anxious about PSA changes to await velocity determinations.

FREE-TO-TOTAL PSA RATIO

The most recent PSA derivative is the comparison of unbound (free) PSA to the total amount of PSA in the serum. In serum, PSA can exist as free PSA and PSA bound to alpha$_1$-antichymotripsin (ACT) or alpha$_2$-macroglobulin (A$_2$M). PSA bound to PSA-A$_2$M is antigenically shielded and not measurable by any PSA assay. PSA complexed to PSA-ACT is immunoreactively unique and can be measured in the serum as a separate moiety. As a result, it is possible to compare the amount of free PSA to the total amount of PSA (free + PSA-ACT). Lilja and coworkers documented that the majority of PSA in the serum is complexed to ACT (PSA-ACT), accounting for approximately 85% of the total serum PSA. They later compared the free:total (F:T) PSA in men with BPH to the F:T PSA of men with prostate cancer. They found that the F:T ratio was significantly lower in men with prostate cancer than men with BPH (0.18 to 0.28, respectively; $P = 0.0001$). Importantly, this difference was present for PSA values above and below 10. They concluded from their initial studies that the use of F:T PSA ratio would allow for a differentiation of elevated PSA levels secondary to BPH and prostate cancer without decreasing the sensitivity of PSA.

The explanation of why PSA elaborated from BPH is less likely to be bound to ACT (higher F:T ratio) may be found within prostate cancer cells. Bjork and colleagues found that prostate cancer cells produce not only PSA but also ACT. This coexpression of PSA

and ACT may allow for an increased likelihood of a PSA-ACT complex when PSA is elaborated from a cancer cell as opposed to a benign or normal cell. However, this is only speculative and the reason or reasons behind the observed F:T differences remain unknown.

Regardless of the reason for the increased PSA-ACT complex in PSA elaborated from prostate cancer cells (lower F:T ratios), F:T PSA ratios improve PSA specificity for patients with serum PSA levels in the 4- to 10-ng/mL "reflex" range (the laboratory goes into a reflex mode of determining the free PSA) (Table 24–3). The use of Hybritech's F:T PSA has recently been granted U.S. Food and Drug Administration (FDA) approval, and F:T ratios from other companies are expected to be granted approval in the near future. However, F:T PSA like the other derivatives is not without controversy. A universal F:T PSA cut-off has yet to be established, and it appears that, like PSAD and age- and race-specific PSA, the resultant increases in specificity are associated with decreases in sensitivity. **Most investigators agree that F:T PSA is best suited for patients with a total PSA in the 4- to l0-ng/mL range, but recent data demonstrate that F:T ratios may allow us to decrease the normal range of PSA for all men, not just those in specific age ranges** (see Table 24–3).

Despite the FDA approval, the appropriate "normal" F:T PSA has not been agreed on. This is in part secondary to numerous individual assays with different performances and selection biases in the populations under study. The normal F:T ratio appears to be a function of prostate volume and may be stratified by age when larger patient popula-

Table 24–3
Percentage of Free PSA and Cancer Probability

F:T Ratio (%)	Probability of Cancer (%)
0–10	56
10–15	28
15–20	20
20–25	16
>25	8

PSA, prostate-specific antigen; F:T, free:total.
Data from Urology Times Vol. 26, #4, 1998.

tions have been studied. If this proves to be the case, F:T PSA may suffer some of the same difficulties of PSAD. In addition, although some investigators have suggested that F:T ratios be used for patients with PSAs less than 4 ng/mL, others have failed to show percent-free PSA to be a useful variable when the total PSA is less than 4.0 ng/mL. At the time of this writing, it is impossible to make any absolute recommendations regarding a normal F:T ratio. We can say that for patients with a normal DRE and a PSA in the reflex range, the suggested F:T ratio is 25%. That is, patients who meet this criteria and have an F:T ratio less than 25% are more likely to have a positive biopsy than those with a ratio greater than 25%. However, no patient should be spared a biopsy based solely on F:T PSA. Age, health, and likely longevity must also be considered. For patients with serum PSA levels less than 4 ng/mL, F:T PSA would appear to be an appropriate addition to age-specific reference ranges. Further, more extensive prospective clinical trials are required to better define the role of F:T PSA ratio.

PSA as a Tumor Marker for Staging

Tumor markers can be used not only for screening purposes but also for staging, prognosis, and follow-up. The role of PSA, alone and in combination with other preoperative markers, has been evaluated extensively as a staging tool for prostate cancer. To understand the role of PSA as a staging tool, one must understand prostate cancer staging. The first step is to assign the prostate cancer a clinical stage (T1 through T4). This is performed solely on the basis of the DRE and is covered elsewhere in this text. Extraprostatic disease (T3 through T4) is clinically detected cancer invading outside the prostatic capsule into the periprostatic tissues (T3A and B), the seminal vesicles (T3C), and the bladder neck or rectum (T4). The differentiation between organ-confined disease (T1 and T2) and T3 and T4 disease is important in both selection of therapy and prognosis. However, clinical assessment of clinical stage is inaccurate since in many instances the prostate feels normal (T1C = PSA-detected cancer) and in other

instances extraprostatic cancer cannot be palpated.

Preoperative staging next consists of determining if the cancer has metastasized. Prostate cancer preferentially metastasizes to pelvic lymph nodes and bone. Traditionally, this is determined by nuclear medicine bone scan and a pelvic computed tomographic (CT) scan. Patients deemed to be at high risk for pelvic lymph node metastases sometimes undergo a laparoscopic pelvic lymph node dissection (PLND). PSA plays a role in all of the above because the patient's PSA level at diagnosis affects the risk of extraprostatic, regional, and metastatic disease.

The likelihood of identifying metastatic disease to bone in asymptomatic men with newly diagnosed prostate cancer by radionuclide bone scanning has been extensively studied as a function of the patient's PSA level. **Analysis of the data has led to the recommendation that bone scans be deferred in asymptomatic men with newly diagnosed prostate cancer if they have a PSA of 10 ng/mL or less.** This recommendation is appropriate for patients with well or moderately differentiated prostate cancer. It has been our approach to perform a bone scan if the cancer is poorly differentiated or anaplastic, since in this setting PSA may be less reliable owing to low PSA production in cells not maturing or differentiating. Even with this caveat, a substantial economic savings may be realized since in our recent experience, 50% to 60% of all patients diagnosed with prostate cancer have a PSA less than 10 ng/mL and a Gleason score of 7 or less.

The routine use of CT of the abdomen and pelvis was controversial even prior to the discovery of PSA. Many have argued that the use of CT imaging is ineffective secondary to its poor sensitivity and specificity in predicting lymph node metastasis and its inability to accurately predict extracapsular prostate cancer extension. Huncharek and co-workers evaluated 425 patients with newly diagnosed prostate cancer undergoing CT imaging for staging. No patient with a PSA less than 4 ng/mL had a positive finding, 2 patients (0.6%) with a PSA between 4 and 10 ng/mL had positive results, and 1 patient (0.3%) with a PSA between 10.1 and 20 had a positive finding. **They concluded that CT** imaging in patients with newly diagnosed prostate cancer and a PSA less than 20 ng/mL was unnecessary and not cost effective. They calculated a potential cost savings in 1996 dollars of up to $50 million per year.

The role of routine PLND in the post-PSA era has also been under investigation. Studies have been ongoing to define a subset of patients that may be spared PLND. These studies are particularly useful in patients wishing to undergo a perineal radical prostatectomy or radiation therapy since in these settings, lymph node dissection requires an additional procedure. Parro and associates evaluated 155 men, all of whom were scheduled to undergo perineal radical prostatectomy. Of the 155, 74 were assigned to the low-risk group (defined as having a PSA < 10 ng/mL and a biopsy revealing moderate to well-differentiated prostate cancer [Gleason score ≤ 6]). None of the 74 patients had positive pelvic lymph nodes compared with 5 (6%) of 81 that did not meet this low-risk criteria. **The authors performed a similar study evaluating the risk factors associated with positive lymph node metastasis and concluded that only patients with a PSA greater than 20 and a poorly differentiated cancer (Gleason score ≥ 7) require PLND.** Other investigators have confirmed these findings, and although not yet universally accepted, many centers are using PSA in combination with other preoperative factors to eliminate PLND in a subset of patients.

One of the most important uses of PSA is in defining which patients are at risk for extracapsular disease (T3 and T4). This determination is important in making treatment decisions and holds prognostic significance. In general, most urologists agree that radical prostatectomy surgery has survival advantages over other modalities in patients with a 15-year or greater life expectancy and localized disease (confined within the prostatic capsule [T2]). Unfortunately, in some studies as many as 40% of patients who are believed to meet this criteria preoperatively and undergo radical prostatectomy are found upon pathologic examination of their prostate to have extracapsular disease. In 1993, Partin and colleagues from Johns Hopkins published a paper that evaluated Gleason score (biopsy histology), PSA, and clinical stage to predict which patients would have extracapsular disease. They found that PSA was the best single predictor of extracapsular disease. However, they also demonstrated that by combining all three in a nomogram table, extracapsular disease could be predicted most accurately. The incorporation of this nomogram into the therapeutic decision tree allows for a better informed consent and will sometimes influence the patient's choice of therapy.

PSA as a Marker of Response to Therapy

PSA can be extremely useful in assessing a patient's response to therapy. But even here, there is not universal agreement on how PSA should always be used and interpreted. For patients with localized disease (T1 and T2), radical prostatectomy should result in an undetectable serum PSA (in general < 0.1 ng/mL). The development of an undetectable PSA does not mean that the patient is cured. PSA production by microscopic residual disease may be too low to be measurable by standard PSA assays. It takes between 4 and 5 years of undetectable PSA levels before the risk of failure plateaus. However, this is far better than the 15 years necessary to assess success if one uses clinical or radiologic endpoints. Failure to achieve an undetectable PSA indicates residual prostate tissue. In most instances, this residual prostate tissue is clinically undetectable (i.e., micrometastatic prostate cancer). In rare instances, however, the residual prostate tissue could be benign, unresected normal prostate either from the apex or base of the gland. Therefore, although the failure to achieve an undetectable PSA almost always indicates residual prostate cancer, each case needs to be individually analyzed. A rising PSA following radical prostatectomy, whether or not there was an undetectable nadir, indicates recurrent prostate cancer.

Following external radiation therapy for T1 to T2 disease, the PSA should fall to levels less than 0.5 to 1.5 ng/mL. The nadir that best correlates with durable response is subject to debate among radiation oncologists. However, there is an agreement that the lower the nadir, the better the prognosis; and also a rising PSA following radiation therapy indicates disease recurrence. The definition of a rising PSA is also subject to controversy in the radiation oncology literature. Some believe that any progressive rise indicates failure, whereas others believe that there must be three sequential rises at least 1 month apart. The reader should be aware that androgen deprivation is frequently used in association with radiation therapy. Androgen deprivation causes a patient's PSA to fall, in some instances to undetectable levels (a function of PSA level, androgen responsiveness, and length of therapy). Following discontinuation of androgen deprivation, a patient's PSA may rise, and this rise is not necessarily an indication of disease recurrence; rather, it may represent a normal return of prostate function.

Patients with advanced disease being treated with continuous androgen deprivation should have a rapid and profound fall in their serum PSA. Like the situation with radiation therapy, the lower the nadir, the better the prognosis. Failure to achieve an undetectable serum PSA following androgen deprivation usually indicates a tumor less responsive to this therapy and translates into a response of shorter duration. A rise in serum PSA while a patient is on androgen deprivation may be the first sign of the emergence of androgen-independent prostate cancer cell growth.

Future Directions: Molecular Staging of Prostate Cancer Using RT-PCR for PSA mRNA

A unique way of preoperative staging and predicting patients with extracapsular disease was introduced by Katz and coworkers from Columbia-Presbyterian Medical Center. This staging tool uses an enhanced reverse transcriptase polymerase chain reaction (RT-PCR) assay that is able to detect messenger RNA (mRNA) for PSA in the peripheral blood. This is a very sensitive blood test that can detect the mRNA coding for PSA production. Since only prostate cells encode for PSA, the detection of mRNA for PSA in the blood implies the detection of prostate cells circulating in the blood. The process of metastasis is complex and composed of multiple steps, invasion, intravasation into vessels, arrest, extrav-

asation out of vessels, and proliferation. The detection of living prostate cells in the circulation is therefore not synonymous with metastasis. Although a positive RT-PCR assay may not be bad, it cannot be good.

The largest trial with the most encouraging results using this form of molecular staging comes from Columbia-Presbyterian Medical Center. In the Columbia experience, the enhanced RT-PCR assay for PSA resulted in better specificity, sensitivity, and odds ratio in predicting which patients would have advanced prostate cancer than pathologic Gleason score, serum PSA, or preoperative imaging. Like other tests of advanced disease, the RT-PCR accuracy could be enhanced by combining it with PSA. For example, a (positive) RT-PCR and a preoperative PSA greater than 10 ng/mL results in a patient having a 90% chance of extraprostatic disease. In contrast, if the RT-PCR were (negative), the chance of organ confined disease is 81%.

The biggest drawback of the assay is the widely disparate reports of its efficacy and accuracy. In some centers, the sensitivity of the RT-PCR technology is sufficiently low that it is unable to detect patients with extracapsular disease, whereas in others the assay creates too many false-positive results in those with organ-confined disease. Unfortunately, although the RT-PCR techniques are relatively standard, the materials used (different primers and DNA sequences) varies significantly from institution to institution. This probably explains the variance in results from different studies. Further research and standardization of materials and methods are necessary before it can be recommended that RT-PCR for PSA be incorporated into the preoperative evaluation of all patients.

SUGGESTED READINGS

The May 1997 volume of the Urologic Clinics of North America is dedicated to serum PSA. It is composed of 24 articles that review in detail all aspects of serum PSA.

1. Prostate-specific antigen: The best prostatic tumor marker. Edited by JE Oesterling. Urol Clin North Am 24:1–270, 1997.

Free:total PSA is an aspect of serum PSA that is in evolution. The reader is advised to review the articles in the Urologic Clinics issue but also to be alert for new publications that would be best discovered using a computer search of the literature.

25 Carcinoma of the Genitourinary System

Donald L. Lamm

Cancer of the genitourinary tract is more common than generally appreciated. Prostate cancer is the most common noncutaneous cancer in Western industrialized countries, and in the United States bladder cancer is the fourth most prevalent malignancy. Genitourinary carcinomas range from the clinically insignificant, such as incidental low-grade prostate cancer in the very aged, to highly aggressive malignancies that can strike in the prime of life, such as renal cell carcinoma and nonseminomatous testis tumors. This chapter provides an overview of the important clinical features, diagnosis, and current management strategies for carcinoma of the prostate, bladder, kidney, testis and penis. Rare urologic malignancies such as urethral carcinomas are mentioned only briefly.

Prostate Cancer

Malignancies other than adenocarcinoma, such as sarcomas, lymphomas and leukemias, are rare and pale in importance for primary care physicians compared with adenocarcinoma. The increase in the incidence of prostate cancer in the last decade approaches epidemic proportions. This increase is in part related to the advent and increased use of prostate-specific antigen (PSA), which detects prostate cancer on average 7 years earlier than other clinical means. But the increase in new cases is above that which can be explained by PSA alone. In 1998 an estimated 184,500 men were diagnosed with prostate cancer and 39,200 men died of the disease. **Presumably as a result of PSA screening, early detection, and effective treatment,** mortality in 1999 is projected to be *down* to 37,000.

Clinical Features

Prostate cancer, which is the second most common cause of cancer death in men in the United States, does not generally cause symptoms until the disease is advanced and often incurable. Prevention of death from prostate cancer is therefore dependent on routine screening of men at risk of dying from the disease. When symptoms from prostate cancer do occur, prostatism, with hesitancy, decreased force of urinary stream, frequency, urgency, and nocturia are seen most frequently. Unfortunately, if PSA evaluation is not done, men may continue to present with back pain or even paraplegia from spinal metastasis as the first symptom of prostate cancer. **Detection of prostate cancer can be made on the basis of routine physical examination, with palpation of the prostate, and with use of PSA.** PSA is the subject of another chapter, but it should be noted that **PSA is superior to digital rectal examination in the detection of prostate cancer, and when used routinely every 1 to 2 years in high-risk men 40 to 75 years of age, the number of men who present with advanced or metastatic disease can be dramatically reduced.** Prostate cancer occurs most commonly posteriorly in the peripheral zone of the prostate, where it can be palpated by rectal examination. To detect prostate cancer one should feel for areas of increased firmness within the gland. Rock-hard diffuse nodularity of the prostate is easy to detect as typical prostate cancer but represents advanced, extracapsular disease that is generally incurable. **The goal**

285

of rectal examination is to detect early-stage, potentially curable disease. About 50% of palpable nodules are cancer, and only a fraction of cancers are within reach of the examiner's finger. Prostate examination has many limitations in the detection of prostate cancer but remains an essential diagnostic procedure because not all prostate cancers increase PSA.

When the PSA is elevated or an area of increased induration is palpated in the prostate, needle biopsy is indicated. Biopsy can be guided by palpation or transrectal ultrasound. Even when a nodule is palpated or a hypoechoic area found on ultrasound, systematic sextant biopsies are performed because the malignancy is typically diffusely distributed within the gland.

The needle biopsy provides information of prognostic importance. The number of positive biopsies and the percentage of cancer in each needle core provide information on the extent or volume of cancer, which is correlated with the risk of metastasis. If only a small focus of low-grade adenocarcinoma is found in a biopsy done for elevation of PSA, it may represent "incidental" carcinoma, that is, the carcinoma that is incidentally found in autopsies of up to 40% of men 50 years of age and older, rather than clinically significant disease. Even clinically diagnosed prostate cancer may, of course, not require aggressive treatment. It is estimated that the lifetime risk of clinical prostate cancer for a 50-year-old man is 9.5%, but the risk of dying from prostate cancer is less than 3%.

Tumor grade has a significant influence of prognosis, and along with tumor stage and patient life expectancy, should be considered when discussing treatment (or nontreatment) options. The Gleason grading system, which evaluates the degree of glandular differentiation on a scale of 1 (well differentiated) to 5 (poorly differentiated) of the primary and secondary components to yield an overall score of 2 to 10, is currently popular and correlates well with tumor-free and overall survival.

Staging and Work-Up

Carcinoma detected incidentally at the time of transurethral resection for presumed benign disease is termed Stage T1 in the TNM system and Stage A in the American system. If less than 5% of the resected tissue is malignant, it is T1a (A1), and further treatment may not be needed if the disease is low grade and/or the patient has a life expectancy of less than 10 years. Life expectancy for these patients is similar to the unaffected population, but disease progression is expected if patients are otherwise healthy and survive beyond 10 years. T1b (A2) carcinoma involves more than 5% of the resected tissue, and these patients have a prognosis similar to or in some reports even worse than Stage T2 (B) patients do. **Stage T1c (B0) disease is that detected on the basis of elevation of PSA. Prostate examination in these patients is normal. Stage T1c is now the most common presentation of prostate cancer, whereas prior to PSA most patients presented with metastatic or locally advanced extracapsular disease.** Management of these patients is controversial. Some argue that PSA screening results in the detection of clinically insignificant disease, and treatment may result in more morbidity and death than the disease. On the other hand, if incidental insignificant disease is defined as less than 0.5 mL of well-differentiated adenocarcinoma, clinical studies have shown that there is no increase in the proportion of incidental tumors found when patients are discovered based on PSA elevation. In fact, extension to the prostatic capsule or beyond the margin of resection is found much more frequently (roughly 60% of cases) than insignificant disease (10% or less) in patients detected by PSA screening. Palpable tumor confined to the prostate is termed *Stage T2 or B*. Stage T2a (B1) involves less than half of one lobe, T2b more than half of one lobe, and T2c (B2) both lobes. These patients are generally considered the optimal stage for complete surgical removal of the prostate and seminal vesicles. Partial prostatectomy is not done because in 80% of cases the disease is multicentric within the gland. In patients with low-grade disease or a life expectancy of less than 10 years (generally considered to be those 70 years of age and older) radiation therapy is generally preferred. Stage T3 (C) disease extends beyond the prostate. Positive margins are most often found at the apex of the gland and at the base, where the nerves and vessels penetrate the gland. When the seminal vesicles are involved (Stage T3C or C2), the prognosis is significantly reduced.

The site of earliest metastasis is to pelvic lymph nodes. Any nodal involvement reduces the survival, but long-term survival is seen in patients with small metastasis (< 2 cm) to a single node (N1 or D1 disease). The next most frequent site of metastasis is to bone (M1b or D2). Locally advanced or metastatic disease was seen in about half of patients prior to the advent of PSA screening, but now less than 5% of screened patients present with lymph node or bone metastasis.

Laboratory and Imaging Studies

In patients with a PSA below 20, little is needed in addition to the standard hematology and chemistry evaluation. An acid phosphatase level can be done as a baseline or as an aid to the diagnosis of metastasis, but it is currently omitted in most patients because of the superior sensitivity of PSA. In patients with a PSA less than 20, the negative predictive value for skeletal metastasis is more than 99%. Since false-positive bone scans occur for many reasons, in the absence of elevation of alkaline or acid phosphatase, bone pain, or poorly differentiated carcinoma (which may not produce PSA), bone scans can safely be deleted. Deletion of unnecessary bone scans would save an estimated $20 million in medical costs in the United States each year. Similarly, computed tomographic (CT) scanning or magnetic resonance (MR) imaging does not significantly add to the staging of patients with PSAs less than 20 and no palpable evidence of extraprostatic extension. In patients with significant obstructive symptoms or physical or ultrasonographic evidence of prostate carcinoma at the base of the gland, cystoscopy and evaluation of the upper urinary tracts with ultrasound or intravenous urography may be needed to exclude invasion of the bladder neck and trigone and accompanying ureteral obstruction.

Treatment

Carcinoma of the prostate confined to the gland is a surgically curable disease. Radical prostatectomy is therefore appropriate treatment for men who are at risk of disease progression and cancer death. The difficulty is in knowing whether or not the cancer is con-fined to the gland, the risk of progression, and the life expectancy of the patient. It has long been recognized, as subsequently confirmed by the Scandinavian studies, that men older than 70 years of age with well-differentiated prostate cancer are likely to die of disease other than prostate cancer, and therefore aggressive therapy is generally not required. Radical prostatectomy is therefore generally reserved for men younger than 70 years of age with organ-confined disease. Men with disease beyond the capsule of the prostate and those with a life expectancy of 10 years or less are generally offered radiation therapy.

Radiation therapy can be accomplished with brachytherapy, most frequently using radioactive iodine 125, or external beam. With brachytherapy, seed implants are typically inserted from the perineal approach using transrectal ultrasound guidance. This is done under anesthesia with hospital stays of 1 day or less. Brachytherapy is sometimes combined with external-beam radiation. Irritative or obstructive voiding symptoms are common for several months after the procedure but typically respond to symptomatic medication. Incontinence is uncommon in patients who have not had or do not receive a transurethral resection of the prostate, and potency is retained in most patients. PSA reduction to less than 0.5 ng/mL is expected in more than 75% of men with T1 to T2b tumors, and 5- and 10-year results are comparable to those of external-beam radiation or surgery.

Patients with advanced or metastatic prostate cancer are treated primarily with hormone therapy, that is, androgen ablation. Early cooperative studies by the Department of Veterans Affairs suggested that orchiectomy or testosterone suppression with estrogen administration provided comparable palliation of symptoms but did not prolong life when early versus late administration were compared. Today combined hormonal blockade, using luteinizing hormone–releasing hormone (LHRH) agonists plus antiandrogens are popular, based on studies suggesting prolonged time to progression (3 months) and survival (7 months) when compared with LHRH agents alone. In these studies maximal prolongation of survival was seen in patients with minimal metastatic disease. This observation plus the use of PSA monitoring has prompted the use of early hormonal therapy in many patients.

Most patients have both an improvement in symptoms and a marked reduction in PSA in response to hormone ablation. Cytotoxic chemotherapy has been relatively ineffective in prostate cancer and is generally reserved for those who fail to respond to hormonal therapy. Combinations currently showing some promise include estramustine phosphate and VP16 or vinblastine, and doxorubicin and cisplatin. The investigational agent suramin, used in the treatment of African sleeping sickness, has also shown some promise with measurable response in up to 50% of patients.

Bladder Cancer

Bladder cancer, one of the first cancers associated with industrialization, is not unexpectedly increasing in incidence in the modern world. In the United States it was estimated that 54,400 new cases were diagnosed and 12,500 people died of the disease in 1998. Despite efforts to decrease cigarette smoking, the most common cause of bladder cancer, the incidence of bladder cancer continues to increase, but we have succeeded in improving the treatment of the disease. The survival of bladder cancer in the past decade has increased by 8% despite a 36% increase in incidence. Improved survival may relate to earlier detection, with fewer patients presenting with invasive disease, improved treatment of superficial and in situ carcinoma with the advent of bacille Calmette-Guérin (BCG) immunotherapy, and improved chemotherapy for advanced disease. Fewer patients are requiring radical cystectomy as the primary treatment, and those who do often can receive bladder replacement and enjoy a better quality of life.

Epidemiology and Etiology

In the United States transitional cell carcinoma accounts for more than 90% of the cases of bladder cancer. In decreasing order of frequency, squamous cell carcinoma, often associated with chronic inflammation, adenocarcinoma, occasionally associated with urachal

remnants, undifferentiated carcinoma, rhabdomyosarcoma, and rare histologic types such as sarcomatoid carcinoma, small cell carcinoma, and lymphoepithelioma occur. Squamous cell carcinoma and adenocarcinoma of the bladder generally present at higher stage than transitional cell carcinoma, are less responsive to chemotherapy, and therefore have a less favorable prognosis.

Transitional cell carcinoma was first associated with aniline dye exposure in Germany in 1895. Since then multiple chemicals and environmental exposures, as listed in Table 25–1, have been implicated. The listed chemicals are highly carcinogenic, but fortunately exposure to these chemicals is limited. **Cigarette smoking carries a relative risk of developing bladder cancer of only 3 to 1 in most studies, but it is estimated that as much as 60% of bladder cancers may result from smoking. The increasing incidence of bladder cancer despite the reduction in smoking in the United States suggests that other environmental factors are playing an increasing role in the development of bladder cancer.** Several reports of increased risk of bladder cancer associated with increased water intake in both industrial and agricultural areas are of concern and suggest that both industrial carcinogens and pesticides have contaminated some water supplies.

Multiple genetic changes are associated with bladder cancer. Studies of X chromosome inactivation suggest that bladder tumors typically descend from a single cell. Genetic changes may confer a growth advantage

Table 25–1
Chemicals and Occupations Associated with Bladder Cancer

Chemicals	Occupations
Alpha and beta naphthylamine	Textile workers
4-Aminobiphenyl	Dye workers
Benzidine	Tire and rubber workers
Chlornaphazine	Leather workers
4-Chloro-o-toluidine	Bootblacks
o-Toluidine	Painters
4,4'-Methylene bis (2-chloroaniline)	Truck drivers
	Drillpress operators
Methylene dianiline	Chemical workers
Benzidine-derived azo dyes	Petroleum workers
Phenacetin-containing compounds	Hairdressers

on the cell, and with continued division and accumulation of genetic damage, overt tumors occur. Genetic studies may explain the well-known clinical dichotomy between low-grade papillary tumors that frequently recur but rarely progress and high-grade in situ or flat tumors that commonly invade and spread aggressively. About 60% of bladder tumors have P16 mutation, and this is associated with low-grade papillary tumors. Mutation of the retinoblastoma (Rb) gene or the well-known tumor suppressor gene *p53* is correlated with increased risk of disease progression.

Grade and Stage

The World Health Organization system for grading transitional cell carcinoma divides tumors into three grades based on the degree of anaplasia. *Grade I tumors* are characterized by minimal variation in nuclear shape and an increase in the number of cells in the epithelium beyond the normal seven layers. In *Grade III tumors* there is marked anaplasia with variation in cell and nuclear size and shape. *Grade II tumors* are between these two extremes and are a heterogeneous group. Grade correlates well with prognosis. In a review of 1009 patients in six reported series, the incidence of progression to muscle invasion or metastasis in patients with Grade I tumors was only 7%, compared with 28% for Grade II and 38% for Grade III.

Bladder cancer is staged by an American system and an increasingly popular international system, as illustrated in Figure 25–1. Prognosis correlates with depth of invasion, with the exception of carcinoma in situ, which is by nature an aggressive, poorly differentiated malignancy. In patients without invasion of the lamina propria (TA), only 9% have disease progression, compared with 29% of patients with lamina propria invasion (T1).

Clinical Features

The most frequent presenting feature of bladder cancer is gross or microscopic hematuria, which occurs in 80% of patients. Delay in referring patients with hematuria for cystoscopic examination remains a too common cause of failure in the management of bladder cancer. Hematuria in bladder cancer is typically intermittent, making it easy to be deceived into believing that an intervention for benign disease, most commonly antibiotics for presumed urinary tract infection, has been effective. Twenty percent or more of patients complain of irritative voiding symptoms such as frequency, urgency, or dysuria, which can further obscure the true diagnosis. **Irritative symptoms are more frequently associated with aggressive bladder tumors, such as Grade III carcinoma or carcinoma in situ. Fortunately, urinary cytology is positive in more than 80% of patients with high-grade transitional cell carcinoma. Urinary cytology is helpful when positive, but two thirds or more of patients with bladder cancer may have a negative urinary cytology.** Newer markers for bladder cancer, including urinary bladder tumor antigen, nuclear matrix protein, and fibrin degradation products, are available, but the mainstay of diagnosis in bladder cancer continues to be cystoscopic examination.

Diagnosis

Cystoscopic examination may reveal papillary tumors that can be missed on imaging studies, or raised, roughened, or reddened areas that suggest carcinoma in situ and are readily biopsied with cupped forceps. Bladder wash cytology done at the time of cystoscopy further increases the detection of transitional cell carcinoma. Visible tumors are resected transurethrally, accomplishing the most important therapeutic and diagnostic steps simultaneously. Transurethral resection done under anesthesia permits deep resection for muscle biopsy as well as thorough bimanual examination, important clinical staging procedures. Random bladder biopsies and biopsy of the prostatic urethra in men provide important prognostic information. Atypia or carcinoma in situ in such biopsies markedly increases the risk of tumor recurrence and stage progression. The prostatic urethra harbors transitional cell carcinoma in up to 40% of patients undergoing cystectomy for bladder cancer. Invasive transitional cell carcinoma within the prostatic urethra is associated with poor prognosis, and noninvasive carcinoma significantly influences treatment planning, since intravesical chemotherapy is

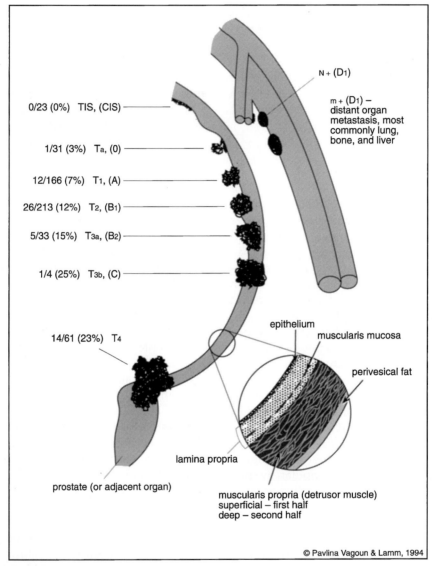

Figure 25-1

TNM and Jewett-Marshall (in parentheses) staging systems for bladder cancer. Stage Ta (0) tumors are limited to the epithelial layer. Invasion begins with stage T1 (A) tumors that extend to the lamina propria and progresses to T2 (B1), less than halfway through the detrusor muscle; T3a (B2), more than halfway through the detrusor muscle; T3b (C), into perivesical fat; and T4, into adjacent organs. Metastasis typically begins with pelvic lymph nodes (N+ or [D1]) prior to spreading systemically (M+ or [D2]). The percentages listed to the left represent typical incidences of nodal metastases according to primary tumor stage. It has recently been proposed that muscle invasive tumors be termed *T2a* and *T2b* rather than *T2* and *T3a*. (From CA Cancer J Clin 46:93–112, 1996. © Pavlina Vagoun & Lamm, 1994.)

generally ineffective in the prostatic urethra and orthotopic bladder replacement carries the risk of urethral recurrence.

Generally, only 2% to 3% of patients with bladder cancer develop upper tract transitional cell carcinoma, but in high-risk patients followed for up to 15 years this incidence may be as high as 25%. Intravenous urography is therefore considered to be an important baseline study, particularly in patients with hematuria, and is repeated at intervals during follow-up. For tumors not invading the detrusor muscle, additional imaging studies such as cystography, CT scanning, MR imaging, ultrasonography, and bone or liver scans are generally neither necessary nor cost effective.

TREATMENT OF SUPERFICIAL BLADDER CANCER

The primary treatment for papillary bladder tumors that do not invade the detrusor muscle, that is Stage Ta, and T1 transitional cell carcinoma, is transurethral resection. Small, low-grade noninvasive tumors can be fulgurated or lasered. These procedures can be done without anesthesia and have minimal morbidity, but pathologic examination may be compromised. Despite complete tumor resection, two thirds of patients develop tumor recurrence within 5 years and by 15 years 88% of patients develop tumor recurrence. The high rate of bladder tumor recurrence provides opportunity to institute chemoprevention or prophylactic therapy.

Intravesical Therapy

INTRAVESICAL CHEMOTHERAPY

Intravesical chemotherapy became popular in the early 1960s, when thiotepa was demonstrated by many investigators to reduce tumor recurrence and eradicate approximately one third of papillary tumors. Since most papillary tumors can be readily resected transurethrally, prophylaxis against tumor recurrence has been the most common use of intravesical chemotherapy. Controlled trials demonstrate that intravesical chemotherapy reduces short-term tumor recurrence by about 20% and long-term recurrence by 7%, but un-

fortunately it does not reduce progression. Currently used drugs include the alkylating agents thiotepa, and mitomycin C and the intercalating agent doxorubicin. Chemotherapy is generally preferred for patients with low-grade, Stage Ta tumors who have a low risk of progression. Single or short-course treatments given weekly for up to 6 weeks, beginning immediately after surgery, provide the best results.

INTRAVESICAL IMMUNOTHERAPY

Despite the checkered past of BCG immunotherapy in other cancers, intravesical BCG immunotherapy is now recognized to be the treatment of choice for carcinoma in situ of the bladder and aggressive superficial transitional cell carcinoma. Although the mechanism of action of BCG is incompletely defined, this tuberculosis vaccine is a potent, nonspecific immune stimulant. Intravesical BCG induces infiltration of a broad range of inflammatory and immune cells in the lamina propria of the bladder and activates macrophages, T and B lymphocytes, natural killer cells, and a variety of other immune surveillance mechanisms, including lymphokine and interferon production.

BCG prophylaxis reduces tumor recurrence by about 40% when compared with surgical resection alone, and several studies suggest that, unlike chemotherapy, protection from tumor recurrence and progression lasts for many years. BCG immunotherapy is particularly effective in transitional cell carcinoma in situ. Prior to the advent of BCG, 54% of patients with carcinoma in situ progressed to muscle invasion within 5 years. Complete response to intravesical chemotherapy in carcinoma in situ ranges from 38% to 53% for thiotepa and mitomycin, respectively. Despite these significant response rates, intravesical chemotherapy has not been demonstrated to alter the long-term aggressive natural history of carcinoma in situ, and in general fewer than 20% of patients remain disease free for 5 years. The overall complete response rate of carcinoma in situ to BCG is more than 70%. Controlled multicenter, randomized comparison of BCG and doxorubicin revealed complete response in 34% of patients in the doxorubicin arm and 70% in the BCG arm. By 5 years only 18% in the doxorubicin arm remained disease free, compared with 45% in the BCG arm ($P < 0.001$). With an improved BCG treatment schedule (three additional weekly instillations at 3 months) the complete response can be increased to more than 80%, and continued maintenance treatments at 6-month intervals results in an increase in 5-year disease-free status from the expected 65% to 83%.

ALTERNATIVE THERAPIES FOR SUPERFICIAL BLADDER CANCER

Intravesical alpha-interferon results in a complete response rate of about 25% in patients with Stage Ta, T1 transitional cell carcinoma and 47% in patients with carcinoma in situ. Oral agents also appear to have promise. Chemoprevention using antioxidant, immune-stimulating, and differentiating agents appear to be remarkably effective. In a randomized double-blind study high doses of vitamins A, B_6, C, and E (Oncovite, Mission Pharmacal) reduced tumor recurrence by 40%.

Photodynamic therapy using intravesical laser light and intravenous administration of the photosensitizer porfimer sodium (Photofrin) has a high response rate in carcinoma in situ and is being investigated as an alternative treatment modality. Photodynamic therapy may be particularly useful in patients who have failed first-line intravesical therapies, especially those who are poor surgical risks for cystectomy.

MUSCLE-INVASIVE BLADDER CANCER

The prognosis and treatment of bladder cancer change radically once invasion of the detrusor muscle occurs since less than half of patients survive 5 years despite aggressive treatment. Unfortunately, more than 80% of patients with muscle-invasive bladder cancer are diagnosed with this locally advanced stage at initial presentation. Further improvement in survival requires earlier detection or improved treatment of advanced disease. There is some evidence that both may be possible. In a study of 1575 men older than 50 years of age serial home reagent strip tests

for hematuria resulted in 1.3% of patients being diagnosed with bladder cancer. Stage at presentation in the screened population and tumor-specific survival were significantly increased.

Advances in the treatment of invasive and metastatic bladder cancer include improvement in the quality as well as the duration of life, through advances in surgical technique with the advent of continent urinary diversion and orthotopic bladder substitution, bladder sparing with combined radiation therapy and chemotherapy, and cisplatin-based combination chemotherapy. Popular surgical alterations of internal plumbing are illustrated in Figure 25–2.

In the United States cystoprostatectomy is the treatment of choice for most patients with Stage T2 to T4 bladder cancer. Improvement in intravesical therapy, particularly BCG immunotherapy, and the advent of effective systemic chemotherapy have also increased interest and success of bladder-sparing techniques, including repeat transurethral resection in patients with Stage T2 disease, partial cystectomy in patients with localized small volume disease, and radiation therapy.

Bladder preservation using chemotherapy and radiation therapy has been evaluated and appears to result in a higher complete response rate than radiation therapy alone. 5-Fluorouracil and cisplatin are considered to enhance the effect of radiation therapy. Patients who are not candidates for radical cystectomy or decline surgery may have an option that appears to be superior to radiation therapy alone.

CHEMOTHERAPY FOR METASTATIC TRANSITIONAL CELL CANCER OF THE UROTHELIUM

Transitional cell carcinoma has been relatively resistant to systemic chemotherapy. About one third of patients with bladder cancer develop metastases during the course of their disease. Patients with metastases have historically survived for less than 1 year, but combination-chemotherapy regimens based on experience with single-agent trials have markedly improved the treatment of advanced bladder cancer. Among single agents evaluated in transitional cell carcinoma of the

Indiana Pouch   ## Neoileal Bladder

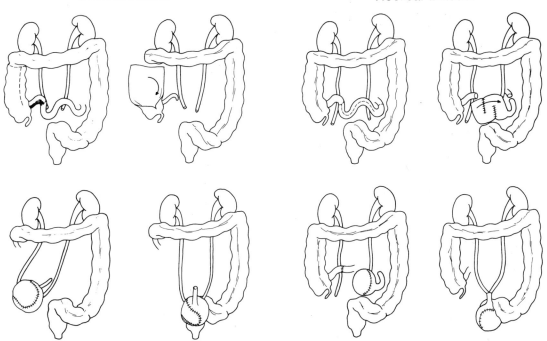

Figure 25-2

Illustrations of the two most common bladder substitutes. The "Indiana pouch" on the left uses the ascending colon as a reservoir, the ileocecal valve as a continence mechanism, and the terminal ileum as a catheterizable conduit that is generally brought to the umbilicus. The neoileal bladder on the right is constructed from ileum folded into a spherical reservoir. The reservoir is then sewn to the urethra, and the patient voids by increasing abdominal pressure. (From Lamm DL, Torti FM: Bladder cancer, 1996. CA Cancer J Clin 46:93–112, 1996.)

bladder, the most effective are cisplatin and methotrexate. With the advent of cisplatin- and methotrexate-based combination chemotherapy in the late 1980s, metastatic bladder cancer has become a moderately chemosensitive malignancy. A number of chemotherapeutic agents have been investigated in detail, including CMV, which consists of cisplatin, methotrexate, and vinblastine, and MVAC, which adds doxorubicin. Using these combinations plus aggressive surgical resection of residual disease about 20% of patients have remained continuously disease free for extended periods, and a number appear to be cured. New combinations including taxol and/or gemcitabine are encouraging.

Kidney Cancer

Tumors originating from urothelial cells lining the renal pelvis and calyces comprise less than 10% of renal malignancies. These transitional cell or squamous cell tumors have many similarities with tumors of the same cell type originating in the bladder and may be considered an extension or variety of those tumors. In fact, when nephrectomy is performed in the treatment of these malignancies, the entire ureter with a cuff of bladder is removed because of the high risk (>50%) that tumors will recur if these structures are retained. Even with complete resection, these patients are followed for recurrence of tumor within the bladder, which occurs in up to 50% of patients.

By far the most important renal tumor is adenocarcinoma of the kidney. This tumor has been termed the "internist's tumor" or the "great masquerader" because of its propensity to cause a wide variety of symptoms, signs, and laboratory abnormalities. These abnormalities are often confused with other diseases, and therefore familiarity with the vagaries of renal cell carcinoma is important for primary care physicians.

Benign renal tumors were once of little clinical significance, but with the increased use of CT scans, these tumors are being diagnosed with increasing frequency. Differentiation of benign tumors such as oncocytoma, angiomyolipoma, and adenomas from renal cell carcinoma is now a much more frequent dilemma.

RENAL PELVIC AND URETERAL CANCERS

Incidence

Less than 4% of urothelial cancers and less than 10% of tumors of the kidney involve the renal pelvis. These tumors are closely related to urothelial tumors of the bladder and have similar etiology, pathology, staging systems, and even treatment. The risk of developing a bladder tumor in these patients is 30% to 50%, but fewer than 5% of patients with bladder tumors develop upper tract tumors. In either case, evaluation is required to confirm that the associated tumors are not present and do not develop in the future.

Diagnosis

The initial symptom in upper tract tumors is gross hematuria in 80% of patients. The passage of wormlike clots, casts of the ureter, is pathognomonic of upper tract bleeding. Obstruction with the passage of clots or tissue may result in renal colic. As many as 10% of patients may have irritative voiding symptoms suggestive of cystitis, so it is important to consider the possibility of transitional cell carcinoma of the upper tract in patients with irritative symptoms who do not have a typical presentation or response to treatment. Urinary cytology, which is highly sensitive and specific for high-grade bladder tumors, is much less sensitive in upper tract tumors. Diagnosis requires intravenous urography, which typically shows a lucent filling defect within the collecting system, followed by cystoscopic examination with ureteral cytology, brush biopsy, and, more frequently today, direct inspection and biopsy using flexible or rigid ureteroscopes.

Treatment

The traditional approach to management of upper tract urothelial tumors, nephroureter-

ectomy with resection of a cuff of bladder, remains the best treatment for most patients. Patients with solitary kidneys, and occasionally other patients such as those with low-grade tumors or high surgical risk, can be treated with transureteral or percutaneous tumor resection followed by topical BCG immunotherapy or chemotherapy.

BENIGN TUMORS OF THE RENAL PARENCHYMA

Benign adenomas of the cortex are found in about 20% of autopsies done in adults, but only recently have they become clinically significant as a result of the increased frequency of detection on CT scan or MR imaging. Unfortunately, we do not presently have a reliable means of distinguishing benign adenomas from renal carcinoma. Therefore, surgical excision is generally required. Partial nephrectomy for small (≤ 3 cm) peripheral tumors is preferred.

Renal oncocytomas are benign adenomas that are composed of large eosinophilic cells packed with mitochondria. A few of these tumors are associated with renal cell carcinoma, and differentiation from malignant renal tumors is difficult and generally unreliable. Therefore, despite the fact that the diagnosis can often be suspected on the basis of the angiographic appearance of typical "spoke-wheel" vessels or other factors, radical nephrectomy is generally done.

The benign renal tumor that can be diagnosed radiographically is angiomyolipoma. These tumors are composed of smooth muscle, blood vessels, and fat. The fat can be readily seen on CT scan and has negative (-20 to -80) Hounsfield units. Angiomyolipoma occurs in up to 80% of patients with tuberous sclerosis, but most occur sporadically. Bilateral lesions are seen commonly in the cases associated with tuberous sclerosis, where preservation of renal parenchyma is of paramount concern. Spontaneous rupture with hemorrhage into the retroperitoneum is common and may require surgery, but in general conservative management, which includes yearly follow-up with ultrasound or CT, is appropriate. Surgery is reserved for those with recurrent bleeding, pain, or actively growing tumors.

Other rare benign renal tumors include lipomas, leiomyomas, hemangiomas, and the exceedingly rare juxtaglomerular cell tumors that secrete renin and cause hypertension. With the exception of juxtaglomerular cell tumors, these benign tumors generally cause no symptoms and are clinically important only in that they must be differentiated from renal cell carcinoma.

RENAL CELL CARCINOMA

An estimated 29,900 patients developed cancer of the kidney in the United States in 1998, and more than 40% of that number died of the disease, making renal cell carcinoma the most lethal of the genitourinary tumors. Surgical excision of all disease remains the only reliable curative treatment, but the increased use of abdominal ultrasound, CT scan, and MR imaging has increased early detection of this tumor, and new immunotherapy and chemotherapy show promise for improving the management of patients with advanced disease.

Incidence and Epidemiology

About 85% of primary malignant renal tumors are renal cell carcinoma. The disease occurs most commonly in the fifth to sixth decade of life but can occur in childhood. The parenchymal renal tumor of childhood is Wilms' tumor. It is twice as common in men than women. The incidence in African Americans and whites is similar, but Hispanics have a one third increased incidence of renal cell carcinoma.

Etiology

Smoking appears to more than double the risk of renal cell carcinoma. In women, but not men, obesity has been reported to be a risk factor, which may relate to increased plasma estrogen. Estrogen has been implicated because it can induce renal tumors in hamsters. Occupational risks include exposure to cadmium, petroleum products, and asbestos. Patients who are on long-term renal dialysis commonly develop acquired renal cystic disease, which markedly increases the risk of renal cell carcinoma. Familial cluster-

ing of renal cell carcinoma occurs. Von Hippel-Lindau disease, an autosomal dominant phakomatosis characterized by hemangioblastomas of the retina, cerebellum, and spinal cord and cysts and angiomas of the visceral organs, is associated with renal cell carcinoma in up to 45% of cases. These cases as well as sporadic cases are found to have deletions and translocations in the short arm of chromosome 3. Multiple other genetic abnormalities are seen as well, including overexpression of proto-oncogenes and underexpression of tumor suppressor genes.

Pathology and Staging

Renal cell carcinoma originates in the proximal renal tubule of the cortex and typically distorts the shape of the kidney and the outline of the calyces. Four histologic variants occur: clear cell, composed of cholesterol, lipids, and glycogen that are extracted during histologic preparation; granular cell; tubulopapillary; and sarcomatoid. Most tumors are composed of a mixture of cell types. Anaplasia and the presence of sarcomatoid variant are associated with a poor prognosis.

Most of these tumors are hypervascular, and early vascular spread as well as direct extension is common. Tumors confined to the parenchyma are termed Stage I (T1 ≤ 2.5 cm, or T2, N0, M0), and have a 5-year survival of 60% to 80%. Tumors that spread beyond the renal capsule but remain confined to the perinephric fascia of Gerota, Stage II (T3A, N0, M0), have a similar prognosis with 5-year survival rates of 50% to 80%. Stage III disease involves the main renal vein or vena cava (Stage IIIA or T3b, N0, M0 in the TNM system), regional lymph nodes (IIIB or N+), or both (IIIC). Lymphatic spread is a poor prognostic sign, reducing 5-year survival to 30% or less, but venous extension, if surgically resectable, appears to have little prognostic significance. Surgical resection is generally indicated even when the tumor extends up the vena cava to the atrium. Such patients often have disease elsewhere, but long-term survival can occur. Extension beyond Gerota's fascia (T4) is more ominous than renal vein extension, reducing 5-year survival to 45%. Distant metastasis occurs most commonly to the lung, liver, and bone. Median survival of patients with metastatic disease (Stage IV, or M+) is only 10 months, but some patients survive many years with metastasis. Poor prognostic features are liver metastasis, multiple sites of metastasis, occurrence of metastasis within 1 year of nephrectomy, weight loss of more than 10%, decreased performance status, no nephrectomy, and erythrocyte sedimentation rate above 100.

Presenting Features

Renal cell carcinoma is recognized as one of the great masqueraders in medicine. Metastasis can occur to virtually any location, and paraneoplastic syndromes can mimic a wide variety of diseases. The "classic triad" of hematuria, flank pain, and abdominal mass occurs late in the course of the disease and fortunately is now seen in less than 10% of patients. **Gross or microscopic hematuria occurs in about 60% of patients, pain in about 40%, and palpable mass in 25%. Other common presenting signs and symptoms include weight loss (36%), hypertension (22%), fever (18%), and hypercalcemia (6%). Vague abdominal symptoms such as abdominal discomfort and change in bowel habits occur in about half of patients, so patients who have persistent abdominal symptoms and a negative gastrointestinal evaluation should have renal cell carcinoma included in the differential diagnosis.** Unfortunately, about 30% of patients have metastatic disease at presentation, with symptoms of metastatic disease such as dyspnea, cough, or bone pain.

Paraneoplastic syndromes occur in 10% or more of patients and are characteristic of renal cell carcinoma. The syndromes are more varied than those of other tumors, and in addition to fever, hypertension, and hypercalcemia, include erythrocytosis (erythropoietin), hepatopathy (10% to 30%), Cushing's syndrome (adrenocorticotrophic hormone), galactorrhea (prolactin), hypoglycemia (insulin), gynecomastia (gonadotropin), decreased libido (gonadotropin), amenorrhea, and protein enteropathy (enteroglucagon).

Laboratory and Imaging Studies

The most common laboratory abnormality in patients with renal cell carcinoma is elevation of the erythrocyte sedimentation rate, which occurs in more than half of patients. **Anemia occurs in more than one third of patients, and abnormal liver function tests are seen in about one sixth.**

The least invasive and most cost-effective imaging study is ultrasonography, and this is the recommended initial screening study in patients who are at relatively low risk of having the disease. Renal cysts can be diagnosed with an accuracy of about 98%, and ultrasonography is sensitive in the diagnosis of renal cell carcinoma.

Intravenous urography is preferred in patients who present with hematuria, because it provides visualization of the renal calyces, pelvis, and ureter that is superior to that of ultrasound, MR imaging, or CT scan. The accuracy of intravenous urography in renal cell carcinoma is only in the range of 75%, so additional studies are generally required.

The anatomic delineation provided by CT scan or MRI imaging is superior to that of other imaging studies, and in addition to confirming the diagnosis of a solid renal mass, can provide clinical staging information. These studies can be used interchangeably in those who have no contraindication for intravenous contrast medium. In patients in whom renal cell carcinoma is highly suspected, either of these studies may be the study of choice and may obviate the need for other studies.

When the diagnosis is inconclusive, angiography may be used. The presence of neovascularity helps to establish the diagnosis, but the diagnosis may remain provisional until surgery. Generally, needle biopsy is avoided because a negative biopsy finding may be falsely negative, and there is concern about seeding the needle tract or spreading the tumor. Vena cavography may be necessary to determine the presence and extent of caval thrombus.

Treatment

The treatment of choice for localized disease is radical nephrectomy, which consists of removal of a wide margin of normal tissue, including Gerota's fascia, local lymph nodes, and renal vessels at their origin. The ipsilateral adrenal gland is generally taken unless the tumor is small or located in the lower renal pole.

With the increased use of abdominal CT scans and ultrasonography, many early-stage tumors are being found. For tumors that are small ($\leq$ 3 cm) and located peripherally, bilateral tumors (about 3% of cases), and tumors in solitary kidneys, partial nephrectomy is an option. The survival of properly selected patients treated with partial nephrectomy is at least as good as that reported for radical nephrectomy. Partial nephrectomy is not a good option for marginal surgical candidates, however, because the surgery is technically more difficult and has more potential complications than radical nephrectomy.

Radiation therapy has not been found to be effective as a primary or adjuvant treatment but can offer important palliation in patients with metastasis to bone, brain, and even lung. Patients who are not candidates for surgery but have continued bleeding or pain from the primary tumor can be treated with renal artery embolization using mechanical devices such as Gelfoam or steel coils or infarction with ethanol. Infarction may also be used in patients with large and vascular tumors to facilitate surgical resection. Infarction is associated with flank pain, fever, and leukocytosis that typically lasts for 3 days.

Metastatic renal cell carcinoma remains a therapeutic dilemma because survival is dependent on systemic therapy of limited efficacy. Surgery continues to play a role in the management of some of these patients, and nephrectomy is appropriate palliative therapy for local symptoms. In the presence of solitary metastasis, nephrectomy and excision of metastasis provides 5-year survival approaching 30% in selected patients. The role of nephrectomy in patients with unresectable metastases is controversial. Spontaneous regression of metastasis has occurred following nephrectomy, but the incidence of spontaneous regression, 0.4% to 0.8%, is less than the operative mortality from nephrectomy, which can be as high as 2%. Nephrectomy in the hope of inducing spontaneous regression may therefore be an unwise bet. Many urologists, including the author, believe that nephrectomy to reduce tumor burden in selected patients improves the results of immunotherapy. Confirmation of the benefit of adjunctive ne-

phrectomy in controlled studies has, however, been elusive.

Chemotherapy has been relatively ineffective in the treatment of metastatic renal cell carcinoma. Although response rates of new drugs or combinations in single-institution trials are often encouraging, larger studies consistently report response rates of less than 10%. Among the most active single agents are bleomycin (16% response in 33 patients), floxuridine (16% response in 238 patients, circadian; 11% response in 46 patients, constant infusion), and vinblastine (8% response in 99 patients). Combination chemotherapy regimens do not appear to significantly increase the response rate, but improved responses may be seen with the combination of chemotherapy plus immunotherapy. We have been impressed with the published response rates with the combination of infusion of circadian 5-fluorouracil plus interferon, which range from 21% to 36%. Using 200 mg/m^2 continuous infusion of 5-fluorouracil daily for 6 months plus 1 million units of alfa$_{2b}$-interferon subcutaneously in 21 consecutive patients we observed a 43% response rate, good palliation of symptoms, and minimal toxicity.

Immunotherapy or biologic response modifier therapy has been somewhat encouraging. Interferon, particularly interferon-alfa, has clear activity with response rates in the 15% to 20% range. Interleukin-2 (IL-2) is specifically approved for the treatment of metastatic renal cell carcinoma. IL-2 with or without concurrent administration of lymphocyte-activated killer (LAK) cells produces responses in the range of 10% to 20%. Early treatment protocols used high IL-2 doses, and most patients required support in the intensive care unit. Lower-dose outpatient regimens, often combined with interferon, are much better tolerated and appear to produce comparable responses.

Alternative treatments for disseminated renal cell carcinoma include autolymphocyte therapy, which uses in vitro activated lymphocytes, cimetidine plus coumarin (12% response in 198 patients), and progesterone.

Testicular Tumors

Germ cell tumors of the testis are rare but are increasing in incidence. About three cases occur yearly per 100,000 men, primarily white men. Germ cell tumors constitute more than 90% of testicular tumors. **The most important etiologic factor in testis tumor is cryptorchidism. Nearly 10% of the cases occur in men who have a history of undescended testis. The risk of tumor formation varies with the location of the undescended testis: about 5% of abdominal testes develop germ cell tumors versus less than 2% of testes within the inguinal canal. Early orchidopexy may lessen, but does not eliminate, the increased risk of tumors. Even the contralateral normally positioned testis has an increased risk of testis tumor.**

Pathology and Classification

Germ cell tumors of the testis are derived from the totipotential germ cells and are divided into two categories: seminomatous and nonseminomatous tumors. Seminomas come in three varieties: classic (85%), anaplastic (5% to 10%), and spermatocytic (5% to 10%). Nonseminomatous germ cell tumors include embryonal carcinoma, teratoma, choriocarcinoma, and mixed tumors. The remarkable sensitivity of seminomas to radiation therapy relative to nonseminomatous tumors, which has traditionally dictated management, provides a rationale for this classification system.

Seminoma is the most common testis tumor, comprising about 35% of cases. Classic seminoma is composed of uniform sheets of large cells. The anaplastic variety has increased nuclear pleomorphism and mitoses. Anaplastic seminoma more commonly presents at a higher stage, but stage for stage has a prognosis equal to that of classic seminoma. Spermatocytic seminoma presents more commonly in older men, half of whom are older than 50 years of age. These tumors are composed of cells that have a characteristic appearance, with round nuclei and densely staining cytoplasm.

Embryonal cell carcinoma is the next most common pure germ cell tumor, comprising about 20% of cases. Hemorrhage and necrosis are common. The yolk sac variant of embryonal cell carcinoma occurs in infants and children and is in fact the most common testicular tumor in this age group. Microscopically, embryoid bodies having the appearance of 1- to 2-week-old embryos may be seen.

Teratoma is seen in both adults, where it is a malignant tumor, and children, where it is benign. Five percent of testicular tumors are pure teratoma and show elements derived from multiple germ cell layers such as squamous epithelium or neural tissue (ectoderm), glandular tissue (endoderm), or cartilage, muscle, or bone (mesoderm).

The most aggressive of testicular tumors, choriocarcinoma, is fortunately rare: less than 1% of testicular tumors are pure choriocarcinoma. These tumors metastasize quickly, and primary tumors are typically small and often hemorrhagic. Microscopically, syncytiotrophoblasts and cytotrophoblasts are seen.

About 40% of germ cell tumors are of mixed cell types. These tumors are managed according to the most aggressive component present, but there is a tendency for tumors that contain seminoma to be less aggressive.

Clinical Features

The most common presenting symptom is a painless enlargement of the testis. A sensation of heaviness or a dull aching may occur, and about 10% present with acute scrotal pain resulting from hemorrhage. Not infrequently the patient attributes these symptoms to trauma, which unfortunately can delay the diagnosis and increase the opportunity for metastasis. About 10% of patients present with symptoms of metastasis, including back pain, pedal edema, or gastrointestinal symptoms from retroperitoneal disease, or symptoms from pulmonary or skeletal metastasis.

On examination enlargement, irregularity, or firmness within the testis is typical. Distinction of true testicular masses from those of the epididymis and cord is key, because masses outside the testis itself are rarely malignant. Infiltration of the epididymis may occur and lead to an incorrect diagnosis of epididymitis. About 10% of testis tumors are associated with hydroceles, and these may limit examination of the testis. In these cases, as in any examination that is uncertain, scrotal ultrasound can be most helpful.

The retroperitoneal origin of the testes results in a unique pattern of metastatic spread. The primary lymphatic drainage of the testes is to the retroperitoneum: the interaortocaval nodes below the testicular vein on the right and the para-aortic nodes at the level of the renal hilum on the left. Crossover metastasis can occur on the right side but does not occur on the left unless multiple metastases are present. **The primary lymphatic drainage of the scrotum is to the inguinal nodes, so the orchiectomy or biopsy of the testis for possible tumor is done using an incision over the inguinal canal to avoid contamination of the scrotum and lymphatic spread to the groin.**

The frequent retroperitoneal lymphatic metastasis of germ cell tumors is reflected in the staging system. Tumors confined to the testis are termed *Stage A,* those with retroperitoneal lymph node spread are *Stage B,* and those with spread beyond the regional nodes are *Stage C.* Stage B is often subcategorized into B1 (nodes < 5 cm in diameter), B2 (5 to 10 cm in diameter), and B3 (> 10 cm in diameter).

Diagnosis

The tumor markers alpha-fetoprotein (AFP) and beta human chorionic gonadotropin (hCG) are often more sensitive indicators of metastatic disease than are imaging studies. Markers also help distinguish the subtypes of testis tumors. For example, even with biopsy showing pure seminoma, elevation of AFP is indicative of nonseminomatous germ cell tumor and management would be based on the assumption, as confirmed by previous autopsy studies, that "pure" seminoma can metastasize as nonseminomatous tumor. hCG elevation is seen in all patients with choriocarcinoma, more than half of those with embryonal carcinoma, and one fourth of those with teratoma. **AFP elevation does not occur in patients with pure choriocarcinoma or seminoma but is elevated in more than two thirds of those with embryonal cell carcinoma and about 40% of those with teratoma. Half-lives of these markers are 1 day for hCG and 5 days for AFP.** Response to treatment can generally be judged by marker response but, following chemotherapy relapse, can occur in the absence of marker elevation. Lactic acid dehydrogenase has also been useful as a marker of tumor burden and may be elevated in seminomatous or nonseminomatous testis tumor.

The most common sites of metastasis, the retroperitoneum and the lungs, are assessed with abdominal and pelvic CT and chest films, respectively.

Treatment

Following inguinal orchiectomy, treatment plans are based on tumor histology, tumor markers, and imaging studies. Low-stage (Stage A) seminoma can be cured in more than 95% of patients with orchiectomy followed by 2500 to 3000 cGy of retroperitoneal radiation. Even with low-volume Stage B disease, radiation therapy completely eradicates seminoma in about 90% of patients, so retroperitoneal lymphadenectomy is not indicated. Patients with bulky seminoma and any patient with an elevated AFP are treated with nonseminomatous regimens.

Patients with Stage A nonseminomatous tumors are treated with retroperitoneal lymphadenectomy or a protocol of surveillance, if they are reliable and free of signs of increased risk for metastasis such as the presence of choriocarcinomatous elements and vascular or epididymal/tunica albuginea invasion. As many as 25% of patients with clinical Stage A testis tumor with negative markers and CT scan have unsuspected lymph node metastasis. Meticulous follow-up with monthly chest films and tumor markers and CT scans every 3 to 4 months for 2 years detects recurrent disease in time to rescue the patients with surgery and/or combination chemotherapy.

Patients found to have limited lymph node metastasis have an excellent prognosis with surgery alone, but those with more extensive disease (i.e., ≥ 5 nodes or nodes > 2 cm in diameter) have nearly a 50% risk for relapse. These patients are treated with adjuvant cisplatin-based combination chemotherapy.

Patients with high-stage germ cell tumors, that is those with pulmonary metastasis or bulky retroperitoneal nodes, are treated with primary chemotherapy. One of the major advances in chemotherapy for nonseminomatous testis tumor was the combination of cisplatin, vinblastine, and bleomycin (PVB). Successful subsequent regimens include bleomycin, etoposide, and cisplatin (BEP), which has equal or superior efficacy and less neurotoxicity, as well as salvage regimens adding ifosfamide. Retroperitoneal lymphadenectomy may be required to remove residual mass and is advocated by some even without evidence of residual disease because about 10% of patients may have positive nodes.

Cancer of the Penis

Cancer of the penis is rare in the United States, accounting for less than 1% of cancers in men. **The most common etiologic factor is poor hygiene. Penile cancer almost never occurs in men who are circumcised at birth, and it is believed that smegma accumulation in the unretracted foreskin results in chronic inflammation that promotes squamous carcinoma.**

Clinical Features

Carcinoma of the penis occurs most frequently in the sixth decade. Related lesions include three precancerous lesions: (1) leukoplakia, which is a white plaque that often involves the meatus and occurs most commonly in diabetics; (2) giant condyloma acuminata (Buschke-Löwenstein tumor), which is a large, chronic cauliflower-like tumor caused by the human papillomavirus; and (3) balanitis xerotica obliterans or lichen sclerosis et atrophicus, an atrophic, depigmented, sclerotic lesion that often involves the meatus and is also more common in diabetics. Carcinoma in situ of the penis (Bowen's disease or erythroplasia of Queyrat) appears as a red, crusted, or velvety lesion that may ulcerate. These lesions may be associated with invasive disease.

Invasive carcinoma of the penis occurs most commonly on the glans but may occur on the prepuce or shaft. Lesions may be papillary or ulcerative and are typically painless. Biopsy of such lesions is imperative.

Carcinoma in situ can be treated with 5-fluorouracil cream or laser fulguration. Tumors that are limited to the prepuce (Stage I, about 20% of penile cancers) are treated primarily with circumcision. Local recurrence occurs in about 30% of lesions so treated, but long-term survival approaches 90%. Mohs' surgery, which uses a chemical fixative and serial excision, is an effective approach for noninvasive squamous cell carcinoma of the penis. Tumors that invade the subepithelial connective tissue (T1) or corpus spongiosum

or cavernosum (T2) generally require partial penectomy, or total penectomy if adequate (generally 2-cm) margins cannot be achieved. Metastatic spread is lymphatic, and primary drainage from the prepuce and skin of the shaft of the penis is to the superficial inguinal nodes. The lymphatic drainage of the glans and corpora is to the superficial and deep inguinal nodes, and then to the external iliac nodes. The urethral lymphatic drainage is to the hypogastric and common iliac nodes. Considering these lymphatic drainage patterns and the observation that lymphadenectomy can be curative in squamous cell carcinoma, patients with invasive carcinoma of the penis often require inguinal and pelvic lymph node dissection. Radiation therapy is an option for treatment of cancer of the penis, and metastatic disease can be palliated, but as yet not cured, with chemotherapy.

Urethral and Scrotal Malignancies

Tumors of the urethra may present with bleeding, obstructive symptoms, associated stricture, mass, or adenopathy. In both men and women, tumors may be squamous cell, transitional cell, or adenocarcinoma. Distal lesions may be treated by surgical resection with preservation of continence, but more advanced tumors or proximal tumors require anterior exenteration. Radiation therapy, lymph node dissection, and in the case of transitional cell carcinoma, adjuvant chemotherapy can be beneficial.

Tumors of the scrotum are rare. Like penile cancer, squamous cell carcinoma is the most common, and both Kaposi's sarcoma and melanoma occur. Tumors spread to the inguinal nodes and are managed similar to carcinoma of the penis.

SUGGESTED READINGS

Prostate Cancer

1. Begun FP: Epidemiology and natural history of prostate cancer in prostate diseases. *In* Lepor H, Lawson RK (eds): Prostate Diseases. Philadelphia, WB Saunders, 1993.
2. Hanks GE, Diamond JJ, Krall JM, et al: Ten-year follow up of 682 patients treated for prostate cancer with radiation therapy in the United States. Int J Radiat Oncol Biol Phys 13:499, 1987.

3. Rosen MA, Goldstone L, Lapin S, et al: Frequency and location of extracapsular extension and positive margins in radical prostatectomy specimens. J Urol 148:331, 1992.

Bladder Cancer

1. Cohen SM, Johansson SL: Epidemiology and etiology of bladder cancer. Urol Clin North Am 19:421–428, 1992.
2. Lamm DL: Carcinoma in situ. Urol Clin North Am 19:499–508, 1992.
3. Lamm DL, Griffith JG: Intravesical therapy: Does it affect the natural history of superficial bladder cancer? Semin Urol 10:39, 1992.
4. Lamm DL, Torti FM: Bladder cancer, 1996. CA Cancer J Clin 46:93–112, 1996.
5. Ro JY, Staerkel GA, Ayala AG: Cytologic and histologic features of superficial bladder cancer. Urol Clin North Am 19:435–453, 1992.
6. Schwalb D, Herr HW: Upper tract disease following intravesical BCG for superficial bladder cancer. J Urol 147:273A, 1992.

Kidney Cancer

1. Droz JP, Rey A, Mahjoubi M, et al: Prognostic factors in metastatic renal cell carcinoma. *In* Klein EA, Bu-
kowski RM, Finke JH (eds): Renal Cell Carcinoma: Immunotherapy and Cellular Biology. New York, Marcel Dekker, 1993, pp 11–24.
2. Fossa SD, Kjolseth I, Lund G: Radiotherapy of metastasis from renal cancer. Eur Urol 8:340, 1982.
3. Logan TF, Trump DL: The role of cytotoxic chemotherapy in the management of renal cancer. *In* Ernstoff MS, Heaney JA, Peschel RE (eds): Urologic Cancer. Cambridge, MA, Blackwell Scientific, 1997, pp 444–463.
4. Paganini-Hill A, Ross RK, Henderson BE: Epidemiology of renal cancer. *In* Skinner DG, Lieskousky G (eds): Diagnosis and Management of Genitourinary Cancer. Philadelphia, WB Saunders, 1988, pp 32–39.
5. Siminovitch JM, Montie JE, Straffon RA: Prognostic indicator in renal adenocarcinoma. J Urol 130:20, 1983.

Testicular Tumors

1. Boden G, Gill R: Radiotherapy and testicular neoplasms. Lancet 2:1195, 1951.
2. Donahue JP, Zachary JM, Magnard BR: Distribution of nodal metastasis in nonseminomatous testis cancer. J Urol 128:315, 1982.
3. Henderson BE, Ross RK, Pike MC: Epidemiology of testicular cancer. *In* Skinner DG, Lieskousky G (eds): Diagnosis and Management of Genitourinary Cancer. Philadelphia, WB Saunders, 1988, pp 46–52.

26

The Role of Primary Health Care Providers in Cancer Prevention

Robin E. Blum
Graham A. Colditz

How We Approach Prevention

A 45-year-old man concludes his annual physical examination, turns to his primary care provider, and asks, "What can I do to reduce my risk of prostate and bladder cancer?" As we show in this chapter, primary prevention is the best answer.

In 1990 the U.S. Department of Health and Human Services, Public Health Service, released *Healthy People 2000: National Health Promotion and Disease Prevention Objectives*, which delineates a national strategy to improve the health of the U.S. population. In general, these objectives have the nation looking forward to the year 2000 as a target date for taking charge of the state of health and the direction of health care in the United States. After a century of biomedical and scientific research, there is now sufficient scientific knowledge to move the focus of health care toward primary prevention in an attempt to reduce the burden of disease and increase the overall well-being of the population. With an abundant and still-growing knowledge base to support prevention and the political will to provide the resources necessary to implement prevention, social strategies such as those outlined in *Healthy People 2000* may be carried out to reduce the burden of cancer in the United States. In this chapter we show how this approach to cancer prevention provides a framework for translation of the emerging scientific evidence on causes of prostate, bladder, and other cancers into prevention strategies that can be implemented by health care providers.

Cancer accounts for approximately 24% of all deaths in the United States. Approximately 75 million, or about one in three Americans now living, will eventually have cancer. As an overwhelming number of Americans are affected by the burdens of cancer, the priorities for health promotion and disease prevention must include a reversal of the rise in cancer deaths through improved screening practices and targeting of other factors such as dietary and environmental exposures (i.e., low fruit and vegetable consumption and excessive sun exposure) that have been linked to cancer incidence. Thus, primary care providers must be prepared to provide answers to questions about cancer prevention. This chapter reviews how the primary health care provider fits into the overall strategy for the prevention of cancer, including prostate cancer, whose incidence continues to rise, accounting for 27.5% of cancers in men, and bladder cancer, which accounts for 6% of all new cases of cancer among men.

Components of Change: Role of the Primary Care Provider

The primary care provider has a central role to play in the social strategy to reduce the burden of cancer in the United States. Three components must be in place for a social strategy to be successful: (1) regulatory change, (2) individual-primary and community-implemented change, and (3) access to counseling and support from primary health care providers. In this section we use the example of tobacco to highlight the role of these three components of cancer prevention.

Since the release of the original Surgeon General's report on the harmful effects of tobacco consumption in 1964, regulation of the advertising and sale of cigarettes has played an increasing role in the reduction of access to nicotine, an addictive drug that is packaged in cigarettes and chewing tobacco. With restrictions in advertising, adult smoking rates decreased through the 1980s. Taxing of cigarettes and limiting of access to cigarette vending machines have been successful in reducing the number of adolescents who experiment with and eventually become addicted to tobacco products. For example, investigators examined the relationship between smoking restrictions and smoking rates among teenagers. **Their analyses showed that restrictive smoking regulations have a significant effect on teenage cigarette consumption that is even stronger than the effect on consumption by adults. They concluded that smoking regulations are more effective in preventing adolescents from starting to smoke than in reducing tobacco consumption by those who are already smokers.**

Although regulations are important in achieving the goals delineated in *Healthy People 2000*, individuals and communities must also make changes that send messages to current smokers and potential adolescent smokers that smoking is not "cool" and will not be accepted as a social norm. Illustrations of such changes abound. For example, a number of communities have begun to support smoke-free public areas. As of 1989, 44 states were exercising some restrictions on smoking in restaurants, while 51% of cities with populations of 25,000 or more had passed local ordinances restricting smoking in restaurants. A number of malls throughout America have adopted smoke-free policies. In Chicopee, Massachusetts, a group of teenagers petitioned for and implemented a smoke-free policy in their local shopping mall with the help of the mall director and the support of the community. A number of university and professional-league sports stadiums and arenas have also enacted smoke-free policies. As of 1994 at least 23 states were restricting smoking in gymnasiums or arenas as part of clean indoor air legislation.

Tobacco accounts for approximately 400,000 deaths in the United States each year, and almost 30% of these deaths are due to tobacco-related cancers. In fact, cigarette smoking has been linked to a twofold to threefold increased risk of bladder cancer and has also been seen to increase the risk of mortality in men with prostate cancer. Bladder cancer accounts for 6% of all new cases of cancer among men and 2% among women in the United States, while prostate cancer is currently the most commonly diagnosed cancer among men, accounting for approximately 27.5% of all cancers in men in the United States. In addition to increasing the risk of cancer, smoking results in a generalized arteriosclerosis that causes impotence early in life and heart disease that often complicates treatment of smoking-related cancer(s). Therefore, any attempt to dissuade youth from using tobacco products will help decrease the burden of cancer in this country. In addition to the regulatory efforts and individual and community changes, the primary care provider is a vital component of the social strategy to alleviate this national burden. As a point of access to the health care system, an authority figure, and a source of information, the primary care provider has a key role in advising, counseling, and prescribing strategies for cancer prevention. For example, primary care providers can mobilize schools and communities to develop strategies to prevent tobacco use and promote its discontinuation. They can also serve as powerful role models who positively influence the health-related behavior of their adolescent and adult patients. Clinic or office visits offer opportunities for the primary care provider to inform individuals about lifestyle changes such as the cessation of tobacco use that reduces the risk of a number of diseases, including cancer. Studies show that such counseling is both a deterrent and a cost-effective approach to the prevention of smoking-related illnesses. Smokers include a physician's advice among the important factors motivating attempts to quit smoking. A number of analyses have demonstrated that treatment that promotes the cessation of smoking is as cost effective as other routine medical interventions such as the treatment of high blood pressure and high cholesterol levels and periodic mammography. In fact, smoking-cessation treatment may be considered the gold standard of preventive interventions.

Figure 26–1 is an algorithm suggesting the critical pathway for smoking cessation. The role of primary health care providers is highlighted in the figure. Their role begins with the initial contact with the patient. At this point, and at every subsequent visit, the primary provider should screen the patient for tobacco use and if the patient is a current user, the health care provider must advise about the detrimental effects of smoking. Some patients will be willing to quit and others will not. If a patient is not willing to quit, the physician should promote motivation to quit in hopes that the patient will change his or her mind. If the willingness is there, the primary care provider needs to assess the level of cigarette smoking and then intervene by suggesting steps that the patient may take to begin to quit. It is also of utmost importance that the primary health care provider follow up the office visit to show the patient the support needed and to continue to motivate him or her to remain smoke-free (Fig. 26–1).

In summary, when, as with smoking, the patient's exposure status is dichotomous (i.e., you smoke or you do not smoke) and exposure is a clear cause of many major illnesses and premature mortality, a social strategy for prevention requires three components. Regulation, community and individual change, and health care support all must be in place if the desired benefit in an overall reduction in the rates of smoking is to be obtained. If any of the three components is missing, then the rate of progress will be substantially slowed. Therefore, primary care providers must recognize their role as a vital component of a social strategy and join the nation in its shift toward primary prevention and increased general well-being.

Counseling: Recommendations from the Preventive Services Task Force

The Preventive Services Task Force recently published a set of recommendations to help health care providers achieve a variety of patient education and prevention counseling

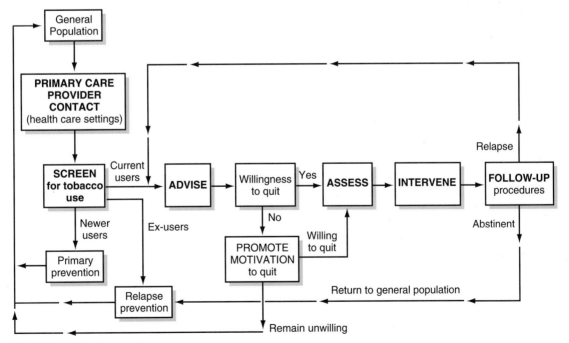

Figure 26-1

Algorithm suggesting the critical pathway for smoking cessation. The role of the primary care provider is highlighted in capital letters. (Modified from Fiore MC, Wetter DW, Bailey WC, et al: Smoking cessation: Clinical practice guideline. Rockville, MD: Agency for Health Care Policy and Research, Public Health Service, US Department of Health and Human Services, 1996.)

goals in areas such as tobacco use, exercise, and nutrition. The strategies presented have two major objectives related to primary prevention: changing health behaviors and improving health status. The principles of counseling presented in Table 26–1 are made because each has been found to be effective in changing certain health behaviors in the primary care setting.

In addition to the 12 recommendations presented in Table 26–1, physicians must "practice what they preach" to foster health within themselves and their patients. The Public Health Service has created a prevention implementation program, "Put Prevention into Practice" (PPIP), to assist clinicians in overcoming barriers to the implementation of counseling interventions. Primary health care providers can use the tools provided by PPIP to deliver appropriate counseling to change patients' personal health practices at each patient visit. PPIP materials can be ordered from the Department of Health and Human Services on the World Wide Web at the following address: http://www.dhhs.gov/PPIP/contact.html#order. There are also several PPIP partner groups that have made these materials available to their members and the general public. These groups include the American Nurses Association, the American Academy

of Family Physicians, the American Academy of Pediatrics (child components only), and the Texas Department of Health.

There is abundant evidence for the effectiveness of physician counseling. For example, a number of clinical trials have demonstrated the efficacy of certain types of counseling by primary care providers in altering patients' smoking behavior and smokeless-tobacco use. The nearly 40 controlled clinical trials examining the different types of clinical smoking-cessation techniques have found that the effectiveness of counseling depends on a number of factors, such as the number of interactions with the patient; the use of personal, face-to-face advice; and the type of counselor (e.g., physician, nurse practitioner, or medical assistant). The most effective techniques were those that involved more than one modality (e.g., primary care provider advice and self-help materials), those that involved the entire staff of a clinic, and those that provided the most motivational messages over the longest period.

The Preventive Services Task Force recommends that clinicians counsel patients to incorporate a program of regular physical activity, appropriate to their health status and lifestyle, into their daily routines. National surveillance programs have documented that about one in four adults in the United States is physically inactive, spending no leisure time engaged in physical activity. Moreover, one third of American adults are not active enough to accrue any of the health benefits of physical activity. Given that the majority of Americans lead sedentary lifestyles, almost anyone could potentially benefit from encouragement by a primary care physician to increase his or her activity level. In fact, Macera and associates assessed the predictors for the adoption of leisure-time physical activity among initially inactive Americans. Their observation that having a physician discuss physical activity was a predictor of adopting leisure-time physical activity among white and African American women and men supports the involvement of primary care providers in the promotion of physical activity among all races and both sexes. In light of the recent U.S. Surgeon General's report emphasizing the health benefits of physical activity and the effectiveness of physician coun-

Table 26-1
Principles Recommended by the Preventive Services Task Force to Induce Behavior Change and Improve Health Status

1. Frame the teaching to match the patient's perceptions.
2. Fully inform the patient of the purposes and expected effects of interventions and when to expect these effects.
3. Suggest small changes rather than large ones.
4. Be specific.
5. Keep in mind that it is sometimes easier to add new behaviors than to eliminate established behaviors.
6. Link new behaviors to old behaviors.
7. Use the power of the profession.
8. Get explicit commitments from the patient.
9. Use a combination of strategies (e.g., one-on-one counseling and self-help material).
10. Involve office staff.
11. Refer the patient appropriately (e.g., to community agencies, national voluntary organizations, instructional references such as books and videos, or other patients).
12. Monitor the patient's progress through follow-up contact.

seling in changing other behavior (such as tobacco use and mammography screening practices), it is clear that primary care providers are a vital component in the attainment of the *Healthy People 2000* goals for physical activity and in the consequent reduction in the burden of cancer in the United States.

These examples illustrate that counseling by primary care providers can be effective as an integral component of cancer prevention. With the three components (regulatory change, individual-primary and community-implemented change, and access to counseling and support from primary health care providers) in place for a successful social strategy, now what might we recommend to our 45-year-old patient? Guidelines for the primary prevention of bladder cancer are provided in Table 26–2 and for prostate cancer in Table 26–3.

Primary Prevention of Bladder Cancer

The most effective way to prevent bladder cancer is the avoidance of cigarette smoking because the proportion of cases attributable to smoking is greater than that for other risk

Table 26-2
Primary Prevention of Bladder Cancer

Recommendations

Avoid cigarette smoking.
Increase fruit and vegetable consumption.
Avoid occupational exposure to certain chemicals and
  substances (such as those listed below).
  Be knowledgeable about the chemicals and
    substances you work with.
  Wear personal protective equipment where indicated.
  Insist that your work environment be designed so as
    to prevent exposure to toxic substances.

Substances or Processes Judged by the IARC to
Be Associated with Bladder Cancer Risk

CARCINOGENIC TO HUMANS

Aluminum production
4-Aminobiphenyl
Auramine manufacture
Benzidine
Magenta (manufacture of)
2-Naphthylamine
Rubber industry

PROBABLY CARCINOGENIC TO HUMANS

Hairdresser, or barber

IARC, International Agency for Research on Cancer.

Table 26-3
Primary Prevention of Prostate Cancer

Eat a varied diet:
  Increase fruit and vegetable intake, consuming at
    least five servings of fruit and vegetables per day.
  Increase tomato consumption.
  Reduce overall fat consumption, emphasizing a
    reduction in saturated fat.
Avoid cigarette smoking.

factors. Currently, approximately 48% to 60% of bladder cancer may be attributed to cigarette smoking. Since the 1950s and the identification of bladder cancer hazards in the British dyestuffs and rubber industries, scores of studies have suggested approximately 40 potentially high-risk occupations. Therefore, it is fair to suggest that the curtailment of occupational exposures will help prevent bladder cancer (see Table 26–2 for a partial list of occupational carcinogens). It has also been suggested that a diet rich in fresh fruit and vegetables, and therefore rich in carotenoids and other antioxidants, may reduce an individual's risk of developing bladder cancer.

La Veccia and Negri reviewed the epidemiologic evidence on the relation between nutrition and bladder cancer and found that 10 case-control studies and 3 cohort studies were published in English between 1979 and 1994. **Six of the seven studies that considered various measures of fruit and vegetable consumption found a reduced risk of bladder cancer with increasing consumption. The reduced risk was more consistent for vegetables, with relative risk (RR) estimates ranging from 0.5 to 0.7.** Vitamin A and particularly carotenoids also showed an inverse relationship with bladder cancer risk in four case-control studies but were not consistently related in two other studies. They found the data on the relationships between bladder cancer and the following dietary components inconsistent: meat and milk, total fat, protein, carbohydrates, vitamins C and E, calcium, and sodium. They concluded that despite limitations, the available data suggest that a diet rich in fruits and vegetables, and therefore possibly in carotenoids, is consistently related to a reduced bladder cancer risk.

Bladder cancer must be ruled out in every case of hematuria, gross and/or microscopic (0 to 3 red blood cells per high-power field).

The patient must undergo imaging studies preferably intravenous pyelogram (IVP) or renal ultrasound of the upper urinary tract, if there is a history of allergy to IVP contrast agent. The patient should then be referred to the urologist for cystoscopy. Retrograde pyelogram is indicated in a patient with history of allergy to IVP contrast agent. Patient's awareness of the significance of hematuria could lead to detection of early type of bladder cancer and prevention of tumor progression and mortality from bladder cancer (see Table 26–2).

Prevention of Prostate Cancer Through Dietary and Other Factors

Epidemiologic evidence suggests that consuming a diet high in fruits and vegetables will reduce the risk of prostate cancer. Recently, researchers conducted a prospective cohort study of fructose intake in relation to prostate cancer among 47,781 men of the Health Professionals Follow-Up Study. Fructose is a simple sugar found primarily in fruits and fruit juices (fresh or canned). The authors observed that high-fructose intake was associated with decreased risk of prostate cancer (RR = 0.77; 95% confidence interval [CI], 0.63 to 0.94; P for trend = 0.002) and of advanced prostate cancer (RR = 0.47; 95% CI, 0.31 to 0.72; P for trend = 0.0007). Fructose from fruit (fresh or canned) and that from other sources (e.g., soda, high-fructose corn syrup) similarly predicted a lower risk of advanced prostate cancer. Fruit intake was inversely associated with risk of advanced prostate cancer (RR = 0.63; 95% CI, 0.43 to 0.93, for >5 vs. <1 serving per day). Overall, these findings support a benefit of increased fruit and fructose consumption on prostate cancer risk.

Emerging evidence suggests an inverse association between the intake of lycopene (a carotenoid with antioxidant but not vitamin A activity) and the risk of prostate cancer. Both food-based studies and blood levels of lycopene support this inverse association. The major source of lycopene is tomatoes. The increased consumption of lycopene in toma-

toes and tomato-based products may prove useful in the prevention of prostate cancer. For example, national food-consumption data indicate that African American men consume approximately half as much tomato-based food as do white men. Given the higher rates of prostate cancer among African American men, an increase in their lycopene consumption through tomato products may be beneficial.

Further evidence suggests that high intake of fat increases the risk of invasive prostate cancer. The relation between total fat intake and prostate cancer has been observed consistently across a number of studies. (In the interpretation of this relation it is important to recognize that a diet high in fat is most likely low in fruit and vegetables.)

As discussed earlier, it has been suggested that smoking may increase mortality from prostate cancer. In 1996 the Australian Reparation Medical Authority convened an international consensus conference to review the issue of the interpretation of the epidemiologic data relating smoking to risk of prostate cancer. After review of the data from a wide range of epidemiologic studies, a Consensus Statement was unanimously endorsed and adopted. In summary, the conference concluded that there is inadequate evidence that smoking is causally linked to the occurrence or incidence of prostate cancer. The conference participants also agreed that there is limited evidence that smoking is associated with increased mortality attributable to prostate cancer. They concluded that smoking may be associated with poorer survival among those with prostate cancer and that additional studies may help to interpret this possible association.

Most recently, Giovannucci and colleagues analyzed data from the Health Professionals Follow-Up Study to better understand the nature of the relationship between smoking and prostate cancer incidence and mortality. They followed 47,781 U.S. males biennially from 1986 to 1994. They calculated multivariate RR and 95% CI for total, distant metastatic, and fatal prostate cancer in relation to early smoking (before 30 years of age), late smoking (within recent 10 years), and cumulative lifetime smoking. All levels of smoking were unrelated to risk or total prostate cancer incidence. Although, they found that men who had smoked 15 or more pack-years of cigarettes within the preceding 10 years were at higher risk of distant metastatic prostate cancer (RR = 1.81; CI, 1.05 to 3.11; P for trend = 0.03) and fatal prostate cancer (RR = 2.06, CI, 1.08 to 3.90; P = 0.02) relative to non-smokers. Excess risk was eliminated within 10 years after quitting smoking. Their results suggest that recent tobacco use may have a direct impact on mortality from prostate cancer, but the excess risk abates after 10 years of cessation from cigarette smoking.

Primary care providers can counsel their patients to change their dietary and cigarette smoking habits in a manner that lowers prostate cancer risk and mortality (see Table 26–1). The Preventive Services Task Force currently recommends that dietary counseling should focus on the intake of fat, complex carbohydrates, fiber, and total calories. Primary care providers should encourage their patients to consume a variety of foods, with an emphasis on whole-grain products, cereals, vegetables, and fruits. This type of dietary plan is in accordance with the Surgeon General's *Healthy People 2000* risk-reduction objectives in which people 12 years of age and older are encouraged to consume five or more daily servings of fruits and vegetables. The Surgeon General also recommends that for people 2 years of age and older, dietary fat intake be reduced to an average of no more than 30% of calories and average saturated fat intake to less than 10% of calories. As presented previously, primary care providers play an important role in counseling patients to stop smoking and can even serve as role models for younger patients by encouraging them not to begin cigarette smoking. Given the power of physician counseling to increase adherence to preventive guidelines, more routine counseling may speed change leading to a lower cancer risk and mortality.

Summary

Counseling by primary health care providers during a routine visit need not stand alone, for as we have seen the most effective smoking-cessation interventions are those that involve more than one modality (e.g., primary care provider advice and self-help materials), those that involve an entire clinic staff, and those that provide the most motivational messages over the longest period. Primary care providers, therefore, are most influential if they offer a combination of one-on-one counseling, referrals when necessary (e.g., to a dietitian), self-help materials, and the commitment of a staff that is dedicated to the long-term follow-up and support of patients trying to alter their lifestyle.

SUGGESTED READINGS

1. Atwood K, Colditz GA, Kawachi I: From public health policy to prevention policy: Placing science in its social and political contexts. Am J Pub Health 87:1603–1606,1997.
2. Colditz GA, DeJong W, Hunter D, et al (eds): Harvard Report on Cancer Prevention, Vol 1: Causes of Human Cancer. Cancer Causes Control 7:S5–S6, 1996.
3. Colditz GA, Frazier AL: Cancer culture: Prescription for prevention. (submitted for publication).
4. Cummings KM, Giovino G, Emont SL, et al: Factors influencing success in counseling patients to stop smoking. Patient Educ Counsel 8:189–200, 1986.
5. Giovannucci E: Epidemiologic characteristics of prostate cancer. Cancer 75:1766, 1995.
6. Giovannucci E, Rimm EB, Ascherio A, et al: Fructose and fruit intake in relation to risk of prostate cancer. Cancer Res 58:442–447, 1998.
7. Giovannucci E, Rimm EB, Stampfer MJ, et al: A prospective study of dietary fat and risk of prostate cancer. J Natl Cancer Inst 85:1571–1579, 1993.
8. Healthy People 2000: National Health Promotion and Disease Prevention Objectives. Publication No. (PHS) 91-50213. Bethesda, MD, U.S. Department of Health and Human Services, 1990.
9. Howe HL: Repeat mammography among women over 50 years of age. Am J Prev Med 8:182–185, 1992.
10. La Vecchia C, Negri E: Nutrition and bladder cancer. Cancer Causes Control 7:95–100, 1996.
11. Le Marchand L, Kolonel LN, Wilkens LR, et al: Animal fat consumption and prostate cancer: A prospective study in Hawaii. Epidemiology 5:276–282, 1994.
12. Lerman C, Rimer B, Trock B, et al: Factors associated with repeat adherence to breast cancer screening. Prev Med 19:279–290, 1990.
13. Macera CA, Croft JB, Brown DR, et al: Predictors of adopting leisure-time physical activity among a biracial community cohort. Am J Epidemiol 142:629–635, 1995.
14. Ockene JK: Smoking intervention: The expanding role of the physician. Am J Public Health 77:782–783, 1987.
15. Ross RK, Schottenfeld D: Prostate cancer. *In* Schottenfeld D, Fraumeni JF Jr (eds): Cancer Epidemiology and Prevention, 2nd ed. New York, Oxford University Press, 1996, pp 1180–1206.
16. Silverman DT, Morrison AS, Devesa SS: Bladder cancer. *In* Schottenfeld D, Fraumeni JF Jr (eds): Cancer Epidemiology and Prevention, 2nd ed. New York, Oxford University Press, 1996, pp 1156–1179.

17. Steinmetz KA, Potter JD: Vegetables, fruit, and cancer: I. Epidemiology. Cancer Causes Control 2:325–357, 1991.
18. U.S. Bureau of the Census: Statistical Abstract of the United States: 1995, 115th ed. Government Printing Office, Washington, DC, 1995.
19. U.S. Department of Health and Human Services: Preventing Tobacco Use Among Young People: A Report of the Surgeon General. Atlanta, U.S. Department of Health and Human Services, Public Health Service, Centers for Disease Control and Prevention, National Center for Chronic Disease Prevention and Health Promotion, Office of Smoking and Health, 1994.
20. Wasserman J, Manning WG, Newhouse JP, Winkler JD: The effects of excise taxes and regulations on cigarette smoking. J Health Econ 10:43–64, 1991.

27

Acute Renal Failure

Filitsa H. Bender
Edward Weinman

Acute declines in renal function, with or without associated symptoms, are a common clinical problem. The term *acute renal failure* is often used to describe a clinical syndrome characterized by rapid deterioration of renal function with accumulation of nitrogenous waste products and abnormalities in fluid, electrolyte, and acid-base homeostasis. A variety of renal disorders can result in acute renal failure, all presenting with the same constellation of signs and symptoms. Acute renal failure and most of its precipitating causes are often encountered in the hospital setting, hence the diagnosis and management of acute renal failure have traditionally been an inpatient process. However, it can be expected that the decreasing need for hospital-based diagnostic evaluation and therapeutic management of many diseases will increase the frequency with which acute renal failure is encountered in the outpatient setting.

Initial Approach to the Patient

Patients may present with symptoms related to renal dysfunction, such as acute decline in urine output, although in many cases the symptom complex is not sufficiently unique to permit a definitive diagnosis without laboratory testing and verification (Table 27–1). Many patients are identified by screening laboratory tests such as concentrations of blood urea nitrogen (BUN), plasma creatinine, serum electrolytes, or urinalysis. When a patient is initially found to have abnormal renal function, it is essential to determine if the

newly identified abnormalities represent an acute change in function or a chronic process that has occurred over months or years. This information is key to assessing the reversibility of the acute renal failure and, as a consequence, the speed and extent of the diagnostic evaluation and therapy. For example, if the newly diagnosed abnormalities are indicative of long-standing chronic and irreversible disease, there is often less need for extensive diagnostic evaluation. The distinction between acute and chronic disease may be apparent from the history. Acute renal failure is often associated with acute medical or surgical illnesses and/or recent introduction of potentially nephrotoxic medications. Rapid increase in plasma creatinine over a period of hours to days usually indicates acute renal injury or acute injury superimposed on chronically diseased kidneys. Previous history of abnormal laboratory tests such as BUN, creatinine, or urinalysis and signs and

Table 27–1
Diagnostic Approach to Patients with Acute Renal Failure

1. Detailed history with emphasis on previous renal function indices and urinalyses and on exposure to possible nephrotoxic insults
2. Physical examination with emphasis on volume status and evidence of systemic illness
3. Examination of the urine (urinalysis, urinary electrolyte excretory indices, urine culture, special tests when indicated)
4. Laboratory tests: measurement of renal functional changes over time, special serologic tests
5. Determination of the anatomy of the kidney
6. Renal blood flow studies (when indicated)
7. Renal biopsy (when indicated)

symptoms such as edema, hypertension, hematuria, polyuria, or nocturia likely reflect chronic disease. Physical examination is not particularly helpful in differentiating between acute and chronic renal failure. Other laboratory abnormalities such as the presence of anemia and hyperphosphatemia are also of limited diagnostic value since these abnormalities may be present in patients with either acute or chronic renal failure. An elevated serum alkaline phosphatase level may reflect the presence of renal osteodystrophy, a complication of long-standing renal disease, hence a finding that would signify chronicity.

As shown in Figure 27–1, initial differential diagnosis includes (1) prerenal azotemia, (2) intrinsic renal disease, and (3) postrenal disease. Prerenal azotemia is a condition in which the kidneys function normally but are inadequately perfused. Intrinsic acute renal failure is defined as the acute development of abnormal renal function due to disease of the renal glomeruli, tubules, and/or the interstitium. *Postrenal acute renal failure* refers to renal dysfunction caused by obstruction of the urinary outflow tract. Evaluation and treatment of obstructive uropathy, which is often reversible, are presented elsewhere in this book.

Diagnostic Evaluation of Patients with Acute Renal Failure

Patients identified as having abnormal concentrations of BUN, plasma creatinine, and electrolytes or discovered as having abnormal urine output usually require diagnostic evaluation. Anatomic evaluation of the kidneys and urinalysis are standard initial tests; additional urinary indices may add information with regard to the functional capacities of the kidneys. Serologic testing and renal biopsy may be indicated in selected patients (see Table 27–1).

Determination of anatomy of the kidneys is a most important test in evaluating patients with renal dysfunction. Renal ultrasound is the preferred initial test. Measurement of the size of the kidneys is important in differentiating acute from chronic renal failure. Kidneys that are small, with thin cortices and increased echogenicity are highly suggestive of chronic disease. The renal ultrasound is also sensitive in detecting ureteral obstruction, bladder size, and parenchymal masses or cysts.

The urinalysis should include both a "dipstick test" and microscopic examination of the sediment; the latter is of great value in the evaluation of patients with renal insufficiency (Table 27–2). Typically, the dipstick is negative or shows only minimal proteinuria in patients with prerenal azotemia. In addition, the sediment is usually unremarkable but may contain a few hyaline casts. By contrast, urinalysis is invariably abnormal in patients with acute tubular necrosis. In such patients, mild proteinuria is present and characteristic pigmented granular casts are seen.

The presence of mild to moderate proteinuria with white blood cells, white blood cell casts, eosinophils, and hematuria characterizes acute interstitial nephritis. Moderate to severe proteinuria with dysmorphic red blood cells and red blood cell casts are present in cases of acute glomerulonephritis or rapidly progressive glomerulonephritis. Urine that tests positive for blood by dipstick but in which no red blood cells are seen on examination of the sediment suggests the presence of myoglobinuria or hemoglobinuria

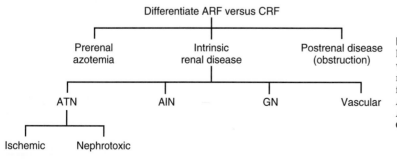

Figure 27–1
Diagnostic algorithm in patients with newly recognized decreased renal function. ARF, acute renal failure; CRF, chronic renal failure; ATN, acute tubular necrosis; AIN, acute interstitial nephritis; GN, glomerulonephritis.

Table 27-2
Urinary Findings in Different Types of Acute Renal Failure

Test	Prerenal Azotemia	ATN	AIN	GN	Postrenal (obstruction)
Urine dipstick	No or trace proteinuria	± Mild proteinuria ± Mild hematuria	Mild to moderate proteinuria; mild hematuria	Moderate to severe proteinuria; hematuria	Variable; may be normal
Urine sediment	Normal or few hyaline casts	Pigmented granular casts	WBCs/WBC casts, eosinophils, RBCs	RBCs/RBC casts	Variable; may be normal
Urine osmolality (mOsm/kg)	>500	<350	<350	>500	Variable; may be <350
FENa (%)	<1	>1	>1	<1	Variable; may be <1

ATN, acute tubular necrosis; AIN, acute interstitial nephritis; GN, glomerulonephritis, FENa, fractional excretion of sodium; WBC, white blood cell; RBC, red blood cell.

and the likely diagnosis of rhabdomyolysis or transfusion reaction, respectively.

Studies of the functional capacities of the kidney provide significant diagnostic information (see Table 27–2).

1. BUN/plasma creatinine ratio: Normally, the BUN:plasma creatinine ratio is 10 to 15:1, and a similar ratio is maintained in acute tubular necrosis. In patients with prerenal azotemia, however, this ratio may be greater than 20:1. The BUN:plasma creatinine ratio must be interpreted in a clinical context. For example, the BUN may be elevated independently of creatinine concentration in patients with gastrointestinal tract bleeding, patients who are catabolic, and patients receiving steroid medications. Patients ingesting little protein may have low BUN concentration, which may confound accurate interpretation of the BUN:creatinine ratio.

2. Urine osmolality: Urine osmolality greater than 500 mOsm/kg is highly suggestive of prerenal disease reflecting both increased secretion of antidiuretic hormone in response to volume depletion and maintenance of normal tubular function. A urine osmolality less than 350 mOsm/kg, particularly after 8 or more hours of water deprivation, reflects loss of renal concentrating ability and is an early and frequent finding in acute tubular necrosis.

3. Urine sodium concentration and fractional excretion of sodium: Urine sodium con-

centration tends to be low in prerenal azotemia (<20 mM/L), reflecting the kidney's attempt to conserve sodium. The urine sodium concentration is high in most patients with acute tubular necrosis (>40 mM/L), reflecting injury to the renal tubules. Because the urine sodium concentration is affected by variations in water reabsorption, fractional excretion of sodium is considered a more reliable index of renal tubular integrity in evaluation of patients with acute declines in renal function.

The fractional excretion of sodium (FENa) measures the fraction or percent of sodium filtered at the glomerulus that is ultimately excreted in the urine. FENa can be readily calculated from the formula:

$$\text{FENa (\%)} = \frac{U_{Na}/U_{Cr}}{P_{Na}/P_{Cr}} \times 100$$

where U_{Na} and U_{Cr} are the urine sodium and creatinine concentrations, respectively, measured in a random urine sample, and P_{Na} and P_{Cr} are the respective concomitant plasma concentrations.

The FENa is probably the most accurate test for differentiating prerenal azotemia and acute tubular necrosis. A value less than 1% suggests prerenal disease, reflecting reabsorption of filtered sodium in response to decreased renal perfusion. A value greater than 2% usually indicates acute tubular necrosis.

Interpretation of the results of the FENa calculation must be done with caution in patients receiving diuretics since these agents increase the urine concentration of sodium and the FENa. Patients with advanced renal failure may also have FENa greater than 2%, regardless of the state of hydration or renal perfusion.

Causes of Acute Renal Failure

PRERENAL AZOTEMIA

Prerenal azotemia causes approximately 70% of community-acquired acute renal failure and 40% of hospital-acquired acute renal failure. A variety of conditions can affect renal perfusion pressure and cause prerenal azotemia (Table 27–3). In most cases, correction of the underlying cause reverses the renal functional abnormalities; however, sustained and severe prerenal azotemia may result in

Table 27–3
Causes of Prerenal Azotemia

Decreased "actual" intravascular volume
  Hemorrhage
  Renal fluid and electrolyte losses
    Diuretics, salt-wasting disorders
  Gastrointestinal losses
    Vomiting, diarrhea, nasogastric suction,
      enterostomy drainage
  Skin losses
    Burns, intense sweating
Decreased "effective" arterial blood volume
  "Third space," capillary leak loss of vascular volume
    (pancreatitis, peritonitis)
  Reduced cardiac output
    Congestive heart failure, myocardial infarction,
      pericardial tamponade, pulmonary embolism,
      arrhythmias
  Cirrhosis
  Nephrotic syndrome
  Peripheral vasodilation
    Sepsis, medications
Primary renal vascular disorder
  Large vessel
    Arterial thrombosis, embolism, severe stenosis,
      clamping
    Venous thrombosis, obstruction
  Small vessel
    Renal vasculitis, hemolytic-uremic syndrome,
      malignant hypertension, scleroderma,
      hypercalcemia
  Hepatorenal syndrome
  Medications
    Angiotensin-converting enzyme inhibitors,
      cyclosporin, tacrolimus, nonsteroidal anti-
      inflammatory drugs

ischemic acute tubular necrosis. The signs and symptoms of prerenal azotemia reflect those of the underlying disorder. Characteristic laboratory abnormalities include an elevated BUN and plasma creatinine level, a BUN:creatinine ratio greater than 20 and a urine sodium concentration and FENa of less than 20 mEq/dL and 1%, respectively. Prerenal azotemia may result from true decrease in extracellular fluid volume. Common clinical conditions associated with prerenal azotemia include fever and sweating, hemorrhage, nausea and vomiting, diarrhea, and administration of diuretics. The intake of fluid is usually inadequate and does not match extrarenal or renal losses. Clinical signs include tachycardia, low-to-normal blood pressure, poor skin turgor, and dry mucous membranes. Postural changes in pulse rate and blood pressure are valuable clinical findings indicative of volume depletion.

Prerenal azotemia may occur in patients in whom there is a redistribution of fluid from the intravascular to the interstitial space secondary to conditions such as overwhelming sepsis, ascites, and pancreatitis. A number of clinical conditions causing prerenal azotemia are characterized by a decrease in the effective (as contrasted with the true) extracellular fluid volume. Such conditions include congestive heart failure, cirrhosis, nephrotic syndrome, and sepsis. Although these patients may appear volume repleted or even volume overloaded due to the presence of ascites and/or edema, renal function responds as if renal perfusion were compromised. Patients with either large- or small-vessel disease, such as renal artery thrombosis and embolism, severe renal artery stenosis, renal vasculitis, malignant hypertension, and scleroderma, can also present with a clinical picture of prerenal azotemia if renal blood flow becomes impaired. Several medications, including angiotensin-converting enzyme inhibitors, cyclosporin, tacrolimus, and nonsteroidal anti-inflammatory drugs (NSAIDs), can diminish renal perfusion by virtue of their effect on the renal vasculature. Often prerenal azotemia is multifactorial in etiology. For example, prerenal azotemia occurs frequently in elderly patients receiving a diuretic and an angiotensin-converting enzyme inhibitor who develop gastroenteritis with vom-

Table 27-4
Medications Associated with Acute Renal Failure

Medication	Possible Mechanism
Nonsteroidal anti-inflammatory drugs, angiotensin-converting enzyme inhibitors, cyclosporin, tacrolimus, amphotericin, radiographic contrast media	Renal vasoconstriction
Aminoglycosides, radiographic contrast media, cisplatin, cyclosporin, tacrolimus, amphotericin, pentamidine	Direct tubular toxicity
Cocaine, ethanol, lovastatin	Rhabdomyolysis
Penicillin, cephalosporins, sulfonamides, nonsteroidal anti-inflammatory drugs, rifampin	Acute interstitial nephritis
Acyclovir, sulfonamides, methotrexate	Intratubular obstruction

iting and diarrhea while continuing to take the prescribed medications (Table 27–4).

INTRINSIC RENAL DISEASE

Renal ischemia and nephrotoxins are the most common causes of intrinsic acute renal failure. A variety of specific medical conditions, however, can affect different parts of the renal parenchyma and cause intrinsic renal disease (Table 27–5). The renal vessels can be affected as described in Table 27–3 and infrequently cause acute renal failure. The glomeruli also can be affected causing acute or sometimes subacute renal failure. The interstitium can be affected by medications, infections, or unknown mechanisms that cause acute interstitial nephritis. The tubular epithelium can be injured by ischemia, toxins, or other insults and cause acute tubular necrosis. Infrequently, intratubular precipitation of compounds such as oxalate, urate, myeloma proteins, or pigments can occur.

Ischemic Acute Tubular Necrosis

Ischemic acute tubular necrosis occurs in patients with severe compromise of cardiovascular function associated with decreased organ perfusion and often hypotension. Acute tubular necrosis is a common complication of cardiac surgery, abdominal aortic aneurysm repair, and surgery to correct obstructive jaundice. Although these conditions are more common in acutely ill hospitalized patients, elderly patients and patients receiving angiotensin-converting enzyme inhibitors, NSAIDs, cyclosporin, or tacrolimus are more susceptible to the development of either prerenal azotemia or ischemic acute tubular necrosis.

The clinical picture of ischemic acute tubular necrosis is often dominated by the primary disease. The urinalysis typically demonstrates mild proteinuria and pigmented granular casts. The urine sodium concentration is greater than 20 mM/L and the FENa is greater than 2%. Acute tubular necrosis may be associated with oliguria (<500 mL

Table 27-5
Causes of Intrinsic Acute Renal Failure

Vascular
  Large vessel
    Bilateral renal artery thrombosis, emboli, severe stenosis
    Bilateral renal vein thrombosis
    Major arterial or venous lesion of solitary kidney
  Small vessels
    Vasculitis
    Malignant hypertension
    Scleroderma
    Thrombotic thrombocytopenic purpura/hemolytic-uremic syndrome
    Atheroembolic disease
Glomerular
  Acute glomerulonephritis
    Postinfectious glomerulonephritis
    Medications—nonsteroidal anti-inflammatory drugs
  Rapidly progressive glomerulonephritis
    Systemic lupus erythematosus, Goodpasture's syndrome, Wegener's granulomatosis, idiopathic
Interstitial
  Medications
  Infections
  Infiltrative disease, hypercalcemia
  Idiopathic
Tubular
  Ischemic acute tubular necrosis
  Nephrotoxic acute tubular necrosis
    Medications—aminoglycosides, amphotericin, cisplatin
    Radiographic contrast media
    Toxins—heavy metals
    Pigment—myoglobin (rhabdomyolysis), hemoglobin (hemolysis)
    Intratubular obstruction—oxalate, myeloma proteins, uric acid, methotrexate, acyclovir, triamterene, sulfonamides

per day); alternatively, urine output may be normal. There is evidence to suggest that subjects with nonoliguric acute renal failure have less severe disease and a better chance for recovery of renal function. It has been suggested that administration of loop diuretics or mannitol may convert oliguric acute tubular necrosis to nonoliguric renal failure. Fluid and electrolyte management is easier in patients with nonoliguric renal failure as compared with patients who are oliguric. Loop diuretics have a number of other theoretical properties that suggest they would be of value in patients with ischemic acute tubular necrosis. Accordingly, loop diuretics are often administered to patients early in the course of ischemic acute tubular necrosis. Nonetheless, it should be remembered that support for administration of diuretics to patients with acute tubular necrosis from clinical studies is lacking or controversial. In addition, once oliguric acute tubular necrosis is diagnosed, administration of diuretics or mannitol neither shortens the duration of renal failure nor decreases the requirement for dialysis.

Discussion of Selected Causes of Acute Renal Failure

RENAL VASCULAR DISEASE

Bilateral renal artery stenosis or ischemic renal disease is a relatively common renal disorder and is potentially reversible. It may be present in as many as 25% of patients with signs of peripheral vascular disease. The urine sediment is bland, and mild to moderate proteinuria may be present. In addition to systemic atherosclerosis, other clinical clues suggesting the presence of renal vascular disease are severe refractory hypertension, acute elevations in blood pressure, asymmetry of kidney size, recurrent episodes of pulmonary edema in patients with normal left ventricular function, or an increase in the plasma creatinine level following the administration of an angiotensin-converting enzyme inhibitor. Although acute increases in the plasma concentration of creatinine following the administration of angiotensin-converting enzyme inhibitors may occur in the absence of renal artery stenosis, the diagnosis of renovascular

disease should be considered when there is a temporal relationship between starting such an agent and renal dysfunction. No single noninvasive screening test is sufficiently sensitive and specific to definitely diagnose the presence or absence of bilateral renovascular disease. The most widely used noninvasive screening test is nuclear renal scan or renogram that is done following administration of an angiotensin-converting enzyme inhibitor. Typically, angiotensin-converting enzyme inhibitors induce a decline in the glomerular filtration rate in the affected kidney accompanied by an increase in the glomerular filtration rate in the contralateral kidney, therefore enhancing the difference in imaging between the affected and the contralateral kidney. The main disadvantage is the lack of sensitivity in cases of bilateral renal artery stenosis and significant renal dysfunction. Duplex Doppler ultrasonography is another noninvasive test in which direct visualization of the main renal arteries is combined with hemodynamic measurements. The main advantage of Doppler ultrasonography is the ability to detect both unilateral and bilateral disease, and the test is not affected by renal function. This test is operator dependent, limiting its usefulness. Patients suspected of having renovascular disease, particularly those in whom a screening test is consistent with the diagnosis, require a renal arteriogram for definite diagnosis and evaluation for amenability to revascularization by angioplasty or surgery.

RENAL ATHEROEMBOLIC DISEASE

Renal atheroembolic disease is increasingly recognized as an important cause of acute or "subacute" renal failure. Renal atheroembolic disease should be differentiated from renal embolization secondary to clot in the main renal artery or large renal vessels. The latter condition is characterized by the presence of renal infarction and clinically by flank pain, hematuria, fever, and an elevation in the concentration of lactic acid dehydrogenase. By contrast, renal atheroembolic disease is the result of incomplete occlusion of small vessels of the kidney (and other organs) caused by lodging of irregularly shaped small cholesterol emboli. The end result is ischemic atrophy as well as foreign body reaction. This foreign body reaction probably contributes to the persistence of renal dysfunction for weeks after the initial insult. Renal atheroembolic disease may occur after an arteriogram or other manipulations of an atherosclerotic aorta or other major vessels. It may also occur spontaneously or after treatment with warfarin or thrombolytic agents. Clinically, the patient may have a bluish discoloration of the toes that can progress to frank gangrene. Other findings include livedo reticularis (i.e., mottled appearance of the skin) and blood in the stools if there is involvement of the gastrointestinal tract. The BUN and creatinine levels increase a few days after the insult and may continue to increase for several weeks. The urinalysis is benign, although non-nephrotic range proteinuria may be present as well as eosinophilia and hypocomplementemia. End-stage renal disease is the most common outcome, although recovery of renal function does rarely occur.

GLOMERULONEPHRITIS

Acute glomerulonephritis and rapidly progressive glomerulonephritis are relatively uncommon causes of acute renal failure, but they may present initially in the outpatient setting. Other entities such as systemic or renal vasculitis, Wegener's granulomatosis, and Goodpasture's syndrome may present as acute declines in renal function associated with inflammation of the glomeruli. Glomerulonephritis of sufficient severity to cause an increase in the plasma creatinine level is often associated with significant proteinuria, hematuria, and the presence of cellular casts, particularly red blood cell casts, in the urine. Specific serologic markers are available to aid in the diagnosis of some of these diseases (Table 27–6). Often a renal biopsy is necessary for a definite diagnosis as a guide for therapy and for assessment of prognosis.

ACUTE INTERSTITIAL NEPHRITIS

Acute interstitial nephritis is an uncommon cause of acute renal failure, but the true incidence is unknown. Acute interstitial nephritis is defined as acute renal failure associated with infiltration of the renal interstitium by inflammatory cells. It has been associated

Table 27–6
Serologic Findings in Glomerulopathies

Glomerulopathy	Finding
Poststreptococcal glomerulonephritis	Antistreptococcal antibodies
Systemic lupus erythematosus	Antinuclear antibodies
Goodpasture's syndrome	Antiglomerular basement membrane antibodies
Wegener's granulomatosis	Antineutrophilic cytoplasmic antibodies
Mixed cryoglobulinemia	Circulating cryoglobulins

with drugs, systemic diseases such as sarcoidosis, and infections such as legionella and leptospirosis, or it can be idiopathic. The typical clinical presentation includes the acute onset of renal failure temporally related to an offending drug or infection. The list of medications associated with acute interstitial nephritis is large and growing (Table 27–7). There appears to be little or no association between the dose of medication and the development of interstitial nephritis, and recurrences or exacerbations of the renal injury may occur whenever the same or similar medications are used again. Some patients may manifest a drug-related rash. Laboratory findings consistent with renal tubular acidosis or Fanconi's syndrome reflect evidence of tubular interstitial damage. The urinalysis dem-

Table 27–7
Selected Causes of Acute Interstitial Nephritis

Medications	Methicillin
	Penicillins/cephalosporins
	Sulfonamides (including furosemide and thiazide diuretics)
	Rifampin
	Phenytoin
	Allopurinol
	Cimetidine
Systemic infection	Diphtheria
	Streptococci
	Legionella
	Leptospira
Immune	Sarcoidosis
	Antitubular basement membrane disease
	Sjögren's syndrome
	Tubular interstitial nephritis/ uveitis syndrome
Idiopathic	—

onstrates minimal to moderate non-nephrotic-range proteinuria. The urine sediment demonstrates evidence of inflammation, including the presence of white blood cells, white blood cell casts, and, perhaps, red blood cells. Eosinophilia and eosinophiluria occur in some of the drug-associated causes of interstitial nephritis. Methicillin is the prototypic drug associated with interstitial nephritis and eosinophilia and eosinophiluria. Methicillin-associated interstitial inflammation occurs in approximately 17% of patients treated more than 10 days.

Although usually the clinical presentation, as described, may be sufficient for the diagnosis of acute interstitial nephritis, gallium scanning can be of value when the diagnosis is obscure. Patients with acute interstitial nephritis typically show diffuse intense bilateral uptake. The scan is almost always negative in acute tubular necrosis, the condition most commonly needed to be differentiated from acute interstitial nephritis. Although a positive scan is highly suggestive of acute interstitial nephritis, a negative scan does not exclude the diagnosis and a renal biopsy may be indicated. The first step for the treatment is to discontinue the offending medication. In patients with more severe and persistent renal insufficiency, steroids may be administered, although the evidence that steroids are of benefit in drug-induced acute interstitial nephritis is controversial.

NONSTEROIDAL ANTI-INFLAMMATORY DRUGS AND RENAL ABNORMALITIES

It has been estimated that about 1% of persons ingesting NSAIDs will develop an abnormality of renal function (Table 27–8). Despite the seemingly low incidence, the widespread use of these medications indi-

Table 27–8
Renal Abnormalities Associated with Nonsteroidal Anti-Inflammatory Drugs

Sodium and water retention
Worsening of hypertension
Hyperkalemia
Hemodynamically mediated acute renal failure
Nephrotic syndrome with acute interstitial nephritis

cates that a significant number of persons will suffer some degree of renal abnormality. There are several distinct syndromes associated with NSAID usage. NSAIDs can cause sodium and water retention as well as abnormalities in the serum concentrations of electrolytes. Sodium and water retention is a common side effect of NSAID therapy. Clinical correlates include edema and difficulties in control of blood pressure in patients with hypertension. If the inability to excrete water is severe, hyponatremia may ensue. Hyperkalemia is also a relatively common complication of NSAID use. Other factors such as renal insufficiency, administration of potassium supplements, potassium-sparing diuretics, or angiotensin-converting enzyme inhibitors given in combination with NSAIDs are usually required for the development of clinically significant hyperkalemia.

NSAIDs may be associated with hemodynamically mediated acute renal failure. Under normal conditions, prostaglandins play a negligible role in maintaining renal blood flow and the glomerular filtration rate. In conditions associated with diminished effective arterial blood volume such as true volume depletion, congestive heart failure, cirrhosis, nephrotic syndrome, and renal insufficiency, the contribution of vasodilatory prostaglandins to maintenance of renal blood flow is increased. Accordingly, because NSAIDs block the effect of vasodilatory prostaglandins and cause significant decrease in renal blood flow, their use can increase the risk of hemodynamically induced acute renal failure. It is recommended that patients who are at risk for development of renal dysfunction with NSAIDs should be identified and monitored closely if it is necessary to administer NSAIDs for intercurrent disease. Acute renal failure typically occurs within 3 to 7 days of therapy and is often reversible on discontinuation of the drug.

A unique complication of NSAID therapy is the development of nephrotic syndrome, due to "minimal change disease," in combination with acute interstitial nephritis, due to an interstitial infiltrate primarily of T lymphocytes. It is characterized by hematuria, pyuria, white blood cell casts, nephrotic-range proteinuria, and acute renal failure while signs of systemic allergic reaction such as fever, rash, eosinophilia, or eosinophiluria are typically absent. Finally, NSAID usage has been implicated in some cases of papillary necrosis.

AMINOGLYCOSIDE-INDUCED ACUTE TUBULAR NECROSIS

Aminoglycoside-induced acute tubular necrosis is the most common cause of antibiotic-associated renal insufficiency in the hospital setting. Ten percent to 20% of therapeutic courses of aminoglycosides may be associated with the development of renal insufficiency. Aminoglycosides are excreted exclusively by the kidney; they are filtered and then partially taken up by and stored in the proximal tubular cells where they induce damage. The storage in these cells is prolonged, which accounts for the fact that renal failure may become clinically evident several days after the drug has been discontinued. The following risk factors have been associated with the development of aminoglycoside nephrotoxicity: duration of treatment greater than 10 days; volume depletion and other causes of renal hypoperfusion; preexisting renal disease; advanced age; concomitant administration of certain cephalosporins, particularly cephalothin; concomitant administration of other nephrotoxic agents; liver disease; potassium depletion; and previous recent aminoglycoside treatment. Careful monitoring of the plasma concentration of the drug is recommended, although acute tubular necrosis may occur despite maintenance of therapeutic nontoxic concentrations. The dose of aminoglycosides needs to be adjusted in patients with renal insufficiency. Clinically, aminoglycoside nephrotoxicity presents as nonoliguric acute renal failure. Other features include the inability to concentrate the urine and polyuria and rarely renal magnesium wasting and enzymuria. Once the medication is discontinued, recovery ensues, although a return of the plasma creatinine to its baseline level may take as long as 3 weeks.

RADIOGRAPHIC CONTRAST MEDIA-INDUCED ACUTE RENAL FAILURE

Although radiographic contrast media–induced acute renal failure is considered a common problem, its exact incidence is not known. This complication of the use of radiographic contrast media appears to be almost negligible in subjects with normal renal function, including diabetic patients with normal renal function. The incidence of radiographic contrast media–induced acute renal failure, however, is increased in patients with renal insufficiency and, at any level of renal dysfunction, diabetics are at higher risk. More than 50% of patients with baseline serum creatinine concentrations greater than 5 mg/dL develop radiographic contrast media–induced nephropathy.

The pathogenesis of radiographic contrast media–induced acute renal failure is not well understood, but both renal vasoconstriction and direct tubular toxicity have been implicated. Acute renal dysfunction typically begins immediately after administration of the contrast agent and, in most cases, the decline in renal function is mild and transient. Patients may be transiently oliguric, but most recover renal function within days. Patients with baseline creatinine concentrations above 5 mg/dL may progress to the point of requiring dialysis. A unique feature of radiographic contrast media–induced acute renal failure is the fact that the fractional excretion of sodium may be less than 1%. The urine sediment also can be either typical of acute tubular necrosis or unremarkable.

In high-risk patients, nonradiographic contrast means of diagnosis (ultrasound, magnetic resonance imaging) should be considered. The use of lower doses of contrast agent is recommended in high-risk patients, although it is not well established that lower doses are associated with a reduced risk of renal injury. The use of newer non-anionic contrast agents may reduce the risk of acute renal failure in selected patient populations such as those with serum creatinine concentration greater than 2 mg/dL and diabetics. It is advisable to avoid or discontinue the use of NSAIDs prior to the administration of contrast media. Finally, hydration with normal or half-normal saline for several hours prior to the study is strongly recommended for high-risk patients. The use of mannitol or furosemide prior to administration of the radiographic contrast dye and the use of dialysis after administration of the dye have not been shown to provide protection from renal injury.

RENAL DISEASE ASSOCIATED WITH MALIGNANCY

A variety of renal diseases may be associated with malignancy and its treatment (Table 27–9). All types of acute renal failure (prerenal, intrinsic renal, obstruction) can be seen in association with malignancy. Some forms of acute renal failure, however, are uniquely associated with malignancy.

A number of glomerular diseases can be associated with solid tumors or lymphomas as well as with multiple myeloma. Membranous nephropathy, minimal change disease, or focal segmental glomerulonephritis can occur; these are usually manifested as the nephrotic syndrome. Acute renal failure secondary to the nephrotic syndrome can occur but is relatively uncommon in any setting.

Multiple myeloma is associated with several specific types of renal disease. Myeloma

Table 27-9
Renal Abnormalities Associated with Malignancy

Prerenal azotemia
   True volume depletion (nausea and vomiting, poor
      dietary intake)
   Hepatorenal syndrome (liver involvement)
   Capillary leak (interleukin-2)
Glomerular diseases
   Membranous nephropathy (solid tumors)
   Minimal change disease or focal glomerulosclerosis
      (Hodgkin's disease)
   Proliferative glomerulonephritis
   Amyloidosis—multiple myeloma
Hemolytic-uremic syndrome
   Mucin-producing tumors
   Certain chemotherapy agents
Tubulointerstitial disease
   Hypercalcemia
   Cisplatin, ifosfamide, nitrosurea
   Tumor lysis syndrome (hyperuricemia,
      hyperphosphatemia)
   Tumor infiltration (lymphoma, leukemia)
Intratubular obstruction
   Uric acid
   Immunoglobulin light chains
   Methotrexate
   Acyclovir
Urinary tract obstruction
Electrolyte disorders
   Hyponatremia (SIADH)
   Hypercalcemia
   Hypophosphatemia

SIADH, syndrome of inappropriate antidiuretic hormone.

kidney results from filtration of toxic light chains leading to direct tubular injury and intratubular obstruction secondary to cast formation. Myeloma kidney can cause acute or chronic renal failure. In addition, light chains may cause tubular dysfunction without obstruction or decrease in the glomerular filtration rate. The major clinical manifestation in these cases is the development of renal tubular acidosis. Multiple myeloma is also associated with the development of amyloidosis, which typically presents as the nephrotic syndrome and chronic progressive renal insufficiency. Hypercalcemia occurs in a significant portion of patients with multiple myeloma. Severe hypercalcemia can cause acute renal failure directly. Hypercalcemia is also associated with nausea and vomiting. The attendant depletion of the extracellular fluid volume renders the patient susceptible to other renal insults, including drug toxicity and toxicity to light chains. Finally, patients with multiple myeloma appear to be more prone to radiographic contrast media–induced acute renal failure.

The hemolytic-uremic syndrome and thrombotic thrombocytopenic purpura occur in association with malignancy. The triad of acute renal failure, thrombocytopenia, and microangiopathic hemolytic anemia characterizes the hemolytic-uremic syndrome. Thrombotic thrombocytopenic purpura is characterized by the same findings but also fever and focal neurologic deficits. Mucin-secreting adenocarcinomas and some chemotherapeutic agents such as mitomycin C, bleomycin with cisplatin, and radiation therapy with high-dose cyclophosphamide have been associated with these syndromes.

Uric acid–induced acute renal failure and tumor lysis syndrome are complications of malignancy and its treatment. The findings are related to the death of a large number of cells and include hyperuricemia, hyperphosphatemia, hypocalcemia, hyperkalemia, and acidosis. Acute renal failure occurs frequently. These syndromes occur more commonly in patients with lymphoma, especially after radiation therapy or administration of chemotherapeutic agents. Hydration and administration of allopurinol prior to therapy can significantly reduce the development of renal injury.

Although infiltration of the kidney with tumor cells is common in some malignancies, acute or subacute renal failure is uncommon. Cases of acute renal failure secondary to infiltration of the kidney with lymphoma or leukemic cells, however, have been reported. These patients present with acute renal failure, a benign urinalysis, and enlarged kidneys with increased echogenicity on ultrasound examination.

A large number of chemotherapeutic agents have been associated with the development of acute tubular necrosis, acute interstitial nephritis, or intratubular obstruction (see Table 27–9). Ifosfamide nephrotoxicity presents an interesting clinical picture characterized by non–gap metabolic acidosis, hypophosphatemia, glucosuria, aminoaciduria, polyuria, and hypokalemia.

HIV INFECTION AND ACUTE RENAL FAILURE

Renal involvement as well as electrolyte disorders are common clinical complications of human immunodeficiency virus (HIV) infection. Acute renal failure occurs in acquired immunodeficiency syndrome (AIDS) patients who are critically ill and/or are receiving nephrotoxic medications. In recent years, a pathologically unique renal disease, the HIV-associated nephropathy, has been described. HIV-associated nephropathy occurs in approximately 5% to 10% of patients with HIV infection. This entity is characterized histologically by the presence of "collapsing" focal segmental glomerulosclerosis with severe interstitial nephritis. Clinically, it is also characterized by the presence of severe nephrotic syndrome. Characteristically, the ultrasound shows large kidneys with increased echogenicity. The disease progresses to end-stage renal disease rapidly within months.

Complications of Acute Renal Failure

The development of acute renal failure is a significant complication and is associated with important losses of normal homeostatic functions of the kidney (Table 27–10). Depending on the severity of the insult, most patients with acute renal failure demonstrate an inability to regulate the extracellular volume. They fail to respond to excessive losses of fluid and electrolytes from the gastrointestinal tract by increasing tubular reabsorption and fail to excrete excessive amounts of fluid and electrolytes ingested or administered systemically. Volume overload is the more common abnormality manifested clinically as hypertension, edema, and congestive heart failure. A significant number of patients with acute renal failure have abnormalities in serum electrolyte concentrations, including hyperkalemia, hypocalcemia, hyperphosphatemia, hypermagnesemia, and hyperuricemia. Acidosis is also a common finding.

The inability of the kidney to excrete urea and other nitrogenous waste products may result in the uremic syndrome constellation

Table 27-10
Clinical Presentation and Complications of Acute Renal Failure

Urine Volume	Volume Status	Organ Symptoms	Electrolytes/Acid Base
Oliguria	Volume overload	Gastrointestinal tract: anorexia, vomiting, gastritis, hemorrhage	Hyponatremia
Anuria	Volume depletion		Hyperkalemia
Polyuria		Central nervous system: lethargy, agitation, asterixis, seizures, coma	Hypocalcemia
Fluctuating urine volume			Hyperphosphatemia
		Cardiovascular system: congestive heart failure, pericarditis, arrhythmias	Metabolic acidosis
		Hematologic system: anemia, platelet dysfunction, WBC dysfunction	
		Skin: pruritus, vasculitis	

WBC, white blood cell.

of signs and symptoms reflecting dysfunction of many organ systems (see Table 27–10). Gastrointestinal abnormalities are common and include anorexia, nausea, vomiting, and erosive gastritis with gastrointestinal hemorrhage. Hematologic disorders occur, including development of anemia and platelet dysfunction. Infection is a common complication in patients with acute renal failure due to alterations in the function of polymorphonuclear leukocytes, lymphocytes, and plasma cells. Neurologic complications can vary from minor changes in mentation to severe lethargy or agitation, asterixis, and seizures. Cardiovascular complications include volume overload, uremic pericarditis, as well as arrhythmias triggered by electrolyte disorders. The exact nature of the uremic toxin is not known, but the BUN level appears to correlate with symptoms and BUN is used as a surrogate marker for the definition of the syndrome.

Outcome and Management of Acute Renal Failure

Despite advances in the treatment of acute renal failure, especially when it occurs in the intensive care unit, this complication continues to be associated with a poor prognosis and a mortality rate of approximately 50% or more. This high mortality rate relates to the multisystem organ failure syndrome often seen in the intensive care unit. With dialytic therapy, patients die of the underlying disease process rather than from uremia. Survivors may regain near-normal renal function. Although animal studies have suggested that substances such as dopamine, calcium channel blockers, natriuretic peptides, and growth factors may be of value in the treatment and prevention of acute renal failure, none have been shown to be associated with meaningful changes in outcome of acute renal failure in humans. A number of potentially beneficial measures, however, should be considered during the different phases of acute renal failure. Some cases of acute renal failure can be prevented by avoiding nephrotoxic drugs in high-risk patients. The state of hydration should be monitored carefully prior to administration of radiographic contrast agents. The

administration of allopurinol before intense chemotherapy should be considered as prophylaxis against tumor lysis–induced renal failure. Volume deficits should be corrected in all patients to reverse prerenal azotemia and to reduce the risk of development of ischemic acute tubular necrosis. Obstruction to the flow of urine should be diagnosed and treated in a timely fashion to prevent irreversible renal damage. The dosage of all medications should be adjusted for the degree of renal failure. Finally, since the most common cause of death in patients with acute renal failure is sepsis, every effort should be made to prevent this complication.

Conservative, nondialytic treatment is available for selected abnormalities in patients with acute renal failure. Diuretics may be of value in patients with signs and symptoms of fluid overload. Hyperkalemia can be a lethal complication of renal failure. The risk of hyperkalemia can be reduced by avoidance of medications that can elevate the serum concentration of potassium and with restriction of potassium intake. Acute hyperkalemia can be treated with calcium gluconate, glucose and insulin, and/or beta-agonists. Potassium-binding resins can be used to promote potassium excretion in the bowel. Finally, severe hyperkalemia unresponsive to these therapeutic interventions is an indication for dialysis. Hyperphosphatemia may be treated with phosphate binders and a low-phosphorus diet. Calcium carbonate is useful as a phosphate binder and also serves to correct hypocalcemia. Metabolic acidosis can be partially prevented by a low-protein diet and treatment with sodium bicarbonate. Severe acidosis refractory to bicarbonate administration is also an indication for dialysis. A low-protein diet may help prevent uremic symptoms by maintaining the BUN at relatively lower levels. Caution is advised since restric-

Table 27–11
Indications for Acute Dialysis

Pulmonary edema*
Hyperkalemia*
Metabolic acidosis*
Uremic pericarditis*
Uremic central nervous system symptoms

*If conservative treatment is unsuccessful or contraindicated.

tion of protein intake may not be desirable in catabolic patients. Anemia can be treated with transfusions if severe. Platelet dysfunction can be treated with transfusion of packed red blood cells, vasopressin analogs, or estrogen if bleeding is problematic and/or the patient requires surgery or biopsy. Dialysis also reverses, in part, the defect in platelet function.

If conservative measures fail, dialysis may be required. The indications for acute dialysis (Table 27–11) are severe volume overload that does not respond to diuretics, hyperkalemia that persists despite conservative treatment, and severe metabolic acidosis. The presence of pericarditis or severe central nervous system abnormalities are also indications for dialysis.

Intermittent hemodialysis, peritoneal dialysis, and various modes of continuous-dialysis therapies are now available for the treatment of acute renal failure. Advances in the dialytic treatment of patients in acute renal failure have been made and newer, more biocompatible dialyzer membranes have been associated with better patient survival. In addition, use of continuous renal replacement therapies may contribute to improved survival.

SUGGESTED READINGS

1. Bennett WM, Henrich WL, Stoff JS: The renal effects of nonsteroidal anti-inflammatory drugs: Summary and recommendations. Am J Kidney Dis 28:S56–S62, 1996.
2. Coffman TM: Renal failure caused by therapeutic agents. In Greenberg A, Cheung AK, Coffman TM, et al (eds): Primer on Kidney Diseases. San Diego, Academic Press, 1994, pp 139–145.
3. Hou SH, Bushinsky DA, Wish JB, et al: Hospital-acquired renal insufficiency: A prospective study. Am J Med 74:243–248, 1983.
4. Humes HD: Aminoglycoside nephrotoxicity. Kidney Int 33:900–911, 1988.
5. Hutchison FN: Management of acute renal disease. In Greenberg A, Cheung AK, Coffman TM, et al (eds): Primer on Kidney Diseases. San Diego, Academic Press, 1994, pp 157–162.
6. Meyers CM: Acute interstitial nephritis. In Greenberg A, Cheung AK, Coffman TM, et al (eds): Primer on Kidney Diseases. San Diego, Academic Press, 1994, pp 153–157.
7. Molitoris B: Ischemic acute renal failure. In Greenberg A, Cheung AK, Coffman TM, et al (eds): Primer on Kidney Diseases. San Diego, Academic Press, 1994, pp 134–139.
8. Rose BD: Acute renal failure—prerenal disease versus acute tubular necrosis. In Pathophysiology of Renal Disease, 2nd ed. Boston, McGraw-Hill, 1987, pp 63–117.
9. Thadhani R, Pascual M, Bonventre JV: Acute renal failure. N Engl J Med 334:1448–1460, 1996.
10. Whelton A: Nonsteroidal anti-inflammatory drugs: Effects on kidney function. In Greenberg A, Cheung AK, Coffman TM, et al (eds): Primer on Kidney Diseases. San Diego, Academic Press, 1994, pp 163–167.

28

Endocrine and Metabolic Disorders

Robert Hoeldtke
Unyime O. Nseyo

The endocrine system directly or indirectly affects the development and physiologic functions of the genitourinary system. The effect of endocrine and metabolic disorders in sexual, micturitional, and renal functions are discussed in other chapters in this book. This chapter reviews primarily the adrenal gland, including highlights of its hypofunctional and hyperfunctional states, malignant degeneration, and algorithms for evaluating incidental adrenal masses.

Adrenal Structure and Function

ANATOMY

The adrenal glands are small, thin yellowish, triangular (right) or elongated (left) endocrine organs. Each adrenal gland is located on top of the kidney. These retroperitoneal organs lie within the specialized Gerota's fascia. The adrenal remains in its retroperitoneal position in a case of ectopic location or congenital absence of the kidney. The adrenals can be ectopically located near the kidneys, celiac axis, testes, or spermatic cord. When the kidneys are absent, the adrenals are always present. The adrenal has two parts: the outer cortex derived from the ectoderm and the inner layer or medulla derived from the mesoderm. The central medulla is composed primarily of chromaffin cells, which have a neuroendocrine function and secrete the catecholamine hormones norepinephrine and epinephrine. The three zones of the outer cortex secrete steroids, weak androgens, and estrogens.

Blood Supply

The adrenal is supplied by three arteries: the renal (inferior), aorta (middle), and inferior phrenic (superior). However, the adrenal is drained by a single vein: A short right adrenal vein drains directly into the inferior vena cava, while the left adrenal vein drains into the left renal vein.

Innervation

The main innervation to the adrenal is the preganglionic sympathetic nerve fibers to the medullary cells. The cortical cells receive sparse adrenergic innervation.

PHYSIOLOGY

In the adrenal cortex conversion of cholesterol to pregnenolone is the first and rate-limiting step in the synthesis of adrenal steroids. The hormones produced in the adrenal cortex are (1) the glucocorticoids, including cortisol, which is involved in carbohydrate and protein metabolism, and (2) mineralocorticoids, including aldosterone, which regulate sodium and potassium balance. These hormones are essential for life. The adrenals secrete a minimal quantity of androgens and estrogens. The adrenal medulla releases catecholamine hormones epinephrine and small quantities of norepinephrine into the circulation.

Adrenal Diseases

ADRENAL INSUFFICIENCY

Adrenocortical insufficiency can result from a variety of adrenal diseases or from decreased secretion of adrenocorticotropic hormone (ACTH) secondary to dysfunction of the hypothalamic-pituitary axis. The classic form of adrenocortical insufficiency, Addison's disease, results in decreased secretion of glucocorticoids and mineralocorticoids, and is also associated with decreased secretion of adrenomedullary catecholamines. This disease is rare. Causes of Addison's disease are tuberculosis, autoimmune disease, amyloidosis, histoplasmosis, blastomycosis, metastatic carcinoma, iatrogenic (including high-dose adrenal steroid therapy), adrenalectomy, and ketoconazole therapy. Adrenal medullary insufficiency has also been recently described in patients with autonomic neuropathy, which typically results in a decreased epinephrine but normal cortisol response to hypoglycemia.

Clinical Features

The signs and symptoms of cortisol deficiency—lethargy, muscular weakness, anorexia, and weight loss—dominate the clinical picture in most patients, but some present with abdominal cramps, nausea, diarrhea, and, rarely, depression. Concomitant aldosterone deficiency leads to hypovolemia and orthostatic hypotension, which may explain the peculiar craving for salt experienced by some patients. Impaired epinephrine secretion in patients with insulin-dependent diabetes mellitus may compromise the warning signals (palpitations and tremor) as well as the metabolic response (glycogen breakdown) that defends them against hypoglycemia.

Diagnosis

The classic and most specific physical finding, hyperpigmentation of the skin and mucosal surfaces, reflects excessive ACTH secretion secondary to decreased cortisol feedback. The pigmentary changes may be localized, however, or absent altogether. Occasionally the dominant cutaneous finding is vitiligo, a marker of autoimmune endocrinopathy in general, and believed to reflect antibodies directed at tyrosinase, a critical enzyme in melanin formation.

Specific Types of Adrenal Insufficiency

PRIMARY ADRENOCORTICAL INSUFFICIENCY (ADDISON'S DISEASE)

Etiologic Factors. These include, in addition to those listed earlier, tuberculosis and related granulomatous diseases, and autoimmune adrenalitis, sometimes seen in association with other autoimmune endocrine disorders, particularly thyroiditis and insulin-dependent diabetes mellitus. Adrenal insufficiency occurs in association with acquired immunodeficiency syndrome (AIDS) in up to 5% of patients in the terminal phases of the disease. Another recently recognized cause of acute adrenal insufficiency is antiphospholipid syndrome, in which circulating antiphospholipid antibodies promote the formation of multiple arterial and venous thromboses.

SECONDARY ADRENOCORTICAL INSUFFICIENCY

Etiology. Although cortisol deficiency dominates the clinical features of primary adrenal insufficiency, this is not the case in secondary adrenal insufficiency in which deficiencies of other pituitary hormones, thyroid-stimulating hormone, follicle-stimulating hormone, luteinizing hormone, or growth hormone (in children) become evident prior to the recognition of a cortisol deficit. Isolated corticotropin deficiency, although uncommon, can cause cortisol deficiency characterized by weakness, fatigue, abdominal complaints, and weight loss. The diagnosis is difficult because the classic physical finding seen in primary adrenocortical insufficiency, hyperpigmentation, is not present because ACTH is deficient. In most patients, there are other indications of pituitary pathology, such as mass effects of a tumor or multisystem involvement by granulomatous disease (sarcoidosis or histiocytosis X). Diabetes insipidus may dominate the clinical picture in patients with hypothalamic tumors or craniopharyngiomas.

The most common cause of secondary adrenocortical insufficiency is suppression of the hypothalamic pituitary axis by chronic glucocorticoid therapy.

Laboratory Assessment of Adrenal Function

The following abnormalities evident on routine laboratory testing support the diagnosis of adrenal insufficiency:

1. Hyponatremia, present in most patients with primary adrenal insufficiency, reflects aldosterone deficiency and sodium wasting. Hyponatremia is less common in secondary adrenal insufficiency because the renin-angiotensin system is intact and aldosterone secretion is normal. When hyponatremia occurs in patients with hypopituitarism, it often reflects deficiencies of thyroid hormones as well as cortisol since both are needed for the excretion of a dilute urine.

2. Hyperkalemia is associated with primary but not secondary adrenal insufficiency (Table 28–1).

3. Confirmation of the diagnosis of adrenal insufficiency is based on the measurement of serum cortisol. The test should always be performed in the morning between 7 and 9 o'clock because diurnal rhythms in adrenal function cause some normal subjects to have low cortisol secretion in the afternoon and evening. Although very low serum cortisol concentrations (<3 µg/dL) are unequivocal, some patients with Addison's disease have a serum cortisol as high as 12 µg/dL, well within the normal range (6 to 24 µg/dL). Critically ill patients, or those who have experienced recent trauma or infections, may have transient elevations of their serum cortisol that mask a chronic deficiency state. Therefore, all diagnostic studies are difficult to interpret in this setting. If chronic primary adrenocortical insufficiency is present, cortisol is low or low normal, but ACTH is invariably elevated (>100 pg/mL or 22 pmol/L) and no additional tests are needed. The widespread availability of corticotropin measurements has obviated the need for provocative tests in most patients with primary adrenal insufficiency, although these tests may be needed to confirm the diagnosis of secondary adrenocortical insufficiency.

Treatment

Patients with adrenocortical insufficiency should be treated with 15 to 25 mg of hydrocortisone daily, 60% to 70% of which should be taken in the morning. Equivalent amounts of less expensive glucocorticoids may be substituted. The smallest dose that alleviates the presenting symptoms should be used, with the understanding that some people will be unusually susceptible to weight gain, hirsutism, or osteoporosis on even the usual replacement dose. In addition, patients with primary adrenocortical insufficiency should be given mineralocorticoid replacement with fludrocortisone, 50 to 200 µg/day. This is generally unnecessary in patients with secondary adrenal insufficiency since the renin-angiotensin system and aldosterone secretion are intact. Patients should be instructed on the importance of wearing a warning bracelet that states their diagnosis. Patients should also be educated on the importance of doubling or tripling the dose of glucocorticoid when they have a systemic infection or have experienced trauma, including surgical procedures. Finally, they must understand the necessity for parenteral therapy if they are experiencing nausea and vomiting or are too ill to take oral medicine. Patients with acute adrenal insufficiency should be administered 100

Table 28–1
Biochemical Abnormalities in Adrenal Insufficiency

| Element | Adrenal Insufficiency | | Isolated Hypoaldosteronism |
	Primary	*Secondary*	
Cortisol	Decreased	Decreased	Normal
ACTH	Increased	Decreased	Normal
Aldosterone	Decreased	Normal	Decreased
Renin	Increased	Normal	Variable
Epinephrine	Decreased	Decreased	Normal
Sodium	Decreased	Decreased or Normal	Normal
Potassium	Increased	Normal	Increased

ACTH, adrenocorticotropic hormone.

mg of hydrocortisone immediately and given another 100 to 200 mg as a 24-hour intravenous infusion. Isotonic saline, at least 2 L per 24 hours, supplemented with glucose, should also be administered emergently. The response to therapy is generally gratifying, although some patients need to be treated for 4 to 7 days before their symptoms are relieved.

Adrenal Insufficiency/ Hypofunction: Highlights

Causes
  Dysfunction of hypothalamic-pituitary axis
  Tuberculosis
  Autoimmune disease
  Amyloidosis
  Histoplasmosis
  Blastomycosis
  Metastatic carcinoma
  Exogenous steroid therapy
  Adrenalectomy
  Ketoconazole therapy
  AIDS
Signs and symptoms
  Lethargy
  Muscle weakness
  Anorexia
  Abdominal cramps
  Nausea
  Diarrhea
  Depression
  Hypotension
  Salt craving
Diagnosis
  Skin hyperpigmentation
  Hyponatremia
  Hyperkalemia
  Elevated ACTH
  Low serum cortisol
Treatment
  Hydrocortisone 15 to 25 mg daily (60% to 70%) in the morning
  Fludrocortisone 50 to 200 µg daily

Note other causes of hyperkalemia include beta blockers, angiotensin-converting enzyme inhibitors, and angiotensin-receptor blockers.

HYPOALDOSTERONISM

Etiology

Hypoaldosteronism is an unusual disease characterized by chronic asymptomatic hy-perkalemia. It is frequently referred to as selective aldosteronism or isolated aldosteronism since cortisol secretion, by definition, is normal. Failure of renin secretion (hyporeninemic hypoaldosteronism) is the most common form. The pathogenesis of the hyporeninemia is poorly understood, and multiple mechanisms have been postulated, possibly including (1) sympathetic neural dysfunction, (2) damage to the juxtaglomerular (JG) cells, and (3) impaired renin biosynthesis.

Clinical Features

Although the hyperkalemia is generally asymptomatic, occasional patients have muscle weakness or cardiac arrhythmias, most often complete heart block. Sexual dysfunction in men or orthostatic hypotension may be indicative of autonomic neuropathy. Elderly patients typically have high blood pressure when supine that normalizes with sitting or standing. Thirty percent to 50% of patients have diabetes mellitus. Amyloidosis, multiple myeloma, sickle cell anemia, cirrhosis, and AIDS have also been associated with hypoaldosteronism.

Evaluation and Diagnosis

The first step in patient evaluation entails excluding other causes of chronic hyperkalemia. It is first necessary to confirm that the hyperkalemia is reproducible and not an artifact caused by technical difficulties or fist clenching during the phlebotomy. Spurious hyperkalemia, such as occurs in patients with thrombocytosis, also needs to be excluded. The diagnosis cannot be made if patients have end-stage renal disease and a glomerular filtration rate of less than 10 mg/min/1.73 m². Normal cortisol secretion is also a sine qua non for the diagnosis of hypoaldosteronism. It is necessary to document that the patient is not ingesting drugs that cause hyperkalemia, most notably potassium-sparing diuretics or converting enzyme inhibitors, or occasionally indomethacin, heparin, or beta-adrenergic antagonists. A definitive diagnosis can be made by documenting a low plasma aldosterone level under circumstances that would normally activate the renin-angiotensin system, such as assuming the upright posture for 3 hours. In typical patients, especially those with diabetic autonomic neuropathy, the clinical diagnosis suffices and aldosterone measurements are unnecessary. The measurement of plasma renin activity, although of academic interest, is not always necessary.

Treatment

Hypoaldosteronism can be treated with orally active mineralocorticoid, fludrocortisone 0.1 or 0.2 mg daily. This may cause dangerous elevations in the blood pressure, however, in patients with moderate renal insufficiency, autonomic neuropathy, and hypertension. Potassium-wasting loop diuretics, such as furosemide, are frequently substituted. Some patients may need to restrict dietary potassium or ingest a resin such as sodium polystyrene sulfonate, which binds potassium in the gastrointestinal tract.

Hypoaldosteronism: Highlights

Causes
    Hyporeninemia secondary to sympathetic neural dysfunction
    JG cell damage
    Impaired renin synthesis
Symptoms
    Cardiac arrhythmias
    Muscle weakness
    Orthostasis
Diagnosis
    Hyperkalemia
    Low plasma aldosterone
Treatment
    Fludrocortisone 0.1 to 0.2 mg daily
    Loop diuretics

ADRENAL HYPERFUNCTION

The major classifications of adrenal hyperfunction are presented in Table 28–2, along with the diagnostic features.

Primary Aldosteronism

Background and Epidemiology. This is also called *Conn's syndrome.* Primary aldosteronism is an unusual cause of hypertension. It accounts for 0.1% to 0.3% of hypertension in the United States. The male-to-female ratio is 1:2.5, and two thirds of the patients are between 30 and 50 years of age.

Clinical Features. Primary hyperaldosteronism should be ruled out in any hypertensive patient. Hypokalemia is present in the vast majority of patients and may lead to fatigue, muscle weakness, or polyuria. A metabolic alkalosis is invariably associated since the aldosterone-stimulated sodium potassium exchange in the distal tubule also causes a concomitant loss of hydrogen ions. In most instances, however, the metabolic abnormality is diagnosed before the patient becomes symptomatic because serum electrolyte measurements are routinely measured in all patients with recently diagnosed hypertension.

Diagnosis. The first step in the laboratory evaluation is to demonstrate inappropriate potassium excretion greater than 30 mEq/day. This requires placing patients on a diet that contains at least 100 mEq of sodium daily, which provides the necessary stimulus

Table 28-2
Evaluation of Adrenal Hyperfunction

	Pheochromocytoma	Primary Aldosteronism	Cushing's Syndrome
Screening tests	Urinary catecholamines Urinary metanephrine and normetanephrine	Serum K Urine K	AM cortisol following 1 mg dexamethasone at midnight
Diagnostic tests	Plasma catecholamines	Plasma aldosterone Urine aldosterone Plasma renin	Urinary cortisol
Assessment of autonomy	Clonidine suppression	Postural stimulation	Urinary cortisol: follow low-dose (0.5 mg every 6 hours) then high-dose (2 mg every 6 hours) dexamethasone
Localization	Abdominal CT or MRI ^{131}I metaiodobenzyl-quanidine imaging	Abdominal CT or MRI	*Plasma ACTH*—low: abdominal CT or MRI; normal or high: pituitary CT or MRI

ACTH, adrenocorticotropic hormone.

to the distal tubular sodium-potassium exchange mechanisms that promote potassium wasting. Diuretics must be discontinued for at least 2 weeks, preferably longer. Definitive diagnosis depends the demonstration of excessive concentrations of aldosterone in serum and urine and suppressed plasma renin activity. A normal or high plasma renin level rules out primary aldosteronism. Hyperreninemia suggests that hypokalemia is the result of secondary hyperaldosteronism, which in the setting of hypertension would most likely indicate the presence of renovascular disease. The presence of edema excludes primary hyperaldosteronism. Serum sodium may be slightly elevated; slight proteinuria may be present; and an electrocardiogram (ECG) may show premature ventricular contractions and depressed ST segments, T waves, and the presence of U waves.

Aldosteronism Secondary to Adrenal Tumor. Although the diagnosis of excess of aldosterone is generally straightforward, differentiation of adenoma from bilateral hyperplasia, which accounts for approximately 40% of cases, is frequently difficult. The usual test for making this differentiation is to determine the effect of postural stress on renin and aldosterone. In patients with hyperplasia, the renin-angiotensin system remains under physiologic regulation, so posture will stimulate the secretion of both hormones, whereas in patients with adenomas, aldosterone secretion is autonomous, and the renin suppression cannot be reversed physiologically. Imaging studies, particularly computed tomography (CT), are frequently employed to diagnose an aldosterone-secreting adenoma, but these tumors are frequently very small and more difficult to diagnose than other hormone-producing adrenal tumors. Misleading findings can result in patients with nonfunctioning adrenal tumors that are common in the general population (as discussed later). Magnetic resonance (MR) imaging studies are no more reliable than CT. Radiolabeled ^{131}I cholesterol scanning frequently makes it possible to differentiate unilateral from bilateral adrenal hyperfunction, but this is estimated to be accurate in only 72% of patients and is useful only in patients with abnormal CT scans.

Treatment. The differentiation between adenoma and hyperplasia is clinically important because they are treated differently. Surgery is generally recommended for those with adenomas even though medical therapy with spironolactone 200 to 400 mg daily may control the blood pressure as well as the hypokalemia. Chronic use of spironolactone may cause gynecomastia in men or menstrual disturbances in women. Patients with hyperplasia are generally treated medically. Although spironolactone corrects the hypokalemia, other antihypertensive drugs, usually calcium channel blocking agents, may need to be added to correct the hypertension. Diuretics can also be added to control hypertension provided that potassium is monitored and supplemented appropriately.

Adrenal Hyperfunction: Highlights

Causes
    Adrenal tumors
    Bilateral adrenal hyperplasia
Symptoms
    Fatigue
    Muscle weakness
    Polyuria
Diagnosis
    Increased urine potassium
    Hypokalemia
    Suppressed plasma renin activity
    Elevated plasma and urinary aldosterone
    Abnormal ECG
Treatment
    Surgery for adenomas
    Spironolactone 200 to 400 mg daily
    Diuretics or calcium channel blocker for hypertension

PHEOCHROMOCYTOMA

Epidemiology

Catecholamine-secreting tumors of chromaffin tissue most typically (95%) occur in the adrenal gland, but they may be found throughout the body from the floor of the pelvis to the carotid body. They have been described in such unusual locations as the pericardium or the urinary bladder. Most extra-adrenal pheochromocytomas develop in the paravertebral sympathetic ganglia, the organ of Zuckerkandl near the aortic bifurcation, or the posterior mediastinum. Approximately 10% of patients with extra-adrenal pheochromocytomas have multiple tumors or bilateral adrenomedullary tumors.

Although pheochromocytomas constitute an uncommon cause of hypertension (0.1% to 0.2%), they frequently appear unexpectedly at autopsy. Some series of patients with incidentally discovered adrenal masses on imaging studies performed for other reasons have included a surprising number of pheochromocytomas (as discussed later). Undiagnosed pheochromocytomas may lead to lethal hypertensive crises, cardiac arrhythmias, congestive heart failure, cardiovascular accidents, cardiomyopathy, and hemorrhage. Surgical removal may cure the hypertension and eliminate the risk of cardiac and other complications. The diagnosis of a pheochromocytoma may lead to the discovery of one of the multiple endocrine neoplasia (Type 2) syndromes or other genetic disorders such as von Hippel–Lindau disease, or neurofibromatosis. These unusual variants should be suspected whenever the diagnosis is made in childhood or bilateral adrenomedullary or multiple extra-adrenal tumors are encountered.

Diagnosis

The urinary excretion of catecholamines or their *o*-methylated metabolites metanephrine and normetanephrine are clearly elevated in the majority of patients, although mild elevations are also seen in essential hypertension. The diagnosis of pheochromocytomas is made by demonstrating elevated levels of catecholamines in the blood or urine. The excretion of vanillylmandelic acid, the major catecholamine metabolite, is a less sensitive test. Plasma catecholamines can also be measured, but the patients must be supine for at least 15 minutes before the test. Aging, cigarette smoking, certain antihypertensive drugs such as alpha-adrenergic blockers or vasodilators increase plasma norepinephrine significantly (by nearly a factor of 2), which must be considered in interpreting test results in these individuals. Many patients being evaluated for pheochromocytomas take multiple antihypertensive drugs, which may obscure the interpretation of the catecholamine studies. If

these cannot be safely discontinued for at least 48 hours, it may be useful to switch the patient to clonidine (0.1 to 0.3 µg three times daily), which may suppress catecholamines slightly but will not lead to a false elevation.

The clonidine suppression test is useful in patients with equivocal catecholamine studies. Clonidine (0.3 µg orally) suppresses plasma norepinephrine into the normal range in patients without pheochromocytomas but fails to do so in most patients with catecholamine-secreting tumors because they function autonomously. The test is simple and reliable and has replaced the glucagon and tyramine stimulatory tests, which occasionally resulted in dangerous blood pressure elevations.

Clonidine may cause hypotension, sedation, or bradycardia in patients taking beta-adrenergic antagonists. If the plasma norepinephrine is markedly elevated (>1500 pg/mL), the clonidine suppression test may be unnecessary. It is most useful when the plasma norepinephrine is not dramatically increased (500 to 1500 pg/mL).

The diagnosis of pheochromocytoma is based on the history, physical examination, and catecholamine studies. Imaging studies are necessary for localization that can be readily accomplished with either CT scan or MR imaging, which will detect nearly all adrenomedullary tumors. Scintigraphy using ^{131}I-metaiodobenzylguanidine (mIBG) is superior for extra-adrenal, recurrent, or metastatic pheochromocytomas. Typically malignant pheochromocytomas secrete elevated dopamine levels with high levels of norepinephrine and low epinephrine.

Treatment

Surgical excision is the cornerstone of therapy for pheochromocytomas, since the vast majority are benign and a successful operation is generally curative. The adrenergic stimulation and concomitant hypertension needs to be suppressed preoperatively with oral phenoxybenzamine 10 to 30 mg twice daily. Concomitant beta-adrenergic blockade is only indicated in patients with tachycardia or arrhythmias. Despite these precautions, patients remain at risk for hypertension during the induction with anesthesia or during the removal of the tumor and pressor crises may need to be treated with the rapid-acting alpha-adrenergic antagonist phentolamine (1 to 5 mg intravenously).

Pheochromocytoma: Highlights

95% of pheochromocytomas occur in the adrenal gland

The organ of Zuckerkandl is the most common extra-adrenal site of pheochromocytoma

Symptoms
Lethal hypertensive crisis
Cardiac arrhythmias
Congestive heart failure
Cardiomyopathy
Hemorrhage

Diagnosis
Elevated urinary or plasma catecholamines
Clonidine suppression test

Treatment
Surgical excision of pheochromocytoma
Preoperative suppression with oral phenoxybenzamine, 10 to 30 mg twice daily

CUSHING'S SYNDROME

Epidemiology

Cushing's syndrome is a rare but classic endocrine disorder characterized by adrenal glucocorticoid overproduction. Most cases (75%) are caused by pituitary microadenomas that secrete excessive ACTH, which is responsible for the glucocorticoid overproduction (Cushing's disease). Adrenal adenoma and carcinoma constitute 25% of Cushing's syndrome with glucocorticoid excess. Cushing's syndrome can also result from exogenously administered glucocorticoid. Rarely, Cushing's syndrome is the result of ectopic production of ACTH, most typically oat cell carcinoma of the lungs. In this instance the patients are wasted rather than obese, and neuropsychiatric features or mineralocorticoid overproduction that manifests as hypokalemia and metabolic alkalosis, dominate the clinical presentation.

Clinical Features

The clinical features—truncal obesity, hypertension, diabetes mellitus, abdominal striae,

and osteoporosis—are widely recognized. A wide variety of signs and symptoms (depression, "moon facies," dorsocervical fat pad, easy bruising, and hirsutism) are frequently suggestive but are rarely secondary to Cushing's syndrome unless accompanied by more specific physical findings such as muscle wasting and weakness, thinning of the skin, and purple abdominal striae.

Screening and Diagnosis

Low-dose dexamethasone testing (1 mg of dexamethasone at midnight followed by the measurement of serum cortisol the following morning) is a commonly used screening test. It is a sensitive but nonspecific test; severe depression or uncontrolled diabetes, for example, can lead to nonsuppressibility (false positivity). On the other hand, unequivocal suppression of serum cortisol following low-dose dexamethasone excludes Cushing's syndrome. Urinary free cortisol is a more reliable test and has largely replaced the less specific assays for 17-hydroxycorticosteroids.

Glucocorticoid overproduction may result from an ACTH-secreting pituitary adenoma, an adrenal tumor, or an ectopic source of ACTH. In adrenal pathology serum ACTH concentrations are suppressed and imaging studies generally confirm the presence of an adrenal lesion. Sampling of the venous drainage of the pituitary via the petrosal sinus veins may establish an ACTH source from the pituitary adenoma. This makes it possible to document the source of the excess ACTH and determine whether it derives from the left or right side of the gland, which is a useful guide to the surgeon.

Treatment

Transsphenoidal resection is the treatment of choice for pituitary microadenomas that cause Cushing's syndrome in adults, whereas radiation therapy is the usual initial therapy in children. A wide variety of pharmacologic therapies are available when these primary treatments are ineffective. Adrenal adenomas generally respond to surgical excision, whereas carcinomas are frequently very large or metastatic at diagnosis, in which case surgery is performed for palliative reasons. Mitotane is a cytotoxic agent that selectively affects the adrenal cortex and is the most useful drug for those patients who refuse an operation or have an unsatisfactory response to surgery. The usual doses of mitotane required to suppress glucocorticoid production (2 to 10 g daily) generally cause gastrointestinal side effects. The alternative pharmacologic agents (metapyrone, ketoconazole, or aminoglutethimide) are often ineffective or tolerated poorly. Bilateral adrenalectomy is reserved as a last resort when the pharmacologic treatment of glucocorticoid excess fails.

Cushing's Syndrome: Highlights

Causes
  75% are caused by pituitary microadenoma
  25% are caused by adrenal adenoma and carcinoma or ectopic ACTH
Symptoms
  Hypertension
  Osteoporosis
  Depression
  Diabetes
  Easy bruising
  Hirsutism
Diagnosis
  Dexamethasone test: low dose
  Urinary free cortisol is most reliable test
  Pituitary venous sampling for ACTH locations
Treatment
  Transsphenoidal resection of pituitary adenoma

INCIDENTALLY DISCOVERED ADRENAL MASSES

The widespread use of noninvasive imaging techniques has led to recognition of a new disease entity, the incidentally discovered adrenal tumor or "incidentaloma," which has been estimated to be present in approximately 0.5% of adults undergoing abdominal imaging. Steps for screening the patient with an incidental adrenal tumor are given in Figure 28–1.

Only 5% to 10% of incidentally discovered adrenal tumors are functional and associated

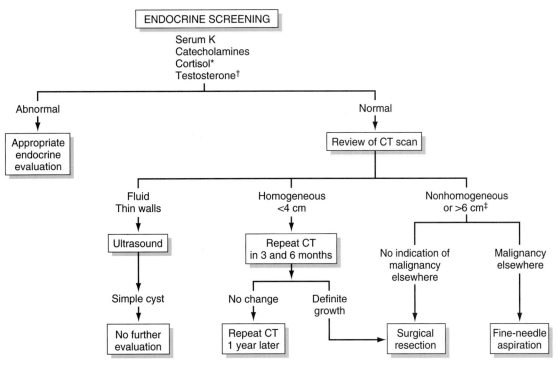

Figure 28-1
Algorithm for evaluation of an adrenal incidentaloma. *Only if there are clinical indications of excess cortisol. †Only in women with hirsutism. ‡Measure dehydroepiandrosterone sulfate, a marker of primary adrenal carcinoma.

with excessive hormone secretion; however, proper follow-up is mandatory. Pheochromocytomas are the most common of the secretory tumors, so catecholamine studies are always indicated since this is a lethal condition if not diagnosed. Some patients with incidental pheochromocytomas do not have hypertension. Aldosteronomas are rarely discovered incidentally; nevertheless serum potassium, a simple and inexpensive test, should be measured in all patients. Cortisol-secreting adenomas are likewise rarely discovered incidentally. Urinary cortisol should therefore be measured only in patients with signs or symptoms of Cushing's syndrome. Androgen-secreting adrenal tumors are likewise rare so the measurement of serum testosterone should be reserved for women with hirsutism. Dehydroepiandrosterone sulfate (a marker of adrenal androgen secretion) should also be measured in patients with hirsutism and in patients suspected of having a primary adrenal carcinoma. Adrenal estrogen overproduction in men is very rare, so estradiol measurements should not be performed unless the tumor is large and there is a new onset of gynecomastia. Finally, the ACTH excess associated with the untreated congenital adrenal hyperplasia may cause adrenal adenomas or nodular hyperplasia. In the most common form of this disorder, 21-hydroxylase deficiency, cortisol synthesis is decreased by the enzymatic defect so ACTH is secreted excessively and leads to hyperandrogenism. The latter is evident in infancy in females who have ambiguous genitalia. Male children may appear normal early in life but then develop precocious puberty. In other children salt wasting as a result of aldosterone deficiency is the predominant clinical manifestation. The diagnosis is missed in some patients who develop hirsutism, oligomenorrhea, or infertility in young adulthood. If these features are present in a patient with an incidentally discovered adrenal tumor, the serum cortisol level will be low and the cortisol precursor 17-hydroxyprogesterone will be elevated or show an exaggerated response to the administration of ACTH.

Occasionally, incidentally discovered adrenal tumors are malignant. Metastatic tumors are more common than primary in most series, particularly if the tumors are bilateral. In most patients with metastatic lesions, the primary will most often have been previously diagnosed. A general malignancy evaluation is not cost effective in those without an obvious primary because the chances of discovering a previously undiagnosed but treatable malignancy are remote. Primary adrenal carcinomas are generally large, so that surgical exploration should be pursued whenever the tumor has a diameter larger than 4 cm. Tumors less than 3 cm in diameter would be followed with repeat imaging study in 3 to 6 months and surgery pursued in those that are enlarging. There are no guidelines for the frequency with which imaging studies should be repeated on long-term follow-up. Most lesions, however, are benign adenomas or myelolipomas and show no evidence of growth.

SUGGESTED READINGS

1. Bravo EL: Pheochromocytoma. *In* Bardin CW (ed): Current Therapy in Endocrinology and Metabolism, 6th ed. St. Louis, CV Mosby, 1997, p 195.
2. DeFronzo R: Hyperkalemia and hyporeninemic hypoaldosteronism. Kidney Int 17:119, 1980.
3. Hoeldtke RD, Boden G: Epinephrine secretion, hypoglycemia unawareness, and diabetic autonomic neuropathy. Ann Intern Med 120:512, 1994.
4. Kloos RT, Gross MD, Fracis IR, et al: Incidentally discovered adrenal masses. Endocrinol Rev 16:460, 1995.
5. Lim RC, Nakayama DK, Biglieri EG, et al: Primary aldosteronism: Changing concepts in diagnosis and management. Am J Surg 152:116, 1986.
6. Nieman LK: Cushing's syndrome. *In* Bardin CW (ed): Current Therapy in Endocrinology and Metabolism, 6th ed. St. Louis, Mosby, 1997, p 1612.
7. Oerkers W: Current concepts: Adrenal insufficiency. N Engl J Med 335:1206, 1996.
8. Redman JF: Anatomy of the genitourinary system. *In* Gillenwater JY, Grayhack JT, Howards SS, et al (eds): Adult and Pediatric Urology, 3rd ed. St. Louis, Mosby-Year Book, 1996, pp 1–61.
9. Werbell SS, Ober KP: Acute adrenal insufficiency. Endocrinol Metab Clin North Am 22:303, 1993.

29

Management of Male Infertility

Joseph J. Del Pizzo
Jonathan P. Jarow

Infertility affects approximately 20% of couples in the United States today. Most of these couples have never had children; this is referred to as *primary infertility*. A significant subset of couples experiences difficulty conceiving despite having had children in the past. This is called *secondary infertility*. Studies of fertile couples reveal that approximately 50% achieve conception within 6 months of initiating unprotected sexual intercourse, whereas 90% conceive within 1 year and 10% take longer than 1 year. Based on this information, the general consensus is to initiate a fertility evaluation only if the couple has not achieved conception after 1 year of unprotected sexual intercourse. The exception to this rule is couples in whom there is a known risk factor for infertility, such as a history of cryptorchidism in the man or advanced age in the woman.

A female infertility factor is present in approximately 70% of couples. The most common etiologies are ovulatory dysfunction, endometriosis, and tubal obstruction. However, studies have shown, as one might anticipate, that the male partner plays a significant role in a couple's inability to achieve conception. Approximately 30% of couples have an isolated male factor as the etiology of their infertility, and an additional 20% have combined male and female factor infertility. Thus, a male-derived factor is present in approximately 50% of infertile couples. Therefore, it is important to begin the male partner's evaluation early in the work-up to avoid unnecessary or inappropriate therapy in the female partner. Many therapeutic interventions depend on the fertility status of both partners, and proper counseling of an infertile couple cannot be performed until both partners have been fully evaluated.

Approximately 1% of men with infertility have a significant underlying medical cause such as testicular cancer, which requires treatment. There are no pathognomonic findings on semen analysis to identify these people. Therefore, it is imperative that men with an abnormal semen analysis undergo a thorough urologic evaluation. Second, performing in vitro fertilization (IVF) via intracytoplasmic sperm injection (ICSI) for all couples with a male factor, regardless of reversibility, is displacing all the risks and intervention on the female partner for the male's problem. Finally, the cost and risk of IVF may be excessive compared with evaluation and treatment of the male partner. There is a small but significant risk associated with hyperstimulation from the hormones given to induce superovulation. In addition, the multiple gestation rates from IVF are greater than 40% in most successful programs. Multiple gestation leads to an increased risk of miscarriage and premature delivery. For all of these reasons, the best medical practice for both partners is to evaluate any male partner with an abnormal semen analysis and to use specific therapies for male factor infertility whenever possible.

Male Reproductive Physiology

To evaluate and treat men with infertility, it is important to have a basic understanding of

335

male reproductive physiology. Although male reproduction may appear quite complicated, it is much easier to understand if one employs an analogy of industrial production. Male infertility can be due to an abnormality in any of the components of industrial production, including management, production, delivery, or product design. These areas are analogous to the endocrine disorders, abnormalities of spermatogenesis, ejaculatory disorders, and poor sperm quality, respectively.

HYPOTHALAMIC-PITUITARY-GONADAL AXIS

The testis is a dual organ in terms of both structure and function. The two products are the hormone testosterone and spermatozoa. The testis is made of many seminiferous tubules, which is where sperm are produced. The space between the seminiferous tubules is called the *interstitial compartment.* The Leydig's cells located in the interstitial compartment produce testosterone. Hormones produced by the anterior pituitary gland control these testicular compartments (Fig. 29–1). Luteinizing hormone (LH) stimulates production of testosterone, and follicle-stimulating hormone (FSH) stimulates spermatogenesis. The pituitary gland is controlled by the hypothalamus, which secretes gonadotropin-releasing hormone (GnRH). GnRH has a stimulatory effect on pituitary release of both LH and FSH. There is feedback inhibition of pituitary gonadotropin secretion by hormones produced in the testis. Inhibin produced by Sertoli's cells inhibits FSH secretion, whereas testosterone inhibits secretion of both LH and FSH.

Testosterone, a steroid hormone, is present in the circulation in both a free and bound form. The principal binding protein for testosterone is steroid hormone–binding globulin (SHBG), which is produced in the liver. Testosterone also binds to albumin. Testosterone is tightly bound to SHBG, but the albumin fraction is less tightly bound and is considered bioavailable. Approximately 2% of circulating testosterone is free, another 30% is loosely bound, and the remainder is tightly bound to SHBG. Once testosterone reaches a target organ, it diffuses into the cell where it may be metabolized into a more potent

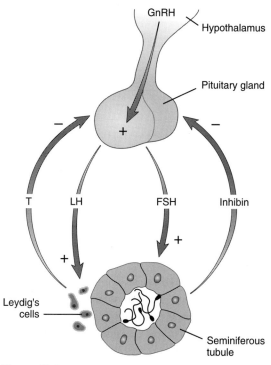

Figure 29–1
Schematic of the hypothalamic-pituitary-gonadal axis. GnRH, gonadotropin-releasing hormone; T, testosterone; LH, luteinizing hormone; FSH, follicle-stimulating hormone.

androgen (known as *dihydrotestosterone*) or a less potent androgen, converted into estradiol, or left intact. Steroid hormones bind to an intracellular receptor molecule, which then interacts with the DNA, influencing transcription. Although small amounts of estradiol are produced in the testis, the primary source of this hormone in men is from the peripheral aromatization of testosterone into estradiol in fatty tissue.

The feedback inhibition of testosterone on the pituitary gland is primarily through estradiol. Clinical evidence suggests that testosterone is converted into estradiol within the pituitary gland and the estradiol inhibits gonadotropin secretion. Thus, systemic administration of estrogens produces hypogonadism by feedback inhibition of pituitary function. Conversely, administration of antiestrogens such as clomiphene citrate increases serum levels of LH, FSH, and testosterone by blocking feedback inhibition of the pituitary gland.

Both testosterone and FSH are required for

the initiation and maintenance of quantitatively and qualitatively normal spermatogenesis. The concentration of testosterone within the human testis is more than 100-fold higher than levels seen in the serum. This is due to both the local production of testosterone within the testis and the high concentration of binding proteins such as SHBG and androgen-binding protein within the testis. Peripheral administration of testosterone actually lowers the intratesticular concentration of testosterone to a level inadequate to support spermatogenesis owing to feedback inhibition of pituitary gonadotropin. Thus, testosterone is a contraceptive agent when administered in routine replacement doses such as 200 mg intramuscularly every 2 weeks. The dosage required to achieve adequate intratesticular concentrations of testosterone by peripheral administration would produce toxic levels of testosterone in the serum.

Spermatogenesis

Spermatogenesis takes place within the seminiferous tubules of the testis that are lined by germ cells and Sertoli's cells. Spermatogenesis has three distinct steps: mitotic division of stem cells (spermatogonia), meiotic division to produce a haploid genotype (spermatocytes), and development of mature spermatozoa by a process of spermiogenesis (spermatids). The Sertoli's cells lining the seminiferous tubules support the process of spermatogenesis. In addition, Sertoli's cells play an important role in the blood-testis barrier, which both protects mature sperm from the immune system and maintains a special environment to support their development. The tight junctions between adjacent Sertoli's cells are first identifiable at the onset of puberty.

The total process of spermatogenesis takes approximately 72 days. Therefore, the effect of any intervention that enhances or is deleterious to fertility may not be seen for several months. Spermatogenesis is also temperature sensitive, requiring a scrotal temperature gradient of approximately 2 or 3° F below the core body temperature. Anything that raises intratesticular temperature, such as a febrile episode, may have a profound effect on spermatogenesis for several months.

Epididymal Sperm Maturation and Transport

Sperm produced in the seminiferous tubules of the testis coalesce in the rete testis, where they then flow through the efferent ductules into the caput epididymis. Spermatozoa that are leaving the testis are fully formed but lack motility and are not capable of fertilizing oocytes. During the 7- to 10-day transit time through the epididymis, sperm acquire normal motility and fertilization capabilities. This is accompanied by metabolic and biochemical changes within sperm called *sperm maturation.* This process of sperm maturation within the epididymis appears to be both time and location dependent within the normal unobstructed epididymis. The pathophysiology of obstruction changes the normal epididymal physiology such that sperm may obtain motility and fertility in more proximal regions of the epididymis. The tail or cauda epididymis acts as a reservoir for sperm prior to ejaculation. Most sperm present in the ejaculate are derived from the cauda epididymis.

Ejaculation

Ejaculation is composed of two events: emission and ejaculation proper. Seminal emission is under autonomic control from the thoracolumbar sympathetic ganglia. These adrenergic nerves stimulate epididymal and vasal peristalsis as well as closure of the bladder neck to allow antegrade ejaculation. Ejaculation proper is under somatic control from the sacral spinal cord and is composed of skeletal muscle contractions of the pelvic muscles, bulbar urethral muscles, and relaxation of the external urethral sphincter. Disorders of ejaculation include retrograde ejaculation and failure of emission. In patients with retrograde ejaculation, sperm are found in bladder urine following ejaculation. In patients with failure of emission, there is complete absence of ejaculate (aspermia) and no sperm are present within the bladder after orgasm.

Sperm Function

In a man with intact spermatogenesis, normal ejaculation, and patent ducts, sperm are normally deposited in the deep vagina near the cervical os during sexual intercourse. Abnormalities of the urethra, such as hypospadias, or abnormal sexual practices may interfere with the delivery of sperm to the cervix. Fertilization normally takes place within the fallopian tubes. The sperm must be able to bind to the zona pellucida of the egg and penetrate the egg cell membrane. Once the sperm and egg have fused, the sperm nuclear material forms the male pronucleus and the centriole of the sperm guides the chromosomal apparatus to form a developing embryo.

Patient Evaluation

The evaluation of a couple having difficulty conceiving is not initiated until they have attempted conception for a minimum of 1 year, unless there are intervening circumstances. Exceptions to this rule include couples with known risk factors for infertility (history of cryptorchidism or prior chemotherapy in the male partner) or advancing age of the female partner. The 1-year time limit is arbitrary but is based on the observation that 50% of fertile couples conceive by 6 months and 90% conceive within 1 year of unprotected sexual intercourse. The typical couple experiencing difficulty achieving conception will initially present to the female partner's physician. This is due to the traditional role of the woman as the bearer of responsibility for procreation and contraception. A semen analysis is obtained from the male partner, and this single test often serves as his entire evaluation. Those men with abnormal semen parameters should be referred for a complete evaluation, including a detailed history, physical examination, and selective laboratory studies.

HISTORY

A complete history and physical examination should be performed on patients being evaluated for infertility. The critical aspects of the history are the sexual history and review of potential risk factors for infertility. The sexual history is often overlooked in the general medical examination because of patient and physician discomfort with the topic. However, normal sexual function and knowledge

of the female partner's ovulatory cycle are critical for conception to occur. It is important to be certain that the couple is engaging in vaginal intercourse and that ejaculation takes place within the vagina. **Studies have shown that conception can occur if sexual intercourse takes place up to 5 days prior to ovulation but does not occur if sexual intercourse is performed 1 day following ovulation.**

Age is an important factor for infertility. Men are normally fertile throughout adult life, with only some decline during late senescence. In contrast, a woman's fertility decreases with age. There appears to be a significant decline in egg quality with age. Although it is arbitrary, most clinical outcome studies divide women into groups based on age greater or less than 40 years old.

Time trying to conceive is an important factor, since most studies demonstrate a significant inverse relationship between duration of infertility and prognosis. A couple who has been able to have children in the past is considered a case of secondary infertility. Prior fertility may rule out certain etiologies such as congenital disorders. Couples with infertility due to recurrent miscarriage undergo a different evaluation from those who are unable to conceive.

Sexual history should include questioning regarding frequency, timing, and type of sexual intercourse. In addition, inquiries regarding use of vaginal lubricants and pain associated with ejaculation are important. Almost all vaginal lubricants have an adverse effect on sperm. Painful ejaculation and/or hematospermia may suggest the presence of prostatic or seminal vesicle pathology.

There are many known risk factors for male infertility, and the history should include questions regarding each one. A history of any congenital urogenital defects, such as cryptorchidism and hypospadias, may be related to infertility in adulthood. Approximately one third of men with a history of unilateral cryptorchidism and two thirds of men with bilateral cryptorchidism are infertile. Developmental disorders such as delayed or precocious puberty may indicate the presence of an endocrine disorder. Viral orchitis may occur after puberty and is a common cause of primary testicular failure.

Testicular torsion and testicular trauma have been associated with infertility, although this relationship is not definitive at this time. Gonadotoxin exposure, such as prior chemotherapy, radiation therapy, or exposure to chemicals in the workplace, may have a transient or sometimes a permanent effect on spermatogenesis. Testicular function is also exquisitely sensitive to temperature. The scrotum is normally 2 or 3° F cooler than intraabdominal temperature. Scrotal hyperthermia due to hot tub use and febrile illnesses may transiently lower sperm count and motility. A more chronic elevation of intrascrotal temperature such as that caused by varicoceles may cause permanent damage to the testis. The type of underwear worn does not appear to significantly affect scrotal temperature. Infections of the male reproductive tract during adulthood may also affect fertility, including venereal disease, prostatitis, and epididymitis. Other potential gonadotoxins are alcohol and tobacco, but their association with male infertility except in cases of alcoholic cirrhosis remains to be fully defined.

A complete medical history is also important. Medical illnesses such as diabetes mellitus and multiple sclerosis can have direct effects on male fertility through neurologic effects on ejaculation. Other medical illnesses, such as hypertension, may have indirect effects through the medications used in treatment. Calcium channel blockers have an adverse effect on sperm function without significantly altering semen parameters. Azulfidine, used in the treatment of inflammatory bowel disease, has a significant adverse effect on sperm motility. Illegal drug use, including marijuana and cocaine, has been shown to have adverse effects on male fertility as well.

A complete surgical history is necessary. Prior surgical procedures can have a significant effect on fertility. Prior scrotal or inguinal surgery, such as hydrocelectomy or herniorrhaphy, may result in inadvertent obstruction of the epididymis or vas deferens, respectively. Retroperitoneal lymph node dissection for testis tumors may cause ejaculatory dysfunction. Transurethral surgery, such as endoscopic stone manipulation, may cause obstruction of the ejaculatory ducts, and bladder neck surgery often results in retrograde ejaculation.

Environmental factors may also affect fertility, although the clinical evidence for this is not strong. Dietary habits such as caffeinated products have been associated with reduced fertility potential, particularly in cigarette smokers and men with varicoceles. Moderate use of alcohol has not been shown to have a deleterious effect, but heavy use leading to hepatic dysfunction can significantly impair male reproduction through endocrine effects. Use of other drugs, including both cocaine and marijuana, has been shown to have deleterious effects. Although moderate use of these recreational drugs probably has little effect on sperm production, patients with abnormal semen analyses should avoid exposure to all known gonadotoxins. Extremely heavy exercise, such as marathon running, has been shown to adversely affect the hypothalamic-pituitary-gonadal axis in women, resulting in amenorrhea, and there is reason to believe that there may be a similar effect in men.

PHYSICAL EXAMINATION

A general physical examination is an integral part of the male infertility evaluation, but the main focus is on the secondary sexual characteristics and genitalia. Normal masculinization rules out the presence of a congenital endocrinologic disorder. This includes the presence of a normal male escutcheon, facial hair, and phallic size. Other signs of congenital hypogonadism, such as Klinefelter's syndrome, include disproportion of extremities versus truncal length. Men with post-pubertally acquired hypogonadism have normal male phenotypic features but often lack the normal receding temporal hairline and develop fine wrinkles of facial forehead skin. The presence of gynecomastia suggests an estradiol-testosterone imbalance usually due to excessive estrogen production. A major source of estrogens in men is peripheral conversion of testosterone to estrogens in fat tissue. Therefore, it is important to note the presence of obesity in men being assessed for infertility.

Examination of the phallus should include assessment of length and urethral meatus position. Hypospadias affects the deposition of sperm in the vagina and could be a cause of infertility of men who have normal semen analyses. The testes should be evaluated for size, position, and consistency. Testes are normally located in the dependent position of the scrotum, and cryptorchidism should be suspected in any adult with inguinal or absent testes since retractile testes is uncommon in adulthood. Testicular volume should be objectively measured using either a ruler or an orchidometer. Normal testicular volume is 4 × 3 cm or larger than 19 mL for whites and African Americans. Normal testicular volume for Asians is smaller. The bulk of testicular volume is involved in spermatogenesis. Therefore, small testes with soft consistency are strongly predictive of abnormal spermatogenesis. However, the converse is not true, because normal-sized testes do not guarantee normal spermatogenesis. In addition, many patients with atrophic testes have normal serum testosterone levels since the interstitial compartment comprises little volume. Normal-sized testes do not rule out the presence of hypogonadism, but patients with reduced testicular volume often have abnormal sperm production.

Examination of the spermatic cord and paratesticular tissues should include assessment of the epididymis, vas deferens, and spermatic veins. Congenital absence of the vas deferens is the most common cause of obstructive azoospermia and is diagnosed by physical examination. However, some patients have segmental atresia of the vas deferens, which may not be detectable on physical examination. The consistency of both the epididymis and vas deferens may be suggestive of the presence of distal obstruction if they feel full and indurated.

Gross inspection and palpation of the spermatic cord with the patient standing in a warm room and performing the Valsalva's maneuver detect varicoceles. Each spermatic cord should be grasped between the thumb and forefingers and palpated while the patient bears down. A varicocele is defined as dilation of the veins of the pampiniform plexus and is graded as small, medium, and large (Table 29–1). Large varicoceles are visible without the Valsalva's maneuver, medium varicoceles are palpable without performing

Table 29-1
Varicocele Grading System

Grade	Description
Small	Palpable with Valsalva's maneuver only
Medium	Palpable
Large	Visible

a Valsalva's maneuver, and small varicoceles are only palpable with the Valsalva's maneuver.

Digital rectal examination (DRE) is performed to assess the size and consistency of the prostate gland as well as to identify any masses located within or cranial to the prostate. Unfortunately, the DRE is not very sensitive. Many abnormalities detected by transrectal ultrasonography, including müllerian duct cysts, are found in men with normal DREs.

LABORATORY STUDIES

Semen Analysis

There is no consensus regarding the minimal acceptable laboratory evaluation of men with infertility. However, most clinicians initially assess subfertile men with a combination of a series of three semen analyses and baseline endocrine studies that include serum testosterone and FSH. Further evaluation is predicated on the results of these initial studies.

The semen analysis is the cornerstone of the male infertility evaluation. The semen analysis is almost always the first and frequently the last test performed on the male partner of an infertile couple. Unfortunately, the accuracy of this test and its prognostic value do not support this practice. Many studies have demonstrated that the coefficient of variation for semen analysis performed even at major fertility centers is unacceptably high, often greater than 50%. Even when performed accurately, the results of a semen analysis do not always predict whether a couple will be able to conceive on their own. Large outcome studies have shown that neither sperm count nor motility is predictive of conception when the sperm concentration is higher than 5 million per milliliter. Yet, semen analysis remains our main diagnostic test used to determine whether there is a significant male factor responsible for a couple's inability to conceive.

It is critical to provide specific instructions to the patient regarding specimen collection. A standardized period of sexual abstinence of 2 or 3 days should be employed since duration of sexual abstinence can have a dramatic effect on the results. A clean, wide-mouthed container should be given to the patient. It is important that the cap not have an absorbent surface on the inside. The specimen should be collected by masturbation and delivered to the laboratory at room temperature within 2 hours of collection. Collection by coitus with a condom is not acceptable since all commercially available condoms contain spermicides. There are specially made condoms called *semen collection devices* for this purpose, but most laboratory technicians prefer not to receive a sample within a seminal collection device because it is difficult to retrieve all of the sample. The amount of time between semen collection and examination should be noted since this may have an impact on the results. Normal sperm can maintain motility for several hours at room temperature, and neither sperm count nor morphology changes with time.

A standard semen analysis includes measurement of physical characteristics; assessment of sperm numbers, quality, and motility; semen volume; and detection of other cellular elements such as white blood cells, red blood cells, and bacteria. Although there has been some controversy regarding the criteria for a "normal" semen analysis, specific criteria have been developed for what is considered an "adequate" specimen (Table 29–2). The normal value for ejaculate volume is from 1.5 to 5 mL. It appears that fertility is affected once the semen volume drops below 1.5 mL;

at this volume, there is inadequate buffering of the normal vaginal acidity. In addition, it is believed that a low volume may result in inadequate interaction between sperm and cervical mucus. The most common cause of low ejaculate volume on semen analysis is failure to collect the entire specimen. Other etiologies of a low-volume semen sample include retrograde ejaculation, ejaculatory duct obstruction, and androgen deficiency.

Sperm motility is characterized by (1) the quality of sperm movement and forward progression (how fast and how straight the sperm move) and (2) the number of motile sperm as a percentage of the total number. The normal motility is at least 50% and the normal forward progression is greater than 2.0 (ranging from 0 for no movement to 4.0 for fast, straight movement). Sperm motility is perhaps the most important measurement of semen quality. Patients who have very low sperm counts (e.g., those with hypogonadotropic hypogonadism) but normal to highly motile sperm seldom have problems with fertility. Conversely, patients with a low count and poor motility (oligoasthenospermia) often have significant problems with fertility.

It is believed that a sperm density of greater than 20 million per milliliter (total of 50 million sperm per ejaculate) is necessary to achieve conception. As stated, duration of abstinence prior to specimen collection can have a dramatic effect on the results. Therefore, consecutive semen samples from the same patient should be collected after equal abstinence periods. The average sperm concentration amongst fertile men is approximately 60 million per milliliter. The exact lower limit that is adequate for conception is unknown. However, 20 million sperm per milliliter is the standard criterion used for a normal semen analysis.

A sample of the ejaculate is air dried and stained to analyze sperm morphology. In normal semen samples, more than 35% of the sperm are morphologically normal. A finding of increased numbers of abnormally shaped sperm is indicative of testicular stress (environmental toxins or varicocele). Relatively new strict criteria for morphologic assessment of sperm have been developed where greater than 14% is normal. These new strict criteria were developed based on the characteristics

Table 29–2
Limits of "Adequacy" for Semen Analysis

Parameter	Adequate Value
Volume	>1.5 mL
Sperm count	>20 million/mL
Motility	>50%
Forward progression	>2
Morphology	>35%
Absence of significant WBCs, RBCs, and bacteria	

WBC, white blood cell; RBC, red blood cell.

Table 29-3
Frequency of Various Categories of Semen Analysis Results Among Men Being Evaluated for Infertility

Category	Frequency (%)
Normal	14
Azoospermia	14
Multiple parameters abnormal	49
Single abnormal parameter	23
Volume	7
Sperm count	4
Motility	6
Morphology	4
Pyospermia	2

of sperm that were able to penetrate cervical mucus. These criteria are highly predictive of the outcome of IVF but have not been adequately tested in the general population.

The ejaculate is also analyzed for the presence of other cells. Leukocytes are normally present in the semen, but elevated numbers (greater than 1 million per milliliter) is considered abnormal. The presence of pyospermia may indicate pathology of the male sex accessory glands, which requires urologic evaluation. The same is true for the presence of red blood cells (hematospermia) and bacteria.

The results of a semen analysis can be grouped into one of five categories: (1) all parameters normal; (2) azoospermia, defined as the lack of any spermatogenic elements in the ejaculate; (3) all seminal parameters abnormal; (4) isolated problem restricted to one parameter of the seminal fluid; and (5) absence of any ejaculate whatsoever (aspermia). Each pattern then dictates the direction of further evaluation. The results of semen analyses performed on more than 1000 men attending an infertility clinic are depicted in Table 29-3.

A distinct subset of male partners of an infertile marriage has normal semen analyses. If the female partner's evaluation is also normal, the couple's condition is labeled as *unexplained infertility*. This is different from where the male partner's evaluation is abnormal but the cause of the abnormality cannot be determined (*idiopathic male factor infertility*). Sperm function tests to determine if the sperm are capable of fertilizing an egg are sometimes

performed in couples with unexplained infertility in a further attempt to define the problem.

Endocrine Evaluation

Primary endocrine defects can be a cause of male factor infertility, with a prevalence of approximately 3%. Endocrinopathies, however, are rare in men whose sperm concentration is greater than 20 million per milliliter. Therefore, an endocrine evaluation becomes an essential part of the assessment of all male partners with an abnormal semen examination or when an endocrinopathy is suspected based on clinical findings. **The hormonal tests that should be obtained on initial endocrine screening are serum testosterone and FSH.** Further testing with a repeat serum testosterone, LH, and prolactin should be obtained if the initial values are abnormal. The patterns of endocrine studies and the resultant diagnosis are depicted in Table 29-4.

Reduction of spermatogenesis, identified as azoospermia or oligospermia on semen analysis, usually occurs in the setting of decreased inhibin production by Sertoli's cells. This diminishes the negative-feedback effect of inhibin on the pituitary gland, resulting in a concomitant increase in FSH production. Elevated serum FSH is indicative of injury to the germ cell epithelium and distinguishes testicular insufficiency from hypothalamic-pituitary disease. Correlation with levels of serum testosterone, LH, and results of semen analysis helps direct the physician's diagnostic assessment of the patient's underlying problem.

Hyperprolactinemia has also been reported to cause oligospermia. Serum prolactin levels should be measured in patients with low serum testosterone levels as well as with symp-

Table 29-4
Endocrine Evaluation of Infertile Men

Diagnosis	T	LH	FSH
Secondary hypogonadism	↓	↓	↓
Primary hypogonadism	↓	↑	↑
Germ cell abnormalities	NL	NL	↑
Obstruction	NL	NL	NL

T, Testosterone; LH, luteinizing hormone; FSH, follicle-stimulating hormone; NL, normal.

toms of decreased ejaculate volume, diminished libido, visual field disturbances, and galactorrhea.

RADIOLOGICAL IMAGING

Diagnostic imaging studies have taken on a major role in the diagnosis of disease entities associated with infertility. Ultrasonography, magnetic resonance imaging, and other radiologic modalities help the physician identify anatomic abnormalities related to male infertility.

Ultrasonography is helpful in the evaluation of scrotal abnormalities found on physical examination. Ultrasonographic examination of the parenchyma of the testis is important in evaluation of male infertility, specifically tumor identification and the measurement of testicular size for retarded growth or atrophy. Testicular tumors are most common in the same age group in which fertility disorders of the male are most prevalent. **A new diagnosis of testicular tumor is seen in approximately 1% of infertile men, which is significantly higher than the general population, where the incidence is 4 in 100,000 men per year.**

Although the mainstay for diagnosis of a varicocele in a male, as stated previously, is physical examination in a warm room, ultrasonography and venography can be used to confirm the presence of a suspected varicocele. These studies can detect subclinical varicoceles in the infertile patient. The management of radiologically identified subclinical varicocele is controversial. Studies have shown that the degree of improvement following varicocele repair is directly related to the size of the varicocele. Therefore, repair of subclinical varicoceles is of dubious benefit.

Transrectal ultrasonography (TRUS) has become the favored imaging modality for the evaluation of the prostate, ejaculatory ducts, seminal vesicles, and the vasal ampulla in the infertile male. TRUS is effective in identifying anatomic abnormalities of the distal genital duct system that can cause male factor infertility and has largely replaced vasography for the evaluation of patients with suspected obstruction of the ejaculatory ducts. Müllerian duct cysts, ejaculatory duct calcification, dilated ejaculatory ducts, and dilated seminal vesicles are findings consistent with obstruction. A müllerian duct cyst (prostatic utricular cyst) may be present under the bladder base between the seminal vesicles and cause extrinsic compression of the ejaculatory duct. The ejaculatory ducts may also be obstructed by extrinsic compression by a large seminal vesicle (wolffian duct) cyst, which can also be diagnosed by TRUS. The seminal vesicles are frequently abnormal, either absent or hypoplastic in patients with bilateral congenital absence of the vas deferens.

Vasography is still considered the gold standard for identification of obstruction of the male reproductive system. Vasography is performed by scrotal exploration of the vas deferens. The vas deferens is opened through a transverse partial-thickness vasotomy and the intravasal fluid is sampled for sperm to confirm more proximal patency of the epididymis. Contrast medium is then injected distally to document distal patency of the vas deferens and ejaculatory ducts. Potential complications of vasal exploration include vasal stricture formation, bleeding, infection, and sperm granuloma formation. For these reasons, routine exploration is not performed in patients with obvious ejaculatory duct obstruction diagnosed with TRUS.

Therapy

The subject of male factor infertility encompasses not only a wide range of causative factors but also treatment options. Management options for male factor infertility fall into four categories. The underlying diagnosis, patient preference, partner preference, and insurance coverage largely dictate the choice of therapeutic management. The frequency of various diagnoses among men being evaluated for infertility is listed in Table 29–5. The first and most effective are specific therapies aimed at correcting the underlying abnormality or cause of infertility. However, specific therapies can be employed only when the specific cause has been identified. The second kind are empiric therapies. These are treatments aimed at improving the fertility status either of men with idiopathic infertility or of men whose infertility is due to a known cause that is irreversible (e.g., cryptorchidism

Table 29-5
Distribution of Diagnoses of Men Being Evaluated for Infertility

Diagnosis	Number	Percentage
Varicocele	203	29
Idiopathic	158	22
Unexplained	84	12
Obstruction	66	9
Testicular failure	33	5
Ejaculatory dysfunction	31	4
Gonadotoxin exposure	27	4
Cryptorchidism	24	3
Autoimmunity	21	3
Torsion	11	2
Infection	9	1
Chromosomal	9	1
Endocrinopathy	9	1
Viral orchitis	7	1
Testicular cancer	7	1
Ultrastructural abnormalities	4	1
Impotence	4	1
Hypospadias	1	0
Total	**708**	**100.00**

or prior gonadotoxin exposure) or who have failed to respond satisfactorily to specific therapies. By their nature, empiric therapies have no proven efficacy and meta-analysis studies of these therapies do not reveal a high success rate. An alternative approach to the management of male infertility is to attempt to increase the probability of conception without improving semen quality. This is performed through the use of assisted reproductive techniques, which is in itself a form of empiric therapy. Assisted reproductive techniques, like other forms of empiric therapy, were not successful until the relatively recent advent of IVF by ICSI. The final form of management is to bypass the male partner's defect by using either donor sperm insemination or adoption. Knowledge of this wide spectrum of therapeutic options provides the clinician with a full armamentarium to treat male infertility.

NONSURGICAL TREATMENT

Specific Therapy

Nonsurgical factors related to male factor infertility include ejaculatory dysfunction, coital timing, exposure to gonadotoxins, testicular hyperthermia, hormonal imbalances, and immunologic events. Recognition of these fac-

tors can lead to institution of simple corrective measures that may dramatically improve a couple's ability to conceive.

Couples unaware of the cyclic changes that are characteristic of the female ovulatory cycle may not be engaging in sexual relations at the proper time of the wife's ovulatory cycle to induce conception. Education of the couple with simple instructions concerning the ovulatory cycle and the optimal timing of sexual relations may have dramatic effects in couples with otherwise normal fertility status. These patients should be counseled that the optimal frequency of intercourse is believed to be every 48 hours starting on day 10 of the ovulatory cycle until day 16. Testicular function is exquisitely sensitive to temperature; therefore, it is advisable that men with reduced semen quality should minimize testicular exposure to heat. Switching from jockey-type underwear to boxer shorts has no effect, but avoiding hot tub use or saunas can be effective. Gonadotoxic agents, such as those discussed earlier, should be completely discontinued. Recognition of these risk factors early on, perhaps even prior to exposure, is crucial in limiting the amount of damage incurred. This may include a change in lifestyle (quitting alcohol or tobacco use) or a change in occupation.

In subfertile men with low-volume ejaculate (< 1.5 ml), a postejaculate urine specimen should be obtained to rule out retrograde ejaculation. This is due to incomplete bladder neck closure at the time of ejaculation. Etiologies include surgical disruption of the muscle fibers of the bladder neck or of the sympathetic fibers that coordinate the processes of emission, ejaculation, and bladder neck closure. Known risk factors are diabetes mellitus, multiple sclerosis, and certain medications, including haloperidol, amitriptyline, and prazosin. The first-line of treatment for patients with ejaculatory dysfunction is administration of an alpha agonist such as pseudoephedrine to stimulate vasal peristalsis and closure of the bladder neck. If medical therapy fails, several techniques can be employed to harvest sperm for artificial insemination, including harvesting sperm from the bladder if the patient has retrograde ejaculation or rectal probe ejaculation if the patient has failure of emission. These techniques are combined with insemination of the spouse.

Autoimmunity to one's own sperm is mediated by antisperm antibodies found in the ejaculate. The prevalence of antisperm antibodies is less than 10% in most series. Standard therapy is immunosuppression with oral steroids, but the efficacy of this treatment is extremely controversial and the potential side effect (avascular necrosis of the hip) is rare but devastating. At present, most couples are referred for assisted reproduction, including intrauterine insemination or IVF.

Endocrine disorders are an uncommon cause of male infertility. Hypogonadotropic hypogonadism may be treated with either gonadotropin replacement or using a GnRH analogue if the pituitary gland is intact. Therapy for more than a year is often required to induce spermatogenesis. Affected patients require testosterone replacement for life to maintain bone mineralization. The success rate for treatment of hypogonadotropic hypogonadism has been better than an 80% pregnancy rate. Prolactin-secreting pituitary adenoma is another endocrine cause of infertility. Men generally present with much larger pituitary tumors than women. The most common symptoms are sexual dysfunction, headache, visual field disturbances, and galactorrhea. The initial treatment is bromocriptine, to which most patients respond. Surgery or radiation may be required if the tumor is unresponsive to medical therapy. Normalization of serum prolactin levels is often readily achieved, but restoration of normal fertility is uncommon.

Empirical Therapy

The only therapy available for men without an identifiable cause of subfertility is empirical. It is believed that the incidence of idiopathic infertility in male fertility clinics ranges from 5% to 66%, with an average of 25%. Some infertile men with a presumed diagnosis, such as a varicocele, do not respond to specific therapy and therefore become candidates for empiric therapy. Therefore, empiric therapy might be offered to any infertile man for whom a specific treatment is unavailable or in whom a specific treatment has failed.

The most common clinical finding for which there is a need for empiric therapy is idiopathic oligospermia (low sperm count). The theoretical basis for most forms of empirical hormonal therapy is that increasing the amount of circulating testosterone and/or FSH will improve testicular function. The most common therapies used are agents such as clomiphene citrate that block the feedback inhibition of testosterone on the pituitary gland. The alternative approach is to give gonadotropins, but this requires injections three times a week. Most uncontrolled studies of these empirical therapies demonstrate improvement in sperm counts of patients treated, and pregnancies occur. In one study, 80% of men treated had an increase in sperm count and 30% initiated a pregnancy. However, almost all controlled studies of these drugs do not show any increased efficacy of these medications over placebo.

Adequate levels of circulating androgens are needed for normal male sexual and reproductive function. However, it has been known for some time that administration of exogenous androgens results in suppressed gonadotropin secretion and hypogonadotropic hypogonadism, despite normal levels of androgens in the serum. As a result, testicular function is actually suppressed. Therefore, therapeutic doses of exogenous androgens have been low to avoid pituitary suppression. The most commonly used synthetic androgen used is mesterolone in dosages ranging from 2 to 25 mg daily. Its ability to improve seminal parameters has not been consistent in clinical trials. Toxicity, including jaundice, peliosis hepatitis, and gynecomastia, appears to outweigh the efficacy of this form of therapy. Testosterone or any other androgens should never be used in the treatment of male infertility.

SURGICAL MANAGEMENT

The subfertile man diagnosed with obstructive azoospermia has, in many instances, a treatable condition. The ultimate result of that treatment is dependent on the site and etiology of the blockage, the duration of time that it has existed, and the skill of the surgeon in bypassing or relieving the obstruction.

Vasectomy is the most common cause of

obstruction of the vas deferens. Millions of men have undergone this procedure, and some, for a variety of reasons, later want restoration of fertility. Inadvertent transection of the vas deferens during an inguinal hernia repair, hydrocelectomy or deep pelvic surgery can cause azoospermia if the injury is bilateral or happens on the side where the patient has only a single functional testis or vas deferens. Vasectomy reversal is accomplished by a vasovasostomy, where the two ligated ends are identified and anastomosed. Most authors report vasal patency rates of greater than 85% and pregnancy rates of 50% following vasectomy reversal.

The epididymis is the most common site of obstruction in patients with obstructive azoospermia due to inflammatory conditions or congenital abnormalities. In addition, epididymal "blow-out" from increased intraluminal pressure from a distal vasal blockage can occur. The obstruction is bypassed by performing an epididymovasostomy. Both the patency and pregnancy rates with epididymovasostomy are lower than vasovasostomy and have been reported to be 80% and 30%, respectively.

Infertility secondary to ejaculatory duct obstruction, once thought uncommon, is now being seen with increasing frequency as transrectal ultrasonography has evolved into a more effective diagnostic modality. Etiologies of ejaculatory duct obstruction include inflammatory conditions, prior transurethral surgery, and congenital abnormalities, as noted earlier. Ejaculatory duct obstruction can be successfully treated with transurethral resection of the ejaculatory duct. Seminal parameters often improve with an increase in ejaculate volume and increased sperm density within the ejaculate.

Varicocele is the most common treatable cause of male factor infertility. A varicocele is defined as a dilation of the veins of the pampiniform plexus that surround the testis and epididymis in the scrotum. The varicosity of these veins is due to absent or deficient valves in the internal spermatic vein. The goal of varicocelectomy is to ligate the abnormal veins draining the testis while sparing the normal venous drainage, lymphatic drainage, and arterial blood supply. Varicocelectomy can be performed surgically on an outpatient basis under local anesthesia or via a percutaneous method by radiologists. The success rate of surgical repair is approximately 98%, whereas percutaneous repair is significantly lower. Semen parameters improve significantly in approximately 65%, and a 40% pregnancy rate has been observed in controlled studies.

ASSISTED REPRODUCTIVE TECHNIQUES

Couples with male factor as a significant component of their infertility often fail to conceive with traditional therapies. These patients may turn to assisted reproductive techniques for further evaluation and treatment. These are techniques that attempt to improve the ability of the sperm to reach and fertilize the ova. IVF became the cornerstone of this technology after the first successful case was described in 1980. Subsequently, other techniques, such as intrauterine insemination (IUI), gamete intrafallopian transfer, and zygote intrafallopian transfer, have been developed. These procedures achieve their therapeutic effect by bringing the gametes together in increased concentrations and thus ultimately rely on the ability of the sperm to fertilize the ova when placed in close proximity. Newer techniques of assisted fertilization have been developed to bypass particular sperm defects, such as poor motility and abnormal sperm morphology. The most successful one to date is ICSI. ICSI involves direct injection of the sperm into the egg cytoplasm.

IUI offers the advantage of placing a concentrated specimen of the male partner's sperm in close proximity to the natural site of fertilization, the fallopian tube. This bypasses the filtering effect of the cervical mucus. Inseminations are performed at the time of ovulation; over-the-counter kits that detect the presence of the preovulatory urinary LH surge are most commonly used for the timing of these inseminations. The overall success rate for IUI in couples with a male factor is only 3% per cycle. Success rates are enhanced with increased hormonal stimulation of the ovaries, which produces multiple follicles during each ovulatory cycle. This is known as *superovulation.* Superovulation can be induced with hormones such as clomiphene citrate given orally or hMG given parenterally. The success rate for IUI combined with hormonal stimulation of ovulation is much better, at around 15% per cycle. This procedure should be reserved for those couples in whom reasonable evidence exists that the male partner's sperm can fertilize the ova.

The technique of IVF involves insemination of preovulatory oocytes under controlled conditions. The female partner undergoes superovulation to stimulate the ovaries to produce more than one egg. The oocytes are retrieved via needle puncture of the ovaries under transvaginal ultrasound guidance. The eggs are then incubated with sperm in the laboratory. In vitro inseminations are performed with 50,000 to 500,000 motile sperm in non–male factor couples. In male factor couples, sperm concentrations of 500,000 to 1 million are often used. The oocyte-sperm mixture is carefully observed; oocytes are examined for the presence of pronuclei, indicating fertilization has occurred. Embryo cleavage can be seen 2 to 4 days following insemination, at which time the embryos are transferred back into the uterus.

Experience has made it clear that couples with male factor infertility have lower fertilization rates than couples with non–male factor infertility. Oocyte fertilization and embryo development occur in approximately 45% to 60% of couples with male factor (when using > 500,000 motile sperm), compared with 70% to 90% in couples with non–male factor infertility, where significantly fewer motile sperm are required. Pregnancy rates vary widely between centers but average around 10% per cycle. Studies have shown that predictors of success of IVF include motile sperm concentration, sperm morphology, presence of antisperm antibodies, and the ability of the sperm to acrosome react.

For those couples in whom IVF does not appear to be effective, there is a new method of fertilization using micromanipulation techniques. ICSI has the highest pregnancy rates among the various methods of IVF for couples with male factor infertility. Fertilization and conception rates appear to be independent of sperm quality. Ongoing pregnancy rates of up to 50% and higher have been achieved in the most severe cases, including

men with surgically unreconstructable obstruction such as congenital absence of the vas, where poor-quality sperm surgically retrieved from the epididymis is used for fertilization. This is an obvious advantage over both IUI and standard IVF, where success rates appear to be highly dependent on the quality of the semen. In men with severe abnormalities of sperm function, IVF alone is often inadequate to allow for fertilization. In these cases, gamete micromanipulation as an adjunctive procedure during IVF can result in high fertilization and pregnancy rates despite highly abnormal seminal parameters.

Conclusion

Infertility is a widespread problem in the United States, affecting approximately 20% of couples attempting to achieve conception. The underlying problem can be attributed to the male partner in 50% of these couples. The primary care physician can become an integral part in the identification and eventual management of these couples. In the evaluation of the subfertile couple, it is important for the physician to have a basic understanding of the physiology and anatomy of the male reproductive system, as well as the initial laboratory testing process and appropriate radiologic evaluation. This will help facilitate prompt referral to a urologic specialist in the field of male reproduction, as well as provide the opportunity for initial counseling of the couple. Once a diagnosis is reached, there now exist many therapeutic options to aid the couple with male factor infertility in their goal of attaining fertilization and pregnancy.

SUGGESTED READINGS

1. Collins JA, Wrixon W, Janes LB, Wilson EH: Treatment-independent pregnancy among infertile couples. N Engl J Med 309:1201–1206, 1983.
2. Gilbert BR, Schlegel PN, Goldstein M: Office evaluation of the subfertile male. AUA Update 13:69–76, 1994.
3. Jarow JP: Life-threatening conditions associated with male infertility. Urol Clin North Am 21:409–415, 1994.
4. Lipshultz LI, Howards SS (eds): Infertility in the Male. St. Louis, Mosby-Year Book, 1995.

5. Sigman M, Jarow JP: Endocrine evaluation of infertile men. Urology 50:659–664, 1997.
6. Sigman M, Howards SS: Male infertility. *In* Walsh PC, Retik AB, Vaughan ED Jr, Wein AJ (eds): Campbell's Urology, 7th ed. Philadelphia, WB Saunders, 1998, pp 1287–1330.
7. Whitehead ED, Nagler HM (eds): Management of Impotence and Infertility. Philadelphia, JB Lippincott, 1994.
8. Wilcox AJ, Weinstein MC, Baird DD: Timing of sexual intercourse in relation to ovulation: Effects on the probability of conception, survival of the pregnancy, and sex of the baby. N Engl J Med 333:1517–1521, 1995.

30 Sexual Dysfunction in the Male

Daniel C. Merrill

Male sexual dysfunction includes *aspermia* (absence of emission), *the loss of sexual desire, premature ejaculation,* and *the absence of orgasm* as well as *impotence.* However, impotence is far more common than all the other male sexual problems combined; thus, this chapter presents a discussion of this condition first and in more depth than the other entities that comprise male sexual dysfunction.

Impotence

Erectile failure, commonly referred to as *impotence,* may be defined as the inability to achieve or maintain an erection sufficiently firm to permit satisfactory sexual intercourse. Erectile dysfunction occurs, at least to some degree, in 10 million to 30 million American males. Although any adult male may develop erectile failure, impotence is primarily a condition of older males as shown by the fact that its prevalence increases from approximately 5% at age 40 to between 15% and 20% by age 65. The observation that approximately 25% of all new urology consultation requests at our Veterans Affairs clinic are for impotence reflects how common erectile failure is in American males and how important sexual function is to their mental and physical well-being.

Before beginning the discussion on erectile failure, I would like to emphasize two important points. First, because the recently developed treatment modalities for impotency are effective in patients with organic, psychogenic, and mixed types of erectile failure, the vast majority of impotent males will receive the same treatment, irrespective of the etiologic factors responsible for their erectile failure. For this reason, most impotent patients do not require a complex, time-consuming, and expensive diagnostic evaluation prior to treatment. Second, since it is now possible to treat most impotent males safely and effectively with a pill or a urethral suppository, there is no reason that the initial treatment of impotent males cannot be carried out by primary care physicians.

By eliminating the costly diagnostic evaluations, which unfortunately are still commonly being performed on impotent males, and by shifting the responsibility for their initial treatment from urologists to primary care physicians, the cost of treating this common medical condition can be reduced substantially.

ETIOLOGY

Arteriosclerosis is by far the most common cause of impotence. A study that I performed in 150 males who had penile implants revealed that 67% of the patients had developed impotence as a result of vascular penile insufficiency secondary to arteriosclerosis or diabetes mellitus (Table 30–1). Many of these impotent men were cigarette smokers, and most of them had hypercholesterolemia. These risk factors undoubtedly contributed to the severity of their arteriosclerosis and the early onset of their erectile failure. In this respect, it is important to realize that the penile arteries are much smaller than the coronary and cerebral arteries; thus, a patient with atherosclerosis may experience erectile failure many years before he develops more serious manifestations of the arterial insufficiency such as an-

Table 30-1
Etiology of Erectile Failure in One Hundred Fifty Patients with Impotence

Diagnosis	No. of Patients (%)
Vascular	
Arteriosclerosis	66 (44)
Diabetes mellitus	35 (23)
Psychogenic	16 (11)
Peyronie's disease	10 (7)
Pelvic surgery	9 (6)
Neurogenic	6 (4)
Radiation	3 (2)
TURP	2
Alcoholism	1
Hormonal deficiency	1

TURP, transurethral resection of the prostate.

gina, myocardial infarction, or a cerebral vascular accident.

The so-called venous leak is another form of vascular penile insufficiency. In this condition, the venous structures that usually impede venous blood flow from the erectile bodies during the erectile process fail. As a result, penile rigidity does not occur even if there is sufficient arterial blood flow to produce an adequate erection. At present, the presence or absence of a venous leak is of more academic interest than practical clinical significance since there is no satisfactory treatment for the condition.

Drug-induced impotence is believed by some investigators to be the most common cause of erectile failure. Medications that may cause or contribute to impotency include many, if not most, of the antihypertensive medications; diuretics, including hydrochlorothiazide; many of the antidepressant and antipsychotic agents; the ulcer medication cimetidine (Tagamet); and alcohol. Unfortunately, changing medications most often either is not feasible or is ineffective in restoring the patient's erectile function; therefore, men with drug-induced impotency usually require treatment for their erectile failure.

Neurologic causes of erectile dysfunction include spina bifida, multiple sclerosis, and spinal cord injury. Major surgical procedures that damage the pelvic nerve innervation of the penis, including abdominoperineal resection, lower abdominal colon surgery, and radical prostatectomy, also may cause impotence.

Hormonal abnormalities are an infrequent cause of impotence. While testosterone is necessary to maintain secondary sex characteristics and libido, its role in maintaining erectile function is less clear. For example, it is not uncommon to encounter potent men who have abnormally low serum testosterone levels. More significantly perhaps, is the observation that testosterone supplementation seldom produces a lasting improvement in the erectile function of impotent males even if it can be demonstrated that they have low normal or abnormally low serum testosterone levels. For this reason, I do not perform a serum testosterone determination on impotent men unless they complain of decreased libido as well as erectile failure. Similarly, I do not believe it is cost effective to perform a routine serum prolactin on impotent men or to evaluate them for a possible abnormality in thyroid function.

Psychological factors play an important role in organic as well as psychogenic impotence. One should entertain the diagnosis of primary psychological impotency in any man younger than 50 to 55 years of age who experiences a relatively sudden onset of erectile failure and who does not have an obvious organic cause for the problem. The "fear of failing" is the primary cause of psychological impotence, and it also may play an important role in patients with organic impotence. In fact, the fear that he will lose his erection prematurely may render a man, with what otherwise might be a tolerable impairment in erectile function as a result of organic disease, totally impotent.

Psychological factors also may explain the observation that men who are beginning to develop organic impotency often seem to benefit, at least initially, from yohimbine, testosterone injections, and patent medications even though these pharmacologic agents are of little or no long-term value in the treatment of impotence.

DIAGNOSIS

The urologic literature is replete with articles describing elaborate protocols for the evaluation of the impotent male. Although diagnostic tests such as nocturnal penile tumescence monitoring, penile duplex and color Doppler sonography, cavernosometry, gravity cavernosometry, angiography, and penile biopsy have expanded our knowledge of normal and abnormal erectile function, their role in clinical practice is questionable for two reasons.

First, in most cases, the etiology of the patient's erectile failure will be obvious after a brief inquiry into his history. Second, as stated previously, most urologists initially treat impotent patients with alprostadil (Muse), sildenafil (subsequently referred to in this chapter by the trade name Viagra), or a pharmacologic erection program (PEP), irrespective of the cause of their impotency, because these treatment modalities are relatively safe and effective in all types of impotency.

With respect to diagnosis, the vast majority of older men who present with a history of slowly progressive erectile failure have organic impotence secondary to arterial disease. Younger males with impotency of recent onset and no obvious organic cause for their erectile failure usually are suffering primarily from a psychological problem, whereas patients with neurologic impotency most often have a readily ascertainable history of spinal cord injury, stroke, multiple sclerosis, or some other obvious neurologic disease. In all of these situations, the diagnosis usually is relatively straightforward and further diagnostic studies are unnecessary.

A serum free testosterone determination should be made in patients who have testicular atrophy or a loss of libido if they are younger than 55 years of age. In younger men who have a low testosterone level, a serum luteinizing hormone (LH) and a serum follicle-stimulating hormone (FSH) also should be obtained to detect hypogonadotropic hypogonadism. If the gonadotropins are low, suggesting a lesion of the pituitary or hypothalamus, appropriate studies are indicated to rule out a pituitary or other brain tumor. If the LH and FSH levels are elevated, the patient has hypergonadotropic hypogonadism or primary testicular failure. As indicated previously, it is not cost effective to routinely evaluate impotent males for possible hyperprolactinemia or an abnormality in thyroid function.

With respect to laboratory tests, I also obtain a serum glycosylated hemoglobin test if the etiology of the patient's erectile failure is not clear and he has not been tested previously for diabetes mellitus. Finally, a serum cholesterol level should be determined in any man with suspected vasculogenic impotence since they may have hypercholesterolemia that requires treatment.

Although a physical examination is an important component of medical care in general, it seldom reveals an etiologic factor for impotency that was not self-evident from the patient's history. Thus, the physical examination may be limited to the penis and testicles to detect testicular atrophy or to confirm the presence of corporal fibrosis in a patient with symptoms suggesting Peyronie's disease.

TREATMENT

At the time I am writing this chapter on male sexual dysfunction it would seem appropriate to reduce the entire section on impotence to one word—*Viagra!* However, experience has shown that most things that seem to be too good to be true are just that. Thus, on the outside chance that Viagra does not prove to be as effective and all encompassing as the preliminary clinical trials suggest it will be, I will describe several alternate forms of therapy that primary care physicians may use to treat their impotent patients.

The advantages and disadvantages of Viagra, Muse, and two medications that are commonly used in PEPs are compared in Table 30–2. I believe it would be appropriate for family physicians to prescribe any of these medications for their impotent patients and therefore describe my protocol for administering these medications in some detail.

Viagra

As stated previously, the field of impotency presently is undergoing a revolutionary change as a result of the recent introduction of long-awaited "pill" for impotency—Pfizer's Viagra. Since Viagra has just been released, I have no personal experience with this novel new treatment modality; however, the clinical trials of the medication suggest that it has no serious side effects and that it will be effective in 80% of impotent men. If this is so, it seems that, at long last, we have a simple, safe, oral preparation that can be

Table 30-2
Advantages and Disadvantages of Four Medications Commonly Used to Treat Impotence

Medication	Advantages	Disadvantages
Viagra (sidenafil)	The only oral drug for impotence Safe and effective in most patients Approved by the FDA	Extremely expensive May not be as effective as the other treatment modalities Cannot be used if patient is on nitrates Must take 1 hour before intercourse
Muse (alprostadil) uretheral suppository	Does not require injection Less likely to cause priapism Approved by the FDA Does not cause corporal fibrosis	Extremely expensive Must be stored <77° F May not be as effective as injectable vasodilators Drug-induced penile pain is common
Papaverine (30 mg/mL, 10 mL)	Effective in many patients and is the cheapest pharmacologic method of treating impotence Injection is not as painful as Caverjet Does not require refrigeration	Requires penile injection Not as effective as Caverjet Not approved by FDA for impotence May induce priapism May cause corporal fibrosis
Caverjet (injectable alprostadil)	May be more effective than papaverine, Viagra, or Muse Approved by the FDA for impotence	Requires injection Injection is more painful than papaverine Must be mixed with water before each use Must be stored <77° F Is extremely expensive May induce priapism May cause corporal fibrosis

FDA, Food and Drug Administration.

used to treat all types of impotency. Viagra is manufactured in three different strengths and is given 1 hour before intercourse. The primary disadvantages of Viagra are its expense ($10 a pill); the fact that it cannot be prescribed in patients who are taking nitrates; and the need to take the medication 1 hour before contemplated intercourse.

Muse

Muse, a urethral suppository containing alprostadil, provides a second relatively safe and effective way to treat impotence. The suppository is inserted into the distal urethra 10 to 15 minutes prior to intercourse. Muse originally was manufactured in four different strengths containing 125, 250, 500, and 1000 µg of alprostadil. The 125-µg suppository is ineffective and has been withdrawn from the market. I follow the guidelines shown in Table 30–3 to determine the required dose of the drug.

The goal of the treatment protocol is to distinguish patients who have significant cardiovascular disease and are extremely unlikely to respond to a low dose of alprostadil from younger impotent men who may develop priapism if given a large initial dose

of the medication. Although priapism is less likely to occur with Muse than it is with the injectable forms of PEP, it is possible to induce a prolonged erection with any of the vasodila-

Table 30-3
Treatment Protocol for Alprostadil (Muse)

Patient Profile	Treatment Protocol
Patients <50 years of age and patients with neurogenic or psychological impotence Patients who complain of intermittent erectile failure, failure to maintain an erection, or that their erection simply is not firm enough	Low-dose treatment protocol: Start treatment with the 250-µg urethral suppository and progressively increase the dose as necessary
Older patents who have been impotent >2 years Patients who have severe insulin-dependent diabetes or significant cardiovascular disease Patients who do not develop night or day erection at any time under any circumstances	High-dose treatment protocol: Begin with a 500-µg suppository and advance to a 1000-µg suppository if necessary

tors employed to treat impotence; thus, for those who are inexperienced in the use of Muse, the safest course of action is simply to begin treatment in all patients with the 250-µg suppository and increase the dose progressively from 500 to 1000 µg if necessary.

In patients who have a venous leak, the effectiveness of Muse may be increased by constricting the penile venous blood flow before the urethral suppository is inserted. To accomplish this goal, the manufacturer has developed an adjustable rubber tube (Actis), which may be applied to the base of the penis prior to insertion of the suppository. The constricting band is left in place for 10 minutes after the medication is inserted. If the patient begins to lose his erection after the device is removed, it is immediately replaced and left on during intercourse.

The most significant complication of Muse is drug-induced penile and/or perineal pain. In my experience, most of patients who use Muse develop some degree of drug-induced pain, and in at least 20% of these men the painful sensation is so severe that they cannot use the medication. The severity of drug-induced perineal pain may be reduced by applying the penile constricting device before the suppository is inserted into the urethra since this maneuver prevents significant amounts of the drug from entering the pelvic veins draining the penis. Unfortunately, the application of the constricting device does not reduce the severity of drug-induced penile pain.

Finally, it is important to point out that the manufacturer of Muse, Vivus, provides excellent instructional material, including a video, which makes it easy to teach patients how to use Muse.

Pharmacologic Erection Program

Prior to the development of Muse and Viagra, most patients with impotence were treated with one of the pharmacologic erection programs, commonly referred to as PEP. Impotent patients undoubtedly prefer to be treated initially with either Viagra or Muse rather than a penile injection; however, there still is a role for PEP in patients who either do not develop a satisfactory erection with Muse or Viagra or cannot afford these expensive medications. In this respect, it is important to realize that PEP with papaverine provides a relatively inexpensive alternative to Muse, Viagra, and Caverject (the injectable form of alprostadil).

Although drug-induced priapism is possible with any vasodilator that is injected into the penis, the risk of this complication is small if the drugs are used judicially. More important, as I will describe presently, this type of prolonged erection can be reversed easily if treated promptly. Thus, even though PEP is somewhat more complicated and time consuming to administer than Muse or Viagra, I believe it would be appropriate for primary care physicians to provide it for their patients if they are inclined to take the time to learn how to administer the drugs. My protocol for administering papaverine and Caverject is shown in Table 30–4.

Injections are made with a 30-gauge 1/2 inch needle at either the 2 or 10 o'clock positions on the base of the penis. I personally

Table 30–4
Papaverine and Alprostadil (Caverject) Treatment Protocol*

Drug Protocol	Dose per Injection					
Papaverine (mL)						
Low-dose	0.1	0.25	0.5	1.0	1.75	2.5
High-dose	0.5	1.0	1.75	2.5		
Alprostadil (Caverject) (µg)						
Low-dose	1.25	2.5	5	10	20	40
High-dose	2.5	5	10	20	40	

*This table shows my treatment protocol for papaverine and alprostadil. Patients younger than 50 years of age and men with psychological or neurogenic impotence are treated with the low-dose protocol. Older patients with arteriosclerosis may receive a higher initial dose of the drugs. If the diagnosis is in question, the low-dose protocol is appropriate. Doses in excess of 2.5 mL of papaverine and 40 µg of alprostadil generally are ineffective and should be avoided.

perform each of the test injections in my office for two reasons. First, to avoid overdosing during the trial injections, it is important to make sure the drug is being injected into the corporal bodies and not the subcutaneous tissue or the urethra. Second, if the test injection inadvertently induces a prolonged erection, I can reverse it promptly and by so doing avoid the possibility of the patient developing prolonged priapism. After determining the dose of medication that must be used to achieve a satisfactory erection, the patient is taught the injection technique and is provided with a prescription for the medication.

PEP has two particularly important side effects: priapism and corporal fibrosis. Priapism is more likely to occur during the initial injections to determine dose than it is during chronic use of the drug. This, of course, is one of the reasons for performing the test injections in the office rather than teaching the patient the injection technique and allowing him to titrate the dose at home.

Any rigid erection that persists for longer than 1 hour is a cause for concern. Fortunately, if treated early, this type of drug-induced priapism can be easily reversed by simply administering an intracorporal injection of 0.5 to 1 mL of phenylephrine (one 10-mg vial of phenylephrine diluted with 9.5 mL of injectable saline) every 5 minutes until the erection has subsided. Patients who develop a rigid erection that lasts longer than 1 to 2 hours after a self-administered injection at home should be instructed to go to the nearest emergency department for treatment.

Any of the injectable drugs that are used to perform PEP may cause corporal fibrosis. Thus, I examine, by palpation, the penis of patients on PEP patients every 6 months to determine if they are developing areas of firmness suggesting fibrosis. If corporal fibrosis is detected, the penile injections should be discontinued.

Before closing this discussion on the pharmacologic agents which may be used to treat impotency, I would like to emphasize again that papaverine injection provides the most cost-effective method of treating erectile dysfunction. I do not believe that because the manufacturer has not gone to the expense and effort to have the drug approved by the U.S. Food and Drug Administration (FDA) for this application we should be dissuaded from using this inexpensive drug to treat impotent patients, especially if they cannot afford the more expensive FDA-approved alternatives.

The effectiveness of papaverine can be increased by combining it with 5 mg of phentolamine (Regitine). Unfortunately, we have not been able to obtain phentolamine from the manufacturer for the past year; thus, I have not included this useful vasodilator in the proposed treatment protocols for PEP.

Vacuum Devices

Vacuum devices have been used to treat impotence for at least 30 years. These devices consist of a plastic cylinder that is placed over the penis. The open end of the cylinder is pressed against the skin surrounding the base of the penis, and the closed end is connected to a pump that is used to generate a vacuum around the penis. The erection generated by the device is maintained by an elastic band that is placed over the base of the penis before the cylinder is removed.

Vacuum erection aid devices cost between $200 and $600, depending on the complexity of the device. These devices are successful in 60% to 70% of impotent men, and they provide a viable alternative to drug therapy for impotence. Unfortunately, these devices are so cumbersome and difficult to use that many patients refuse to consider them.

Penile Prosthesis

From a historical perspective, it is of interest to note that the present-day interest in impotence began in the early 1970s as a result of the development of the Small-Carrion semirigid and the Scott inflatable penile prostheses. Prior to this time, the medical community had relatively little interest in either the diagnosis or treatment of impotence, in large part because erectile failure was believed primarily to be a psychological condition for which there was no practical medical treatment.

A comprehensive discussion of the complex field of penile prosthetic surgery is beyond the scope of this dissertation; however, primary care physicians should understand the indications for a penile implant and have some knowledge about the advantages and disadvantages of the various devices so that they can give meaningful advise to patients who are considering a penile prosthesis. With this in mind, I would like to share with the reader some of the biases I have developed as a result of having specialized in this field of urologic surgery for the past 25 years.

First, obviously, no patient should consider or be offered a penile prosthesis before he has tried and failed to benefit from the relatively simple and safe treatment modality now readily available for treating impotency.

Second, an inflatable penile prosthesis produces a far more satisfactory erection from both a physiologic and functional standpoint than does a semirigid prosthesis. Thus, a patient who is considering a penile prosthesis should be encouraged to select an inflatable device. In this respect, it is important to realize that the modern inflatable devices manufactured by Mentor are nearly as reliable as the semirigid devices. Thus, the possibility of device failure should not dissuade a patient from having an inflatable penile prosthesis.

Third, the three-piece inflatable prosthesis, which includes a separate large capacity reservoir, is far more likely to provide a satisfactory result than is a device that includes a small-volume reservoir as a component of either the penile cylinders or the pump. This is so because the small reservoirs of the two-piece devices often either do not contain enough fluid to allow adequate inflation of the penile cylinders or do not have enough capacity to allow full deflation of the cylinders following intercourse. For these reasons, I believe it would be preferable for a patient to have a semirigid device than a two-piece inflatable device.

Fourth, I have an extremely strong bias against any penile prosthesis that has inflatable cylinders manufactured from silicone rubber. The failure rate of these devices as a result of wear-induced cylinder leaks is, in my opinion, unacceptably high, just as it was for silicone breast implants. A patient who is contemplating an inflatable penile prosthesis should give strong consideration to a device that has cylinders manufactured from polyurethane since these cylinders are virtually indestructible.

Finally, and possibly most important, the implantation of an inflatable penile prosthesis is a rather complicated surgical procedure, and the results achieved, as with coronary bypass surgery, are directly related to the skill and the experience of the surgical team implanting the device. Thus, a prospective implant patient, with the aid of his referring physician, should seek out a surgeon who has extensive experience in the implantation procedure. The manufacturers of penile prostheses can provide the names of surgeons throughout the country who have acquired the expertise necessary to implant their device correctly, and they will readily provide this important piece of information on request.

Impotence Treatments to Avoid

TESTOSTERONE INJECTIONS

The most common mistake made by family physicians who treat impotency is to give a testosterone injection before determining that the patient has a testosterone deficiency. As stated previously, a deficiency in testosterone is an infrequent cause of impotency. Furthermore, patients with normal serum levels of free testosterone do not benefit from testosterone supplementation unless they are receiving a placebo effect from the drug. For these reasons an impotent male should not be treated with testosterone unless his testosterone level is abnormally low, not just low to normal.

Many older impotent men have abnormally low serum testosterone levels. However, these patients most often do not benefit from testosterone since the primary cause of their erectile failure is vascular penile insufficiency and not a hormonal deficiency. Thus, although a testosterone injection may increase their sex drive and level of frustration, it usually does not improve their ability to obtain or maintain an erection.

Before deciding to recommend a series of testosterone injections, one also should consider the fact that the incidence of prostate cancer increases significantly with age, and early prostate cancer may be exacerbated by testosterone. Thus, it is potentially dangerous to prescribe testosterone to any older man irrespective of his serum testosterone level.

YOHIMBINE

Double-blind studies have confirmed my personal clinical experience, which suggests that yohimbine has no significant effect on erectile function and should not be prescribed for patients with organic impotency. Because of the placebo effect, yohimbine may be useful in some patients with psychological impotency.

PENILE REVASCULARIZATION SURGERY

Because of the complexity of penile revascularization surgery and its low long-term success rate, I do not believe that penile revascularization procedures provide a viable alternative to the other simpler and more effective options for treating erectile dysfunction. A patient who fails to benefit from Viagra, Muse, PEP, or a vacuum device and is willing to consider a surgical procedure should be encouraged to have an inflatable penile prosthesis rather than a revascularization operation.

VENOUS LIGATION PROCEDURES

Procedures designed to interrupt the venous outflow of the penis by ligating the dorsal vein or the more proximal penile venous structures invariably fail and, in my opinion, do not have a role in the treatment of impotency.

Loss of Libido

A decrease of libido usually is the result of a deficiency in testosterone. If a serum free testosterone determination confirms the diagnosis of hypogonadism, the patient is initially treated with an intramuscular injection of 200 to 300 mg of testosterone. If the testosterone injection solves the problem, chronic testosterone supplementation may be achieved with sublingual testosterone or testosterone patches.

Aspermia (absence of emission)

The volume of the ejaculate normally decreases with age. Failure to ejaculate or a decrease in the volume of the ejaculate also may result from a testosterone deficiency that decreases or eliminates the secretions produced by the prostate and seminal vesicles. Most often, however, a failure to ejaculate is a result of retrograde ejaculation. Retrograde ejaculation occurs because the bladder neck fails to contract during orgasm, allowing the ejaculate to enter the bladder. Transurethral resection of the prostate, which destroys the bladder neck, is the most common cause of retrograde ejaculation; however, conditions that produce sympathetic denervation of the bladder neck such as diabetes mellitus and retroperitoneal lymphadenectomy also can produce retrograde ejaculation. Finally, alpha-adrenergic blockers that produce sympathetic blockade can cause retrograde ejaculation.

Many patients will not request treatment for retrograde ejaculation once they have been provided with an explanation for the problem. This is fortunate because there is no treatment for the retrograde ejaculation resulting from surgical resection of the bladder neck. Imipramine hydrochloride, 25 mg twice daily, may be useful in some cases of sympathetic denervation resulting from diabetes or retroperitoneal surgery. If the lack of emission is the result of androgen deficiency, it may be alleviated by testosterone supplementation. Finally, drug-induced retrograde ejaculation usually subsides if the offending medication can be discontinued.

Premature Ejaculation

Premature ejaculation primarily is a result of supersensitivity of the glans penis. Most young men experience some degree of premature ejaculation, and in some patients the condition is disabling.

Premature ejaculation may be treated with either the "freeze" or the "squeeze" technique. Both procedures require a cooperative partner and a good deal of patience and practice. With the freeze technique, the patient's sexual partner stops all movement when he gives a prearranged signal that orgasm is eminent. To apply the "squeeze" technique, the male withdraws when ejaculation is eminent and applies a firm squeeze to his glans penis.

This maneuver causes the sensation of imminent orgasm to subside.

Premature ejaculation also may be controlled in some patients by ingesting 50 mg of clomipramine 1 hour before intercourse. If none of these treatment modalities are effective, the patient can only be reassured that the problem will become progressively less severe with age.

The Absence of Orgasm

Most older males find it progressively more and more difficult to achieve orgasm even if they can maintain an erection for a reasonable period. This problem, which ultimately may become so severe that the patient cannot reach a climax under any circumstance, seems to be an inevitable result of aging. I know of no satisfactory treatment for the condition.

Summary

Sexual dysfunction may result from erectile failure, the loss of sexual desire, an inability to ejaculate, premature ejaculation, and the inability to achieve orgasm. Vascular disease is the most common cause of erectile failure, and it often is complicated by the administration of antihypertensive medications and the psychological "fear of failing." Because of the availability of safe and effective treatment options for impotency, a comprehensive diagnostic evaluation is not necessary and most patients with erectile dysfunction may be treated by their primary care physician with Viagra, Muse, or PEP without a urologic consultation. Patients who fail to benefit from one of these safe and effective treatment options may be referred to a urologist for further evaluation and consideration of a penile prosthesis.

SUGGESTED READINGS

1. Bar-Moshe O, Vandendris M: Treatment of impotence due to perineal venous leakage by ligation of cura penis. J Urol 139:1217, 1988.
2. Bookstein JJ, Valji K, Parsons L: Pharmacoarteriography in the evaluation of impotence. J Urol 137:333, 1987.
3. Lue TF: Treatment of venogenic impotence. *In* Tanagho EA, Lue TF, McClure RD (eds): Contemporary Management of Impotence and Infertility. Baltimore, Williams & Wilkins, 1988, p 175.
4. Lue TF, Hricak H, Marich KW, et al: Evaluation of arteriogenic impotency with intracorporal injection of papaverine and duplex ultrasound scanner. Semin Urol 3:21, 1985.
5. Lydston GF: The surgical treatment of impotency. Am J Clin Med 15:1571, 1980.
6. Merrill DC: Clinical experience with Scott inflatable penile prosthesis in 150 patients. Urology 22:371, 1983.
7. Merrill DC: Mentor inflatable penile prosthesis. Urol Clin North Am 16:51, 1989.
8. Miller JB, Howards SS, McLeod RM: Serum prolactin in organic and psychogenic impotence. J Urol 123:862, 1980.
9. Nadig PW, Ware JC, Blumoff R: Noninvasive device to produce and maintain an erection-like state. Urology 27:126, 1986.
10. Rubin A, Babbott D: Impotence and diabetes mellitus. JAMA 168:498, 1958.
11. Scott FB, Bradley WF, Timm BW: Use of implantable inflatable prosthesis. Urology 2:80, 1973.
12. Small MP, Carrion HH: A new penile prosthesis for treating impotence. Contemp Surg 7:29, 1975.

Superficial Lesions of the Male External Genitalia

Unni M. M. Mooppan

Superficial lesions of the penis can have a variety of causative factors. Although traditionally these lesions have been diagnosed and treated by either urologists or dermatologists, in the present changed environment of U.S. health care, it is important that primary care physicians be well versed in the diagnosis and treatment of these lesions. If not for their ability to accurately diagnose and treat these lesions as the primary care physicians, they should at least be able to recognize these lesions and make appropriate referrals to the specialists. If proper provisional diagnoses are made and necessary investigations are planned in time, these lesions can be effectively treated, saving time and money. At times, accurate diagnosis of certain lesions of external genitalia can be quite challenging in spite of the availability of all the sophisticated tests.

Infection by human immunodeficiency virus (HIV) has produced added significance to these lesions. It has been shown by statistics that the presence of penile sores or lesions due to any etiology can enhance the chance of infection by HIV. In addition, patients can have an obvious lesion by a particular sexually transmitted disease (STD) and at the same time be infected by various other organisms as well as HIV. At times, the same person can have more than one type of lesion on the penile shaft, and if this fact is not appreciated, the physician may treat the obvious lesion and miss treating the accompanying infections or lesions.

Recent knowledge of the various subtypes of human papillomavirus (HPV) and their association with malignant lesions of the penile shaft have created added significance to the

need for their prompt diagnosis and treatment and proper counseling of the patient.

Lesions of External Genitalia as Part of Generalized Skin Disease

Conditions such as psoriasis, chickenpox and lichen planus can affect the external genitalia as part of the generalized skin disease. While examining the external genitalia, if any of these lesions are seen, or if the patient complains of a lesion on the external genitalia and the lesion looks suspicious for one of these conditions, exposing the entire body and examining the skin for more such lesions may help establish the diagnosis (Fig. 31–1). Lichen planus may present as a solitary lesion on the penis (Fig. 31–2) or may have multiple lesions on the penile shaft. It is extremely rare for a patient to present with lichen planus or

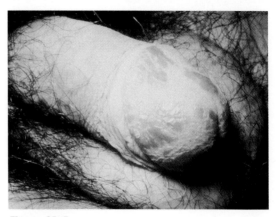

Figure 31–1
Glans penis showing multiple lesions of psoriasis.

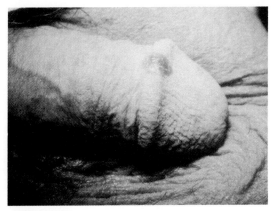

Figure 31–2
Solitary lesion of lichen planus on the corona of the glans penis.

psoriasis lesions only on the external genitalia. However, the characteristic nature of these lesions should be kept in mind, and if suspected, appropriate consultations should be made.

Lesions Found with Sexually Transmitted Diseases

SYPHILIS

Syphilis is the third most frequently reported communicable disease, the first being gonorrhea and the second being chickenpox. The causative organism is *Treponema pallidum,* a spirochete. Although the increased awareness about HIV and acquired immunodeficiency syndrome (AIDS) and the increased use of condoms resulted in a decrease in the incidence of syphilis during the last decade, recent publications have once again shown an alarming increase in its incidence. Syphilitic lesions on the penis can depend on the stage of the disease—primary, secondary, or tertiary.

Primary Syphilis

Lesions of primary syphilis usually appear on the penile shaft after an incubation period of 9 to 90 days. The initial lesion is a papule, and after 3 to 7 days, it breaks down to form the classic "primary chancre" or "hard chancre." It is a clean-cut ulcer, painless, with hardly any exudate. The primary chancre

may be a solitary lesion or multiple ulcers (Fig. 31–3). The character of the ulcer changes when it gets secondarily infected with other suppurative organisms. Once this happens, there is copious discharge from the ulcers and the margins can change from the clean-cut nature to a shaggy appearance. By this time, inguinal lymphadenopathy may be appreciated. Whether treated or not, the primary chancre can heal spontaneously. This clinical course can vary from patient to patient, depending on the immune status, current antibiotic treatment, or the presence of secondary infection.

Serological tests for syphilis and darkfield identification of *T. pallidum* are the usual diagnostic modalities. The commonly performed serologic test for syphilis is the one known as VDRL (Venereal Disease Research Laboratory) test. Another, known as RPR (rapid plasma reagin) also depends on the circulating antibodies. The most sensitive test is known as FTA-ABS: fluorescent treponemal antigen absorption test. All the serologic tests include quantitative dilution techniques to determine the seriousness of the positive test and also to monitor treatment and follow-up.

Treatment of primary syphilis is by intramuscular injection of benzathine penicillin, a single-dose administration of 2.4 million units. Doxycycline, erythromycin, and ceftriaxone also are effective agents. Coexistence of other commonly encountered STDs should be suspected and investigated for. Patients

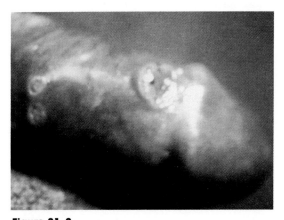

Figure 31–3
Primary chancre of syphilis. (From Mooppan UMM: Cutaneous lesions of the penis. *In* Hashmat AI, Das S [eds]: The Penis. Media, PA, Williams & Wilkins, 1993, p 70.)

should be counseled on HIV infection and advised on "safe sex" practices.

Secondary Syphilis

Secondary syphilis is a systemic disease. Hence, the lesion that is seen on the external genitalia is only a part of the manifestation. Secondary syphilis starts about 6 weeks to 6 months after the initial infection. The skin lesions are usually maculopapular and can be present throughout the body. In addition, there can be mucous patches in the oral cavity, condyloma lata lesions found in the anal region, and generalized lymphadenopathy. The maculopapular lesions can be hypopigmented or hyperpigmented. Serologic tests help establish the diagnosis. Treatment, again, is benzathine penicillin, 2.4 million units as a single dose intramuscularly.

Tertiary Syphilis (Gumma)

Lesions of tertiary, or late, syphilis can either be proliferative or destructive. The lesions can appear anywhere in the body, usually on skin and bone. The nodular lesions can have a central, coagulative necrosis resulting in a gummy material—thus its classic name "gumma." The penis can be one of the sites where these lesions can appear. Diagnosis is by clinical suspicion, confirmed by serologic tests. Treatment is by intramuscular injection of benzathine penicillin, 2.4 million units given at weekly intervals for 3 weeks—a total of 7.2 million units. Doxycycline, 100 mg orally twice daily for 4 weeks, or tetracycline, 500 mg orally four times a day for 4 weeks, is an alternative treatment.

CHANCROID

The causative organism of chancroid, a sexually transmitted lesion, is *Haemophilus ducreyi*, a gram-negative bacillus. The mode of transmission is almost exclusively sexual contact. The lesions, known as "soft chancre," appear when the initial papular lesions break down. Compared to the "clean-looking," painless lesions of syphilis, the lesions of chancroid are "dirty looking," with plenty of purulent discharge and slough, and the edges are undermined (Fig. 31–4). The lesions can be single

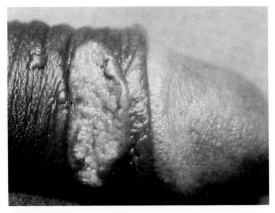

Figure 31–4

Large solitary lesion of the chancroid. Multiple papular lesions are seen by the side. (From Mooppan UMM: Cutaneous lesions of the penis. *In* Hashmat AI, Das S [eds]: The Penis. Media, PA, Williams & Wilkins, 1993, p 74.)

or multiple. They can appear on the prepuce, glans, penile shaft, or anywhere on the external genitalia. If the patient used a condom while having sexual intercourse with an infected partner, the lesion may be seen only at the base of the penis (Fig. 31–5). The lesions are more commonly seen on the uncircumcised penis, as compared to one that has been circumcised. Increased chances of trauma to the penile skin of the uncircumcised penis and the moisture between the prepucial sac and glans penis may be factors contributing to this increased susceptibility. The presence of more lesions on or around the frenulum,

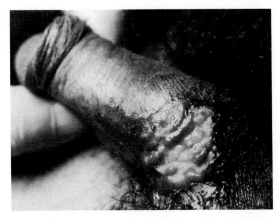

Figure 31–5

Lesion of chancroid at the base of the penis. The rest of the penile shaft was apparently protected by condom. (From Mooppan UMM: Cutaneous lesions of the penis. *In* Hashmat AI, Das S [eds]: The Penis. Media, PA, Williams & Wilkins, 1993, p 75.)

which is the most common area vulnerable to trauma during sexual activity, may add credence to this argument. The penile lesions and the secondary lymphadenopathy are painful. The "bubo" from lymphadenopathy may rupture to form ulcers in the groin.

Diagnosis is by clinical suspicion while noticing the characteristic lesions on the genitalia and confirmed by identification of the organism. *H. ducreyi* is difficult to grow on culture media, hence, the best method to identify the organism is to scrape the edges of the ulcer, prepare a slide, and stain to identify the gram-negative bacilli seen as pairs. Treatment is by oral administration of erythromycin, 500 mg four times daily for 7 days, or ceftriaxone, 250 mg given as a single intramuscular injection. Trimethoprim-sulphamethoxazole, one double-strength tablet twice daily for 1 week, or ciprofloxacin, 500 mg orally twice daily for 3 days, are alternative medications that can be used. The patient and his sexual partner should be tested for other STDs, and preventive measures should be emphasized.

LESIONS FROM GONORRHEA

The causative organism of gonorrhea is *Neisseria gonorrheae*. The classic manifestation of gonorrhea is urethritis with purulent, yellowish discharge and dysuria. However, rarely, superficial lesions on the penile shaft can occur. Gonococcal tysonitis, abscesses on the penile shaft and ulcerative lesions on the penile median raphae, have been reported. Since these lesions are rare, coexistence of classic signs and symptoms of gonorrhea may help make the provisional diagnosis, and it can be confirmed by observation of gram-negative intracytoplasmic diplococci on the slide preparation. The recommended treatment is by single injection of ceftriaxone, 250 mg intramuscularly, followed by a 7-day course of doxycycline, 100 mg orally once a day. Patients who cannot have ceftriaxone can have spectinomycine, 2 g, as a single intramuscular injection. As in all cases of STD, coexistence of other sexually transmitted ailments must be suspected, and the patient should be tested by serologic test for syphilis. In addition, the importance of safe-sex practices should be stressed, and testing and counseling for HIV infection should be offered.

LYMPHOGRANULOMA VENEREUM

Lymphogranuloma venereum (LGV) is sporadic in the United States and other western countries. The disease is endemic in parts of Africa, India, Southeast Asia, and South America. The causative organism is *Chlamydia trachomatis*, and it is sexually transmitted. The organism cannot penetrate healthy, intact skin or mucosa. Therefore, unhealthy skin or mucosa, or a break in these linings, are a prerequisite for this infection.

The most important presenting lesion is inguinal lymphadenopathy. This is because the initial penile lesion is very small, transient and painless and heals spontaneously, without any treatment. The incubation period from the time of exposure to the appearance of a penile lesion is variable—from 3 days to 6 weeks. The lesion goes from papule to pustule and heals spontaneously. By the time the patient presents with the bubo (inguinal lymphadenopathy), it is a systemic disease and the patient has headache, general weakness, weight loss, erythemas, urticarias, and arthralgia. Bubo is painful, unilateral in two thirds of patients, and bilateral in one third. In about one third of cases, the bubo may go through the stages of abscess formation and ulceration.

The most widely used tests for the diagnosis are serologic. Although the organism can be cultured from the aspirate of the lesion, this process can be difficult and costly. There is a skin test known as *Frei's test* for LGV. However, this has been found to be of low sensitivity and specificity. The widely used serologic tests are LGV complement-fixation test and the microimmunofluorescent test for *C. trachomatis* antibody.

Doxycycline, 100 mg by mouth twice daily for 21 days, is the commonly used treatment. Other treatment choices are tetracycline, 500 mg orally four times a day for 21 days; erythromycin, 500 mg orally four times a day for 21 days; sulfisoxazole, 500 mg orally four times a day for 21 days; or any equivalent sulfonamide agent for 21 days.

GRANULOMA INGUINALE (Donovanosis)

Granuloma inguinale is caused by the organism *Calymmatobacterium granulomatis,* an intracytoplasmic gram-negative bacillus. The disease is sexually transmitted. The intracellular inclusion body was described by Donovan, hence the name *Donovanosis.* As in the case of LGV, Donovanosis is also rare in western countries but is one of the common STDs in developing countries.

The incubation period varies from 8 to 80 days. The lesion can be over the penis, groin, or anal region. The lesion starts as a small nodule that later ulcerates and becomes a granulomatous lesion (Fig. 31–6). The lesion can be large and may resemble epithelial malignancy until biopsy proves otherwise. Stained preparation from the lesion shows the classic intracytoplasmic Donovan bodies, which have a characteristic resemblance to a safety pin. Treatment is doxycycline, 100 mg twice daily for 2 weeks. Alternative antibiotics can be ampicillin, 250 to 500 mg orally four times a day for 2 weeks, or trimethoprim-sulphamethoxazole, double-strength orally twice a day for 2 weeks.

HUMAN PAPILLOMAVIRUS INFECTIONS

Genital HPV infection is one of the most common viral STDs in the United States. The Centers for Disease Control and Prevention

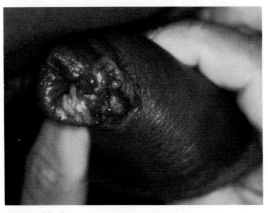

Figure 31–6
Granuloma inguinale over the prepuce. (From Mooppan UMM: Cutaneous lesions of the penis. *In* Hashmat AI, Das S [eds]: The Penis. Media, PA, Williams & Wilkins, 1993, p 77.)

reported in 1994 the incidence of genital warts as 250,000 new cases per year.

HPV has more than 50 subtypes. This STD has to be taken seriously because of the relationship between malignancy in men as well as women. HPV subtypes 16, 18, 31, 33, and 35 have been shown to possess the potential to induce malignancy. In a few cases of penile intraepithelial malignancy as well as in giant condyloma acuminatum (also known as *Buschke-Lowenstein tumor*), both with the potential to develop carcinoma of the penis, association with HPV infection has been established.

Mainly, there are three types of penile lesions produced by HPV infection: condyloma acuminata, Buschke-Lowenstein tumor (giant condyloma), and penile horn (verruca vulgaris).

Condyloma Acuminata

Condyloma acuminata lesions, commonly known as venereal warts, are the most common type of lesions associated with HPV infections. These are sexually transmitted lesions, and only one third of the infected individuals show these lesions. The majority of the lesions are subclinical and can be detected as white patches only after applying 3% to 5% acetic acid on the normal-looking penile skin. Therefore, if the female partner continues to have recurrent lesions and examination of the male partner does not reveal any lesion on the external genitalia, the penile shaft should be wrapped in 3% to 5% acetic acid–soaked gauze for 5 minutes and then examined using a magnifying lens for white patches.

The lesions of condyloma acuminata are usually multiple, seen in the sulcus, along the corona of the glans penis (Fig. 31–7). Although these warty lesions can be seen anywhere on the external genitalia, groin, perineum or perianal region, the common sites are within the prepucial sac or near the urethral meatus (Fig. 31–8). This may be due to the fact that the organism prefers moist areas. Rarely, the urethra and bladder can also be involved.

Diagnosis is usually clinical and confirmed by histopathology of the excised lesion. When clinical suspicion is high, as described earlier,

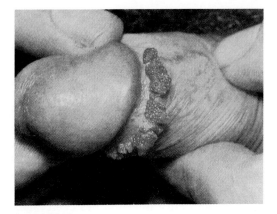

Figure 31-7
Condyloma acuminata. (From Mooppan UMM: Cutaneous lesions of the penis. *In* Hashmat AI, Das S [eds]: The Penis. Media, PA, Williams & Wilkins, 1993, p 77.)

acetic acid treatment may be needed to visualize the subclinical lesions. In uncircumcised men, unless the prepuce is retracted or the external urethral meatus is carefully examined, the lesions in the prepucial sac and fossa navicularis may be easily missed. Since intraurethral lesions are rare (3% to 5%), routine urethrocystoscopy is not recommended unless there is hematuria or positive cytology.

The treatment is aimed at the exophytic lesion, and there is no agent, so far, to eradicate HPV infection. A variety of treatment options are available, and the choice may depend on the treatment pattern set up by the physician or the patient's preference. Topical agents include trichloracetic acid, bichlora-

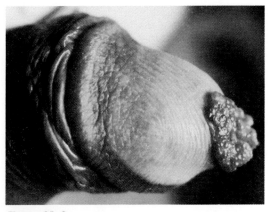

Figure 31-8
Condyloma acuminata at the external urethral meatus. (From Mooppan UMM: Cutaneous lesions of the penis. *In* Hashmat AI, Das S [eds]: The Penis. Media, PA, Williams & Wilkins, 1993, p 78.)

cetic acid, 5-fluorouracil, cantharidin, podophyllin, podophyllotoxin, or imiquimod. Podophyllin is commercially available in liquid form, and imiquimod (an immune-response modifier) is available as a topical cream. Local excision, circumcision, cryotherapy using liquid nitrogen or dry ice, CO_2 laser vaporization, and electrocautery desiccation are some of the other choices. Combination of any of these local treatments with systemic therapy with alpha$_{2b}$-interferon also have been tested with some reported benefits. The most important component of treatment is advising the patient's sexual partner to undergo physical examination for detection of HPV infection, vigorous treatment of the lesions, if any, and the use of condoms until both partners are completely free of lesions. In addition, as usually recommended for any STD, counseling on other possible associated STDs (especially HIV infection) and the practice of safe sex should be provided for all patients.

Buschke-Lowenstein Tumor (Giant Condyloma)

The causative organism for Buschke-Lowenstein tumor is the same HPV. Types 6 and 11 of the HPV have been isolated from these lesions. The characteristic differences between these lesions and the common venereal warts are their size, clinical behavior, and the potential for malignancy. The lesion can attain large size, disfiguring or destroying the external genitalia and groin. Whereas some believe that these are premalignant lesions and only a few develop malignancy, others believe that these are well-differentiated low-grade carcinomas from the beginning. Because of this, the commonly recommended treatment is early surgical removal.

Penile Horn (Verruca Vulgaris)

Penile horn (verruca vulgaris) is associated with HPV type 16. The name derives from its characteristic hornlike outgrowth. The lesion is usually single but can be multiple. Since malignant changes have been reported in some cases, the recommended treatment is early excision of the lesion.

GENITAL HERPES (Herpes Simplex Virus Infections)

The causative organism of genital herpes is a virus. Although herpes simplex virus I (HSV-I) is commonly associated with oral lesions and HSV-II is commonly associated with genital lesions, the reverse is also possible. There have been observations linking HSV infection and cervical cancer in women. HSV infection is mainly seen in the upper- and middle-class socioeconomic strata, especially on college campuses. During the last 2 or 3 decades, the incidence at times reached epidemic proportions. The clinical picture varies depending on the type of infection—whether it is the first-time infection or one of the several recurrent infections. The incubation period for the first-time infection is usually 2 to 10 days. Before the first-time infection lesions appear on the genitalia, the patient experiences headache, low-grade fever, and general weakness. The lesions go through stages of multiple vesicles, pustules, and crusts (Fig. 31–9). In approximately 2 to 3 weeks, these stages may be completed. Dysuria and painful, palpable lymph nodes are sometimes accompanying conditions. The clinical course is shorter during recurrent infections; the area involved may be smaller and dysuria as well as systemic symptoms are usually absent.

The virus stays permanently along the dorsal nerve root ganglia. Sacral nerve root radiculopathies producing urinary retention, impotence, constipation, and other sensory or motor deficiencies have been associated with a primary HSV infection. Prior to the appearance of recurrent lesions, itching, paresthesia, or a burning sensation may be experienced over the previously infected areas.

Clinical picture, viral culture, staining of the dry preparation slides, and serologic tests are the tools to establish the diagnosis. Viral culture is expensive and difficult. Observation of classic lesions; findings of multinucleated, giant epithelial cells on stained preparation; and serologic tests showing high titer of HSV-I and/or HSV-II usually aid the diagnosis. When the lesions are secondarily infected, the typical clinical picture may be missing. In addition, coexistence of other STDs, especially HIV infection, should be suspected.

HSV infection is incurable. The treatment is mainly aimed at reducing the frequency at which the lesions recur and to reduce the clinical course of lesions. Acyclovir is the most commonly used antiviral agent. For the first-time episode, the recommended dosage is 200 mg orally five times daily for 7 to 10 days, or until the lesions subside. Acyclovir is also available in the form of 5% topical preparation, which has been shown to be effective against the local lesions.

Acyclovir capsules or topical cream, if started during the prodromal stage of the re-infection, may reduce the severity and shorten the duration of the recurrences. In addition, continued use as prophylaxis has been shown to be effective against recurrent lesions, especially in increasing the interval between the recurrences, shortening their course, and reducing the severity of lesions and symptoms. The recommended dose is 200 mg orally two to five times a day, or a regimen that is comfortable for the patient to avoid the side effects for many months, or even 1 to 3 years. However, if prolonged use of more than 1 year is needed, it is better to stop for a short period and reassess the status.

Counseling the patients and their partners is an important aspect of management. It should be emphasized that treatment is against the lesions only and that there is no permanent cure against the virus infection. Maximum precaution, preferably abstinence, should be used during the presence of lesions, which is the most contagious period. Use of a condom during sexual intercourse should

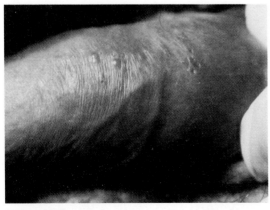

Figure 31-9
Genital herpes, with vesicles intact and ruptured. (From Mooppan UMM: Cutaneous lesions of the penis. *In* Hashmat AI, Das S [eds]: The Penis. Media, PA, Williams & Wilkins, 1993, p 80.)

be stressed, preferably even in the absence of lesions, by patients with recurrent lesions. Since a reduced immune status of the individual may be associated with infections such as HSV, counseling regarding HIV infection should be provided.

MOLLUSCUM CONTAGIOSUM

Molluscum contagiosum lesions are caused by the molluscum contagiosum virus (MSV). The lesions seen in adults are usually sexually transmitted, and the usual sites are the external genitalia and surrounding areas, such as the pubic region, lower abdomen, and thighs. In children, the lesions are usually seen on the exposed regions of the body, and the lesions are usually the result of nonsexual contact.

The incubation period can vary from 1 week to 6 months, but the usual range is from 2 to 7 weeks. Average size of the lesion is about 3 to 5 mm. They appear as white, discrete, rounded lesions (Fig. 31–10). Some of them may show "umbilication," which is the characteristic depression at the top of these rounded lesions. The lesions may spontaneously disappear in 6 to 12 months. Virus from the lesions can autoinoculate other parts of the body by touching. Occasionally, the lesions can produce itching and discomfort ("molluscum dermatitis"). Diagnosis is made by the typical clinical appearance of the lesions and can be confirmed either by histology of a removed lesion or staining of the crushed material from the lesion.

Removal of the lesion by scraping or curettage, topical application of podophyllin, phenol, silver nitrate, or laser vaporization are the modes of treatment. Although the lesions may disappear spontaneously if one waits for 6 to 12 months, it is preferable to remove the lesions to prevent spread to the rest of the body by autoinoculation and to others by sexual or nonsexual contact. As in all other STDs, the sexual partner should be examined and counseling regarding other STDs, and preventive measures should be given.

Lesions of External Genitalia in Patients with AIDS

LESIONS PREDISPOSING THE PATIENT TO HIV INFECTION

Any type of penile ulceration can enhance the chance of HIV infection. Since intact skin is more resistant to HIV infection as compared to unhealthy skin or skin with cuts or ulcerations, presence of lesions such as hard or soft chancre, condyloma, or any type of ulceration can be an added factor predisposing the patient to HIV infection when he has unprotected sexual intercourse with an infected partner. Therefore, even if the lesion seen on the penis is typical for a particular type of lesion, it is important to test the patient for other commonly seen STDs and to counsel the patient regarding HIV infection and testing for it.

LESIONS SECONDARY TO AIDS

As a result of reduced immunity in patients with HIV infection and AIDS, they are more prone to cutaneous lesions due to infections by HSV, HPV, fungus, herpes zoster virus, and MCV. These lesions can be present on the external genitalia, and in the presence of HIV infection, these are more resistant to the usual treatment. Increased dosage of medications over a prolonged period may be needed.

MALIGNANT LESIONS IN AIDS PATIENTS

Kaposi's sarcoma is the most common cutaneous malignant lesion associated with AIDS,

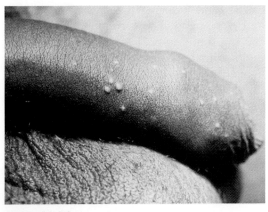

Figure 31–10
Multiple lesions of molluscum contagiosum. (From Mooppan UMM: Cutaneous lesions of the penis. *In* Hashmat AI, Das S [eds]: The Penis. Media, PA, Williams & Wilkins, 1993, p 81.)

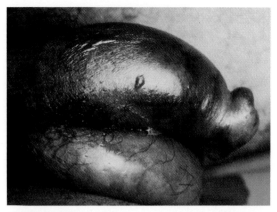

Figure 31-11
Penile skin showing ischemic changes in a patient with human immunodeficiency virus. Histopathology showed intraepithelial squamous cell carcinoma. (From Mooppan UMM: Cutaneous lesions of the penis. *In* Hashmat AI, Das S [eds]: The Penis. Media, PA, Williams & Wilkins, 1993, p 83.)

and this condition can be present on the external genitalia also. There has been an increased incidence of squamous cell carcinomas in HIV-infected patients. In our institution, we have encountered three patients with carcinoma in situ of the penile skin and one patient with squamous cell carcinoma of the penis associated with HIV infection (Figs. 31–11 and 31–12).

When cutaneous lesions from AIDS patients are submitted for histopathologic examination, care must be taken while interpreting

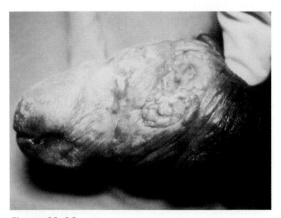

Figure 31-12
Healed lesion on the glans penis (primary chancre) and nonhealing ulcer on the inner surface of the prepuce in a patient with human immunodeficiency virus infection. A nonhealing ulcer showed intraepithelial squamous cell carcinoma on biopsy. (From Mooppan UMM: Cutaneous lesions of the penis. *In* Hashmat AI, Das S [eds]: The Penis. Media, PA, Williams & Wilkins, 1993, p 83.)

the results. There has been a report of "pseudo-Hodgkin's disease" from a lesion of molluscum contagiosum excised from a patient with AIDS. The report cautioned against confusing this picture with true lymphoma. Another report illustrated a case of cutaneous cryptococcosis in a patient with AIDS, mimicking molluscum contagiosum. These are isolated case reports, but gradually a pattern may emerge if attention is paid to all the reported cases.

PENILE ULCERATION IN PATIENTS WITH AIDS RECEIVING FOSCARNET TREATMENT

When treating HSV infection or cytomegalovirus infection in patients with AIDS, the commonly used agents such as acyclovir or ganciclovir may be ineffective. Foscarnet (trisodium phosphonoformate hexahydrate) is the alternative agent commonly used in these circumstances. One of the side effects of this medication has been the appearance of penile ulcers, which are painful and localized to the glans penis. Histologically, they do not resemble fixed drug eruptions. They seem to disappear on discontinuation of the medication.

Fungal Infections

CANDIDAL BALANITIS/ BALANOPOSTHITIS

Infection of the prepuce and glans penis by *Candida* is the most common form of fungal infection of the penis. This usually occurs in uncircumcised men, especially in patients with diabetes mellitus. The common organism is *Candida albicans*. In uncircumcised men, the lesion appears as multiple cracks at the opening of the prepuce (Fig. 31–13). If an adult comes to the physician seeking circumcision because of the above mentioned condition of the prepuce, undiagnosed diabetes mellitus must be suspected and the patient should be investigated for the same prior to circumcision. In addition to controlling the diabetes and treating any other predisposing conditions, the local lesion can be treated by nystatin, clotrimazole, miconazole, or econazole. Once the diabetes and active infection

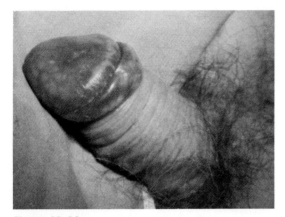

Figure 31-13
Candidal balanitis. (From Mooppan UMM: Cutaneous lesions of the penis. *In* Hashmat AI, Das S [eds]: The Penis. Media, PA, Williams & Wilkins, 1993, p 84.)

are controlled, circumcision may be needed, especially if there is phimosis.

TINEA VERSICOLOR

The causative organism of tinea versicolor is *Pytyrosporum orticulare.* The usually involved areas are the trunk and upper half of the body. Treatment is by topical application of sodium thiosulphate, clotrimazole, or miconazole.

TINEA CRURIS

The organisms responsible for tinea cruris are epidermophytons or trichophytons. The usually involved areas are the groin, but, rarely, the scrotum and penile shaft may be involved. Treatment is by topical antifungal agents. If topical agents alone cannot control the condition, griseofulvin or ketoconazole may be added as oral agents.

In all the fungal infections, the easiest way to establish the diagnosis is to scrape the lesion and examine the scrapings, mixed with 10% potassium hydroxide under the microscope. In addition to the above-mentioned conditions, rare lesions such as penile cryptococcosis and blastomycosis have been reported in the literature. Important things to keep in mind while dealing with fungal infections is to suspect and rule out immunocompromised conditions.

Tuberculosis of the Penis

In spite of the increased incidence of tuberculosis in the United States, penile involvement remains extremely low. However, there are reported cases of primary as well as secondary tuberculosis of the penis. In countries where genitourinary tuberculosis is common, scrotal involvement and chronic sinus formation are more common than penile involvement because of increased incidence of tuberculous epididymitis and secondary abscess formation. In cases of primary tuberculosis of the penis, there is usually a history of sexual contact, but it is not always forthcoming. Biopsy of the lesion helps distinguish the lesion from malignant ulcers. Treatment is the usual multidrug antitubercular therapy, and the lesions usually respond to the treatment.

Parasitic Lesions

AMEBIASIS

Amebiasis of the external genitalia is extremely rare in the United States. The causative agent is *Entamoeba histolyticum.* Anal intercourse with an infected individual is the usual mode of transmission. Review of world literature revealed only nine reported cases so far. Treatment is with emetine hydrochloride and metronidazole, when the diagnosis is established.

SCABIES

The causative organism of scabies is *Sarcoptes scabiei,* commonly known as the "human itch mite." The lesions can vary in nature—flat, red, scaly patches, papules, nodules, or excoriation. Prolonged contact with an infected person is the source of infection. Examination of scrapings from the lesion under the microscope and identification of the organism establishes the diagnosis. Treatment is aimed at the patient as well as to his close contacts. The medication used is 1% gamma benzene hexachloride lotion or cream to the entire body.

PEDICULOSIS PUBIS ("Crabs" or "Pubic Lice")

The lesions on the genitalia in pediculosis pubis, if present, are due to the bite by the causative organism: *Phthirus pubis*. Itching and scratching may produce secondary infection, and pustules may be present. The condition is fairly common, even in Western countries, and transmission is by close contact with infected persons or by sharing contaminated clothing. Treatment should be aimed at the personal contacts also. The agent used to treat the condition is 1% gama-benzene hexachloride in the form of shampoo.

Lymphedema of the External Genitalia

LYMPHEDEMA OF THE PENIS

Any condition producing lymphatic obstruction to the penis can produce lymphedema (Fig. 31–14). In tropical countries, filariasis is one of the most common causes. Trauma, inflammatory conditions, lymphadenectomy, any surgical procedure of the pubic or pelvic region producing interruption of lymphatic drainage, malignancy in the drainage area, radiation therapy of the pubic or pelvic region, and congenital absence of lymphatic drainage (Milroy's disease) are some of the other causes. Complete excision of the edema-

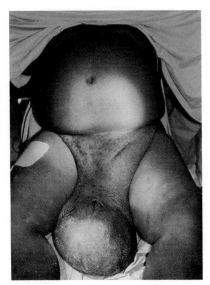

Figure 31–15
Lymphadema of the scrotum. The huge size, reaching below the knee, engulfed the penile shaft.

tous skin and replacement with split-thickness skin graft can be tried, but recurrence of the condition is not unusual.

LYMPHEDEMA OF THE SCROTUM

In tropical countries, filariasis is the most common cause of lymphedema of the scrotum, and it is usually associated with lymphedema of the penis. The causative organism, *Wuchereria bancrofti*, produces lymphatic obstruction and the lymphedema is usually the sequela of the disease. Therefore, medical treatment of filariasis by diethylcarbamazine does not always prevent the development of edema. In countries where filariasis is not common, all the conditions enumerated for the development of lymphedema of the penis can produce that of the scrotum also. When lymphedema is of huge size, the penile shaft is engulfed by the condition and a reduction serotoplasty may be needed to rectify the situation (Fig. 31–15). Recurrence after surgery is not uncommon, especially when the condition responsible for the lymphedema is not correctable.

Gangrene of the External Genitalia

GANGRENE OF THE SCROTUM

Fournier's gangrene is the most common form of gangrene that involves the scrotum.

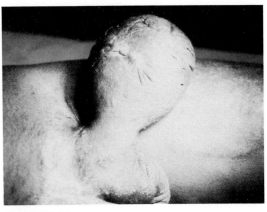

Figure 31–14
Lymphedema of the penis with normal scrotum. A scar at the base of the penis and pubic region from previous surgery produced the lymphatic obstruction. (From Mooppan UMM: Cutaneous lesions of the penis. *In* Hashmat AI, Das S [eds]: The Penis. Media, PA, Williams & Wilkins, 1993, p 86.)

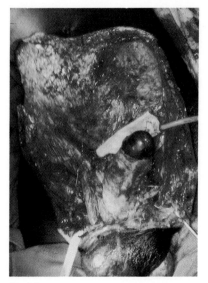

Figure 31-16
Extensive Fournier's gangrene extending from the scrotum to the abdominal wall and penile shaft, after débridement.

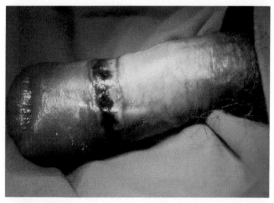

Figure 31-17
Circumferential ischemic change produced by the external urinary drainage device. (Reprinted from Urology, vol 25. Jayachandran S, Mooppan UMM, Kim H: Complications from external [condom] drainage devices, p 33. Copyright 1985, with permission from Elsevier Science.)

The patient presents with fever, toxicity, and scrotal swelling with shiny and, at times, ischemic patches. If the patient presents with the above-mentioned condition of the scrotum, but without fever or leukocytosis, suspicion should arise regarding immuno-compromised conditions, especially HIV infection. Immediate drainage, débridement, antibiotic treatment, urinary diversion, when needed, are the initial steps in treatment (Fig. 31–16). Skin graft may be needed, if there is extensive skin loss. This should wait until healthy granulation is present. The testes and spermatic cord are not usually involved in the process.

GANGRENE OF THE PENIS

Gangrene of the penis may involve only the skin or the entire penile shaft, depending on the mechanism and the blood supply that is jeopardized. Extension of Fournier's gangrene into the pubic region and penile shaft may result in loss of skin cover to the penile shaft (see Fig. 31–16). Strangulation of the glans penis or penile shaft by hair, by the constriction caused by external (condom) urinary drainage devices (Figs. 31–17 to 31–19), and vascular occlusion in renal failure (Fig. 31–20) are some of the other causes. Rare

cases of ischemia produced by vascular occlusion by cholesterol embolism, lymphoproliferative diseases, and in patients with AIDS have also been encountered (see Fig. 31–11). Treatment of the primary condition, local débridement and/or amputation, antibiotics, and other supportive measures form the main components of management.

Premalignant Lesions

Carcinoma of the penis may develop after prolonged existence of the premalignant lesions, or it may coexist with any of these

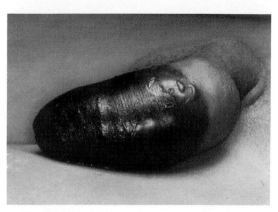

Figure 31-18
Necrosis of the penile skin caused by external urinary drainage devices. (Reprinted from Urology, vol 25. Jayachandran S, Mooppan UMM, Kim H: Complications from external [condom] drainage devices, p 33. Copyright 1985, with permission from Elsevier Science.)

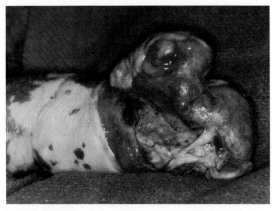

Figure 31-19
Depigmentation, ulceration, and gangrene from prolonged use of an external urinary drainage device. (Reprinted from Urology, vol 25. Jayachandran S, Mooppan
UMM, Kim H: Complications from external [condom]
drainage devices, p 33. Copyright 1985, with permission
from Elsevier Science.)

conditions: Bowen's disease, erythroplasia of
Queyrat, carcinoma in situ of penile skin, leukoplakia, Paget's disease, balanitis xerotica
obliterans and HPV infection (condyloma
acuminata or giant condyloma) are the commonly mentioned premalignant conditions.
Controversy exists among experts regarding
the nature of carcinoma in situ of penile skin,
erythroplasia of Queyrat, and Bowen's dis-

ease. Few believe that these are separate conditions, whereas others believe that these are
varying clinical expressions of one and the
same disease.

ERYTHROPLASIA OF QUEYRAT

Usually, erythroplasia of Queyrat is seen in
uncircumcised men. The lesion, a red, velvety,
moist area, usually involves the inner surface
of the prepuce and the glans penis (Fig. 31–
21). Histologically, the picture is that of intraepithelial malignancy. In 10% of cases, local
invasion is seen. Treatment varies from topical application to local excision. The agent
used for topical application is 5-fluorouracil.
A wide variety of other forms of local ablative
therapies have also been reported.

BOWEN'S DISEASE

Bowen's disease, when it appears on the external genitalia, presents as a scaly, reddish-
brown plaque (Fig. 31–22). It can be present
on the glans penis or penile shaft or on
the prepuce, and the form of the lesion may
vary: polypoid, nodular, ulcerated, verrucous,
or leukoplakic. Whereas erythroplasia of
Queyrat is typically present only on the penis,
Bowen's disease can be present anywhere on
the body. However, the histologic picture of
both are the same. Wide excision is the preferred treatment. Search for internal malignancy should be part of the treatment plan

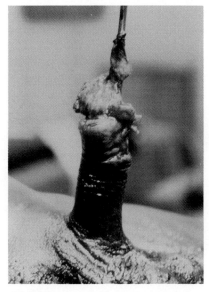

Figure 31-20
Gangrene of the penis in a patient with diabetes and
chronic renal failure. (From Mooppan UMM: Cutaneous
lesions of the penis. *In* Hashmat AI, Das S [eds]: The
Penis. Media, PA, Williams & Wilkins, 1993, p 89.)

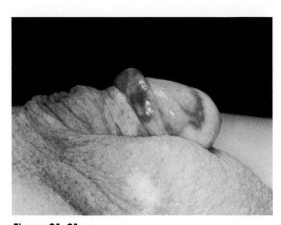

Figure 31-21
Erythroplasia of Queyrat. (From Mooppan UMM: Cuta-
neous lesions of the penis. *In* Hashmat AI, Das S [eds]:
The Penis. Media, PA, Williams & Wilkins, 1993, p 91.)

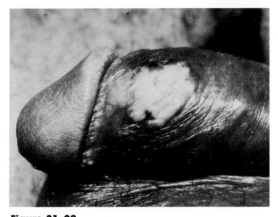

Figure 31-22
Bowen's disease. (From Mooppan UMM: Cutaneous lesions of the penis. *In* Hashmat AI, Das S [eds]: The Penis. Media, PA, Williams & Wilkins, 1993, p 90.)

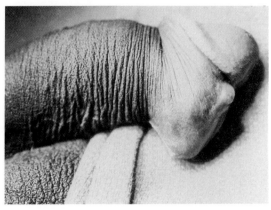

Figure 31-23
Sebaceous cyst involving penile skin. (From Mooppan UMM: Cutaneous lesions of the penis. *In* Hashmat AI, Das S [eds]: The Penis. Media, PA, Williams & Wilkins, 1993, p 92.)

because of the association of visceral malignancies with this condition.

LEUKOPLAKIA

Chronic irritation such as recurrent balanoposthitis in uncircumcised men is one of the causes of leukoplakia. The lesion appears as white plaques. In addition to excisional biopsy and close follow-up, circumcision removes the lesion as well as the cause when the lesion is confined to the prepuce alone.

BALANITIS XEROTICA OBLITERANS

Balanitis xerotica obliterans is also known as *lichen sclerosus et atrophicus*. The lesion mainly involves the glans penis but may also extend into the proximal urethra, producing narrowing of the meatus and difficulty in voiding. The patient may also complain of constant itching and irritation of the involved area. Treatment varies from topical application of steroid preparations to surgical correction of the obstructed urethral opening. Close follow-up is needed because of the premalignant nature of the lesion.

PAGET'S DISEASE

Extremely rare, the lesion in Paget's disease appears as an erythematous, well-circumscribed area. Histology shows carcinoma in situ. As in all premalignant lesions, local excision and follow-up are the treatment options.

Cystic Lesions of the External Genitalia

CYSTS OF THE PENIS

Congenital inclusion cysts, acquired inclusion cysts, and retention cysts are the common varieties of cysts on the penile shaft. Acquired cysts resulting from trauma, circumcision, or entrapment of smegma form the most common group. Retention cysts arising from the sebaceous glands form sebaceous cysts (Fig. 31–23). Congenital inclusion cysts, depending on the lining epithelium, can be either epidermoid cysts or mucoid cysts (Fig. 31–24). In addition to posing a cosmetic problem, they can also become painful if they get trauma-

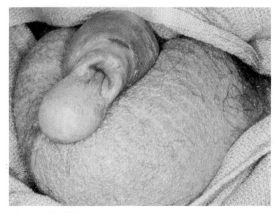

Figure 31-24
Pedunculated cyst from prepuce.

tized, ulcerated, or infected. Excision is the treatment of choice.

CYSTS OF THE SCROTUM (Superficial)

The most common type of cysts seen as superficial lesions on the scrotum are sebaceous cysts. They can be either solitary or multiple. Other than cosmetic concerns, these lesions are usually asymptomatic, unless infected. Excision is the treatment of choice when the lesion is solitary or localized to a limited area, when it is symptomatic or infected. However, when the entire scrotum is involved, elimination of all the lesions can pose a problem.

Other types of acquired or congenital cysts of the scrotal lining are possible, but are extremely rare.

Fixed Drug Eruptions

Tetracycline, sulfonamides, phenolphthalein, analgesic antipyretics, barbiturates, and penicillins are some of the drugs associated with fixed drug eruptions. It is a form of drug allergy. The eruption appears as a well-circumscribed area on the skin and subsides on cessation of the drug. The same area erupts each time the same drug is taken, and hence, the term *fixed drug eruption*. The glans penis and inner surface of the prepuce are the areas most commonly involved on the genitalia. The lesion goes through various stages of well-defined, edematous area, erythema, bullae formation, and hemorrhage prior to healing.

Vitiligo

Vitiligo are hypopigmented or depigmented areas on the skin. Another name for these lesions is *leukoderma*. The etiology is not known. Production of autoantibodies to melanocytes, chemicals used in the manufacture of devices such as condoms, are some of the explanations. The usually affected area is the inner surface of the prepuce and glans penis (Fig. 31–25). The lesion can be a single, large area or a conglomeration of small lesions over a wide area (Fig. 31–26).

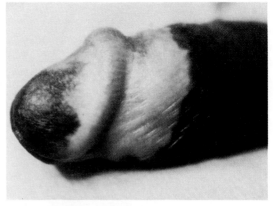

Figure 31–25
Vitiligo. (From Mooppan UMM: Cutaneous lesions of the penis. *In* Hashmat AI, Das S [eds]: The Penis. Media, PA, Williams & Wilkins, 1993, p 93.)

Lesions from Certain Forms of Social Behavior

Body piercing is more commonly seen recently, especially in metropolitan areas. So-called "pierceatoriums" and "tattoo parlors" are popping up with increasing numbers. In addition to the commonly seen areas such as ear lobes or nostrils, a variety of odd sites of the body are being pierced for insertion of "rings" and "rods." In addition to body parts such as eyebrows, nasal septum, tongue, and navel, the external genitalia is being chosen by young adults in increasing numbers for this custom (Fig. 31–27). In addition to the trauma caused to the organ by the process of piercing itself, these patients are more susceptible to STDs because of the continuous pres-

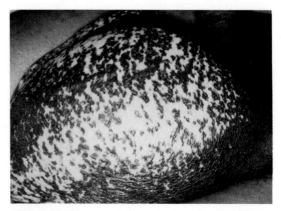

Figure 31–26
Depigmented areas over a large area of the scrotum.

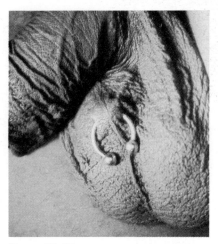

Figure 31-27
Horseshoe-shaped "ring" on the scrotum.

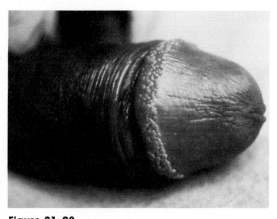

Figure 31-28
Pearly penile papules. (From Mooppan UMM: Cutaneous lesions of the penis. *In* Hashmat AI, Das S [eds]: The Penis. Media, PA, Williams & Wilkins, 1993, p 94.)

ence of a break in the skin barrier. There has been implication that hepatitis B and C may be transmitted in the process of tattooing. Insertion of plastic material under the penile skin to form what is known as "penile spherules" is another odd habit that has been reported.

Miscellaneous Lesions

LESIONS FROM INJECTIONS OF VASOACTIVE AGENTS

Intracavernous injection of papaverine, prostaglandin, and phentolamine mesylate (Regitine), either as single agents or as mixtures, is one of the treatment modalities of erectile dysfunction. Repeated injections of these agents can result in subcutaneous hematomas, nodules, penile ulcers, and pyogenic granulomas.

PEARLY PENILE PAPULES

It is important to distinguish pearly penile papule lesions from condyloma acuminata because many times the patients seek treatment for these lesions thinking that they are venereal warts. About 20% of healthy, uncircumcised men may have these lesions, appearing as uniform, small, whitish papules in one or multiple rows along the corona of the glans penis (Fig. 31–28). They are also known as *papillomatosis coronae penis* and *hirsutoid*

papillomas. Histologically, these are not glands, and there is no evidence of any association with HPV infection. Reassurance is the only treatment that is needed when patients seek advice.

ANGIONEUROTIC EDEMA

Angioneurotic edema is an allergic condition, usually secondary to food, a drug, or a new clothing material used (Fig. 31–29). Antihistamines or a short course of steroid hastens its disappearance. The patient should be reassured, and an attempt should be made to find the causative agent, if possible.

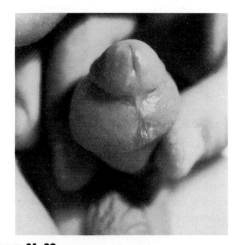

Figure 31-29
Angioneurotic edema. (From Mooppan UMM: Cutaneous lesions of the penis. *In* Hashmat AI, Das S [eds]: The Penis. Media, PA, Williams & Wilkins, 1993, p 94.)

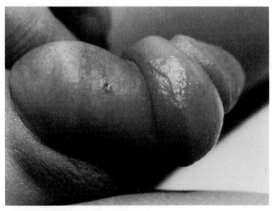

Figure 31–30
Penile swelling due to insect bite. Note the bite mark on the side of the shaft. (From Mooppan UMM: Cutaneous lesions of the penis. *In* Hashmat AI, Das S [eds]: The Penis. Media, PA, Williams & Wilkins, 1993, p 95.)

INSECT BITE

For an insect bite, the clinical picture is exactly that of angioneurotic edema, except that on close observation, a bite mark may be seen (Fig. 31–30). The swelling is the allergic reaction to the material injected during the bite or the material left at the bite site. Treatment is mainly on the same lines as that for angioneurotic edema. In addition, the bite mark should be closely observed to remove any material that was left by the insect.

PENILE SPHERULES

Penile spherules are rare lesions. Plastic spheres, single or multiple, are implanted in the subcutaneous plane of the dorsum of the penis. These lesions, along with tattooing, have been reported in certain international gangs involved in organized crime.

LIPOGRANULOMATOSIS

Lipogranulomatoses are granulomas resulting from exogenous injection of paraffin into the penile shaft, presumably to enhance the size of the penis. Excision of the lesion is the only treatment.

CONTACT DERMATITIS

The usual agents producing skin allergy and lesions of contact dermatitis on the external genitalia are condoms, spermicidal or lubri-cating jellies, and natural or synthetic material used in garments. Constant itching, rash, and swelling may be seen. In addition to short courses of antihistamines or steroids, elimination of the causative agent is important.

HEMANGIOMA

Hemangioma can be capillary or cavernous. Usually, the condition is congenital, but it can be acquired secondary to trauma. Skin discoloration, swelling, and bleeding are the common symptoms. When it is well-circumscribed and cavernous, the classic sign of emptying and blanching on pressure can be demonstrated (Fig. 31–31).

LYMPHANGIECTASIA

Lymphangiectasia is a rare lesion. Classically, it appears in the coronal sulcus, as a painless, nodular, translucent swelling (Fig. 31–32). The pathogenesis is not well understood but is most probably due to lymph stasis. Most of the time, the lesion subsides spontaneously.

LYMPHANGIITIS

As opposed to lymphangiectasia, lymphangiitis is painful. Usually seen as a red, longitudinal streak along the shaft, the lesion represents acute inflammation of the lymphatic channels. Antibiotic treatment is needed, and the lesion usually responds to the treatment promptly.

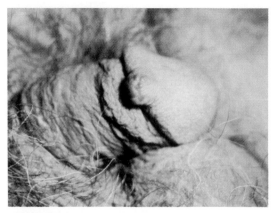

Figure 31–31
Cavernous hemangioma of the glans penis.

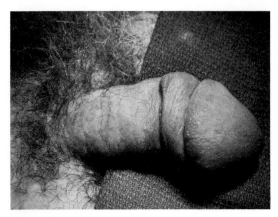

Figure 31-32
Lymphangiectasis. (From Mooppan UMM: Cutaneous lesions of the penis. *In* Hashmat AI, Das S [eds]: The Penis. Media, PA, Williams & Wilkins, 1993, p 95.)

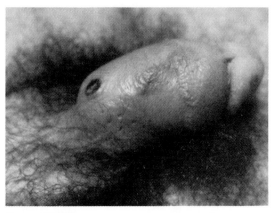

Figure 31-33
Penile abscess secondary to human bite. (From Mooppan UMM: Cutaneous lesions of the penis. *In* Hashmat AI, Das S [eds]: The Penis. Media, PA, Williams & Wilkins, 1993, p 96.)

PENILE VEIN THROMBOSIS

Penile vein thrombosis usually occurs as a result of trauma during sexual intercourse. In addition, an infective process as well as visceral malignancies have been mentioned to cause this condition. The patient feels the thrombosed vein as a "rope" or a "cord" on the surface of the penile shaft. Usually, the condition does not require any treatment and the lesion subsides gradually.

ABSCESS

With increased use of intracavernous injection of vasoactive agents in the treatment of impotence, abscess is seen as one of the rare complications. This can be a sequela to penile irrigation for treating priapism. Any injury to the penis that gets secondarily infected can result in a deep or superficial abscess (Fig. 31–33). Incision and draining, along with antibiotic therapy, is the treatment.

PILONIDAL SINUS

Almost all the cases of pilonidal sinus of the penis have been seen in patients with an uncircumcised penis. Poor hygiene is another contributory factor. Circumcision, along with complete excision of the lesion, resolves the situation.

PLASMA CELL BALANITIS

Plasma cell balanitis may mimic erythroplasia of Queyrat and candidal balanitis. Another

name for the lesion is *Zoon's balanitis*. The condition usually involves the glans penis and/or the inner surface of the prepuce (Fig. 31–34). Excision biopsy distinguishes the condition from erythroplasia of Queyrat. Improvement of hygiene, topical steroids, and circumcision are the components of treatment.

CIRCINATE BALANITIS (Reiter's Syndrome)

Along with the classic triad of urethritis, conjunctivitis, and arthritis, circinate balanitis is seen as superficial, red, erosive areas on the

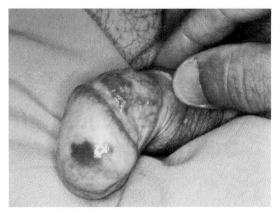

Figure 31-34
Plasma cell balanitis (Zoon's balanitis). Note the red velvety areas on the glans penis and inner aspect of the prepuce. This condition mimics the clinical picture of erythroplasia of Queyrat, but the histology is distinctly different.

corona of the glans penis. Topical steroid application provides relief.

TRICHOMONAL BALANITIS

The causative organism of trichomonal balanitis, *Trichomonas vaginalis*, is sexually transmitted. The patient is usually uncircumcised, and the lesion appears as a superficial ulcer. The patient, as well as his sexual contact, should be treated with metronidazole.

BOWENOID PAPULOSIS

HPV subtypes 6, 16, and 39 have been associated with bowenoid papulosis. These multiple, papular, asymptomatic lesions can regress spontaneously, and this marks the distinguishing feature between bowenoid papulosis and Bowen's disease. Excision or destruction by electrocautery or laser is the treatment option.

VERRUCIFORM XANTHOMA

Verruciform xanthoma is an extremely rare condition on the external genitalia. The usual site for this lesion is the oral cavity. Etiologic factors are not known.

ANGIOMYOLIPOMA

Only one case of angiomyolipoma involving the penile shaft has been reported in literature. The usual site for this lesion is the kidney.

AMYLOIDOSIS

Involvement of the external genitalia by amyloidosis is extremely rare. Excision is the treatment, and histopathology alone can give the diagnosis.

METASTATIC CROHN'S DISEASE

Genital cutaneous lesions by Crohn's disease have been reported, although they are extremely rare. Usually, the scrotal and penile skin are involved together. However, there has been a single case report of isolated penile skin involvement.

ACKNOWLEDGMENTS

Without the color illustrations provided in this section, this chapter would not have much meaning. I am extremely grateful to the excellent work of Mr. Gideon Kedem and Mr. Alan Kaufman, the photographers. I owe a great deal to all my patients, the residents, and staff of our department. I am thankful to Dr. Frederick A. Gulmi, my colleague, and Dr. Hong Kim, the director of the department, for their encouragement and some of the clinical materials. I wish to express my gratitude to Dr. Sandor H. Wax, the previous director of the department, who has always been a source of inspiration and encouragement.

SUGGESTED READINGS

1. Coldison BM, Johnson C: Common penile lesions. Urol Clin North Am 15:671, 1988.
2. Jayachandran S, Mooppan UMM, Kim H: Complications from external (condom) urinary drainage devices. Urology 25:31, 1985.
3. Judson FN: Infectious syphilis: Primary, secondary and early latent. *In* Feldman YM (ed): Sexually Transmitted Diseases. New York, Churchill Livingstone, 1986, pp 23–27.
4. Kaplan MH, Sodick N, McNutt NS et al: Dermatologic findings and manifestations of acquired immunodeficiency syndrome (AIDS). J Am Acad Dermatol 16:485, 1987.
5. Korting GW: Practical Dermatology of the Genital Region. Philadelphia, WB Saunders, 1981.
6. Mooppan UMM: Cutaneous lesions of the penis. *In* Hashmat AI, Das S (eds): The Penis. Media, PA, William & Wilkins, 1993, pp 69–102.
7. Pervez NK: Penile spherules. Am J Forensic Med Pathol 3:9, 1982.
8. Raab B: Genital herpes. *In* Feldman YM (ed): Sexually Transmitted Diseases. New York, Churchill Livingstone, 1986, pp 129–152.
9. Rosenberg SK, Herman G, Elfont E: Sexually transmitted papilloma viral infection in the male: VII. Is cancer of the penis sexually transmitted? Urology 37:437, 1991.
10. Stein BS: Sexually transmitted diseases: Cutaneous lesions. Semin Urol 9:2, 1991.
11. U.S. Department of Health and Human Services: Sexually transmitted diseases: Treatment guidelines. Semin Urol 9:40, 1991.
12. Witherington R: Penile lesions: A generalist's guide. Postgrad Med 70:82, 1981.

Index

Note: Page numbers in *italics* indicate figures; those with t indicate tables.

A

Abortion, septic, 228
Abscess, penile, *376*
  perinephric, 4, 135–136, *136,* 142
ACE inhibitors. *See* Angiotensin-converting enzyme
  (ACE) inhibitors.
Acetaminophen, 220t
Acetazolamide, 98t
Acetohydroxamic acid (AHA), 105
Acidosis, metabolic, 321t
  acute renal failure and, 321t
  dialysis for, 322t
  urolithiasis and, 98t
Acquired immunodeficiency syndrome (AIDS). *See also*
  Human immunodeficiency virus (HIV) disease.
  acute renal failure in, 321
  adrenal insufficiency with, 326
  Fournier's gangrene and, 55
  genital lesions with, 359, 366–367, *367*
  hematuria with, 62
  Kaposi's sarcoma with, 128, 300, 366–367
  sexually transmitted diseases with, 366–367, *367*
Actinomycin D, 270
Acute renal failure (ARF), 311–323. *See also* Prerenal
  azotemia.
  blood urea nitrogen in, 322
  causes of, 314–321, 315t–317t, 320t
  chronic vs., *312*
  complications with, 321t, 321–322
  contrast media and, 319–320
  diagnosis of, 311t, 311–312
  dialysis for, 322t
  evaluation of, *312,* 312–314, 313t
  HIV infection and, 321
  intrinsic, 312
  management of, 322–323
  NSAIDs and, 318t
  postrenal, *312*
  uric acid–induced, 320
  urinalysis for, 312–314, 313t
Acyclovir, for genital herpes, 114, 115t, 365
  prerenal azotemia and, 315t
  renal abnormalities with, 315t, 320t
Addison's disease, 97t, 326
Adenoma, adrenal, 332–333
  aldosteronism and, 330
  bladder, 7, 288

Adenoma *(Continued)*
  cortisol-secreting, 334
  incidental, 334
  mucin-secreting, 320
  pituitary, 332–333, 345
  renal, 4, 293, 294
Adolescents. *See also* Children.
  sexually transmitted diseases in, 110–111, 122–123
    treatment of, 115t–117t, 119
Adrenal glands, anatomy of, 1, *2,* 325
  cysts of, 2
  diseases of, 1–3, 325–334
  ectopic, 1
  function tests for, 327
  hyperfunction of, 329t, 329–333
  hyperplasia of, 239
  physiology of, 325
  tumors of, 2, 333–334
  vasculature of, 325
Adrenal insufficiency, 328
  biochemical abnormalities in, 327t
  causes of, 325–326
  clinical features of, 326
  diagnosis of, 326, 328
  treatment of, 327–328
  types of, 326
African Americans, prostate cancer among, 308
  prostate-specific antigen in, 278t, 279
  renal cell carcinoma among, 295
  sexually transmitted diseases among, 109–110
  urolithiasis among, 93
African sleeping sickness, 288
AHA (acetohydroxamic acid), 105
AIDS. *See* Acquired immunodeficiency syndrome
  (AIDS).
Albumin, urine, 19
Albuterol, 42t
Alcohol use, bladder dysfunction with, 211t
  Fournier's gangrene and, 55
  impotence and, 350
  infertility and, 339
  LUTS with, 198t
  neurogenic bladder and, 184t
  prerenal azotemia and, 315t
Aldosterone, adrenal insufficiency and, 327
  deficiency of, 326
Aldosteronism, 329t, 329–330
  clinical features of, 329

Aldosteronism (*Continued*)
   treatment of, 330
Alkalosis, respiratory, 223t
Allopurinol, for urolithiasis, 104
   interstitial nephritis and, 317t
   pregnancy and, 232
Alpha-adrenergic blockers, for BPH, 193t, 203–204, 214, 215
   for outlet resistance, 193t
   LUTS with, 200t
   retrograde ejaculation with, 356
Alpha$_1$-antichymotrypsin (ACT), 280
Alpha-fetoprotein (AFP), testicular tumor and, 297
   yolk sac tumor and, 267
Alpha$_2$-macroglobulin (A$_2$M), 280
Alport's syndrome, hematuria with, 61
   symptoms of, 66
Alprostadil, 351–353, 352t, 353t
ALS. *See* Amyotrophic lateral sclerosis (ALS).
Aluminum, bladder cancer and, 307t
Aluminum hydroxide, for urolithiasis, 105
Alzheimer's disease, 184t
Ambiguous genitalia, 238–240
Amebiasis, 368
Amenorrhea, infertility and, 339
   renal cell carcinoma and, 296
Amikacin, 137t, 148t
4-Aminobiphenyl, 65–66, 288t, 307t
Aminoglycosides, acute renal failure and, 315t
   hematuria and, 63
   pregnancy and, 218t
   prerenal azotemia and, 315t
   tubular necrosis from, 319
Aminophylline, 42t
Aminosalicylic acid, 59t
Amitriptyline, for voiding dysfunction, 191t
   infertility and, 344
Amniotic fluid embolus, 228
Amoxicillin, for chancroid, 116t
   for children, 148t
   for *Chlamydia* infection, 117t
   for cystitis, 167
   for lower UTI, 159
   pregnancy and, 230t
Amphetamines, 200t
Amphotericin, for aspergillosis, 178
   for renal candidiasis, 140
   prerenal azotemia and, 315t
   side effects of, 140
Ampicillin, for children, 148, 148t
   for granuloma inguinale, 363
   for lower UTI, 159
   for upper UTI, 137t, 138
Ampulla of vas, 7, 9
Amyloidosis, Addison's disease and, 326
   genital lesions from, 377
   malignancy with, 320t
Amyotrophic lateral sclerosis (ALS), neurogenic bladder with, 184t
   syphilis and, 118
Anaphylactoid reactions, 42t, 43
Anemia, acute renal failure and, 321t
   amphotericin and, 140
   renal cell carcinoma and, 296
   urolithiasis and, 98t
Aneurysm, abdominal, 97t
   aortic, 81
   renal infarction with, 56
Angiography, 56
Angioma, renal, 4
Angiomyolipoma, 4, 39, 294, 377

Angioneurotic edema, 374
Angiotensin, 200t
Angiotensin II receptor antagonists, 225t
Angiotensin-converting enzyme (ACE) inhibitors,
      pregnancy and, 225t
   prerenal azotemia and, 314t, 315t
   renal vascular disease and, 316
Aniline dye, 187t, 288
Aniridia, 263t
Anorexia, 321t
Anthraquinone laxatives, 59t
Anticholinergics, 211t
Anticoagulants, 64
Antidiuretic hormone, 254
Antihypertensive drugs, 225t
Antiphospholipid syndrome, adrenal insufficiency with, 326
   preeclampsia and, 225t
Antituberculous drugs, 173t
Antitubular basement membrane disease, 317t
Appendicitis, pyelonephritis vs., 135t
   urolithiasis vs., 97t, 219t
Appendix, epididymal, 9
ARF. *See* Acute renal failure (ARF).
Arrhythmias, acute renal failure and, 321t
   pheochromocytoma and, 331
Arteriosclerosis, erectile dysfunction with, 9
   impotence and, 349–350, 350t
Arthritis, syphilis with, 118
Asbestos, 295
Ascites, 82
Asian Americans, prostate-specific antigen in, 278t, 279
   sexually transmitted diseases among, 109
Aspergillosis, 177–178, *178*
   clinical features of, 177
   diagnosis of, 177–178, *178*
   epidemiology of, 177
   management of, 178
   pathogenesis of, 177
   prognosis of, 178
Aspermia, 337, 349, 356
Aspirin, hematuria and, 64
   pregnancy class of, 220t
Assisted reproduction, 335, 344, 346–347
Asterixis, 321t
Asymptomatic macroscopic hematuria. *See also* Hematuria.
   algorithm for, *72*
   follow-up surveillance for, 73
   imaging studies for, 69–71, *69–71*
   renal biopsy for, 71–73
   work-up for, 65t, 65–73, *69–72*
Atenolol, 225t
Atheroembolic disease, 315t, 316–317
Atropine, 42t
Auramine, 307t
Azithromycin, for chancroid, 115t
   for chlamydial infection, 117t
   for nongonococcal urethritis, 123
Azo dyes, 288t
Azoospermia, 342
Azotemia, prerenal, *312*, 314–315
   causes of, 314t
   drug-induced, 314t, 315t
   in pregnancy, 228
   urinalysis for, 313t
Azulfidine, 339

B

Bacille Calmette-Guérin (BCG), for bladder cancer, 288, 291–292

Bacille Calmette-Guérin (BCG) *(Continued)*
  sepsis from, 174
Baclofen, 200t
Bacteriuria, 131. *See also* Urinary tract infection (UTI).
  of pregnancy, 141, 217–219, 218t, 228–230, 230t
Balanitis, 8
  candidal, 367–368, *368*
  circinate, 376–377
  plasma cell, *376*
  trichomonal, 377
  xerotica obliterans, 300, 371
  Zoon's, *376*
Balanoposthitis, 367–368
BCG. *See* Bacille Calmette-Guérin (BCG).
Beauticians, bladder cancer among, 288t, 307t
Beckwith-Wiedemann syndrome, 263t
Bedwetting. *See* Enuresis.
Behavioral therapy, for voiding dysfunction, 188–190,
  189t
Bell-clapper deformity, 52, *52*
Bence Jones proteins, 19
Bendroflumethiazide, 103
Benign prostatic hypertrophy (BPH), 197–206, 209–216
  algorithm for, *210*
  alpha blockers for, 193t, 203–204, 214, 215
  catheterization for, 214–215
  causes of, 209–211, 211t
  complications with, 210–211
  cost analysis for, 215
  critical pathway for, *210*
  doxazosin for, 204
  evaluation of, 201
  finasteride for, 214
  hematuria with, 49t, 60, 64
  history for, 211–212
  hormones for, 204
  incidence of, 197, 209
  incontinence with, 201
  lasers for, 206, 215
  management of, 203–206
  microwave thermotherapy for, 205–206
  outcomes with, 215, 216t
  pathophysiology of, 197–201
  physical examination for, 201–202, 212–213
  referrals for, 216
  stents for, 206
  surgery for, 215
  symptoms of, 201
    score for, 212t
  tamsulosin for, 204
  terazosin for, 203–204
  tests for, 202–203
  transrectal ultrasonography for, 202–203
  transurethral electrovaporization for, 205
  transurethral incision for, 206
  transurethral needle ablation for, 205, 215
  treatment of, 213–215
  TURP for, 204–205
  voiding dysfunction with, 197–207
Benzidine, bladder cancer and, 288t, 307t
  hematuria and, 65–66
Benztropine, 200t
Bertini, columns of, 3
Beta-adrenergic blockers, bladder dysfunction with, 211t
  LUTS with, 200t
Bethanechol, 193, 193t, 200t
Bichloracetic acid, 364
Bilharzial ulcerations, 175
Biperidin, 200t
Bladder, activity of. *See* Bladder activity.
  anatomy of, 6–7, *7*

Bladder *(Continued)*
  blood clot in, 49, *85*
  BPH and, 210–211
  calcification of, *176*
  cancer of. *See* Bladder cancer.
  capacity of, 37–38
  diseases of, 7
  dysfunction of, 211t, 213
  examination of, 14
  fibrosis of, 12
  function of, 183–184
  HIV disease and, 128
  hypersensitivity of, 185
  inflammation of, 12
  innervation of, 183
  Kaposi's sarcoma of, 128
  neoileal, 293
  neurogenic. *See* Neurogenic bladder.
  obstruction of, 234
  pain in, 122
  rupture of, 83–84, *84*
  surgical substitutes for, 292, *293*
  "tear-drop," *86*
  trauma to, 83–84, *84*
  tuberculosis of, 171–172
  ultrasonography for, 40
Bladder activity, altered, 184–185
  electrical neuromodulation for, 195
  plugs for, 194–195
  surgery for, 195
  therapy for, 188–190, 189t
    pharmacologic, 190–193, 191t–193t
    physical, 190
Bladder cancer, 7, 49, 288t, 288–293, *290, 293*
  adrenal metastasis from, 3
  BCG for, 188, 291–292
  clinical features of, 289
  diagnosis of, 289–291
  epidemiology of, 288
  etiology of, 288t, 288–289
  hematuria with, 66, 289, 292
  interferon for, 292
  intravesical therapy for, 291–292
  muscle-invasive, 292
  occupational hazards for, 288t, 307t
  photodynamic therapy for, 292
  prevention of, 303, 307t, 307–308
  relapsing UTI with, 157t
  rhabdomyosarcoma as, 270
  schistosomiasis and, 174
  staging of, 289, *290*
  superficial, 291–292
  surgery for, 292, *293*
  survival with, 288
  tobacco use and, 288, 304
Blastomycosis, 326
Bleeding dyscrasias, 61
Bleomycin, for renal cell carcinoma, 297
  for testicular tumor, 299
Blood urea nitrogen (BUN), in acute renal failure, 322
  in prerenal azotemia, 314
  tests for, 22
Blue cell tumor, 265
Body piercing, 373–374, *374*
Bone scan, for prostate cancer, 32
Bowenoid papulosis, 377
Bowen's disease, 300
Boyarsky questionnaire, 201
BPH. *See* Benign prostatic hypertrophy (BPH).
Breast cancer metastases, adrenal, 3

Breast cancer metastases *(Continued)*
  renal, 4
  urolithiasis vs., 97t
Bromocriptine, 200t
Brucella, 128
Brushite stones, 94
BUN. See Blood urea nitrogen (BUN).
Buschke-Löwenstein tumor, 300, 363, 364, 371

C

Cadmium, 295
Caffeine, bladder dysfunction with, 211t
  infertility and, 339
Calcium channel blockers, bladder dysfunction with, 211t
  for aldosteronism, 330
  infertility and, 339
  pregnancy and, 225t
  urolithiasis and, 98t
Calcium metabolism, 98t
Calcium oxalate crystals, 21
Calcium oxalate stones. *See also* Urolithiasis.
  incidence of, 94t
  treatment of, 104
Calcium phosphate stones, 18, 94t
Calymmatobacterium granulomatis, 363. *See also* Granuloma inguinale.
Cancer. *See also under anatomy, e.g.,* Prostate cancer.
  prevention of, 303–309
Candida infection, fluconazole and, 140
  in urine sediment, 141
  penile lesions from, 367–368, 368
  renal infections from, 141, 141–142
    drugs for, 140
  UTI with, 132
Candidemia, 131
Cantharidin, 364
Captopril, 105
Carbachol, 200t
Carbamazepine, 200t
Carbonic anhydrase inhibitors, 64
Carcinoma. *See specific type, e.g.,* Squamous cell carcinoma.
Cardiomyopathy, pheochromocytoma and, 331
Caruncle, urethral, 8
Casts, hematuria and, 24
  urinary, 21, 21
Catecholamine-secreting tumor, 330
Catheterization. *See also* Foley catheter.
  chronic, cancer risk with, 187t
    indications for, 194
  for acute urinary retention, 48
  intermittent, for BPH, 214–215
    indications for, 194
Caverject, 352t, 353t, 353–354
Cefixime, 116t, 155t
Cefotaxime, 148t
Cefpodoxime proxetil, 155t
Ceftazidime, 137t
Ceftriaxone, for chancroid, 115t
  for children, 148t
  for gonorrhea, 116t, 362
  for syphilis, 115t, 360
  for UTI, 137t, 138, 143
Cellulitis, 56
Cephalexin, for children, 148t
  pregnancy and, 230t
Cephalosporin, hematuria with, 64
  interstitial nephritis and, 317t
  pregnancy and, 218t

Cephalosporin *(Continued)*
  prerenal azotemia and, 315t
Cerebral palsy, 184t
Cerebrovascular accident (CVA), LUTS and, 197, 198t
  neurogenic bladder after, 184t
Cervical carcinoma, 109
Cervicitis, 120, 121
Chancre, 360, 360–361. *See also* Syphilis.
Chancroid, 361, 361–362. *See also* Sexually transmitted diseases (STDs).
  diagnosis of, 119, 362
    differential, 112t
  incidence of, 119
  lymphadenopathy from, 362
  treatment of, 115t–116t, 119–120, 362
Chemotherapy, intravesical, 291–292
CHF (congestive heart failure), 321t, 331
Chickenpox, 359, 360. *See also* Herpes.
Children. *See also* Neonates.
  chlamydial infections in, 110
  cryptorchidism in, 243–245, 244
  cystinuria in, 106
  cystitis in, 147–148, 148t
  cystourethrogram for, 147
  epididymitis in, 117t, 128
  genitourinary malignancies in, 263–271
  gonorrhea in, 121
  hypertension in, 246
  molluscum contagiosum in, 366
  neuroblastoma in, 265–266, 266t, 268t–269t
  nonfunctioning kidney in, 251
  perinatal herpes in, 114–118
  pyelonephritis in, 145
  renal anomalies in, 77
  renal trauma in, 77
  rhabdomyosarcoma in, 268t–269t, 270
  sexually transmitted diseases in, 110–111, 119, 122–123
    treatment of, 115t–117t, 119
  testicular tumors in, 267, 267t–269t
  urolithiasis in, 100, 106
  UTI in, 145–149
    case study on, 149
    causes of, 145
    clinical features of, 146
    epidemiology of, 145
    laboratory tests for, 146–147
    prophylaxis for, 148–149
    risks for, 145–146
    treatment of, 147–148, 148t
    work-up for, 147, 147
  vesicoureteral reflux in, 145–149, 245–247
  Wilms' tumor in, 263t, 263–265, 265t, 268t–269t
Chlamydia infection, 123–124
  adolescents with, 111, 123
  children with, 117t
  diagnosis of, 123–124
  epididymitis from, 128, 163
  incidence of, 123
  laboratory tests for, 22
  neonates with, 123
  nonspecific urethritis from, 122
  penile lesions from, 362
  pregnancy and, 110
  prevention of, 124
  treatment of, 117t, 124
  urethritis from, 165
Chlordiazepoxide, 200t
Chlornaphazine, 288t
2-Chloroaniline, 288t
4-Chloro-*o*-toluidine, 288t
Cholecystitis, pyelonephritis vs., 135t

Cholecystitis (Continued)
  renal infarction vs., 57
  urolithiasis vs., 97t, 219t
Cholelithiasis, 97t
Cholestyramine, 104
Chordee, 14, 247
Choriocarcinoma, 298
Chromaffin tumor, 330
Chyluria, filariasis with, 179–180
  treatment of, 181
Cimetidine, for anaphylaxis, 42t
  impotence and, 350
  interstitial nephritis and, 317t
Ciprofloxacin, for chancroid, 116t
  for lower UTI, 155t
  for upper UTI, 137t, 138
Circinate balanitis, 376–377. See also Balanitis.
Circumcision, for penile cancer, 300
  Fournier's gangrene and, 55
Cisplatin, acute renal failure and, 315t
  for bladder cancer, 292–293
  for prostate cancer, 288
  for rhabdomyosarcoma, 270
  for testicular tumor, 299
  prerenal azotemia and, 315t
  renal abnormalities with, 320t
Clavulanic acid, 230t
Clear cell sarcoma, 264
Clindamycin, 218t
Clomipramine, 356
Clonazepam, 200t
Clonidine, 200t
Clonidine suppression test, 331
Clotrimazole, 367
CMV. See Cytomegalovirus (CMV).
Cocaine, 57
  infertility and, 339
  prerenal azotemia and, 315t
Codeine, 231
Colic, renal, 13
Colitis, 219t
Colon cancer metastasis, 3
Colporrhaphy, 89
Computed tomography, 40–41. See also Imaging
    study(ies).
Condyloma, giant, 300, 363, 364, 371
Condyloma acuminatum, 124–127, 300, 363–364, 364. See
    also Human papillomavirus (HPV).
  causes of, 125, 363
  diagnosis of, 125, 363–364
  incidence of, 124–125
  lasers for, 364
  lesions of, 363, 364
  treatment of, 125–127, 126t, 364
Congenital adrenal hyperplasia, 239
Congenital anomalies, 243–249
Congestive heart failure (CHF), acute renal failure with,
    321t
  pheochromocytoma and, 331
Conn's syndrome, 2, 329t, 329–330
  clinical features of, 329
  treatment of, 330
Contrast media, 41–45, 42t
  anaphylaxis from, 42t, 42–45
  nephrotoxicity of, 41–42
  properties of, 41
  renal failure from, 319–320
Corpora cavernosa, 7, 8
Corporal fibrosis, 354
Cortisol, 327
Costovertebral angle, 3

Cowper's duct, 38
Creatinine, serum, 22
  urine calcium and, 68
Creatinine clearance test, 22
Crohn's disease, metastatic, 377
  urolithiasis and, 98t
Cryoglobulinemia, 317t
Cryptococcus infection, 128
Cryptorchidism, 14. See also Testes.
  algorithm for, 244
  anomalies with, 244
  complications with, 244
  germ cell tumor and, 298
  hormone therapy for, 244–245
  hypospadias and, 247
  incidence of, 243
  infertility and, 335, 338
  neonates with, 243–245, 244
  physical examination for, 243–244
  testicular tumor with, 268t
  Wilms' tumor with, 263t
Crystals, urinary, 21
Cushing's disease, 2, 332
Cushing's syndrome, 1–2, 332–333
  clinical features of, 332
  diagnosis of, 332
  epidemiology of, 332
  evaluation of, 329t
  renal cell carcinoma and, 296
  treatment of, 332–333
CVA. See Cerebrovascular accident (CVA).
Cyclophosphamide, for rhabdomyosarcoma, 270
  hemorrhagic cystitis with, 64
  urothelial malignancy with, 64
Cycloserine, 173t
Cyclosporin, 314t, 315t
  hematuria and, 63
Cycrimine, 200t
Cystectomy, 292, 293
Cystic renal disease, 60–61
Cystine, 21, 94t
  stones of, 94–95
Cystinuria, in children, 106
  treatment of, 104–105
Cystitis, 7, 166t, 166–167
  children with, 147–148, 148t
  classification of, 166
  clinical features of, 132–133
  definition of, 151
  diagnosis of, 166t, 167
  during pregnancy, 217
  etiology of, 166
  fibrosis with, 12
  hematuria from, 49–50
  hemorrhagic, 64
  HIV disease and, 128
  incidence of, 166, 166t
  men with, 166t, 166–167
  noninfectious, 151
  pyelonephritis vs., 133t
  radiation, 63, 185
  risks for, 132, 132t
  symptoms of, 166
  tuberculosis with, 172
  UTI and, 131, 166
  vesicoureteral reflux and, 246
Cystopathy, autonomic, 198t
Cystoscopy, for children, 71
  for hematuria, 25, 70–71, 71
  for recurring UTI, 158t
  of transitional cell carcinoma, 71

Cystourethrogram, voiding, 30, *37*, 37–38
Cytomegalovirus (CMV), cystitis from, 128
  foscarnet for, 367
  nongonococcal urethritis from, 122
Cytoxan, 66

D

Dalfopristin, 143
Dantrolene, 200t
Deferoxamine mesylate, 59t
Dementia, LUTS with, 198t
  neurogenic bladder with, 211t
Denys-Drash syndrome, 263t
Desmopressin acetate, 254, 258–259, 261
Detrusor hyperactivity, 184, 198t
Detrusor instability, case study on, 261–262
  enuresis with, 260
Dexamethasone test, 332
Diabetes mellitus, adrenal insufficiency with, 326
  aspergillosis with, 178
  balanitis with, 367
  erectile dysfunction with, 9
  Fournier's gangrene and, 55
  gestational, 221
  impotence and, 349–350, 350t
  infertility and, 339, 344
  LUTS and, 197, 199t
  nephropathy with, 227
  neurogenic bladder and, 184t
  penile cancer and, 300
  penile gangrene from, *371*
  preeclampsia and, 225t
  pregnancy and, 227
  urolithiasis vs., 97t
  UTI with, 142, 144, 157t, 158–159
Dialysis, Fournier's gangrene and, 55
  pregnancy and, 227
  renal cell carcinoma and, 295
Diatrizoate, 41
Diazepam, 200t
Dicyclomine, 200t
  bladder dysfunction with, 211t
  for voiding dysfunction, 191t
Diethylcarbamazine citrate, 180–181
Digital rectal examination (DRE), 31
  for infertility, 340
  for prostate cancer, 285–286
  PSA levels and, 276
Digitalis, 200t
Diltiazem, 211t
Dimethyl sulfoxide, 191t
Diphenhydramine, 42t, 43
Diphtheria, 317t
Distigmine, 200t
Diuresis, postobstructive, 49
Diuretics, action sites of, *5*
  for aldosteronism, 330
  for hypoaldosteronism, 328
  for hypocalciuria, 103–104
  impotence and, 350
  interstitial nephritis and, 317t
  pregnancy and, 225t, 232
  urolithiasis and, 95, 98t
Diverticulitis, pyelonephritis vs., 135t
  urolithiasis vs., 97t
Donovanosis. *See* Granuloma inguinale.
Dopamine, 42t
Doxazosin, for BPH, 193t, 2041
  for prostatitis, 169
  side effects of, 204

Doxorubicin, for bladder cancer, 291, 293
  for prostate cancer, 288
  for rhabdomyosarcoma, 270
  red urine with, 59t
Doxycycline, 116t
  for *Chlamydia* infection, 117t
  for epididymitis, 165
  for granuloma inguinale, 363
  for lymphogranuloma venereum, 362
  for syphilis, 115t, 360, 361
DRE. *See* Digital rectal examination (DRE).
Drug(s). *See named drug or drug group.*
Drug eruptions, 373
Duodenal ulcer, 97t
Duplication anomalies, 235–237
Dyscrasias, hematuria with, 61
Dysuria, algorithm for, *121*

E

Eclampsia, 226t. *See also* Preeclampsia.
Econazole, 367
Ectopic pregnancy. *See also* Pregnancy.
  gonorrhea and, 120
  sexually transmitted diseases and, 109
  urolithiasis vs., 97t, 219t
Edema, angioneurotic, *374*
  pulmonary, 322t
Ejaculation, 337
  premature, 356–357
  retrograde, 356
Elderly patients, lower UTI in, 160
  upper UTI in, 133
    management of, 140–141
Electrical neuromodulation, 195
Elephantiasis, 179, *180*. *See also* Filariasis.
  treatment of, 181
Embryonal cell carcinoma, 298
Emphysematous pyelonephritis, 4, 142
Endocarditis, gonococcal, 116t
  hematuria with, 62
Endometriosis, urinary tract, 65
  urolithiasis vs., 97t
Endometritis, gonorrhea and, 120
Entamoeba histolyticum, 368
Enterobacter spp., prostatitis from, 168
  UTI with, 132
Enterococci, vancomycin-resistant, 143
Enuresis. *See also* Incontinence.
  case studies on, 261–262
  definition of, 251
  detrusor instability with, 260
  diurnal, 260–261
  nocturnal, 112, 221, 251–260
    antidiuretic hormone and, 254
    assessment of, 254–257, *255*, *256*
    complicated, 257, 259
    desmopressin acetate for, 258–259
    epidemiology of, 252–253
    etiology of, 253–254
    family history of, 253
    imipramine for, 258
    oxybutynin for, 258
    psychological factors for, 254
    sleep disorders and, 253
    treatment of, 257–259
    UTI and, 254
  pediatric, 251–262
  UTI with, 260
Ephedrine, 42t
Epidermoid cyst, 267t

Epididymis, anatomy of, 9
  anomalies with, 244
  attachment of, *52*
  classifications of, 163–164, 164t
  diseases of, 10
  etiology of, 163
  examination of, 14–15, *15*, 340
  spermatogenesis and, 337
  tuberculosis of, 172
  tumor of, 14–15
Epididymitis, 128–129, 163–165
  acute, 52–54, 128
  causes of, 52–53, 128
  children with, 128
    treatment of, 117t
  chronic, 128
  diagnosis of, 53, 128–129, 164, 164t
    differential, 51t
  hospitalization for, 54
  incidence of, 128
  noninfectious, 163–164
  physical examination of, 163t, 164t
  symptoms of, 128
  testicular torsion vs., 128–129
  treatment of, 53–54, 129, 164t, 164–165
  tuberculous, 368
Epididymovasostomy, 346
Epinephrine, adrenal insufficiency and, 327
  for anaphylaxis, 42t, 43–44
  for priapism, 55
Epispadias, 14. *See also* Hypospadias.
Epithelial cells, in urine, *20*, 20–21
EPS (expressed prostatic secretion), 168
Erectile dysfunction. *See* Impotence.
Erythromycin, for chancroid, 115t
  for *Chlamydia* infection, 117t
  for gonorrhea, 116t
  for lymphogranuloma venereum, 116t, 362
  for nongonococcal urethritis, 117t, 123
  for syphilis, 115t, 360
  pregnancy and, 218t
Erythroplasia of Queyrat, 113, 300, *371*
  plasma cell balanitis vs., 376
Escherichia coli, epididymitis from, 128
  prostatitis from, 168
  pyelonephritis from, 4
  UTI with, 131–132
Esophageal cancer, 3
Estradiol, for voiding dysfunction, 191t
Estramustine phosphate, 288
Estrogen, renal cell carcinoma and, 295
Ethambutol, 173t
Ethanol. *See* Alcohol use.
Ethionamide, 173t
Etoposide, 299
Excretory urography. *See* Intravenous pyelography
    (IVP).
Expressed prostatic secretion (EPS), 168
Extracorporeal shock-wave lithotripsy (ESWL), 93, 105
  for children, 106

F

Famotidine, 42t
FENa (fractional excretion of sodium), 313–315
Fetal alcohol syndrome, 268t
Fetal hydrops, 225t
Fibroma, renal, 4
Filariasis, 178–181, *179*, *180*
  clinical features of, 179, *180*
  diagnosis of, 179–180

Filariasis *(Continued)*
  elephantiasis with, 179, *180*
  epidemiology of, 178
  genital lymphedema from, 369
  management of, 180–181
  pathogenesis of, 178–179, *179*, *180*
  prognosis of, 181
Finasteride, for BPH, 204, 214
  PSA levels and, 274t, 275
  side effects of, 204
Flank pain, as urologic emergency, 50–51
Flavoxate, for voiding dysfunction, 191t
  LUTS with, 200t
Floxuridine, 297
Fluconazole, for renal candidiasis, 140
  side effects of, 140
5-Flucytosine, 140
Fludrocortisone, 327–328
Flunarizine, 200t
5-Fluorouracil, for bladder cancer, 292
  for condyloma acuminata, 364
  for genital warts, 125–127, 126t
  for penile cancer, 300
  for renal cell carcinoma, 297
Foley catheter. *See also* Catheterization.
  for bladder rupture, 84
  indwelling, 194
  pelvic fracture and, 76
  urethra injury and, 87
Follicle-stimulating hormone (FSH), infertility and, 342
  spermatogenesis and, *336*
Formaldehyde, in urine, 19
Foscarnet, 367
Fournier's gangrene, 55–56, *370*
  causes of, 55
  diagnosis of, 56
  treatment of, 56
Fractional excretion of sodium (FENa), 313–315
Free-to-total PSA ratio, 280t, 280–281
Frei's test, 362
FSH. *See* Follicle-stimulating hormone (FSH).
Functional bladder capacity, 255–257
Fungus balls, 178
Funiculitis, 179
Furosemide, hematuria with, 64
  interstitial nephritis and, 317t
  LUTS with, 200t

G

Galactorrhea, renal cancer and, 296
Gallbladder cancer, 3
Ganglioneuroma, 265
Gangrene, Fournier's, 55–56, *370*
  genital, 369–370, *370*, *371*
Gastritis, renal failure with, 321t
Genital herpes. *See* Herpes, genital.
Genital warts, 124–127, 300, 363–364. *See also* Human
    papillomavirus (HPV).
  causes of, 125, 363
  diagnosis of, 125, 363–364
  incidence of, 124–125
  lesions of, 363, *364*
  treatment of, 125–127, 126t, 364
Genitalia, abscess on, 376
  ambiguous, 238–240
  angioneurotic edema of, *374*
  Bowen's disease as, 371–372, *372*
  dermatitis of, 375
  gangrene of, 369–370, *370*, *371*
  hemangioma of, *375*

Genitalia (Continued)
  insect bite of, 375
  lesion(s) of, 111–120, 359–377
    algorithm for, 113
    amyloidosis as, 377
    Buschke-Lowenstein tumor as, 364
    candidal, 367–368, 368
    chancre as, 360, 360–361
    chancroid as, 361
    Crohn's disease as, 377
    diagnosis of, 112t, 113
    drug eruption as, 373
    erythroplasia of Queyrat as, 371
    foscarnet and, 367
    gonorrhea as, 362
    granuloma inguinale as, 363
    herpes as, 365, 365–366
    human papillomavirus as, 363–364, 364
    Kaposi's sarcoma as, 366–367
    leukoplakia as, 372
    lichen planus as, 359–360, 360
    lymphogranuloma venereum as, 362
    molluscum contagiosum as, 366
    Paget's disease as, 372
    parasitic, 368–369
    premalignant, 370–372, 371, 372
    psoriasis as, 359, 359–360
    syphilis as, 360, 360–361
    tineal, 368
    tubercular, 368
    verruca vulgaris as, 364
    vitiligo as, 373
  lipogranulomatosis of, 375
  lymphangiectasis of, 376
  lymphangiitis of, 376
  lymphedema of, 369
  malformations of, 240–241
  trauma to, 90–92, 91
Genitourinary tract. See also Urinary tract.
  anomalies of, 233
  aspergillosis of, 177–178, 178
  cancer of, 263–271
  carcinoma of, 285–300
  during pregnancy, 217
  filariasis of, 178–181, 179, 180
  HIV disease and, 127t, 127–128
  physiology of, 335–338, 336
  schistosomiasis of, 174–177, 175, 176
  trauma to, 75–92
    classification of, 76
    complications with, 75
    evaluation of, 75–76
    renal injuries as, blunt, 77–80, 78t, 79
      penetrating, 80t, 80–81
  tuberculosis of, 171–174, 172, 173, 173t
Gentamicin, for children, 148, 148t
  for UTI, 137t, 138
  pregnancy and, 141–142
Germ cell tumor. See Testicular tumor.
Gerota's fascia, 1, 3
  perinephric abscess and, 135–136
Giant condyloma. See Buschke-Löwenstein tumor.
Gleason score, 282
Glomerular filtration rate (GFR), during pregnancy, 217,
  223t, 223–224
Glomerulonephritis, acute, 315t, 317
  hematuria with, 60, 62
  malignancy with, 320t
  poststreptococcal, 317t
  renal failure with, 312, 315t
  serologic markers for, 317t

Glomerulonephritis (Continued)
  urinalysis for, 313t
Glomerulopathy, serology of, 317t
Gonadal biopsy, 238–239
Gonadoblastoma, 267t
Gonadotropin-releasing hormone (GnRH), 336
Gonorrhea, 120–122, 121
  adolescents with, 111
  children with, 121
    treatment of, 117t
  complications with, 120
  diagnosis of, 121–122
  incidence of, 120–121, 360
  lesions of, 362
  nongonococcal urethritis with, 122
  pelvic inflammatory disease and, 109, 120
  pregnancy and, 110
  prevention of, 122
  symptoms of, 120
  treatment of, 116t, 122, 362
Goodpasture's syndrome, acute renal failure and, 315t
  glomerulonephritis with, 317t
Gorlin's basal cell nevus syndrome, 268t
Gout, treatment of, 104
  urolithiasis and, 98t
Granuloma inguinale, 120
  cause of, 363
  diagnosis of, 112t
  lesions of, 363
  treatment of, 363
Guanethidine, 200t
Gubernaculum, 3
Guillain-Barré syndrome, 211t
Gumma, 118, 361. See also Syphilis.
Gynecomastia, infertility and, 339
  renal cell carcinoma and, 296

H

Haemophilus ducreyi, 361–362. See also Chancroid.
Haemophilus influenzae, 128
Hairdressers, bladder cancer among, 288t, 307t
Haloperidol, infertility and, 344
Hamartoma, renal, 4
Healthy People 2000, 303
Heavy metal intoxication, 97t
HELLP syndrome, 228
Hemangioma, hematuria with, 61
  penile, 375
  renal, 295
Hemangiopericytoma, 4
Hematuria, 4, 22–25, 59–73. See also Urolithiasis.
  anticoagulants and, 64
  bladder cancer with, 289, 292
  bladder rupture with, 83
  blood tests for, 24, 68
  congenital, 60–61, 61t
  cyclic, 65
  cystoscopy for, 70–71, 71
  definitions of, 59–60
  detection of, 60
  diagnosis of, 49
  drug-induced, 59t, 63–64
  etiology of, 22–24, 49t, 60–65, 61t
    age and, 65t
  evaluation of, 13, 66–67
  exercise-induced, 62
  familial, 61
  follow-up surveillance for, 73
  gross, 49–50, 59
  history for, 65–66

Hematuria *(Continued)*
　iatrogenic, 65
　imaging studies for, 24–25, 69–71, *69–71*
　　algorithm for, *43*
　inflammatory, 61t, 62–63
　kidney stones with, 26
　kidney trauma and, 80
　laboratory tests for, 20, *20*, 67–69
　loin pain with, 64
　management of, 49–50
　metabolic, 61t, 63
　microscopic, 60
　neoplastic, 63
　oral contraceptives and, 64
　physical examination for, 22–23
　renal cell carcinoma with, 296
　renal trauma and, 77
　significant, 20, 24
　traumatic, 61t, 61–62
　urinalysis for, 23–24
　urolithiasis with, 63
　UTI and, 133
　work-up of, 65t, 65–73, *69–72*
Hemodialysis. *See* Dialysis.
Hemoglobinuria, 19
　red urine with, 18, 24, 59t
Hemolytic-uremic syndrome, 62
　acute renal failure and, 315t
　in pregnancy, 228
　malignancies with, 320, 320t
Henoch-Schönlein purpura, 62
Hepatitis, 110, 374
Hepatorenal syndrome, 320t
Hermaphroditism, 238–240
Hernia, inguinal, 55
　neonatal, 241
　physical examination of, 163t
Herpes, foscarnet for, 367
　genital, acyclovir for, 114, 115t, 365
　　counseling for, 365–366
　　diagnosis of, 112t, 114, 365
　　incidence of, 113–114
　　incubation period for, 365
　　lesions of, *365*, 365–366
　　pregnancy and, 110
　　prevention of, 114–118
　　symptoms of, 365
　　treatment of, 114, 115t, 365
　LUTS with, 198t
　neurogenic bladder and, 184t, 211t
　penile lesions with, 359
　perinatal, 114–118
Hinman's syndrome, 48t, 262
　enuresis with, 259
Hippocrates, 17
Hirsutoid papillomas, *374*
Hispanics, renal cancer among, 295
Histamine, LUTS with, 200t
Histoplasmosis, 326
Hodgkin's disease, glomerulonephritis with, 320t
　pseudo, 367
Holmium laser ablation, 206. *See also* Lasers.
HPV. *See* Human papillomavirus (HPV).
Human chorionic gonadotropin (hCG), for
　cryptorchidism, 244–245
　testicular tumor and, 297
Human immunodeficiency virus (HIV) disease, 127–128.
　　See also Acquired immunodeficiency syndrome
　　(AIDS).
　acute renal failure with, 321
　adolescents and, 111

Human immunodeficiency virus (HIV) disease
　　(Continued)
　aspergillosis with, 178
　chancroid with, 119
　genital lesions in, 359, 366–367, *367*
　genitourinary tract and, 127t, 127–128
　pregnancy and, 110
　prevention of, 111
　sexually transmitted diseases with, 366–367, *367*
　tuberculosis with, 171
Human papillomavirus (HPV), adolescents with, 111
　bowenoid papulosis from, 377
　genital lesions of, 363
　genital warts from, 125
　incidence of, 363
　penile lesions with, 359
Hyaline cast, *21*
Hydralazine, LUTS with, 200t
　pregnancy and, 225t, 225–226
Hydramitrazine, 200t
Hydrocele, 10
　examination for, 14
　neonatal, 241
　physical examination of, 163t
　testicular cancer and, 14
Hydrocephalus, 198t
Hydrochlorothiazide, for hypocalciuria, 103
　impotence and, 350
Hydrocolpos, 260
Hydrocortisone, for adrenal insufficiency, 327–328
　for anaphylaxis, 42t
Hydronephrosis, hematuria with, 64
　neonatal, 39
　prenatal, 233–237
　schistosomiasis with, 175
　ultrasonography for, 27
　ureteropelvic junction obstruction with, 233
Hydroureter, of pregnancy, 223t
Hydroureteronephrosis, 39–40
Hydroxamic acids, for struvite stones, 105
5-Hydroxytryptamine, 200t
Hyoscyamine, 191t
Hypercalcemia, malignancies with, 320t
　renal abnormalities with, 320, 320t
Hypercalciuria, causes of, 63
　hematuria with, 63
　management of, 103–104
　symptoms of, 63
　types of, 27, 95–96
Hyperkalemia, acute renal failure and, 321t
　adrenal insufficiency and, 327
　dialysis for, 322t
　hypoaldosteronism with, 328
　NSAIDs and, 318t
Hyperoxaluria, treatment of, 104
　urolithiasis and, 96, 98t
Hyperparathyroidism, brushite stones and, 94
　hypercalciuria with, 63
　urolithiasis and, 98t
Hyperphosphatemia, acute renal failure and, 321t
　renal abnormalities with, 320t
　renal failure and, 312
Hyperprolactinemia, 342
Hypertension, aldosteronism and, 329
　children with, 246
　diuretics for, *5*
　infertility and, 339
　NSAIDs and, 318t
　pheochromocytoma and, 331
　preeclampsia vs., 226t
　pregnancy and, 224–226, 225t, 226t

Hypertension (*Continued*)
  treatment for, 226
  renal cell carcinoma with, 296
  renovascular, 4
  transient, 226t
  vesicoureteral reflux and, 246
Hyperuricalciuria, 96
Hyperuricemia, 320t
Hyperuricosuria, 104
Hypoaldosteronism, 328–329
  biochemical abnormalities in, 327t
  clinical features of, 328
  diagnosis of, 328–329
  etiology of, 328
Hypocalcemia, 321t
Hypocitruria, treatment of, 104
  urolithiasis and, 96
Hypoglycemia, renal cancer and, 296
Hyponatremia, acute renal failure and, 321t
  adrenal insufficiency and, 327
  renal abnormalities with, 320t
Hypospadias, 14, 247–249, *248*
  ambiguous genitalia with, 239–240
  chordee and, 247
  cryptorchidism and, 247
  incidence of, 247
  infertility and, 338, 340
  neonates with, 239–240
  treatment of, 247–248
  types of, 247, *248*
  Wilms' tumor with, 263t
Hypothalamic-pituitary axis, dysfunction of, 326
  male fertility and, *336*, 336–337
Hysterectomy, ureter injury with, 81

I

Ibuprofen, 59t. *See also* Nonsteroidal anti-inflammatory
  drugs (NSAIDs).
ICSI (intracytoplasmic sperm injection), 335, 344,
  346–347
Ifosfamide, 321, 320t
IgA nephropathy, 62
Ileitis, urolithiasis vs., 97t, 219t
Imaging study(ies), agents for, 41–45, 42t
  computed tomography as, 40–41
  contrast media as, 41–45, 42t
  for bladder rupture, 83–84, *84–86*
  for genitourinary tract trauma, 76
  for hematuria, 24–25, *43*, 69–71, *69–71*
  for infertility, 343
  for kidney stones, 27–28
  for prostate cancer, 31–32, 287
  for recurring UTI, 158t
  for renal cell carcinoma, 296
  for renal trauma, 77–78
  for urolithiasis, 99
    of pregnancy, 220
  for UTI, 30
  principles of, 35–41
  ultrasonography as. *See* Ultrasonography.
Imipramine, bladder dysfunction with, 211t
  for enuresis, 258
    case study on, 261
  for retrograde ejaculation, 356
  for voiding dysfunction, 191t
  LUTS with, 200t
Imiquimod, 364
Immunotherapy, intravesical, 291–292
Impotence, 349–356
  after urethral trauma, 88

Impotence (*Continued*)
  causes of, 8–9
  diagnosis of, 350–351
  drug-induced, 350
  etiology of, 349–350, 350t
  priapism and, 54
In vitro fertilization (IVF), 335, 344, 346–347
Incidentaloma, 333–334
Incontinence. *See also* Enuresis; Voiding dysfunction.
  BPH with, 201
  causes of, 13
  definition of, 251
  difficult urination with, 211t
  LUTS with, 198t–199t
  stress, 221
  therapy for, behavioral, 188–190, 189t
    pharmacologic, 190–193, 191t–193t
    physical, 190
  urge, 184
    causes of, 13
    LUTS with, 198t
Indiana pouch, *293*
Indinavir, 98t
Infants. *See* Children; Neonates.
Infertility, 335–347
  age and, 338
  causes of, 344t
  cryptorchidism and, 335, 338
  evaluation of, 338–343, 340t–342t
    endocrine, 342–343
  female, 335
  history for, 338–339
  hypospadias and, 338, 340
  imaging studies for, 343
  incidence of, 335
  physical examination for, 339–340
  primary, 335
  risks for, 338–339, 344
  secondary, 335, 338
  surgery for, 345–346
  testicular cancer and, 335
  treatment of, 343–347, 344t
Interferon, for bladder cancer, 292
  for condyloma acuminatum, 364
  for renal cell carcinoma, 297
Interleukin-2 (IL-2), for renal cell carcinoma, 297
  renal abnormalities with, 320t
Intermittent self-catheterization (ISC), 214–215. *See also*
  Catheterization.
  indications for, 194
International classification of reflux, *246*
International Prostate Symptom Score (IPSS), 201
Intersexual conditions, 238–240
Interstitial nephritis, acute, 317t, 317–318
  nephrotic syndrome with, 318t
  drug-induced, 64
Intracorporeal lithotripsy, 105
Intracytoplasmic sperm injection (ICSI), 335, 344,
  346–347
Intrarenal abscess, 135–136, *136*
Intrauterine growth retardation, 225
Intrauterine insemination (IUI), 346–347
Intravenous pyelography (IVP), contrast agent for,
  35–36
  during pregnancy, 231
  findings with, *36*, 36–37, *37*
  for hematuria, 24–25, 69–70, *70*
  for kidney stones, 27
  for recurring UTI, 158t
  for renal trauma, 77–78
  for urolithiasis, 51

Intravenous pyelography (IVP) (*Continued*)
  for UTI, 30
  for Wilms' tumor, 264
  indications for, 35
  of nonfunctioning kidney, *251*
  perinephric abscess and, 135–136
  prostate cancer and, 32
  technique of, 35–36
Intravesical chemotherapy, 291
Intravesical immunotherapy, 291–292
Iohexol, 41
Iopamidol, 41
Iothalamate, 41
IPSS (International Prostate Symptom Score), 201
Irritative symptoms, 12
ISC (intermittent self-catheterization), 194, 214–215
Isoniazid, 173t, 200t
Isoproterenol, for anaphylaxis, 42t
  LUTS with, 200t
Itraconazole, 178
IVF (in vitro fertilization), 335, 344, 346–347
IVP. *See* Intravenous pyelography (IVP).

J

Jewett-Marshall staging system, 289, *290*
Juxtaglomerular cell tumor, 295

K

Kanamycin, 173t
Kaposi's sarcoma. *See also* Acquired immunodeficiency
      syndrome (AIDS).
  genital lesions of, 300, 366–367
  of bladder, 128
Ketoconazole, 326
Kidney(s). *See also* Renal *entries*.
  abscess of, 4, 135–136, *136*, 142
  anatomy of, 2, 3–4
  biopsy of, 25, 311t
  blood supply to, 2, 3
  calyx of, 5–6
  candidiasis of, *141*, 141–142
  congenital anomalies of, 77
  contusion of, 78t
  diseases of, 4, 320t, 320–321. *See also specific disease,*
      e.g., Nephritis.
    intrinsic, 315t, 315–316
    pregnancy and, 226–228
  during pregnancy, 224
  ectopic, 1
  examination of, 14
  hematoma of, 79, *79*
  hematuria and, 71–73
  infectious susceptibility of, 131–132
  laceration of, 78t, *79*
  lymphatics of, 4
  motheaten, *173*
  multicystic dysplastic, 237
  nerves of, 2, 3–4
  oncocytoma of, 294
  pain in, 11, 13, 50–51
  prenatal, 233
  scarring of, 246
  shattered, 78, 78t
  trauma to, 77–81
    blunt, 77–80, 78t, *79*
      imaging studies for, 77–78
      management of, 78–80, *79*
    classification of, 78t
    penetrating, 80t, 80–81

Kidney(s) (*Continued*)
    evaluation of, 80, 80t
      management of, 80–81
  tuberculosis of, *172, 173*
  ultrasonography for, *39*, 39–40
Kidney cancer, 4, 293–297. *See also* Renal cell carcinoma.
  algorithm for, *44*
  benign tumors vs., 294–295
  imaging of, 39, *39*
  incidence of, 293
  metastasis from, 3
  renal abnormalities with, 320t, 320–321
  types of, 293
Kidney stones, 25–28, 26t. *See also* Urolithiasis.
  analysis of, 21, 27
  blood tests for, 27
  hydroureteronephrosis vs., 40
  imaging studies for, 27–28, 69, 69–70, *70*
  intravenous pyelography for, 357
  physical examination for, 25
  renal infarction vs., 57
  staghorn calculi as, 11, 94, 101
  urinalysis for, 25–27
  urine pH and, 18
Klebsiella spp., 98t
  prostatitis from, 168
  pyelonephritis from, 4
  UTI with, 132
Klinefelter's syndrome, 339

L

Labetalol, 225t, 225–226
Laboratory tests, 17–33
Lasers, for BPH, 206, 215
  for condyloma acuminatum, 364
  for molluscum contagiosum, 366
  for prostatectomy, 65
Legionella infection, 317t
Leiomyoma, renal, 4, 295
Leptospira infection, 317t
Lesch-Nyhan syndrome, 98t
Leukemia, priapism and, 54
  prostate cancer and, 285
  renal abnormalities with, 320t
  testicular tumor with, 267t
  urolithiasis and, 98t
Leukocytes, in semen, 33, 342
  in urine, 19, 20
  urinary cast of, *21*
Leukocyte esterase test, 19
Leukoplakia, penile, 300, 372
Levodopa, 200t
Levofloxacin, 155t
Leydig's cells, *336*
  tumor of, 267t
LGV. *See* Lymphogranuloma venereum (LGV).
Libido. *See also* Impotence.
  loss of, 356
Lichen planus, 359–360, *360*
Lichen sclerosis et atrophicus, 300, 372
Li-Fraumani syndrome, 268t
Lipogranulomatosis, 375
Lipoma, renal, 295
Lithium, 200t
Lithotripsy, intracorporeal, 105
  shock-wave, 93, 105
    for children, 106
Liver cancer metastasis, 3
Loin pain hematuria syndrome, 64
Lovastatin, 315t

Lower urinary tract symptoms (LUTS), 197
  causes of, 198t–200t
  men with, 197
Lung cancer metastasis, 3, 4
Luteinizing hormone, infertility and, 342
  spermatogenesis and, *336*
Luteinizing hormone–releasing hormone (LHRH),
    chemotherapy for, 288
  for cryptorchidism, 244–245
  for prostate cancer, 287–288
LUTS. *See* Lower urinary tract symptoms (LUTS).
Lymphadenopathy, from chancroid, 362
Lymphangiectasia, *376*
Lymphangiitis, 376
Lymphedema, genital, *369*
Lymphocyte-activated killer (LAK) cells, 297
Lymphoepithelioma, bladder, 288
Lymphogranuloma venereum (LGV), 120
  diagnosis of, 112t, 362
  Frei's test for, 362
  incidence of, 362
  lesions of, 362
  symptoms of, 362
  treatment of, 116t, 362
Lymphoma, prostate cancer and, 285
  renal abnormalities with, 320t

M

Magnesium ammonium phosphate. *See* Struvite *entries.*
Magnesium oxide, for urolithiasis, 104
Malaria, 62
Melanoma metastases, 3–4
Meningitis, gonococcal, 116t
α-Mercaptopropionylglycine, 104–105
Mesterolone, 345
Metabolic acidosis, 321t
  acute renal failure and, 321t
  dialysis for, 322t
  urolithiasis and, 98t
Metaproterenol, 42t
Methadone, 200t
Methicillin, hemorrhagic cystitis with, 64
  interstitial nephritis and, 317t, 318
Methocarbamol, 200t
Methotrexate, acute renal failure and, 315t
  for bladder cancer, 293
  prerenal azotemia and, 315t
  renal abnormalities with, 320t
Methyldopa, LUTS with, 200t
  pregnancy and, 225t
  red urine with, 59t
Methylenedianiline, 288t
Metoclopramide, 200t
Metoprolol, 225t
Metriphonate, 177
Metronidazole, for amebiasis, 368
  for trichomoniasis, 124
  pregnancy and, 218t
Miconazole, 367
Milroy's disease, 369
Mitomycin C, 291
Mitotane, for Cushing's syndrome, 332–333
  hemorrhagic cystitis with, 64
Mohs' surgery, 300
Molluscum contagiosum, *366*
  HIV disease with, 367
  lasers for, 366
Monosodium urate, 94
Morphine. *See* Narcotics.
Mucin-secreting adenocarcinoma, 320

Multicystic dysplastic kidney, 237
Multiple sclerosis, impotence and, 350
  infertility and, 339, 344
  LUTS and, 197, 199t
  neurogenic bladder with, 184t, 211t
Muse, 351–353, 352t, 353t
Myasthenia gravis, 211t
Mycobacterium tuberculosis, 171. *See also* Tuberculosis.
Mycoplasma infection, 22
Myelodysplasia, 184t
Myelolipoma, 334
Myeloma, multiple, 320t
Myelomeningocele, 237–238
Myocardial infarction, renal infarction vs., 57
  urolithiasis and, 98t
Myoglobinuria, acute renal failure and, 315t
  red urine with, 18, 23, 59t

N

Naphthylamine, bladder cancer and, 288t
  hematuria and, 65–66
2-Naphthylamine, 307t
Narcotics, 231–232
  LUTS with, 200t
  pregnancy class of, 220t
Neisseria gonorrhoeae, 120
  bladder dysfunction with, 211t
  drug-resistant, 122
  epididymitis from, 128
  lesions of, 362
  urethritis from, 165
Neonates. *See also* Children.
  bladder obstruction in, 234
  Chlamydia infection in, 123
  cryptorchidism in, 243–245, *244*
  gonorrhea in, 121
  hernia in, 241
  herpes infection in, 114–118, 115t
  hydrocele in, 241
  hypospadias in, 239–240
  posterior urethral valves in, 234–235
  sexually transmitted diseases in, 115t–117t
  testicular torsion in, 240–241
  ureteropelvic junction obstruction in, 233–234
  UTI in, 145, 146
Neostigmine, 200t
Nephrectomy, 297
Nephritis, acute, 317t, 317–318
  drug-induced, 64
  radiation, 63
Nephrolithiasis. *See* Kidney stones.
Nephroma, mesoblastic, 264
Nephron, transport processes in, *5*
Nephropathy, diabetic, 227
  reflux, 227–228
Nephrostomy, UTI and, 143
Nephrotic syndrome, NSAIDs and, 318t, 318–319
  syphilis with, 118
Neuroblastoma, children with, 265–266, 266t, 268t–269t
  diagnosis of, 266, 269t
  epidemiology of, 265
  genetics of, 265, 268t
  metastasis from, 266
  pathology of, 265, 268t
  presentation of, 265, 268t
  staging of, 266, 268t–269t
  survival with, 266t, 269t
  treatment of, 266, 269t
Neurofibromatosis, 4
  adrenal tumor with, 3

Neurofibromatosis *(Continued)*
   neuroblastoma with, 268t
   rhabdomyosarcoma with, 268t
Neurogenic bladder. *See also* Bladder.
   causes of, 184t, 211t
   children with, 145
   enuresis with, 260
   myelomeningocele with, 237–238
   nonneurogenic, 185
Neurologic examination, 15
Neuromodulation, electrical, 195
Neurosyphilis. *See also* Syphilis.
   symptoms of, 118
   treatment of, 115t, 119
Neutropenia, pyuria and, 133
Newborns. *See* Neonates.
NGU. *See* Nongonococcal urethritis (NGU).
Nicotine. *See also* Tobacco use.
   addiction to, 304
   LUTS with, 200t
Nifedipine, 200t
Nitrites, in urine, 19
Nitrofurantoin, for children, 148, 148t
   for cystitis, 167
   for lower UTI, 155, 155t, 159
   pregnancy and, 218t, 230t
Nitrosourea, 320t
Nocturia. *See* Enuresis, nocturnal.
Nongonococcal urethritis (NGU), 122–123, 165
   adolescents with, 122
   causes of, 122
   diagnosis of, 122
   gonorrhea with, 122
   incidence of, 122
   prevention of, 123
   symptoms of, 122
   treatment of, 117t, 123
Nonsteroidal anti-inflammatory drugs (NSAIDs), acute
    renal failure and, 315t
   hematuria with, 64
   pregnancy and, 220t, 232
   prerenal azotemia and, 314t, 315t
   renal abnormalities with, 318t, 318–319
Norfloxacin, for lower UTI, 155t
   pyelonephritis and, 138
NSAIDs. *See* Nonsteroidal anti-inflammatory drugs
   (NSAIDs).
Nutcracker syndrome, 64
Nystatin, 367

O

Ofloxacin, for *Chlamydia* infection, 117t
   for epididymitis, 165
   for gonorrhea, 116t
Oncocytoma, renal, 4, 294
Oncovite, 292
Oral contraceptives, hematuria and, 64
   renal artery thrombosis and, 56–57
Orchidopexy, 244. *See also* Testes.
Orchiectomy, 299
Orchitis, epididymis with, 163
   infertility and, 338
Orgasm. *See also* Impotence.
   absence of, 357
Osteoporosis, 98t
Outlet resistance, altered, 185–186, 186t
   drugs for, 192t, 192–193, 193t
   seals for, 194–195
   electrical neuromodulation for, 195
   surgery for, 195

Ovarian cyst, 97t, 219t
Oxalate metabolism, 98t
Oxybutynin, for enuresis, 258
   for voiding dysfunction, 191t
   LUTS with, 200t
Oxytocin, 200t

P

Paget's disease, 98t, 372
Pampiniform plexus, 9
Pancreatitis, 97t
Papaverine, 352t, 353–354
Papillary necrosis, from analgesics, 64
   pyelonephritis with, 142
   relapsing UTI with, 157t
Papillary tumors, 291
Papillomatosis coronae penis, *374*
Papulosis, bowenoid, 377
Paraphimosis, 8, 14
   Fournier's gangrene and, 55
Parasites, 368–369
Parkinson's disease, LUTS and, 197, 198t
   neurogenic bladder with, 184t, 211t
Patient education, 305–307, 306t
Pearly penile papules, *374*
Pediculosis pubis, 369
Pelvic floor, electrical stimulation of, 195
   pathology of, 183
Pelvic fracture, bladder rupture with, 83–84, *84*
   Foley catheters and, 76
   impotence after, 88
   urethral trauma with, 86
Pelvic inflammatory disease (PID), gonorrhea and, 120
   pyelonephritis vs., 133, 135t
   sexually transmitted diseases and, 109
   urolithiasis vs., 219t
Pelvic lymph node dissection, 281–282
Penectomy, 300
Penicillamine, for cystinuria, 104
   pregnancy and, 232
Penicillin, for syphilis, 115t, 360, 361
   hematuria with, 64
   interstitial nephritis and, 317t
   pregnancy and, 218t
   prerenal azotemia and, 315t
Penile horn, 364
Penile vein thrombosis, 377
Penis, abscess of, *376*
   amputation of, 90
   anatomy of, 8
   angioneurotic edema of, *374*
   cancer of, 300
    clinical features of, 300
    incidence of, 300
    squamous cell, 367
    treatment for, 300
   chancre of, *360*, 360–361
   chancroid of, *361*, 361–362
   condyloma acuminatum of, 363–364, *364*
   corporal fibrosis of, 354
   cysts of, *372*, 372–373
   dermatitis of, 375
   diseases of, 8–9
   elephantiasis of, 179, *180*
   examination of, 14
   gangrene of, 370, *370, 371*
   gonococcal tysonitis of, 362
   granuloma inguinale of, *363*
   hemangioma of, *375*
   hematoma of, 90

Penis *(Continued)*
  herpetic lesions of, *365,* 365–366
  human papillomavirus lesions of, 363–364, *364*
  insect bite of, *375*
  intracavernous injections of, 374
  lesions of, 359–377
    candidal, 367–368, *368*
    foscarnet and, 367
    parasitic, 368–369
    premalignant, 370–372, *371, 372*
  leukoplakia of, 372
  lichen planus of, 359–360, *360*
  lipogranulomatosis of, 375
  lymphangiectasis of, *376*
  lymphangiitis of, 376
  lymphedema of, *369*
  lymphogranuloma venereum of, 362
  molluscum contagiosum of, *366*
  Paget's disease of, 372
  pearly papules of, *374*
  prosthesis for, 354–355
  psoriasis of, *359*
  revascularization of, 356
  spherules of, 375
  tinea of, 368
  trauma to, 90
  tuberculosis of, 368
  venous leak of, 350, 353
  verruca vulgaris of, 364
  vitiligo of, *373*
Pentamidine, 315t
Pentosan polysulphate sodium, 191t
Pericarditis, acute renal failure with, 321t
  uremic, 322t
Perinatal urologic consultation, 233–238
Perinephric abscess, 4
  diabetes and, 142
  UTI with, 135–136, *136*
Peritonitis, gonorrhea and, 120
Perlmann syndrome, 263t
Pessaries, 194
Petroleum products, bladder cancer and, 288t
  renal cell carcinoma and, 295
Peyronie's disease, 8, 14
Pharmacologic erection program (PEP), 353–354
Phenacetin, bladder cancer and, 288t
  red urine with, 59t
  urothelial malignancy with, 64
Phenazopyridine, for voiding dysfunction, 191t
  red urine with, 59t
Phenol, 366
Phenolphthalein, 18, 24, 59t
Phenothiazine, LUTS with, 200t
  red urine with, 59t
Phenoxybenzamine, 200t
Phensuximide, 59t
Phentolamine, 331
Phenylephrine, 354
Phenylpropanolamine, 191t
Phenytoin, interstitial nephritis and, 317t
  LUTS with, 200t
  red urine with, 59t
Pheochromocytoma, 265, 330–332
  adrenal, 3
  diagnosis of, 331
  epidemiology of, 330–331
  evaluation of, 329t
  incidentally discovered, 334
  renal artery thrombosis and, 57
  treatment of, 331–332
  urolithiasis vs., 97t

Phimosis, 8, 15
Photodynamic therapy, for bladder cancer, 292
Physical examination, urologic, 13–15, *15*
PID. *See* Pelvic inflammatory disease (PID).
Piercing, body, 373–374, *374*
Pilonidal sinus, 376
Piperacillin, 137t
Pituitary adenoma, 2, 332–333
Pityrosporum orbiculare, 368
Placenta previa, 228
Plasma cell balanitis, *376*
Plasmacytoma, 98t
Podofilox, 125, 126t
Podophyllin, 125, 126t, 366
  for condyloma acuminatum, 364
Poliomyelitis, 211t
Polycythemia, priapism and, 54
Polymerase chain reaction, reverse transcriptase, 283
Popcorn effect, 206
Porphyria, red urine with, 18, 23, 59t
  urolithiasis vs., 97t
Postobstructive diuresis, 49
Postvoid residual (PVR) urine, for bladder dysfunction, 213
  for BPH, 202
Potassium citrate, for urolithiasis, 104
Praziquantel, for schistosomiasis, 176–177
  side effects of, 177
Prazosin, for BPH, 193t
  infertility and, 344
  LUTS with, 200t
Preeclampsia, 224–225
  hypertension vs., 226t
  risks for, 225t
  thrombocytopenia with, 228
  treatment of, 225–226
Pregnancy. *See also* Ectopic pregnancy.
  abdominal pain during, 219t
  antibiotics during, 218t, 229–230, 230t
  antihypertensive drugs and, 225t
  bacteriuria of, 217–219, 218t
    risks for, 218
    treatment for, 218t, 218–219
  cystitis during, 217
  genital herpes and, 110
  genital warts and, 125
  genitourinary tract changes during, 217
  glomerular filtration rate during, 217, 223t, 223–224
  HELLP syndrome during, 228
  HIV testing during, 110
  hydroureter of, 223t
  hypertension in, 224–226, 225t
    classification of, 226t
    treatment of, 226
  intravenous pyelogram during, 231
  physiologic changes during, 223t, 223–224
  pyelonephritis during, 141–142, 217, 229
  renal disease during, 226–228
  renal failure during, 228
  renal function during, 223–232
  renal plasma flow during, 217
  sexually transmitted diseases during, 110t
  stress incontinence during, 221
  syphilis and, 118
  thrombocytopenia during, 228
  urinary frequency and, 221
  urolithiasis during, 106, 219t–221t, 219–221, 230–232
    diagnosis of, 219t, 219–220
    etiology of, 219
    hospitalization for, 221t
    imaging studies for, 220

Pregnancy *(Continued)*
    physical examination for, 220t
    symptoms of, 219
    treatment for, 220t, 220–221, 221t
    UTI during, 159–160, 217–219, 218t, 228–230, 230t
    vesicoureteral reflux during, 246
Prehn's sign, 53
Premature ejaculation, 356–357. *See also* Impotence.
Prematurity, cryptorchidism and, 243
    hypertension and, 225
Prerenal azotemia, *312,* 314–315. *See also* Acute renal
        failure (ARF).
    BUN in, 314
    causes of, 314t
    drug-induced, 314t, 315t
    malignancy with, 320t
    urinalysis for, 313t
Pressure-flow studies, synchronous, 203
Preventive Services Task Force, 305–307, 306t
Priapism, 54–55
    diagnosis of, 54, 54t
    from impotence drugs, 352–354
    treatment of, 54–55, 55t, 354, 376
Procyclidine, 200t
Progesterone, 200t
Propantheline, 191t
Propranolol, 211t
Prostate, anatomy of, *7,* 7–8
    biopsy of, 32, 276, 286
    high-riding, 76, 86
    infection of. *See* Prostatitis.
    opportunistic infections of, 127–128
    pain in, 122, 169
    size of, PSA levels and, 274t
    stones in, 8
    thermotherapy for, 205–206
    tuberculosis of, 172
    ultrasonography for, *40*
Prostate cancer, 285–288
    biopsy for, 286
        TRUS for, 276, 286
    clinical features of, 285–286
    digital rectal examination for, 276, 285–286
    HIV disease and, 127
    hormone therapy for, 287–288
    imaging studies for, 287
    incidence of, 285
    laboratory tests for, 30–32
    location of, 7–8
    metastasis from, 3
    pelvic lymph node dissection for, 281–282
    prevention of, 303, 307t, 308–309
    race and, 308
    rhabdomyosarcoma as, 270
    screening for, 275–277
    staging of, 286–287
        Gleason score for, 282
        molecular, 283
        PSA for, 281–282
    tobacco use and, 304, 308–309
    treatment of, 287–288
    tumor markers for, 32
Prostatectomy, BPH and, 215
    for prostate cancer, 287
    laser for, 65
Prostate-specific antigen (PSA), 273–283
    age-specific, 278t, 278–279
    assay for, 273–274
    concentration of, 274t, 274–275
    derivatives of, 273, 277–281, 278t, 280t
    finasteride and, 204

Prostate-specific antigen (PSA) *(Continued)*
    for staging, 281–282
    for therapy response, 282–283
    imaging studies with, 287
    screening with, 275–277
        pitfalls of, 277
    testing for, 30–31
Prostatic massage specimen, 21
Prostatitis, 7–8, 167t, 167–169
    calculi and, 169
    chronic, 167–168
    classification of, 167t, 167–168
    cultures for, 168
    diagnosis of, 167t
    etiology of, 167
    hematuria from, 49t
    PSA levels and, 274t
    treatment of, 167t, 168–169
    urinary retention from, 168
Prostatodynia, 122, 169
Protease inhibitors, urolithiasis and, 98t
Proteinuria, 19
    hematuria with, 4, 24, 67–68
    tests for, 19
Proteus spp., 98t
    pyelonephritis from, 4
    struvite stones with, 94
    urine pH and, 18
    UTI with, 132
Providencia infection, 18
PSA. *See* Prostate-specific antigen (PSA).
PSA density, 277–278
PSA ratio, free-to-total, 280t, 280–281
PSA velocity, 279–280
Pseudodyssynergia, 185
Pseudoephedrine, 191t
Pseudohermaphroditism, 238–240
Pseudo-Hodgkin's disease, 367
Pseudomonas spp., prostatitis from, 168
    urine pH and, 18
    UTI with, 132
Psoas abscess, 97t
Psoriasis, penile lesions with, *359*
Pulmonary edema, 322t
Purine metabolism, 98t
Pyelogram. *See also* Intravenous pyelography (IVP).
    accuracy of, 77
    antegrade, *82*
    retrograde, for hematuria, 71
    two-shot, 78
Pyelonephritis, algorithm for, *138*
    children with, 145
        treatment of, 148, 148t
    clinical features of, 132–133
    cystitis vs., 133t
    diagnosis of, 134–135
        differential, 135t
    emphysematous, 4, 142
    flank pain with, 50
    hematuria from, 49t
    hospitalization for, 137
    medications for, 137t137–138
    nephrostomy and, 143
    obstructive, 96
        evaluation of, 98
    pain with, 11
    papillary necrosis from, 142
    pregnancy and, 141–142, 217, 227, 229
    reflux nephropathy with, 227
    renal infarction vs., 57
    renal transplant and, 143

Pyelonephritis *(Continued)*
  septic shock from, 131
  signs of, 4
  UTI and, 131
  vesicoureteral reflux and, 246
  xanthogranulomatous, 98
Pyonephritis, 4
Pyrazinamide, 173t
Pyridoxine, 104
Pyuria, children with, 146
  neuropenia and, 133
  UTI with, 131, 133

Q

Queyrat, erythroplasia of, 113, 300, *371, 376*
Quinolones, 218t, 230t
Quinupristin, 143

R

Radiation nephritis, 63
Radiographic contrast media allergy, 319–320
Ranitidine, 42t
Rectal examination, 15. *See also* Digital rectal
  examination (DRE).
Red diaper syndrome, 59t
Red urine. *See under* Urine.
Reflux. *See also* Vesicoureteral reflux (VUR).
  nephropathy, 227–228
  vaginal, 260
Reiter's syndrome, 376–377
  urethritis with, 165
Renal. *See also* Kidney(s).
Renal atheroembolic disease, 315t, 316–317
Renal cell carcinoma, 4, 295–297. *See also* Kidney cancer.
  children with, 264
  diagnosis of, 294
  epidemiology of, 295
  etiology of, 295
  imaging studies for, 296
  incidence of, 295
  metastatic, 297
  multicystic dysplastic kidney and, 237
  nephrectomy for, 297
  presentation of, 296
  staging of, 295–296
  tobacco use and, 295
  treatment of, 296–297
  ultrasonography of, *39, 39,* 70
Renal colic, 11
  acute, 50–51
  hematuria with, 13
Renal disease, 4, 320t, 320–321. *See also specific types, e.g.,*
  Nephritis.
  intrinsic, 315–316
  causes of, 315t
  pregnancy and, 226–228
Renal failure, acute, 311–323
  causes of, 314–321, 315t–317t, 320t
  chronic vs., *312*
  complications with, 321t, 321–322
  diagnosis of, 311t, 311–312
  dialysis for, 322t
  drug-induced, 314t, 315t
  evaluation of, *312,* 312–314, 313t
  from contrast media, 319–320
  HIV infection and, 321
  intrinsic, *312*
  management of, 322–323
  NSAIDs and, 318t
  postrenal, *312*

Renal failure *(Continued)*
    uric acid–induced, 320
    urinalysis for, 312–314, 313t
  pregnancy and, 228
Renal function, during pregnancy, 223t, 223–232
  tests of, 22
Renal hamartoma, 4, 39, 294, 377
Renal infarction, 56t, 56–57
Renal pelvic cancer, 294. *See also* Kidney cancer.
Renal plasma flow (RPF), 217
Renal scarring, 246
Renal transplants, 55, 143
Renal tubular disorders, brushite stones and, 94
  hematuria with, 61
  urine pH and, 18
Renal tumors. *See also* Kidney cancer; Renal cell
    carcinoma.
  algorithm for, *44*
  benign, 294–295
  types of, 4
  ultrasonography for, 39, *39*
Renal vascular disease, 316
Renal vein thrombosis, acute renal failure from, 315t
  hematuria with, 64
  urolithiasis vs., 97t
Renin, adrenal insufficiency and, 327
  hypoaldosteronism and, 328
Renovascular pedicle injury, 81
Reproduction, assisted, 335, 344, 346–347
Respiratory alkalosis, 223t
Retrograde urethrogram, 38, *38*
Retroperitoneum, anatomy of, *2*
Reverse transcriptase polymerase chain reaction, 283
Rhabdoid tumor, 264
Rhabdomyolysis, 315t
Rhabdomyosarcoma, anomalies with, 268t
  children with, 268t–269t, 270
  diagnosis of, 269t, 270
  enuresis with, 260
  epidemiology of, 270
  etiology of, 270
  of bladder, 288
  pathology of, 268t, 270
  staging of, 268t–269t, 270
  testicular, 267t
  treatment of, 269t, 270
Rhodamine B, 59t
Rifampin, 173t
  interstitial nephritis and, 317t
  prerenal azotemia and, 315t
  red urine with, 59t
Rind sign, *136*

S

Salpingitis, 120
Sarcoidosis, brushite stones and, 94
  interstitial nephritis with, 317t
  urolithiasis and, 98t
Sarcoma, bladder, 7
  clear cell, 264
  prostate, 285
  renal, 4
Sarcomatoid carcinoma, 288
Scabies, 368
Schiller-Duval bodies, 267
Schistosoma haematobium, egg of, *176*
  life cycle of, 174–175, *175*
Schistosomiasis, 174–177, *175, 176*
  bladder calcification with, *176*
  cancer risk with, 187t
  clinical features of, 175

Schistosomiasis (Continued)
  diagnosis of, 176
  drugs for, 176–177
  epidemiology of, 174
  hematuria with, 62
  management of, 176–177
  pathogenesis of, 174–175, 175
  prognosis for, 177
Scleroderma, 315t
Scrotum, acute, 51–54, 53
  diagnosis of, 51t
  anatomy of, 10, 10
  cysts of, 373
  elephantiasis of, 179, 180
  examination of, 14–15, 15
  gangrene of, 369–370, 370
  hypospadias and, 248
  layers of, 10
  lymphedema of, 369
  malignancies of, 300
  physical examination of, 163t
  trauma to, 90–92, 91
  ultrasonography for, 40, 343
  vitiligo of, 373
Seizures, renal failure with, 321t
Semen. See also Sperm.
  analysis of, 340–342, 341t, 342t
  composition of, 32–33
  leukocytes in, 33, 342
  pH of, 33
Seminal vesicles, 9
Seminoma, alpha-fetoprotein and, 297
  types of, 298
Septic shock, from UTI, 135
  pyelonephritis with, 131
Sertoli's cell(s), 337
Sertoli's cell tumor, 267t
Sexual dysfunction, 349–357. See also specific types, e.g., Impotence.
Sexually transmitted diseases (STDs), 109–129. See also specific types, e.g., Syphilis.
  adolescents with, 110–111, 122–123
  children with, 110
  comorbidity with, 362
  complications with, 109
  counseling for, 111
  epididymitis and, 117t
  gender and, 109
  genital lesions with, 111–120, 360–366
  incidence of, 109
  pregnancy and, 110, 110t
  prevention of, 111
  race and, 109
  risks for, 109–110
Shingles, 184t, 211t. See also Herpes.
Shock-wave lithotripsy (SWL), 93, 105
  for children, 106
Shy-Drager syndrome, 198t
SIADH (syndrome of inappropriate antidiuretic hormone), 320t
Sickle cell disease, hematuria with, 61
  priapism and, 54, 55
Sildenafil, 351–352, 352t
Sjögren's syndrome, 317t
SLE. See Systemic lupus erythematosus (SLE).
Sleep disorders, 253
Small cell carcinoma, 288
Smoking cessation program, 303–305, 305. See also Tobacco use.
Sodium nitroprusside, 226
Spectinomycin, 116t
Sperm. See also Semen.

Sperm (Continued)
  absence of, 337, 349, 356
  function of, 337–338
  morphology of, 32
  motility of, 32, 341
Spermatic cord. See also Testicular torsion.
  anatomy of, 9
  physical examination of, 163t, 164t, 340
  trauma to, 91
Spermatocele, 10, 14
Spermatogenesis, 336, 336–337
  endocrine abnormalities and, 342–343
Spinal cord injury, impotence and, 350
  LUTS with, 198t
  neurogenic bladder with, 184t, 211t
Spinal dysraphism, enuresis with, 260
  impotence and, 350
Spinal stenosis, LUTS with, 198t
  neurogenic bladder with, 184t
Spironolactone, 330
Spondylosis, 198t
Squamous cell(s), in urine, 20, 20–21
Squamous cell carcinoma, bladder, 7, 187, 288
  genital ulcer with, 113
  penile, 8, 300, 367
  renal, 293
  schistosomiasis and, 174
  scrotal, 300
  urethral, 300
Staghorn calculus. See also Kidney stones.
  management of, 101
  pain with, 11
  Proteus mirabilis and, 94
Staphylococcal infection, renal abscess from, 4
  urine pH and, 18
  UTI with, 131–132, 132
Steinstrasse, 105
Stevens-Johnson syndrome, 165
Stomach cancer, 3
Storage dysfunction, 184
  therapy for, 189t
Straddle injury, 88
Streptococcal infection, 317t
Streptomycin, 173t
Streptozyme test, 68
Struvite crystals, 21
Struvite stones, 94
  incidence of, 94t
  management of, 105
  urine pH and, 18
Sulfa drugs, hematuria with, 64
Sulfamethoxazole, 160. See also Trimethoprim-sulfamethoxazole.
Sulfisoxazole, for Chlamydia infection, 117t
  for lymphogranuloma venereum, 116t, 362
  pregnancy and, 230t
Sulfonamides, acute renal failure and, 315t
  interstitial nephritis and, 317t
  pregnancy and, 218t
  prerenal azotemia and, 315t
  urolithiasis and, 98t
Sulfosalicylic acid test, 19
Suramin, 288
SWL (shock-wave lithotripsy), 93, 105
  for children, 106
Sympathoblastoma, 265
Synchronous pressure-flow studies, 203
Syndrome of inappropriate antidiuretic hormone (SIADH), 320t
Syphilis. See also Sexually transmitted diseases (STDs).
  bladder dysfunction with, 211t
  chancre of, 360, 360–361

Syphilis *(Continued)*
  chancroid with, 119
  children with, 117t, 119
  congenital, 118
  diagnosis of, 118–119
    differential, 112t
  incidence of, 118
  neurogenic bladder and, 184t
  penile lesions of, 360360–361
  pregnancy and, 110
  prevention of, 119
  renal artery thrombosis and, 57
  secondary, 361
  symptoms of, 118
  tertiary, 361
  treatment of, 115t, 119, 360–361
Systemic lupus erythematosus (SLE), acute renal failure
    and, 315t
  glomerulonephritis with, 317t
  hematuria with, 62
  symptoms of, 66

T

Tacrolimus, 314t, 315t
Tamsulosin, for BPH, 193t, 214, 2041
  for prostatitis, 169
  side effects of, 204
TCAs (tricyclic antidepressants), 200t, 211t, 258
Teratoma, testicular, 267t, 298
Terazosin, for BPH, 193t, 203–204
  for prostatitis, 169
  side effects of, 204
Terbutaline, for anaphylaxis, 42t
  LUTS with, 200t
Terodiline, 200t
Testes. *See also* Cryptorchidism.
  anatomy of, 9
  biopsy of, 299
  diseases of, 9–10
  ectopic, 243
  examination of, 14–15, *15*
  measurement of, 340
  pain in, 122
  physical examination of, 163t, 164t
  physiology of, *336*, 336–337
  retractile, 14, 243–244
  suspension of, *52*
  trauma to, 90–92, *91*
    infertility after, 339
  tuberculosis of, 172
  ultrasonography for, *40*
Testicular torsion, 9–10, 52, *52, 53*
  diagnosis of, 51t, 52
  epididymitis vs., 128–129
  incidence of, 52
  infertility and, 339
  laboratory tests for, 52
  neonatal, 240–241
  outcomes with, 52
  treatment of, 52
Testicular tumor, 297–300
  children with, 267, 267t–269t
    diagnosis of, 267, 269t
    pathology of, 267t, 268t
    presentation of, 267, 268t
    staging of, 267, 268t–269t
    survival with, 269t
    treatment of, 267, 269t
    types of, 267t
  classification of, 298
  clinical features of, 298–299

Testicular tumor *(Continued)*
  cryptorchidism with, 244, 268t, 298
  diagnosis of, 51t
  hydrocele and, 14
  incidence of, 297–298
  infertility and, 335
  metastases from, 298–299
  physical examination for, 164t
  risks for, 298
  treatment of, 299–300
Testis Determining Factor *(TDF)* gene, 243
Testosterone, impotence and, 350, 355
  infertility and, 342
  LUTS with, 200t
  spermatogenesis and, *336*
Tethered cord syndrome, 260
Tetracycline, for gonorrhea, 116t
  for syphilis, 115t, 361
  pregnancy and, 218t
Theophylline, LUTS with, 200t
  urolithiasis and, 98t
Thermotherapy, for BPH, 205–206
Thiacetazone, 173t
Thiazide diuretics. *See* Diuretics.
Thin basement membrane nephropathy, 61
Thioridazine, 200t
Thiotepa, 291
Thrombocytopenia, 278
Thrombosis, penile vein, 376
  renal artery, 56–57, 64, 97t, 315t
Thrombotic thrombocytopenic purpura (TTP), acute
    renal failure and, 315t
  in pregnancy, 228
Thyroiditis, 326
Tinea infection, 368
Tobacco use, bladder cancer and, 288, 304
  bladder dysfunction with, 211t
  impotence and, 349
  infertility and, 339
  LUTS with, 200t
  mortality with, 304
  preeclampsia and, 225t
  prostate cancer and, 304, 308–309
  renal cell carcinoma and, 295
  smoking cessation program for, 303–305, *305*
  transitional cell carcinoma and, 187
Tobramycin, for children, 148t
  for UTI, 137t
Tolterodine, 191t
Toluidine, 288t
Toxoplasmosis, 128
Transitional cell carcinoma, 288, 289–291
  cystoscopy of, *71*
  occupational hazards for, 65–66
  renal, 293
  tobacco use and, 187
  treatment of, 291–292, 292–293
Transrectal ultrasonography (TRUS), 31
  for BPH, 202–203
  for infertility, 340, 343
  for prostate biopsy, 276, 286
Transurethral electrovaporization (TUEVP), 205
Transurethral incision of prostate (TUIP), 206
Transurethral needle ablation (TUNA), 205, 215
Transurethral resection of prostate (TURP),
    complications with, 215
  for BPH, 204–205, 215
  for prostatitis, 169
  hematuria after, 65
  radical, 169
  retrograde ejaculation after, 356
  VaporTrode vs., 205

Transvaginal ultrasonography, 231. *See also*
    Ultrasonography.
Treponema pallidum, 118. *See also* Syphilis.
    penile lesion from, *360*
    tests for, 118–119, 360
Triamterene, acute renal failure and, 315t
    urolithiasis from, 64, 95, 98t
Trichlormethiazide, 103
Trichloroacetic acid, 364
Trichomoniasis, 124
    balanitis from, 377
    diagnosis of, 124
    incidence of, 124
    treatment of, 124
    urethritis from, 165
Tricyclic antidepressants (TCAs), bladder dysfunction
        with, 211t
    for enuresis, 258
    LUTS with, 200t
Trimethoprim-sulfamethoxazole, for children, 148, 148t
    for cystitis, 167
    for granuloma inguinale, 363
    for lower UTI, 155t, 155–156, 159
    for upper UTI, 137t, 143
    pregnancy and, 218t, 230t
    teratogenicity of, 160
Triple-phosphate. *See* Struvite *entries.*
Trisodium phosphonoformate, 367
TRUS. *See* Transrectal ultrasonography (TRUS).
TTP (thrombotic thrombocytopenic purpura), 228, 315t
Tuberculosis, Addison's disease and, 326
    calcified lesions of, 171, *172*
    clinical features of, 172
    diagnosis of, 172–173, *173*
    drugs for, 173t
    epididymitis from, 128
    hematuria with, 62
    LUTS with, 198t
    of genitourinary tract, 171–174, *172, 173,* 173t
    pathogenesis of, 171–172, *172*
    penile, 368
    prognosis for, 174
    secondary, 174
    treatment of, 173, 173t
Tubular necrosis, 315–316
    aminoglycosides and, 319
    hematuria with, 65
    renal failure and, *312,* 315t
Tubulointerstitial disease, 320t
TUEVP (transurethral electrovaporization), 205
TUIP (transurethral incision of prostate), 206
Tumor(s). *See specific type, e.g.,* Wilms' tumor.
Tumor lysis syndrome, 320t
TUNA (transurethral needle ablation), 205, 215
Tunica vaginalis, 10
TURP. *See* Transurethral resection of prostate (TURP).
Tysonitis, gonococcal, 362

U

Ulcerative colitis, 98t
Ultrasonography, for abdominal masses, 264
    for ambiguous genitalia, 239
    for bladder, 40
    for prostate, 40
    for recurring UTI, 158t
    for renal cell carcinoma, *70,* 296
    for urolithiasis, 99
    for voiding dysfunction, 188
    prenatal, 233
    renal, *39,* 39–40
    scrotal, 40, *91,* 343

Ultrasonography *(Continued)*
    testicular, *40*
    transrectal, 31
        for BPH, 202–203
        for infertility, 340, 343
        for prostate biopsy, 276, 286
    transvaginal, 231
Urachus, 6
Urate crystalluria, 59t
Ureaplasma prostatitis, 168
Urease inhibitors, 105
Uremic pericarditis, 322t
Ureter, anatomy of, 5–6
    bowel segments for, 83
    cancer of, 294
    duplication of, 235–236
    ectopic, 235–236
    pain in, 12
    trauma to, 81–83, *82*
        delayed presentation of, 83
        evaluation of, 81–82
        iatrogenic, 82
        imaging for, *82*
        management of, 82–83
    tuberculosis of, 171
Ureterocele, 235–237, 260
Ureteropelvic junction obstruction, 61, 233–234
Ureteropyelocaliectasis, 217
Urethra. *See also* Hypospadias.
    anatomy of, *7, 8*
    cyst of, 260
    discharge from, algorithm for, *121*
    diseases of, 8, 63
    duplication of, 260
    female, trauma to, 89–90
        evaluation of, 76
    male, trauma to, 84–90, *87–89*
        evaluation of, 76
    malignancies of, 300
    straddle injury to, 88, *89*
    valves of, 234–235
        voiding cystourethrogram of, *252*
Urethritis, 165t, 165–166
    classification of, 165
    definition of, 151
    diagnosis of, 165t, 165–166
    etiology of, 165
    hematuria from, 49t
    lower UTI with, 160–161
    nongonococcal, 122–123, 165
        treatment of, 117t, 123
    sexually transmitted, 120, *121*
    symptoms of, 165t
    treatment of, 165t, 166
Urethrogram, retrograde, 38, *38*
Urethrorrhagia, idiopathic, 64
Urge incontinence, 184. *See also* Incontinence.
    causes of, 13
    LUTS with, 198t
Urgency, urinary, 12, 199t
Uric acid crystals, 21
Uric acid stones, 94, 107
    incidence of, 94t
    urine pH and, 18
Uricosurics, 98t
Urinalysis, 18–22, *20, 21*
    for acute renal failure, 312–314, 313t
    for BPH, 202
    for children, 146–147
    for glomerulonephritis, 313t
    for hematuria, 23t, 23–24
    for kidney stones, 25–27, 26t

Urinalysis *(Continued)*
  for prerenal azotemia, 313t
  for urolithiasis, 100t
  for UTI, 28t, 28–29, 134
Urinary retention, 13
  acute, 47–49, 48t
    causes of, 47, 48t
    diagnosis of, 47
    management of, 47–48
    physical examination for, 47
  HIV disease and, 128
  LUTS with, 198t–199t
  rhabdomyosarcoma with, 270
Urinary tract. *See also* Genitourinary tract.
  anatomy of, 183–184
  during pregnancy, 221, 224
  endometriosis of, 65
  fistula of, 13
  neoplasms of, 63
  obstruction of, BPH and, 211t
    children with, 147
  trauma to, 61–62, 75–92
Urinary tract infection (UTI), 28–30. *See also* Bacteriuria.
  aspergillosis as, 177–178, *178*
  cancer risk with, 187t
  children with, 145–149
    case study on, 149
    clinical features of, 146
    epidemiology of, 145
    etiology of, 145
    laboratory tests for, 146–147
    prophylaxis for, 148–149
    risks for, 145–146
    treatment of, 147–148, 148t
    work-up for, 147, *147*
  during pregnancy, 217–219, 218t, 228–230, 230t
  enuresis with, 254, 260
  filariasis as, 178–181, *179, 180*
  hematuria with, 62, 133
  imaging studies for, 30
  lower, algorithm for, *161*
    catheterized patient with, 160
    complications with, 151t, 158–161
    definition of, 151t, 151–152
    diabetes with, 158–159
    diagnosis of, 152t, 152–154
    elderly patients with, 160
    epididymitis as, 163–165, 164t
    follow-up for, 157–158, 158t
    health care costs of, 151
    men with, 163t–167t, 163–169
    pathophysiology of, 152
    physical examination for, 153, 154t
    pregnancy and, 159–160
    recurrent, 152, 156–157
      causes of, 157t
      tests for, 158t
    symptoms of, 152t
    treatment of, 154–161, 155t–158t, *161*
    urethritis and, 160–161
    urinalysis for, 153–154
    women with, 151–161, 152t–158t, *161*
      elderly, 160
  neonates with, 145, 146
  physical examination for, 28
  schistosomiasis as, 174–177, *175, 176*
  tuberculosis as, 171–174, *172, 173,* 173t
  uncommon, 171–181
  upper, 131–144
    case studies on, 143–144
    clinical features of, 132–133, 133t
    complications with, 135–136, *136,* 139–143

Urinary tract infection (UTI) *(Continued)*
    diabetes mellitus and, 142, 144
    diagnosis of, 133–135
    elderly patients with, 133
      management of, 140–141
    epidemiology of, 131–132
    management of, 136–143, 137t, *138*
    nephrostomy with, 143
    nosocomial, 132, 142–143
    pathogenesis of, 131
    pregnancy and, 141–142
    pyuria and, 133
    renal candidiasis with, *141,* 141–142
    renal transplant and, 143
    risks for, 132, 132t
  urinalysis for, 28t, 28–29, 134, 153–154
Urination. *See* Voiding dysfunction.
Urine, appearance of, 13
  bacteria in, 20, *20*
  Candida albicans in, *141*
  casts in, 21, *21*
  collection of, 16–17
  crystals in, 21, *21*
  cultures of, 21
  cytology for, 68, 187
  epithelial cells in, 20, 20–21
  formaldehyde in, 19
  glucose in, 19
  hemoglobin in, 19
  leukocytes in, 19, 20
  microscopic examination of, 19–21, *20, 21*
  nitrites in, 19
  pH of, 18
    kidney stones and, 25–26
  protein in, 19
  red, 18, 59t, 59–60
  specific gravity of, 18, 67
  storage of, 18
  storage problems with, 184
Urine calcium, 68
Uroflowmetry, for BPH, 202
Urolithiasis, 93–107. *See also* Kidney stones.
  as urologic emergency, 50–51
  children with, 106
  colic with, 96, 97t
    management of, 100–101
  comorbid conditions with, 98–99
  diagnosis of, 50t, 97t
  diet recommendations for, 102t
  drug-induced, 64
  evaluation of, algorithm for, *100*
    emergency department, 98–99
    metabolic, 100t
    office, 98–99
  fictitious, 106–107
  health care cost of, 106
  hematuria with, 63
  history for, 96–97, 98t
  imaging studies for, 99
  incidence of, 93–94, 106
  intravenous pyelogram for, 51
  laboratory tests for, 99–100, *100,* 100t, 101t
  management of, 51, 100–105, 102t
  of pregnancy, 106, 219t–221t, 219–221, 230–232
  pathogenesis of, 95–96
  physical examination for, 97–98
  presentation of, 96–99
  preventive measures for, 102t, 102–103
  pyelonephritis with, 96
  race and, 93
  recurrence rates for, 101–102
  regional influence on, 93

Urolithiasis *(Continued)*
  schistosomiasis and, 174
  surgery for, 105
  types of, 94t, 94–95
Urologic emergencies, 47–57
Urologic evaluation, 11–15, *15*
Uroscopy, 17–18
Uterine cancer, 3, 4
UTI. *See* Urinary tract infection (UTI).
Uveitis syndrome, 317t

V

Vagal reactions, 44
Vaginal discharge, 120, *121*
Vaginal reflux of urine, 260
Valproic acid, 200t
Vancomycin, enterococci resistant to, 143
  for children, 148, 148t
VaporTrode, 205
Varicella, 184t, 211t. *See also* Herpes.
Varicocele, definition of, 340
  grading of, 340t
  infertility and, 339
  physical examination of, 340
  surgery for, 346
Vas deferens, anatomy of, 9
  diseases of, 9
  segmental atresia of, 340
Vasculitis, acute renal failure and, 315t, 321t
  glomerulonephritis with, 317t
Vasectomy, 345–346
Vasography, 343
Venereal warts. *See* Condyloma acuminatum.
Verruca vulgaris, penile, 364
Verruciform xanthoma, 377
Vesicoureteral reflux (VUR), children with, 145–149,
    245–247
  classification of, 245–246, *246*
  cystitis and, 246
  diagnosis of, 245, *245*
  hypertension and, 246
  incidence of, 245
  pregnancy and, 246
  prognosis for, 246–247
  pyelonephritis and, 246
  sequelae with, 246
  treatment of, 247
  UTI with, 132, 157t
  voiding cystourethrogram for, *37*, 245, *245*
Viagra, 351–352, 352t
Videourodynamics, for BPH, 203
Vinblastine, for bladder cancer, 293
  for prostate cancer, 288
  for renal cell carcinoma, 297
  for testicular tumor, 299
Vincristine, 270
Virchow's nodes, 15
Virilization, 2
Vitamin B$_{12}$ deficiency, 198t
Voided bladder 3 (VB-3) specimen, 168
Voiding cystourethrography (VCUG), 30, 37–38
  for multicystic dysplastic kidney, 237
  for recurring UTI, 158t
  for vesicoureteral reflux, 245, *245*
  indications for, 37
  of posterior urethral valves, 234, *252*
  retrograde, 147
  technique of, *37*, 37–38
Voiding dysfunction, 183–195. *See also specific types, e.g.,*
    Incontinence.
  algorithm for, *255*

Voiding dysfunction, 183–195 *(Continued)*
  assessment of, 254–257, *255*, *256*
  BPH with, 197–207
  cancer and, 187t
  catheterization for, 194
  classification of, 184t
  diagnosis of, 186–188
  diurnal, 260–261
  electrical neuromodulation for, 195
  enuresis and, 251–262
  history for, 186t
  laboratory tests for, 187
  LUTS with, 199t
  men with, 197–207
  pessaries for, 194
  physical examination for, 186–187, 187t
  plugs for, 194–195
  surgery for, 195
  symptoms of, 12–13
  therapy for, 188–195
    behavioral, 188–190, 189t
    pharmacologic, 190–193, 191t–193t
    physical, 190
  urinary tract symptoms with, 197–207
Von Hippel-Lindau disease, adrenal tumor with, 3
  renal cell carcinoma and, 295
VP16 (drug), 288
VUR. *See* Vesicoureteral reflux (VUR).

W

WAGR syndrome, 263t
Warfarin, 64
Weddellite stones, 94
Wegener's granulomatosis, acute renal failure and, 315t
  glomerulonephritis with, 317t
  urethritis with, 165
Whewellite stones, 94
Whiff test, 124
White blood cells. *See* Leukocytes.
Wilms' tumor, 263t, 263–265, 265t, 268t–269t
  congenital anomalies with, 263t
  diagnosis of, 264, 269t
  epidemiology of, 263
  management of, 264, 269t
  multicystic dysplastic kidney and, 237
  pathology of, 264, 268t
  presentation of, 263–264, 268t
  renal cell carcinoma and, 295
  staging of, 264, 268t–269t
  survival with, 264–265, 265t, 269t
Wilson's disease, 98t
Wuchereria bancrofti. See also Filariasis.
  drugs for, 180–181
  life cycle of, 178–179, *179*
  lymphedema with, 369
  photomicrograph of, 181

X

Xanthoma, verruciform, 377

Y

Y chromosome, in dysgenetic gonads, 239
Yohimbine, 356
Yolk sac tumor, 267t, 298

Z

Zoon's balanitis, *376*